D1190179

Digestive Physiology and Nutrition of Ruminants

Volume 2- Nutrition

by
D.C. Church, Ph.D.
Ruminant Nutritionist
Senior Author & Editor

ISBN 0-9601586-5-0

Published and Distributed by **O & B BOOKS, Inc.**
1215 N.W. Kline Place
Corvallis, Oregon 97330
United States of America

Printed by Oxford Press
1427 S.E. Stark
Portland, Oregon 97214

TABLE OF CONTENTS

Tables of Contents for other Volumes in this Series

Other Volumes Distributed by O & B Books, Inc.

BASIC ANIMAL NUTRITION AND FEEDING

by D.C. Church and W.G. Pond, 1974

This book is intended as a basic introductory text for the field of animal nutrition. Relatively detailed chapters are included on all of the major nutrients and information is included on nutrient metabolism, requirements and deficiency symptoms. Less detailed information is presented on some more applied topics such as composition of feedstuffs, ration formulation and related subject matter. It is amply illustrated with graphs, photographs and tabular data. Many NRC tables on nutrient requirements are included.

LIVESTOCK FEEDS AND FEEDING

by D.C. Church et al, 1977

This volume is intended as a text book on applied animal nutrition for university level classes at the sophomore-junior level. Only very brief information is given on the nutrients. Major emphasis is placed on description of feedstuffs, ration formulation, feed processing, feed additives and feeding practices for all of the common domestic animal species. Chapters are also included on dogs, rabbits and hatchery fish. It is amply illustrated with graphs, pictures and tabular data. Many of the NRC tables have been included in the appendix.

Chapter 1 - Introduction

In this chapter the intent is to point out and discuss briefly some of the factors related to nutrient utilization by ruminant animals. Many of these factors will be discussed in succeeding chapters, thus this chapter is intended only to bring them to the reader's attention and to set the stage for the material to follow.

ACCURACY OF NUTRIENT REQUIREMENTS

Over the past 50 years there have been thousands of man hours spent on experimental studies where the object was to define or refine nutrient needs for ruminant animals. This has resulted in the various publications put out by the NRC (National Research Council), the ARC (Agricultural Research Council in England) and other feeding standards which have been developed in other countries. Even though this information exists, it is well recognized by nutritionists that the nutrient requirements of broilers, layers and growing and fattening swine are defined with more precision and accuracy that those for ruminants. There are several reasons why this is so.

One of the important reasons is related to variability encountered in rations. Two types of variability are involved—variation in nutritive content of feedstuffs and variation in the proportions of ingredients used in rations. The standard broiler diet in the USA is based on corn and soybean meal with small amounts of other ingredients. Variability in nutrient composition of corn and soybean meal is generally less extreme than that encountered in many ruminant feeds, particularly most roughages. Variability in nutrient composition of diet ingredients adds to the problems in evaluating nutrient needs simply because scientists often do not recognize that it occurs (or it may not be feasible to sample and analyze enough batches of feed), and they may think that the nutrient consumption was different than it actually was. This could result in misleading data. In addition to this problem, ruminant diets are generally more variable from area to area with regard to the feedstuffs utilized. Changes in the amounts (%) of feedstuffs in a ration, even though nutrient composition might not change, creates problems. For example, the major protein in corn, zein, is less soluble than protein in most other cereal grains. More of it is likely to pass into the gut without digestion in the rumen than proteins from barley or wheat, and this probably alters animal response. Similarly, there appear to be differences in the rate at which rumen microorganisms degrade starch from the different cereal grains. Also, unknown or unexplained interactions occur between feed ingredients which alter utilization by animals, and changes in feed ingredients may mask changes in nutrient content. The fact that ruminant diets may vary from 100% forage or roughage to 90-95% concentrates contributes to this problem.

Secondly, the ability to evaluate animal response is enhanced in poultry and, to a lesser extent in swine, by the availability of large numbers of similar animals. With broilers, for example, all of the experimental animals might be half or full sibs, thus genetic variability can be reduced to almost nothing compared to cattle or sheep experiments. In addition, the large numbers of birds or pigs that can be used for a given experimental cost enhance the statistical predictibility of experimental results, allowing more precise estimates of nutrient requirements in a given situation.

A third factor is that broilers, for instance, are maintained in rather standard conditions from the time the chick is hatched until it is marketed. The temperature is controlled as well as other environmental factors. The same situation prevails, although to a lesser extent, for layers and growing and fattening pigs. In contrast, the age that calves are marketed may range from a few days of age for some veal to over 2 years of age for some market beef. In the meantime the animals may be managed in many different ways, depending on the objectives of the owner. Calves may be put into the feedlot and finished directly after weaning. They may be carried through the winter at a low rate of gain, pastured during the summer, and either finished on grass or put into the feedlot after the end of the normal pasture season. Similar methods are applied to lambs. Thus, this variability in management methods makes it more difficult to be precise in establishing nutrient requirements since there are greater age and environmental differences with ruminants.

A fourth factor is that the broiler industry has developed and utilized rather specific breeds or cross breeds for broiler production. This practice reduces variability in performance and nutrient needs that might otherwise occur because of breed differences. Contrast this to the many different beef and sheep breeds being used at the present time. Included are breeds which mature at different sizes and rates and have other characteristics which alter nutrient needs.

Last but certainly not least the environment for poultry and swine is normally controlled to a much greater extent than for most ruminants. Broilers are often maintained in heated buildings in cold weather, whereas this is unheard of for ruminants except for very young animals. In addition a very high percentage of poultry and swine spend their entire life in confinement, whereas ruminant animals are confined much less, usually only feedlot animals and young veal calves or, to a lesser extent, lactating dairy cows. Confinement under rather standard conditions contributes to more uniformity in animal requirements. Thus, it is unlikely that nutrient requirements for ruminant animals will ever be as well defined as for swine and poultry.

ANIMAL FACTORS AFFECTING NUTRIENT REQUIREMENTS

Even if we could resolve the problems in ration and nutrient variability just discussed, there are many other factors which are known to alter requirements or utilization of feed. These include such things as body size and surface area, basal metabolic rate, age, sex, breed, species, environment, level of production, diseases and parasites, and natural toxins found in feeds. Many of these are discussed in different chapters which follow. However, quantitative data are difficult to obtain and a number of these items are not built into the NRC tables of nutrient requirements for this reason.

It has been recognized for some time that energy requirements are related to body size, but the relationship is much higher if it can be related to body surface area. Studies with inanimate objects show clearly the high relationship between heat loss and surface area, and all of our current feeding standards relate energy requirements and, sometimes requirements for other nutrients, to body surface area as estimated by multiplying body weight by a fractional power (0.7-0.77). However, this still leaves some room for improvement. For example, the surface area

of an irregular shaped object like an animal body is difficult to calculate, and it may change with posture. To take an extreme example, the relationship between body weight and surface area of an Aberdeen Angus bull must be quite different than that of an animal with a long neck and long legs such as a giraffe, although both are ruminants. Thus, the profile of an animal may alter its effective surface area as will insulation (such as wool) and other physiological factors (see Ch. 18 and 16). In addition to this, the basal metabolic rate (BMR) varies considerably between highly excitable animals and slow moving, quiet animals and these differences are reflected in different energy requirements.

It is recognized that young animals have different nutrient requirements than older or mature animals, and this is reflected in feeding standards. No adjustments are made, however, for old animals. Likewise, some differences in requirements as affected by sex are reflected in feeding standards but rarely are breed differences given consideration, although there is information showing appreciable differences in energy metabolism between different breeds of cattle.

Hot or cold temperatures (outside the comfort zone) may have a pronounced effect on energy requirements. Since other factors affect chilling or heat stress, these are difficult to quantitate and adjustment factors are not normally included in feeding standards. Level of production alters requirements, of course, but the efficiency of feed utilization also changes, partly because digestibility declines as consumption increases. The ARC standards include an adjustment factor for increased consumption but the NRC standards usually do not. The effect of diseases and parasites are usually recognized, but there is no attempt to adjust animal requirements accordingly. Thus, we see that many factors may alter requirements but it is difficult or impossible to quantitate many of them and to include appropriate adjustments into feeding standards.

DEFICIENCIES IN NUTRITIONAL KNOWLEDGE

Knowledge about the nutrient needs of ruminant animals has increased tremendously in the past two decades but much still remains to be learned. Of current interest is the relationship between requirements and solubility of proteins and non-protein nitrogen components in feedstuffs or added ingredients such as urea and the need for essential amino acids by high producing animals (see Ch. 3). Although many research papers have been published on these topics, the problems are still not resolved. For example, it has been recognized for many years that urea must be fed with some readily available carbohydrate if good utilization is to be achieved. However, the amount and kind of carbohydrate needed is still not quantitated' with any accuracy and arguments continue as to the feasibility of using non-protein nitrogen in the rations of high producing animals.

Very little effort has been expended on evaluating nutrient needs of goats, buffalos and most of the wild species, a few of which show some promise for more intensive use by man. Although goats are used extensively in many underdeveloped countries, in particular, very few research reports have been published on this topic in the past 10 years.

Nutrient and feed interactions remain a largely unknown and unexplained factor which affects digestibility as well as efficiency of utilization of feedstuffs. A number of examples may be found in the literature illustrating interactions in digestiblity, but the information is so limited that it is impossible to apply it in practice.

There are many other factors that need further study, particularly interactions between nutrient needs and environmental factors, nutritional and genetic interactions, etc. The specific items that were mentioned here by no means complete the relatively long list that could be given.

Thus, we see that there are many problems remaining which need clarification or refinement. Certainly, animals vary from day to day in their physiology and functions such as digestibility undoubtedly vary considerably during a given period of time, even in "normal" animals. We should not expect to develop the field of ruminant nutrition with the same degree of precision that might be accomplished with monogastric species such as broiler chicks for reasons that have been given. However, it is certain that we can improve the current knowledge considerably with concerted effort on some of these areas that have been mentioned. New instrumentation allowing the collection of more complete data on nutrient composition of feeds and animal biochemistry, and careful utilization of computer simulation techniques and other new technology should improve our understanding and ability to quantitate nutrient needs of ruminant animals.

Chapter 2 - Water

Water is an extremely important compound (nutrient) for livestock since it makes up about two thirds of the fat-free animal body. It has numerous functions and the various compartments in which it abounds in the body have been well documented elsewhere. Thus, the material covered in this chapter will not be concerned primarily with body function.

A substantial number of research papers have been published on different topics related to water utilization by ruminant animals since the first edition of this volume. For the readers wishing more detail, the following articles or books would be recommended: A book by Schmidt-Nielsen (1964); a discussion on water requirements in the ARC (1965); a chapter by Roubicek (1969) in a book and an NRC report (1974).

BODY WATER

Water content of the animal body varies considerably, being influenced over the long run by age and the amount of fat in the tissues. However, the water content of the fat-free adult body is relatively constant for many species, averaging from 71-73% of body weight (Reid et al, 1955; Mitchell, 1962). Reid et al demonstrated that composition of the animal body can be estimated with reasonable accuracy if either the fat or water content is known.

A variety of different methods have been developed to estimate body water in animals. These methods depend upon dilution of a compound in body water following intravenous administration of the compound. Following injection of the test compound, serial samples of blood (or other body tissue) are taken, and the concentration can then be determined after equilibration with body tissues and then extrapolated to zero time. In most cases a given compound is not restricted completely to a given water "compartment" since there may be some metabolism of the compound or diffusion into other tissues at an irregular rate.

On the basis of published data, Mannery (1954) concluded that about one third of total body water is extracellular (17-30% of BW) of which about 6% is plasma water, and that cellular water amounts to about 40% of BW. Data of Bensadoun et al (1963) indicate that water in the GIT of sheep represents from 9-21% of total body water although values

approaching 25% have been reported when sheep were deprived of both feed and water for 24 hr (Smith and Sykes, 1974). Wade and Sasser (1970) concluded that total body water in sheep amounted to 64.7% of BW and that water in plasma and erythrocytes amounted to 7.43% of BW.

Age has an important effect on water content as demonstrated by Wellington et al (1956). When body water was estimated in cattle differing in age from 16 to 80 weeks, data showed that body water decreased as the animals aged and as the level of feeding went from low to high. Body water of 16-wk-old heifers ranged from 78.3 to 67.3% of BW and body fat increased from 2.0 to 8.4%. In 48-wk-old heifers body water ranged from 70.6 to 56.3% and fat from 4.2-21.4%. In bulls trends were comparable. An equation, $Y = 388.44 + 0.5366X - 227.37 \log X$ (where X = % body water), could be used to calculate body fat with relatively good precision. In contrast Garrett et al (1959) made 45 direct comparisons with cattle between body fat calculated from antipyrine body water and from specific gravity methods and found that the results were too variable to be very useful. Sheep were used to determine the effect of GIT contents on total water as estimated with antipyrine and again, results were quite variable. Bensadoun et al (1963) used a combination of antipyrine (AP) and N-acetyl-4-amino-antipyrine (NAAP) to measure body water in sheep. NAAP is excreted rather slowly into the GIT and gives an estimate of ingesta-free empty BW. These studies showed that a combination of these compounds allowed a good estimate of body water. The NAAP space was not affected by level of feed intake, kind of feed, or age of the sheep. The AP space was significantly larger for 15-mo.-old sheep (more body water) than for 27-mo.-old sheep. Sheep fed chopped hay had larger AP space than those fed corn-hay pellets, thus indicating differences in water in the GIT which were affected by age and type of feed.

Aschbacker et al (1965) used tritiated water to measure body water in dairy cows. They found 69.8-71.9% for two lactating cows, 69.0 and 67.6% for two nonlactating cows, and 56.3 and 56.2% for two "fat" nonlactating cows. In growing calves Wrenn et al (1962) used sodium thiocyanate to measure extracellular body water; they found that extracellular water decreased rapidly from

Table 2-1. Water metabolism in sheep and black tailed deer.[a]

Item	BW, kg	Total body water, l.	% of BW as water %	Water turnover l./day	Water turnover ½ life, days
Sheep					
Winter	50.7	26.3	53.3	5.17	3.52
Summer	55.1	25.4	46.0	7.70	2.30
Deer					
Winter	33.3	21.3	63.4	1.75	8.52
Summer	32.0	23.5	73.5	3.33	4.92

[a] From Longhurst et al (1970)

about 48% of BW at birth to about 30% at 1 yr of age. This decrease occurred during the first 4 mo. in heifers and in the 5th to 7th mo. for bulls. Thiocyanate space of young bulls tended to be higher than in heifers of the same weight.

There is evidence that total body water may vary considerably between different species. Note in Table 2-1 that body water content of sheep (Corriedale-Targhee breed) was considerably less than for black-tailed deer when animals were given similar diets, and body water was measured during the winter or summer months. The authors (Longhurst et al, 1970) found that water content of thigh muscles was similar for the two species (73.6 and 73.1%, respectively, for deer and sheep) and suggest that the lower body water content of sheep was a result of greater fat content together with the added weight of wool. The values given by Longhurst et al for black-tailed deer agree reasonably well with other data reported on mule deer (Knox et al, 1969).

WATER TURNOVER IN THE TISSUES

When using tritiated water, Black et al (1964) found that the half life of water averaged 3.5 days for cows (no effect of lactation), 3.4 for males, 2.8 for a 7-day-old calf, and 3.5 days for a 6-mo.-old calf. Argenzio and co-workers (1968) reported a somewhat longer time for lactating cows (5.5 days). Rumen water turnover averaged 10 hr in a cow and 17 hr in a goat. In studies with grazing twin cattle, Wright and Jones (1974) found that water half life was 2.0-2.4 days for lactating cows and 2.8-3.3 days for dry cows. With young calves Sekine et al (1972) found that the half life of body water was 4.8, 6.9

and 6.4 days for male Holstein calves at 2, 7 and 12 weeks of age.

With aged ewes (2.5-14 yr of age) it has been estimated that the half life ranged from 4.4-7.0 days with an average of 5.4 days (Anand et al, 1966). With ewes 3-8 yr of age, Longhurst et al (1970) reported values of 2.3 to 3.5 days (Table 2-1). Other data in the literature are: black-tailed deer, 4.9-8.5 (Table 2-1); camels during winter, 12.2 and 6.4 in summer (Siebert and MacFarlane, 1971).

MacFarlane and co-workers have probably spent more effort than anyone in looking at water turnover in a variety of ruminant species in various situations. Some of their research with sheep (MacFarlane et al, 1966) indicated a half life of 3.3 to 4.5 days, the longer half lives being in dry periods of the year. When expressed as ml/kg·82 BW, the values ranged from 174 to 259. As compared to other ruminant species, the turnover rates in a tropical environment were (ml/kg·82): banteng, 348, Brahman, 350; Santa Gertrudis, 373; Shorthorn, 461; buffalo, 535 (Siebert and MacFarlane, 1969); these values correspond to half lives of 2.6 in buffaloes to 3.9 days in the banteng. When comparing camels to other species (MacFarlane et al, 1963), values were (ml/kg/24 hr): camels, 61; Merino sheep, 110; and Shorthorn cattle, 148. Other research (MacFarlane and Howard, 1966) has shown that stall-fed cattle used about one third (74-132 ml/kg·82) of the water turned over by grazing cattle (261-364). The male Oryx was shown to be able to conserve water. Marked differences were noted between individual sheep of the same breed (MacFarlane et al, 1967).

Based on detailed studies with feral African ruminants, MacFarlane et al (1972) point out that water turnover in the suckling young is a direct measure of milk intake. In adult animals, water turnover is highly related to the wetness of the environment and the capability of a particular species to conserve water. In the equatorial desert Boran cattle had about twice the rate of turnover as Ogaden sheep and Somali goats and dromedaries had a slightly lower rate than the sheep. In hot-wet equatorial pastures, Karakul sheep had greater turnover rates than Merino or Dorper sheep. In upland equatorial grasslands Boran cattle and eland were similar but wildebeest and hartebeest were much lower. In equatorial temperate upland pastures, *Bos taurus* cattle used 16-38% more water than *Bos indicus* cattle.

Thus, data from a variety of sources show marked species differences, effect of age, lactation, temperature and humidity, seasonal differences related to water content of forage, and effects due to consumption of plants high in salt.

WATER SOURCES

Water available to an animal's tissues comes from (1) drinking water, (2) water contained in or on feed, (3) metabolic water produced by oxidation of organic nutrients, (4) water liberated from polymerization reactions such as condensation of amino acids to peptides, and (5) preformed water associated with the tissues which are catabolized during a period of negative energy balance.

The importance of these different sources of water is believed to differ from species to species, depending upon diet and habitat, and on ability to conserve body water. Some species of desert rodents are said not to require drinking water except in rare situations; this is not the case with most ruminant species, although some, such as sheep, do not require water as frequently as others. Taylor (1968) reports that desert antelopes such as the Oryx (*Oryx beisa*) and Grant's gazelle (*Gazella granti*) are apparently able to obtain all water needed by consuming desert plants which are capable of rehydrating themselves from the night air. The American pronghorn antelope has been thought not to consume much free water. However, recent quantitative observations show that drinking water is readily taken in the summer in desert areas (Sundstrom, 1970).

Water in the feed and on the feed (precipitation, dew) is quite variable and may range from a low of 5-7% to as high as 80% or more in lush young grass. Consequently, the amount available differs markedly from season to season, in different geographical areas, and on the diet.

Metabolic water from oxidation of organic nutrients is also quite variable depending upon the diet. Oxidation of carbohydrates results in the production of about 60 g of water/100 g of carbohydrate; fat yields about 108 g of water, and protein about 42 g. Ruminants do not normally consume diets containing more than 2-4% fat, however oxidation of the volatile acids resulting from rumen and gut fermentation would yield 67-93+ g of water/100 g of acid. Metabolic water from fat and protein would be of more relative importance during periods of negative energy balance when depot fat and tissue protein are likely to be catabolized to supply energy. This would be especially true during the winter months and for animals such as male deer which markedly reduce their voluntary feed intake during the rutting season. Schmidt-Nielsen (1964) aptly points out that the differences in yield of metabolic water between fats and carbohydrates such as starch are misleading. He shows clearly that fats, being less oxidized compounds, require more oxygen for complete oxidation in the body; thus, more oxygen must be respired as well as more water expired. The consequence being that starch yields more net water than fat for a given energy intake, at least where air humidity is low.

Mitchell (1962) cites data from the Pennsylvania Experiment Station (work) of Forbes and Swift on the water metabolism of steers fed a maintenance ration of alfalfa hay in calorimeter trials. In this case drinking water accounted for 89.4% of available water, water in the hay accounted for 3.4%, and calculated values for metabolic water amounted to 7.2% of the total. When evaluating dry diets with sheep, Wallace et al (1972) found that free water accounted for 88-90%, water in the feed for 1.9-2.9% and metabolic water for 7.2-10.1% of total water.

In studies with Dorcas gazelles, Ghobrial (1970) determined that free water accounted for 68.9% and 81.4% of total water in winter and summer, respectively. Preformed water accounted for 4.4 and 2.7% and water from oxidation of nutrients accounted for 26.7 and 15.9%, respectively, during these different seasons. Thus, it is apparent the relative amount consumed as drinking water or as water in the feed or from oxidation will vary considerably depending on many different factors.

Table 2-2. Water metabolism of sheep maintained indoors at 20-26°C.[a]

Item	Month	
	June	December
Water input, g/day		
Free water consumed	2,093	1,732
Water in feed	51	56
Metabolic water[b]	240	138
Total input	2,384	1,926
Water output, g/day		
Fecal water	328	552
Urinary water	788	502
Vaporized water	1,268	872
Total output	2,384	1,926
Water in feces, %	57	56
Water in urine, %	92	94

[a] From Wallace et al (1972); diets were dried samples collected during June or December from esophageal fistulated steers.
[b] Calculated values.

WATER LOSSES

Losses of water from the animal body occur by way of urine, feces, vaporization from the lungs and skin (insensible water) and water lost via sweat from the sweat glands during warm or hot weather.

Urinary water losses are usually in excess of the amount needed to excrete body wastes (obligatory losses) unless water intake is restricted by some means. If an animal is conditioned to reduced consumption of water, urinary losses can usually be reduced to some extent without ill effects. There are tremendous differences between species in urinary losses since some desert dwellers normally drink much less water, but they are also capable of concentrating urine to a much greater extent than species adapted to wet climates.

There are a number of factors which have a marked effect on urinary losses. Probably the most important factor is temperature. Naturally if animals consume large quantities of water during hot weather, urinary losses will be increased greatly. Other factors which have an important effect on urinary losses include: dry matter and digestible dry matter in the diet, N consumption and urinary N production, and consumption of fat, K, P and Cl (Paquay et al, 1970).

Fecal water losses are normally considerably higher in ruminants than in many other species, being about equal to urinary losses (see Table 2-2), whereas in man the fecal loss is about 7-10% of urinary water (Mitchell, 1962). There are appreciable differences between species in the percentage of water found in feces. Those species such as sheep, which form fecal pellets, usually excrete feces with less water than other species which do not form pellets. Sheep feces, for example, may be expected to have 50-70% water with mean values on the order of ca. 65%. Cattle, on the other hand, excrete feces with considerably more water; values would usually be on the order of 68-80% water depending on the diet. Presumably, species which form fecal pellets and thereby reabsorb more water from the gut, are better adapted to drier climates and to more severe water restriction.

Fecal water is, of course, highly related to total water intake, but many other factors contribute to total excretion. Dry matter consumption is an important factor (see section on water requirements). Other factors include: fecal dry matter and N, fibrous components in the diet (pentosans, crude fiber), fecal fat, energy consumption and K and Cl consumption (Parquay et al, 1970).

Water vaporized from the body represents a rather large amount of the total water loss

Table 2-3. Effect of 50% water restriction on water metabolism of dairy cows at 18 and 32°.[a]

Measurement	18°		32°	
	Ad lib.	Restricted	Ad lib.	Restricted
Body wt, kg	641	623	622	596
Feed consumed, kg	36.3	24.9	25.2	19.1
Urine volume, l./day	17.5	10.1	30.3	9.9
Feces weight, kg	27.8	14.7	15.1	10.9
Fecal water, %	76.6	71.7	77.2	75.7
Metabolic water, kg	2.5	2.0	2.1	1.9
Vaporized water, kg	27.2	14.0	28.2	23.0
Total water loss, kg[b]	65.1	34.1	68.6	40.7

[a] Data taken from Seif et al (1973)

[b] Estimated from data

(see Tables 2-2, 3), primarily because of the large loss from the lungs, especially in a very hot atmosphere. Inhaled air may be very dry, but expired air is about 90% saturated with water. Consequently, the loss can be large, particularly during periods of hyperventilation that occur during hot weather. Respiratory water losses have been reported to range from about 23 ml/m^2 of body surface/hr at 27°C to 50 ml at 41° (Kibler and Brody, 1952). More recent information for lactating cows showed losses averaging 1133 and 1174 g/hr for cows at 18 and 32°C, respectively (Seif et al, 1973). Maximum loss in sheep is said to be about 95 ml/m^2/hr (Roubicek, 1969).

Sweat losses by ruminants have been measured, among other ways, by placing capsules over a small skin area in order to trap excreted water. Murray (1966) found that ¾-blood Santa Gertrudis cattle had about 1,610 sweat glands/cm^2 as compared to 1,280 for Hereford cattle; although sweat production was not statistically different between breeds. Under laboratory conditions sweat production ranged from 1.73-2.20 g/m^2/5 min. During field conditions sweating rates were considerably higher, ranging from 2.99-5.06 g/m^2/5 min. Murray's data led him to conclude that solar radiation leads to a marked increase in sweat production as compared to hot temperatures in the laboratory where lighting was with artificial light.

Kibler and Brody (1952) suggested that maximum dissipation of water from the skin of cattle is ca. 3X the maximum from the lungs in a variety of different breeds. MacFarlane (1964) found that sheep respired about 8X as much water as was lost through sweating; whereas in Zebu cattle sweating loss was about 6X respiratory losses. In Shorthorn cattle, which have less efficient sweating mechanisms, the ratio was 3 or 4 to 1. The high ratio of respiratory to sweat losses by sheep is because sheep sweat very little.

DRINKING HABITS

The drinking habits of various ruminant species have been investigated to a limited extent. Although there are many qualitative observations in the literature, quantitative observations are rare. Since environmental influences are such an important factor, it is difficult to describe the drinking habits of a given species.

Warner and Stacy (1968) observed that sheep with restricted access to water normally drank 90-100% of their total intake immediately after eating at a rate of 0.5 l./min. and, if they drank any more, they usually did so within the next 15-30 min. In studies with sheep where food was provided at distances ranging from 2.4 to 5.6 km from water, it was observed that sheep would normally eat and then walk to water and drink before 1000 hr. If a second drink was taken, it was between 1730 and 2000 hr (Squires and Wilson, 1971; Daws and Squires, 1974). The distance to water and temperature had an effect on whether the sheep drank 1 or 2 times daily. There was also a breed effect. Merinos made one walk to water daily at 4.8 km and an average of two walks every 3 days at 5.6 km. When maximum temperatures were in excess of 38°C, the afternoon drink was abandoned. Border Leicesters walked to water once daily at 5.6 km and normally made two trips daily at shorter distances. Total water consumption ranged from 3-6 l./day for Merinos and 3-9 for Border Leicesters. Temperatures above 38°C caused a reduction in water consumption, drinking frequency and reduced feed intake.

Schmidt-Nielsen (1964) points out that free-ranging camels, which were observed to go as long as 6 days between waterings, drink large quantities of water very rapidly; the amounts being equivalent to as much as one third of their normal weight or one half of their dehydrated weight. The frequency of watering was observed to be highly related to the type of diet consumed. Plants high in salt resulted in more frequent drinking.

With regard to cattle Hancock (1953) observed that when water was readily available to grazing cows, they usually drank from 2-5X daily and probably never more than 7X daily. These values were similar to those reported by Castle et al (1950) who found that dairy cows drank from 2-7X/day with an average of 3.8X/day. In studies with dairy cows in England, Thomas (1971) found that most cows drank 3-4X/day but an average of 7X was observed on one farm in June. Castle and Thomas (1975) observed that cows on winter rations drank 40% of total daily intake between 1500 and 2100 hr. Drinking time ranged from 2.0-7.8 min./cow/day and the rate of drinking varied from 4.5-14.9 kg/min.

Observations of numerous investigators indicate that confined cattle tend to drink frequently if water is readily available, particularly during warm weather. Ragsdale et al (1950, 1951) pointed out that until the ambient temperature exceeds 80°F, cattle tend to do most of their drinking in the forenoon and late afternoon and evening, while very little water is consumed at other times. At 90°F and above, the periods during which no water is consumed tend to be shortened and the animals may drink every 2 hr or more. During warm weather cattle in the feedlot drink more frequently during the late afternoon and night (Ray and Roubicek, 1971). In one experiment it was observed that water consumption was as follows (time, % of total water): summer time with shelter, 0900-1200, 10.9%; 1200-1500, 24.7%; 1500-1800, 23.3%; and 1800-2100, 19.3%; in the winter, values for the same times were: 13.3, 20.4, 30.6 and 17.3% (Hoffman and Self, 1972). In studies with confined steers on different types of diets, Bond et al (1976)

found that 60-65% of total time at the waterer was spent between 0600 and 1800 hr.

In many situations it is obvious that animals grazing semidesert ranges cannot drink as often as studies would indicate with cattle in confinement. Depending upon the given situation and distance from water, it is more common for range beef cattle to drink no more than once daily during the warmer months and less frequently during cooler weather. Sheep may go several days without drinking in cool weather.

WATER REQUIREMENTS

Water requirements have been expressed in a number of different ways. For example: per unit of body weight or metabolic size (surface area), per unit of dry matter intake or in relationship to energy, protein or salt consumption, and in relationship to ambient (environmental) temperature. It was noted many years ago that free water consumption is highly related to dry matter consumption (Ritzman and Benedict, 1924), but there are marked differences between species such as cattle and sheep because of differences in fecal and urinary water excretion. Probably the best overall relationship would be between water consumption and heat production by the animal (Mitchell, 1962), but this method also has shortcomings when heat production is very high at low temperatures or at hot stressing temperatures when animals tend to drink water to cool their bodies (Razdan et al, 1971; Bond and McDowell, 1972).

Winchester and Morris (1956) have used the data of a number of investigators who collected information on cattle under defined environmental conditions and have made estimates of water consumption and requirements as influenced by temperature and dry matter intake for different classes of cattle. Data from calorimeter trials were used to interpolate dry matter consumption at different temperatures. Winchester and Adams developed a graph from which values were derived (Fig. 2-1).

When water consumption per unit of dry matter was plotted, Winchester and Morris found intake to be as follows (temperature in F, kg water intake/kg dry matter consumed): 40°, 3.09; 50°, 3.35; 60°, 3.84; 70°, 4.51; 80°, 5.17; and 90°, 7.34. As shown in the figure, water consumption was slightly higher for *Bos taurus* than for *Bos indicus* species. Since the values of Winchester and Morris were derived primarily from cattle in calorimeter trials, it might be questioned if the

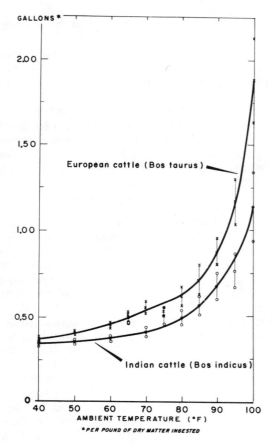

Figure 2-1. Water intake expressed as a function of dry matter consumption and ambient temperature. From Winchester and Morris (1956).

reduced activity of confined cattle would result in lower values than for cattle in an outdoor environment. The exposure to radiant heat has also been shown to increase sweating and respiratory effort in hot weather when compared to animals maintained in equivalent temperatures in the shade, thus this might result in an additional error for cattle in an outdoor environment. More recent data on consumption by heifers during the summer in Nevada (Weeth et al, 1968) indicated intake of ca. 4-5 kg of water/kg of hay consumed and data of Waldo et al (1965) indicate an intake of 3.2-4.9 kg of water/kg of dry matter by Holstein heifers consuming a variety of rations. Thus, these values may be appropriate for farm or ranch conditions although exact comparisons to field conditions are not possible.

The difficulty in relating water needs to feed intake is partially illustrated by the previous facts, i.e., that feed intake will be depressed at the higher ambient tempera-

tures while water intake will continue to rise. Thompson et al (1949) found that non-lactating cows consumed about 6% of their body weight/day of water. In a hot environment this quantity will increase tremendously, far past the added amount needed for increased respiratory and sweat losses. For example, data reported by Kelly et al (1955) show that steers in a hot environment consumed about 12.5% of their mean body weight daily. As a result of this added consumption, urinary excretion increases tremendously. Thompson et al (1949) mentioned one cow that increased urinary volume from 25 to 125 l./day, indicating that the cow was drinking water (at 15°F) to cool her body. The relationship between dry matter and water consumption for non-lactating cows in a moderate European climate is illustrated in Fig. 2-2.

The ARC committee (1965) summarized literature on water consumption from a variety of sources on cattle as related to environmental temperature and made recommendations for moderate tempeatures typical of those in Britain. They recommend 6.5 kg of water/kg of DM intake for calves (up to 5-6 wk of age) and from 3.5 to 5.5 kg of water/kg of DM intake for older cattle when temperatures range from -17° to above 27°C.

The water requirements of calves have not been well evaluated in many situations. Pettyjohn et al (1963) found that preruminant calves took in a maximum DM intake when receiving liquid diets with 25% DM (range 4-25%). Maximum gain occurred at a concentration of 15% DM. Total water intake —

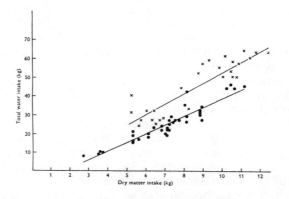

Figure 2-2. The correlation between total water intake and dry matter intake in dry dairy cows. The x value refers to feeds (silage, grass) with high moisture content; the • values refer to dry rations. These equations show that 5.5 kg of water was consumed for each kg of DM on the wet rations and 4.6 kg with dried feeds. From Paquay et al (1970).

that in the liquid diet and additional water consumed — ranged from 4.6 to 18.7 kg water/kg of DM. The apparent optimum concentration of 15% DM resulted in a total intake of 6.4 kg of water/kg of DM consumed. In another example, calves 3-20 days of age were allowed fluid intakes of 7.5, 10 or 12.5% of their BW (Stiles et al, 1974). No data were given on gain or efficiency, but the information on scours suggested that the low level (7.5% of BW) adversely affected well being of the calves.

In a study with calves which had been weaned at 28 days of age, Hodgson (1973) found that water consumption ranged from 2.9 to 3.6 kg/kg of DM. The basal diet was dried, chopped grass. Water consumption/kg of DM was increased when the diet was ground and pelleted. With older Holstein bulls (7.5 mo.) in Israel, Holzer et al (1976) found that the cattle consumed 3.71 kg of water/kg DM when the diet (straw, concentrate) contained 10% moisture. Total water consumption was increased to 3.82 and 5.09 kg/kg DM when moisture content of the ration was increased to 50 or 75%, respectively. Increasing roughage in the diet from 25-45% or particle size of the straw in the diet both resulted in slight increases in water consumed/kg of DM consumed. Data from India show total water consumption of 5.9 and 6.4 g/g DM for Zebu cattle and buffalo, respectively, on a variety of diets (Razdan et al, 1971).

The water needs of lactating cows were derived by Winchester and Morris by subtracting 87% of the weight of milk produced from the water ingested and by calculating appropriate values at different temperatures. For a cow producing milk with 4% fat, the following values are suggested at the various temperatures (°F; kg water/kg milk): 40°, 0.98; 50°, 1.01; 60°, 1.13; 70°, 1.25; 80°, 1.36; and 90°, 1.79. These amounts of water are required over that normally required for non-lactating animals. These authors pointed out that temperature was found to have more effect on feed intake of lactating cows since feed intake began to decline at about 70°F as compared to about 90°F for non-lactating animals.

It might be mentioned that a rule of thumb used for water consumption of dairy cows is that lactating cows will consume about 20 gal (76 kg) per head/day. Obviously, this value is subject to many modifications.

The average intake of water of lactating cows during winter months in England was 3.70 kg/kg DM after subtracting the amount of water in the milk (Castle and Thomas, 1975). The mean consumption of drinking water was 49.9 kg/cow when milk production was 16.8 kg/day and mean temperature was 8.2°C and relative humidity was 84.8%. Water drunk was positively related to milk yield and DM content of the ration but not to air temperature or humidity. The range in water consumption was from 20.1 to 87.1 kg for cows with DM intakes of 10.0 to 21.7 kg/day.

In a study with water consumption of grazing dairy cows, it was shown that average consumption of water was 23.0 kg when DM content of the herbage was 17.8% and mean air temperature 13.4%C. Water consumption was positively related to daily milk yield and DM percentage of the herbage and negatively related to rainfall and relative humidity (Castle, 1972). Additional studies with grazing cows demonstrated that water consumption could be limited to about 3 hr/day without adverse effects on milk production (Castle and Watson, 1973).

Some of the earlier information on water requirements of sheep have been summarized by the ARC (1965) resulting in conclusions that requirements vary from 1.4 kg of water/kg of DM for sheep with short fleeces at cool temperatures (46°F) to about 5 kg of water/kg of DM at warmer temperatures. In studies with sheep on native grasslands in the summer in Australia, Wilson (1974) found that maximum intakes were 3-3.5 l./sheep/day. When shade was available, consumption decreased by 0.3-0.5 l./day.

Pregnancy has an important effect on water consumption of ewes. Head (1953) demonstrated that water intake of pregnant ewes increased from 1.9 kg/kg of DM in the first month of pregnancy to 4.3 kg in the 5th month. In other studies in England, water intake of pregnant ewes was higher than for non-pregnant ewes, particularly after the 14th week of pregnancy (Forbes, 1968). Twin-carrying ewes required more water than those carrying a single fetus. The water intake of ewes carrying singles and twins was increased to 138 and 212%, respectively, of that for non-pregnant ewes by the 5th month of pregnancy. Water intake of lactating ewes, when corrected for water in the milk, ranged from 100 to 164% of non-lactating ewes. Forbes suggests that the greater water need of pregnant ewes is due to greater heat production, resulting from increased metabolic activity, and to greater urinary excretion. He further points out that the high water requirements, if not met, would result in reduced feed intake and possible consequences of ketosis. Additional information on this topic was published by Davies (1972). Water consumption of ewes carrying single fetuses amounted to 2.5-3.7 kg/kg DM from 134 days on of pregnancy. Corresponding consumption of ewes with twins was 3.4-4.7 kg/kg of DM. During lactation, ewes with singles and twins consumed 3.0 and 3.3-3.5 kg/kg of DM, respectively.

Under simulated desert conditions water consumption of African goats and haired sheep amounted to ca. 8% of BW/day (Maloiy and Taylor, 1971). Limited data are also available on captive impala (Jarman, 1973).

OTHER FACTORS AFFECTING WATER CONSUMPTION

Dietary Factors

The previous discussion has shown that water consumption, for a given ration and temperature, is highly related to the amount of feed consumed; thus, an animal needs water in direct relationship to the amount of feed. Information on other dietary factors, other than NaCl, are rather scarce in the literature. In a statistical study of water metabolism of lactating cows fed 37 different rations over several years, Paquay et al (1970) found the following nutritional items to be highly correlated (items with $r>0.4$ are given): pentosans, .707; digestible crude fiber, .626; dry matter intake, .610; Cl, .545; K, .486; Ca, .428; starch intake, -.419.

It has been known for some time that cattle on a high protein intake consume more water (up to 26% more) than similar animals on low protein rations (Ritzman and Benedict, 1924). Other more recent information shows that feeding urea increased urinary flow (Thornton, 1970) and feeding of increasingly soluble proteins resulted in increased water consumption and urinary excretion (Wohlt et al, 1976). In addition reducing protein consumption resulted in reduced consumption and excretion of water (Utley et al, 1970). Razdan et al (1971) also noted that feeding urea (vs. peanut meal) to cattle or buffalo resulted in greater water consumption.

The influence of other types of rations is shown in Table 2-4. Data in Table 2-4 show clearly that the physical form of feed or the consumption of silage influenced the amount of total water intake. In experiment 2

Table 2-4. Effect of some rations on water intake of Holstein heifers.[a]

Item	Experiment 1			
	Hay	Pellets	Hay-grain	Silage
Water consumed, kg/kg feed dry matter				
Water in feed	0.14	0.14	0.14	1.40
Water drank	3.57	3.10	3.16	2.84
Total water intake	3.71	3.24	3.30	4.24

	Experiment 2			
	Hay		Silage	
	Ad lib.	Maint.	Ad lib.	Maint.
Water consumed, kg/kg feed dry matter				
Water in feed	0.11	0.12	3.38	3.38
Water drank	3.36	3.66	1.55	1.38
Total intake	3.48	3.79	4.93	4.76
Urine, kg/kg feed dry matter	0.93	1.14	1.85	1.68

[a] Data from Waldo et al (1965)

the same crop of forage was made into hay or silage, but it is evident that the silage resulted in a considerably higher water intake. Calder et al (1964) and Forbes (1968) have also reported that silage feeding resulted in a greater water intake as compared to other types of feed. In Forbes' work he points out that the silage used had a considerably higher amount of soluble ash than the hay but even so the ewes consumed more of a self-fed mineral lick, thus increasing the soluble ash intake even further. The figures in Table 2-4 show a higher urinary excretion/unit of DM intake by heifers consuming silage. Whether this is related to soluble ash intake is unknown since no information on feed composition was presented.

With respect to NaCl there are quite a number of good research reports which show that increasing consumption of NaCl in a dry diet will result in increased consumption and excretion of water. With saline waters experiments generally show that a moderate degree of salinity (1%) will be tolerated by sheep or cattle without a marked change in feed or water intake. However, as the concentration of salt increases, especially in warm or hot weather, then adverse effects are likely to occur. Also, consumption of salt or saline water results in more frequent watering. Refer to Ch. 4 for more information on salt toxicity.

It is frequently suggested that the high water content of feeds such as silage or succulent young grass may restrict the intake of dry matter by ruminants. Although research on this subject is limited, it might be of interest to mention several papers. Campling and Balch (1961) found that pouring 100 lb of water into the rumen during the daily meal did not affect intake of dry matter by cows, although the same amount of water in bladders in the rumen did reduce intake. Baile et al (1969), using goats, observed that injections of water into the rumen during feeding reduced intake of feed although not the frequency of feeding when an average of 1,250 ml of water were introduced. A volume of 900 ml did not reduce intake. Duckworth and Shirlaw (1958) investigated the intake of dairy heifers which were fed silage and partially dried grass. They observed that maximum dry matter intake occurred when the dry matter in the herbage was above 24-28%. On diets below 24% dry matter, the weight of wet matter consumed apparently controlled feed intake. These authors further point out that wetter diets were more bulky and required more bites/unit of dry matter consumed.

Data in Table 2-5 illustrate that addition of water to a dry diet is likely to increase DM consumption. When total moisture was increased to 50%, dry matter intake was increased. At the 75% level DM intake was the same as the original diet (10% water). Thus, information from these various papers does not prove the point, pro or con, but the author is inclined to go along with observations of Duckworth and Shirlaw and conclude that water, per se, is unlikely to be a limiting factor on intake. The fact that water is readily excreted by the kidney in large amounts and the high excretion that may occur via feces indicate that excretion should not be limiting. Plant material containing more water may require more rumen volume and fill in other parts of the GIT, although information from Holzer et al (1976) indicates very little change when water

Table 2-5. Effect of added water on feed and water consumption of Holstein bulls.[a]

Item	Moisture content of ration, %		
	10	50	75
DM intake, kg/day	10.24	10.96	10.24
Water drunk, kg/day	36.9	31.3	21.5
Water in feed, kg	1.14	10.6	30.6
Total water, kg/kg DM consumed	3.71	3.82	5.09

[a] Data from Holzer et al (1976)

was added to dry diets. Plant material which contains water in the plant cells should be readily fermented in the rumen.

Environmental Effects

Relative humidity has been shown to have only a negligible effect on water consumption at temperatures below 75°F (Ragsdale et al, 1953; Castle and Thomas, 1975), and wind up to 9 mph did not influence water intake by dairy cattle (Brody et al, 1954). Water consumption is also reduced when cattle (Garrett et al, 1960) or sheep are provided with shade (Wilson, 1974). Providing cooled water (65° vs. 88°F) resulted in a reduced consumption of water and greater daily gain of Hereford cattle when the maximum mean temperature was 100.5°F (Ittner et al, 1951). Later work from this same experiment station (Lofgreen et al, 1975) confirmed these findings for British breeds of cattle. Brahman x British crossbred cattle did not do any better on the cooled water. At somewhat lower temperatures (31°C), Harris et al (1967) did not find any appreciable response by providing cooled water for finishing steers.

Cunningham and others (1964) carried out some research during the fall and winter months in which cows were given water at temperatures ranging from 34° to 103°F. Their data indicated that less water was consumed at the 34° temperature and more at the higher temperatures. The range in consumption varied from 47-54 kg/head/day in one trial and from 42-48 kg/head/day in a second trial. With sheep Bailey et al (1962) found that a reduction in environmental temperatures from 15° to -12°C caused a reduced water intake from about 1,600 to 800 ml/day. At an environmental temperature of -12°C the temperature of the drinking water (0-30°C) did not influence the amount of water consumed. Williams (1959) studied the water intake in feedlot steers when temperatures ranged from -35° to 45°F. He reported that water intake was correlated with air temperature on the same day and with feed intake on the previous day.

The effect that consumption of cold water has on rumen temperature has been shown by Cunningham and co-workers (1964). They reported that ingestion of 21 kg of water at 34°F depressed the lower, middle and upper rumen temperatures by 23, 10 and 2 degrees, respectively, within 10 min. Sims and Butcher (1966) observed that consumption of snow or water at 1 or 20°C resulted in a drop in temperature of sheep's rumens of 4.5, 15

and 7°C, respectively. Snow resulted in a slower drop as well as a longer recovery time.

The consumption of cold water should be beneficial to animals which are subject to heat stresses as the cooling effect would be considerable. Likewise, when exposed to cold stress, it is obvious that an appreciable amount of dietary energy will be required to warm cold water to body temperature. However, when attempting to show the response in terms of liveweight gain or some other productive function, it has been difficult to show statistical differences.

EFFECT OF WATER RESTRICTION

It is obvious that the fluid intake of animals is intermittent while the loss of water from the body is continuous, although variable, in amount or rate. The body does not have a mechanism for storing water in the strict sense that fat is stored. However, many of the tissues can give up some water for a time without adverse effects. A degree of dehydration is a normal thing. The animal's reaction to water restriction which continues for any length of time is to restrict losses from the body or to reduce the need for water by cutting back on feed intake, as will be illustrated later. Dehydration results in loss of plasma water and both extra- and intra-cellular water. The rumen and other parts of the GIT also can give up some water for a time, but all of these must be replenished or the normal physiological functions will suffer.

The first noticeable effect of moderate water restriction is a reduced intake of feed; consequently, it is to be avoided if maximum feed intake is desired (Balch et al, 1953; French 1956; Bianca et al, 1965; Weeth et al, 1967). Bianca and others (1965) have studied some of the physiological responses in Ayrshire bulls during periods of water deprivation lasting 4 days at ambient temperatures at 15°C and for 2 days at 40°C. When water intake was not restricted at the 40° temperature, the cattle exhibited mild heat stress as evidenced by increased water consumption and evaporation, volume of urine, respiration rate, depressed feed intake and output of feces and a possible isotonic increase in plasma volume. When deprived of water, the cattle had lost about 12% of their BW by the end of the period, but the weight was regained in the first day of rehydration. At both temperatures the chief means of water conservation was a reduction in fecal water loss which was associated with

Table 2-6. Effect of water deprivation on Hereford heifers.[a]

Item	Days of Deprivation				
	0	1	2	3	4
Hay consumption, kg					
Controls			av.6.6		
Deprived	7.6	4.2	2.2	0.9	0.5
Water consumption, kg					
Controls	32	30	31	31	26
Deprived	34	0	0	0	0
Urine excreted, kg					
Controls	7.3	6.4	7.0	7.5	8.2
Deprived	6.6	7.2	4.7	2.9	2.3
Feces excreted, kg					
Controls	14.7	14.9	16.0	16.9	17.8
Deprived	16.0	10.4	4.7	2.5	1.6
Fecal water, %					
Controls	85.1	85.6	84.9	85.0	85.6
Deprived	84.8	83.4	79.5	75.2	71.9

[a] From Weeth et al (1967)

reduced feed intake and fecal output. Smaller reductions in evaporative and urinary water loss took place. At 15° the dehydrated animals were able to maintain normal body temperature, although there was a slight fall in heat production. At 40° the rectal temperature of dehydrated steers had increased slightly with no change in heat production.

Weeth et al (1967) assessed the changes in Hereford heifers resulting from complete deprivation of drinking water for 4 days. Some of their results are shown in Table 2-6. As shown in the table, the feed intake declined rapidly to a value of 0.5 kg/day by the 4th day. Likewise, urinary excretion declined but to a lesser extent than feed intake. Fecal excretion declined and the feces excreted were considerably drier resulting in more water saving than by reduced urine output. Other data presented indicated that urine was markedly concentrated, the osmolality increasing to 1,196 Mosmol/kg on the 4th day as compared to 780 Mosmol/kg for the control heifers. In addition plasma volume decreased, there was hemoconcentration, and the thiocyanate space (extracellular water) decreased.

Some data that have been published on sheep (Gordon, 1965; MacFarlane et al, 1961) indicate that sheep will consume very little food after the second day of water deprivation although Ruckebush et al (1967) found little difference in feeding behavior until the 4th and 5th day when intake decreased 80 and 90%, respectively. In the research reported by Mac Farlane et al, Merino wethers were deprived of water and subjected to temperatures of 29-42°C in tropical latitudes. Urine volume fell after 2 days without water, and in a hot season less than 100 ml/24 hr were excreted on the 4th or subsequent days. Urinary concentrations increased over the first 4 to 5 days. During rapid dehydration more Na was excreted than K. More than half of the weight loss appeared to come from intracellular sources; plasma and extracellular volume decreased up to 45% while a hemoconcentration up to 60% occurred. It was found that control of body temperature failed when 31% of body weight was lost by the end of 10 days without water. In hotter weather 5 days without water caused a 25% loss of body weight and in some sheep, irreversible circulatory failure. English (1966) found that water restriction in sheep resulted in negative balances of Na and Cl, but that of K remained positive.

When sheep are deprived or restricted in water intake, weight losses tend to be related to the degree of restriction and significant losses apparently occur only when water is restricted to half or less of ad libitum intake (Taneja, 1965, 1966). Severe restriction results in reduced urine volume accompanied by a marked increase in urinary Na concentration and a reduced glomerular filtration rate (Ghosh et al, 1976). Desert sheep begin to decrease total body water, total blood and plasma volumes and extracellular, intracellular and interstitial fluid volumes when water intake is reduced below 75% of normal requirements (Purohit et al, 1972).

In studies with cattle in a desert climate, Siebert and MacFarlane (1975) found that Shorthorn cows lost ca. 6% of BW per day. One third of the loss was body solids, a third was fluid from the gut and intracellular fluids and the remainder was interstitial fluid and plasma.

Studies on the camel indicate that this animal is very resistant to water deprivation as indicated previously. Schmidt-Nielsen (1964) points out some of the reasons that this species is resistant to water deprivation are: the camel's body temperature may vary considerably with the result that it can dissipate some body heat at night when the temperature is cooler and, secondly, the warmer body takes on less heat from the environment. The body fur is an important insulator, sweat being evaporated on the skin surface rather than at the tips of the fur. The camel does not pant, thus reducing respiratory losses, and it has the capacity to greatly concentrate urinary excretions (an 8:1 concentration as compared to blood), at least twice that of cattle. Apparently the camel does not have a greater hemoconcentration with moderate water deprivation, thus facilitating circulatory functions.

In addition to the camel, a number of desert antelopes are quite tolerant of water restriction or have a low requirement for water (Taylor, 1969; Schoen, 1972; Maloiy, 1973; Siebert and MacFarlane, 1975). These various species are capable of reducing urinary water losses by concentrating urine, sometimes to as high as 5000 Mosmoles/l. Feces are drier, evaporative losses of water are reduced, and losses from the lungs may be reduced. The eland accomplishes this by reducing its body temperature at night along with a decreased respiratory rate accompanied by an increased efficiency of extraction of oxygen from inspired air. During the day-time, body temperatures rise above normal values, allowing accumulation of body heat. Most domestic ruminants do not show this response in body temperature (Maloiy and Taylor 1971; Siebert and MacFarlane, 1975). In species such as reindeer which are adapted to arctic climates, water deprivation results in marked weight losses and there appears to be little adaptation of the body to conserve body water (Rosemann and Morrison, 1967).

Recovery of weight losses in dehydrated sheep is relatively rapid (Taneja, 1966). With a moderate water deficit (7-10% of BW), sheep may replenish lost water in a single act of drinking (Bott et al, 1965). When sheep were given restricted water for several weeks and then given 5 l./day, they drank almost all of the allotment for 6-10 days. After 10-20 days BW became constant at about 1-2 kg above that at maximum dehydration and only slightly below initial BW (Warner, 1971).

Cattle do not, apparently, recover BW losses as rapidly as sheep. After short-term deprivation, it may take as long as 24 hr to recover weight losses (Weeth et al, 1970), although Siebert and MacFarlane (1975) found that cattle deprived of water for up to 4 days were able to replace one third of their hydrated body water in 20 minutes. Bond et al (1976) found that feeding and drinking patterns of steers were similar before and after deprivation of feed, water or both. Water intake was reduced when steers were deprived of a high roughage diet but not when deprived of a 100% concentrate diet. Feed intake was reduced about 50% regardless of type of diet when water was withheld from steers for up to 48 hrs.

In studies with sheep which were given water every 3-4 days, Wilson (1970) observed that Border Leicesters drank more water (20-40%) and ate more food per unit of BW (15-28%) than Merinos. The Border Leicesters lost more water in their feces but similar amounts in urine. Urine volume appeared to be related to amount of K and Na excreted.

In long term studies in Australia with sheep which were given no water for 12-22 months, lambs from ewes without water had lighter birth weights. Body water turnover rates were lower in sheep without water in the summer. Lactation and heat stress resulted in 25% mortality of ewes without drinking water and subsequent death of their lambs, but there were no deaths in ewes without lambs (Lynch et al, 1972). Sheep without water were observed to lick the dew from forage and fences in early morning while sheep with water grazed normally. There was a tendency for more grazing activity during the night and predawn period by sheep without water. These sheep also weighed less, presumably because of reduced feed consumption (Brown and Lynch, 1972).

When lactating cows were given 60-100% of ad libitum water consumption, the 60% level resulted in a 16% decrease in DM and 16% decrease in milk yield but only minor changes in milk composition. There was no marked reduction in urine output but fecal water was reduced. Serum Na, urea and osmolality increased with increasing water deprivation (Little et al, 1976).

Weeth and Lesperance (1965) have studied intermittent watering of Hereford cattle which were watered ad libitum, once daily, and on alternate days with tap and 0.5% NaCl water during the summer. They concluded that once daily watering was adequate providing the water was of good quality and that watering only every 48 hr was inadequate under the conditions imposed even with water of high quality. Solovyh (1959) concluded that digestibility by sheep was more nearly optimum when they were watered 3 times daily than when watered only once daily.

A variety of responses to water deprivation has been observed by various authors in recent years. Water deprivation resulted in a decrease in rumination after 4-5 days, both in terms of time spent chewing (30%) and the number of boli regurgitated (46%) (Gordon, 1965). In addition to a decrease in rumen motility (Ruckenbusch et al, 1967), fermentation rates were restricted when water intake was reduced 50% (Phillips, 1961). In one case it was shown that varying degrees of water restriction resulted in some increase in percentage of DM and fiber digestibility by Zebu cattle when water was available every 72 hr (Thornton and Yates, 1968). If it was available every 48 hr, there was no effect. With moderate restriction feed intake was reduced and there was a higher digestibility of fiber. Asplund and Pfander (1972) also observed higher digestibility by sheep fed pelleted hay and restricted in water, but they suggested that this was probably an artifact due to DM accumulation in the GIT rather than to an increase in digestion. When sheep were given a high level of feed (1200 g) and low water (1200 g), the rumen rapidly became impacted and defecation was decreased greatly.

With respect to N retention, Balch et al (1953) found no effect of water restriction. In contrast, Thornton and Yates (1969) reported that water restriction decreased N retention when compared with cattle taking in a similar amount of digestible energy but unrestricted water. The reduced N balance was due to a combination of more fecal excretion and urinary urea excretion. Utley and others (1970) observed that water restriction increased digestibility of DM and N by steers and N retention tended to increase and their data suggested increased N recycling. Weeth et al (1968) found that watering once/day or once every 2nd day as compared to ad libitum intake resulted in an increased excretion of urinary urea when only a moderate decrease in feed intake occurred. Other research from this laboratory (Weeth et al, 1970) has shown that water deprivation of cattle resulted in an increase in plasma globulins and a marked increase in urinary excretion of proteins, including albumin and globulin, following 2-4 days of water deprivation. Thus, it would seem that water restriction is very likely to result in reduced N retention.

It is apparent that ruminant species can tolerate some degree of water restriction without a drastic depression in performance, particularly if the water is of good quality. If heat stress is not involved, it is likely that a slight restriction of water will reduce wasteful production of relatively dilute urine (Schmidt-Nielsen, 1964). However, the precise amount of restriction that can occur without detriment to the animal remains undetermined and would, of course, be affected by numerous other variables such as temperature and type of diet, to mention only two factors. Taneja (1965) reported that weight loss of sheep watered on the 2nd, 3rd and 4th days was 5.5, 9.3 and 12.3%, respectively, and he calculated that 169 sheep could be maintained on the water ration required for 100 animals if watering was done every 3rd day. Numerous other examples are available to show that total water intake is lowered by reducing the frequency of watering. However, the results on N retention and feed intake mentioned elsewhere would indicate that such restriction and loss of body weight must be detrimental to production. It would seem that body weight losses must be held to less than 10% in order to avoid reduced production. A 5% value might be a more appropriate value.

WATER INTOXICATION

Water intoxication has been reported in calves in a number of clinical reports, and it has been produced experimentally in two laboratories (Hannan, 1965; Kirkbride and Frey, 1967). Calves appear to be particularly susceptible since they can and often will consume as much as 35-50% of total body water within a half hr period. This is particularly true when they are dehydrated and are fed in a manner in which milk is normally given. A second reason is that cattle which have been deprived of water for a time are unable to adjust quickly to large quantities of water in the tissues.

The common symptoms seen include: hemoglobinura (red urine), colic, diarrhea, irregular heart beat and distension of surface veins; the body hair tends to stand on end and excessive salivation occurs. Fluid tends to collect in soft tissues beneath the skin and is often noticeable in the eyelids which become swollen. In more severe cases nervous signs become evident. A wobbly gait

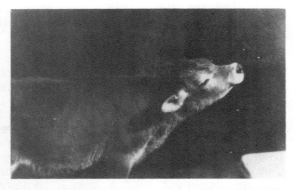

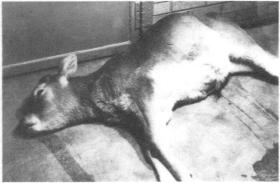

Figure 2-3. Water toxicity in the calf. Upper. 2 hr after ingesting 14 l. of water. Notice abnormal position of the head and neck. Lower. Same calf 4 hr after ingesting water. Calf is comatose. Distension of the abdomen is evident and saliva is on the floor. Courtesy of C.A. Kirkbride.

may develop and excessive rubbing and licking of the body is common. Animals often assume a position with head and neck extended. The lethargy and depression progress to a coma. Some cattle with severe symptoms recover completely although extremely dehydrated animals which have consumed large quantities of water usually die. Treatment generally involves intravenous administration of hypertonic glucose or saline in an attempt to remove excess water from the tissues (Kirkbride and Frey, 1967; Kirkbride, 1970). An example of an affected calf is shown in Fig. 2-3.

WATER QUALITY

There is relatively little information relating quality of water to production of domestic livestock. Generally, it has been assumed that water safe for human consumption may be used safely by stock but it appears that animals can tolerate higher salinity than humans; thus, it is probable that tolerances for other substances may be different, also. For additional reviews on this topic, a compilation edited by McKee and Wolf (1963) and an NRC (1974) report would be recommended.

Water quality may directly affect feed consumption since low quality water will normally result in reduced water consumption and, hence, lower feed consumption and production. Substances which may reduce palatability of water include various saline salts. At "high" rates of consumption, these salts may be toxic, of course (see Ch. 4). Substances which may be toxic without much affect, if any, on palatability include nitrates and F as well as salts of other heavy metals. Other materials which may affect palatability or be toxic include pathogenic microorganisms of a wide variety, algae and/or protozoa, hydrocarbons and other oily substances, pesticides of various types and many industrial chemicals which sometimes pollute water supplies. For the purposes in this chapter, the discussion will be limited to natural mineral compounds and nitrates normally found in water supplies.

Salts

Studies in Australia (Anon., 1950) point out that total salts include chlorides, sulfates and bicarbonates of Na, Ca and Mg with NaCl constituting as much as 75% of total salinity. Natural stream waters in the USA have been classified into 4 chemical types based on the most common components. These are Ca-Mg/CO_3, Ca-Mg/SO_4-Cl, Na-K/CO_3-HCO_3, and Na-K/SO_4-Cl. In the USA 87% of the water contains high percentages of Ca and Mg while only 13% is of the Na-K type. Ca and Mg usually occur with carbonates and bicarbonates and to a lesser extent with sulfate and chloride. Na and K are more likely to be combined with sulfates and chlorides than with carbonates and bicarbonates (Rainwater, 1962). Open lakes may have 100-200 ppm of dissolved solids but closed lakes tend to be much higher and some may even be in excess of 100,000 ppm. Most shallow ground waters have less than 3,000 ppm and, thus, should be satisfactory for livestock. Values for surface water are shown in Table 2-7.

Table 2-7. Mineral composition of surface waters in the USA.[a]

Element	Mean (range)
P, mg/l.	0.087 (0.001-5)
Ca, mg/l.	57.1 (11.0-173)
Mg, mg/l.	14.3 (8.5-137)
Na, mg/l.	55.1(0.2-7, 500)
K, mg/l.	4.3 (0.06-370)
Cl, mg/l.	478.0 (0.0-19,000)
Sulfate, mg/l.	135.9 (0.0-3,383)
Cu, mcg/l.	13.8 (0.8-280)
Fe, mcg/l.	43.9 (0.1-4,600)
Mn, mcg/l.	29.4 (0.2-3,230)
Zn, mcg/l.	51.8 (1-1, 183)
Se, mcg/l.	0.016 (0.01-1)
I, mcg/l.	46.1 (4-336)
Co, mcg/l.	1.0 (0-5)

[a] Data from Dantzman and Breland (1969) and Durum et al (1971).

The tolerance of animals to salts in water depends on factors such as water requirements, species, age, physiological condition, season of the year and salt content of the total diet as well as the quality and quantity of salts present in the water (McKee and Wolf, 1963). Water with high loads of salts generally causes injury due to the osmotic effect rather than a specific toxic reaction of any constituent. Alkali salts are rated somewhat more injurious than neutral salt, sulfates are more harmful than chlorides and $MgCl_2$ is more harmful than $CaCl_2$ or NaCl (Heller, 1933). Sheep generally are more tolerant than cattle of most saline salts, perhaps partly because they normally consume less water per unit of feed than cattle. Excessive salts may result in various disturbances such as reduced water and feed consumption, gastrointestinal disturbances, diarrhea, cessation of lactation, dehydration and death.

Although animals will not normally choose to drink saline water if given a choice of good quality (low salt) water, within limits they can adjust and will drink saline waters that will be refused at first. Sudden changes in water quality may cause acute salt poisoning and rapid death.

Limiting Levels of Solids and Salts

Based on research from a variety of laboratories, the following levels of solids or salts appear to be limiting for ruminants (Herrick, 1971; NRC, 1974).

Total dissolved solids. Most animals can tolerate levels of 1.3-1.7% total dissolved solids, although the tolerance depends on what components make up the dissolved solids in the water. Some recommendations go as high as 2.5% for beef cattle.

Chlorides. The tolerance depends on age and water requirements. For young animals and lactating dairy cows, an upper level of 0.7% appears to be appropriate. Older non-lactating beef cows may tolerate 1% or more depending on season of the year and nature of the diet. Sheep tolerate 1% salt but levels of 1.5% are apt to result in reduced feed consumption, rate of gain and other disturbances such as diarrhea. In experiments where total salts are 1-1.3% of the water, $MgSO_4$ or $MgCl_2$ or $CaCl_2$ have little adverse effect when total salts are ca. 1%. At higher levels (1.3-1.5%) there may be some adverse effects on both ewes and lambs.

Sulfates. Sulfates over 0.1% may cause diarrhea, particularly in younger animals, although animals develop a tolerance to constant levels (.2-.25%) after a period of time. Young animals can tolerate 0.4-0.7% Na_2SO_4 but levels of ca. 2% of Na or Na and Mg sulfate are apt to cause severe problems and some death in cows. Sheep can exist on 2% $MgSO_4$ but not without problems.

Toxic Substances

Naturally occurring compounds of concern in water are nitrates and fluorides. With regard to fluorides, available data suggest that cattle and sheep can tolerate up to 10 mg/l. without severe effects other than mottled teeth or, perhaps, some decrease in wool production. A level of 20 mg/l. caused poor health and severe mottling in the teeth of sheep (McKee and Wolf, 1963).

Nitrates are frequently found in surface and well waters, often as a result of accumulation from feedlots or because of heavy applications of fertilizer or manures. Levels of nitrates and nitrites in water fluctuate greatly during the year, and it is difficult to define a toxic level since toxicity is affected by adaptation, type of diet, age, species and water consumption. Some veterinary practitioners suggest that nitrate may begin to be a problem between 50 and 100 ppm in water supplies (Herrick, 1971).

Recommended limits of some substances in water for livestock are shown in Table 2-8. Data are relatively limited, however, on most of these for ruminants since most toxicity studies have been done with feed or by dosing in other ways.

Table 2-8. Recommended limits of some potentially toxic substances in drinking water for livestock.[a]

Substance	Safe upper limit, mg/l.
Arsenic	0.2
Cadmium	0.05
Chromium	1.0
Cobalt	1.0
Copper	0.5
Fluoride	2.0
Lead	0.1
Mercury	0.01
Nickel	1.0
Nitrate-N	100.0
Nitrite-N	10.0
Vanadium	0.1
Zinc	25.0

[a] From NRC (1974)

MINERAL NUTRIENTS IN WATER

When thinking about water, it is much more customary to think in terms of requirements, excretions, hardness, salinity, toxins, or pollution than to consider water as a source of some of the soluble minerals needed by animals. However, the amount of water consumed is considerable and, when the mineral content is high, an appreciable amount of the daily requirement may be consumed in water. This information may be of particular concern in areas where mineral imbalances are a problem. Note in Table 2-7 that there may be a tremendous range in concentration of mineral elements in surface water. If these mean values from Table 2-7 are used along with some assumed values for water consumption, then the percentages of the daily requirement (according to NRC) consumed in the form of soluble salts in water are as shown in Table 2-9. The maximum consumption is not given in Table 2-9. However, for some of the major elements, water might supply 2-5X the daily requirement of NaCl, 20-85% of the Ca requirement, 50-91% of the Mg requirement, 24-49% of the K requirement and 5-11X of the sulfur requirement (NRC, 1974). Consequently, if there is any thought that mineral imbalance may be a problem, water analyses should be done along with analyses on appropriate feed samples.

CONCLUSIONS

In a given environmental situation water requirements are highly related to dry matter intake with the result that an increased consumption of dry matter will increase water consumption and vice versa. At an environmental temperature which causes no heat stress, water intake tends to be about 3-5 units/unit of dry feed intake in adult cattle. Optimum water intake of preruminant calves is indicated as being higher than for adults, probably on the order of 6-7 kg/kg of dry matter intake. Consumption is increased during late pregnancy. In cattle additional requirements for water over and above that secreted in the milk are on the order of 0.24-0.30 kg/kg of milk produced. In the case of sheep, water intake appears to be somewhat lower than for cattle.

There are marked species differences in water turnover rates as indicated by the half life of tritiated water. Species such as desert antelopes have the ability to conserve water while others adapted to wet climates have high turnover rates. The camel, a pseudoruminant, probably has the greatest ability of animals in the ruminant class to conserve water.

In addition to dry matter, other dietary factors may affect water requirements.

Table 2-9. Nutrient intake from water.[a]

Item	Cattle					Sheep	
	Young Animals		Adults			Fattening lamb	Lactating ewe
	Growing Heifer	Steer in feedlot	Maintenance	Beef, lactating	Dairy, lactating		
Assumed water consumption/day, l.	60	60	60	60	90	4	6
NaCl							
requirement, g	21	24	21	25	66	10	13
from water, %	40	35	40	34	19	6	7
Ca							
requirement, g	15	21	12	28	76	3	7
from water, %	23	16	28	12	7	8	5
P							
requirement, g	16	21	12	22	58	3	5
from water, %	<1	<1	<1	<1	<1	<1	<1
Mg							
requirement, g	9	9	9	14	14	1.1	1.5
from water, %	10	10	10	6	9	5	6
K							
requirement, g	70	70	45	90	99		
from water, %	<1	<1	<1	<1	<1		
Sulfur							
requirement, g	10	9	6	10	20	2	3
from water, %	27	29	45	27	20	10	11

[a]From NRC (1974)

Compounds associated with increased water consumption include: salts of various types, protein or N, pentosans, fiber and silage.

Water restriction results in a rapid decrease in excretion, particularly via the feces, and a rapid decrease in feed consumption, especially in hot environments which accelerate body water losses. Ruminants can tolerate a degree of water restriction without harm since they can conserve water by reducing losses via feces and urine and some species can reduce respiratory losses from the lungs. If restriction is severe enough, water loss from the tissues prohibits normal function. N retention is reduced with only moderate restriction. Infrequent watering can result in lowered water intake, but probably reduces the performance of most species.

Water quality is of great importance in many areas, particularly arid range lands where the soil and water are saline. Excess salts will cause greater excretion, but eventually the kidney reaches its capacity to concentrate the salts sufficiently and they become toxic. Domestic ruminants can tolerate about 1.3-1.5% total dissolved solids without much if any harm. Higher levels will usually reduce production.

In areas where mineral imbalances may be a problem, consideration should be given to the mineral content of water. Surface waters, in particular those from closed lakes, may be very high in some mineral elements. Toxins of various types, both naturally occurring and those from industrial pollution, will probably become an increasing problem for livestock in many areas.

REFERENCES CITED

Anand, R.S., A.H. Parker and H.R. Parker. 1966. Amer. Vet. Res. 27:899.

Anon. 1950. J. Agr. W. Aust. 27:156.

ARC. 1965. The Nutrient Requirements of Farm Livestock. No. 2 Ruminants. Agr. Res. Council, London.

Argenzio, R.A., G.M. Ward, J. E. Johnson. 1968. J. Animal Sci. 27:1121 (abstr).

Aschbacker, P.W., R.H. Kamal, R.G. Cragle. 1965. J. Animal Sci. 24:430.

Asplund, J.M. and W.H. Pfander. 1972. J. Animal Sci. 35:1271.

Baile, C.A., J. Mayer, C. McLaughlin. 1969. Amer. J. Physiol. 217:397.

Bailey, C.B., R. Hironaka, and S.B. Slen. 1962. Can. J. Animal Sci. 42:1.

Balch, C.C., D. A. Balch, V.W. Johnson and J. Turner. 1953. Brit J. Nutr. 7:212.

Bensadoun, A., B.D.H. Van Niekerk, O.L. Paladines, and J.T. Reid. 1963. J. Animal Sci. 22:604.

Bianca, W., J.D. Findlay and J.A. McLean. 1965. Res. Vet. Sci. 6:38.

Black, A.L., N.F. Baker, J.C. Bartley, T.E. Chapman and R.W. Phillips. 1964. Science 144:876.

Bond, J. and R.E. McDowell. 1972. J. Animal Sci. 35:820.

Bond, J., T.S. Rumsey and B.T. Weinland. 1976. J. Animal Sci. 43:873

Bott, E., D.A. Denton and S. Weller. 1965. J. Physiol. 176:323.

Brody, S., A.C. Ragsdale, H.J. Thompson and D.M. Worstell. 1954. Missouri Agr. Exp. Sta. Res. Bul. 545.

Brown , G.D. and J.J. Lynch. 1972. Aust J. Agr. Res. 23:669.

Calder, F.W., J.W.G. Nicholson and H.M. Cunningham. 1964. Can. J. Animal Sci. 44:266.

Campling, R.C. and C.C. Balch. 1961. Brit. J. Nutr. 15:523.

Castle, M.E. 1972. J. Brit. Grassld. Soc. 27:207.

Castle, M.E., A.S. Foot and R.J. Halley. 1950. J. Dairy Res. 17:215.

Castle, M.E. and T.P. Thomas. 1975. Animal Prod. 20:181.

Castle, M.E. and J.N. Watson. 1973. J. Brit. Grassld. Soc. 28:203.

Cunningham, M.D., F.A. Martz and C.P. Merilan. 1964. J. Dairy Sci. 47:382.

Dantzman, C.L. and H.L. Breland. 1969. Proc. Soil Crop. Sci. Fla. 29:18.

Davies, P.J. 1972. Animal Prod. 15:307.

Daws, G.T. and V.R. Squires. 1974. J. Agr. Sci. 82:383.

Duckworth, J.E. and D.W. Shirlaw. 1958. Animal Behavior 6:147.

Durum, W.H., J.D. Hem and S.G. Heidel. 1971. USGS Geol. Surv. Cir. 643.

English, P.B. 1966. Res. Vet. Sci. 7:233.

Forbes, J.M. 1968. Brit. J. Nutr. 22:33.

French, M.H. 1956. J. Expt. Agr. 24:128.

Garrett, W.N., T.E. Bond and C.F. Kelly. 1960. J. Animal Sci. 19:60.

Garrett, W.N., J.H. Meyer and G.P. Lofgreen. 1959. J.Animal Sci. 18:116.

Ghobrial, L.I. 1970. Physiol. Zoo. 43:249.

Ghosh, P.K., M.S. Khan and R.K. Abichandani. 1976. J. Agr. Sci. 87:221.

Gordon, J.G. 1965. J. Agr. Sci. 64:31.

Hancock, J. 1953. Animal Breed. Abst. 21:1.

Hannan, J. 1965. Irish Vet. J. 19:211.

Harris, R.R., H.F. Yates and J.E. Barnett. 1967. J. Animal Sci. 26:207 (abstr).

Head, M.J. 1953. J. Agr. Sci. 43:214.

Heller, V.G. 1933. Oklahoma Agr. Exp. Sta. Bul. 217.

Herrick, J.B. 1971. Feedstuffs 43(8):28.

Hodgson, J. 1973. Animal Prod. 17:129.

Hoffman, M.P. and H.L. Self. 1972. J. Animal Sci. 35:871.

Holzer, Z., H. Tagari, D. Levy and R. Volcani. 1976. Animal Prod. 22:41.

Ittner, N.R., C.F. Kelly and N.R. Guilbert. 1951. J. Animal Sci. 10:742.

Jarman, P.J. 1973. East African Agr. For. J. 38:343.

Kelly, C.F., T.E. Bond and N.R. Ittner. 1955. Agr. Eng. 35:173.

Kibler, H.H. and S. Brody. 1952. Missouri Agr. Expt. Sta. Res. Bul. No. 497.

Kirkbride, C.A. 1970. Animal Nutr. & Health. Nov. 1970, p. 3.

Kirkbride, C.A. and R.A. Frey. 1967. J. Amer.Vet. Med. Assoc. 151:742.

Knox, K.L., J.G. Nagy and R.D. Brown. 1969. J. Wildl. Mgmt. 33:389.

Leitch, M.A. and J.S. Thompson. 1944. Nutr. Abstr. Rev. 14:197.

Little, W., B.F. Sansom, R. Manston and W.M. Allen. 1976. Animal Prod. 22:329.

Lofgreen, G.P., R.L. Givens, S.R. Morrison and T.E. Bond. 1975. J. Animal Sci. 40:223.

Longhurst, W.M., N.F. Baker, G.E. Connolly and R.A. Fisk. 1970. Amer. J. Vet. Res. 31:673.

Lynch, J.J., G.D. Brown, P.J. May and J.B. Donnelly. 1972. Aust. J. Agr. Res. 23:659.

Mac Farlane, W.V. 1964. In: Handbook of Physiology. Amer. Physiological Soc., Washington, D.C.

MacFarlane, W.V. and B. Howard. 1966. J. Agr. Sci. 66:297.

MacFarlane, W.V., B. Howard and R.J.H. Morris. 1966. Aust. J. Agr. Res. 17:219.

MacFarlane, W.V., B.Howard and B.D. Siebert. 1967. Aust. J. Agr. Res. 18:947.

MacFarlane, W.V., G.M.O. Maloiy and D. Hopcraft. 1972. Int. Atomic Energy Agency. 156:83.

MacFarlane, W.V., R.J.H. Morris and B. Howard. 1963. Nature 197:270.

MacFarlane, W.V., et al. 1961. Aust. J. Agr. Res. 12:889.

Maloiy, G.M.O.1973. Proc. Royal Soc. London. B 184:167.

Maloiy, G.M.O. and C.R. Taylor. 1971. J. Agr. Sci. 77:203.

Manery, J.F. 1954. Physiol. Rev. 34:334.

McKee, J.E. and H.W. Wolf. 1963. Water Quality Criteria, 2nd ed. Pub. No. 3-A, Resources Agency of Cal., State Water Quality Control Board.

Mitchell, H.H. 1962. Comparative Nutrition of Man and Domestic Animals. Vol.1, Academic Press.

Murray, D.M. 1966. J. Agr. Sci. 66:175.

NRC. 1974. Nutrients and Toxic Substances in Water for Livestock and Poultry. Natl. Acad. Sci., Washington D.C.

Paquay, R., R. De Baere and A. Lousse. 1970. J. Agr. Sci. 74:423; 75;251.

Pettyjohn, J.D., J.P. Everett and R.D. Mochrie. 1963. J. Dairy Sci. 46:710.

Phillips, G.D. 1961. Res. Vet. Sci. 2:209.

Purohit, G.R., P.K. Ghosh and G.C. Taneja. 1972. Aust. J. Agr. Res. 23:685.

Ragsdale, A.C., H.J. Thompson, D.M. Worstell and S. Brody. 1950. Missouri Agr. Expt. Sta. Res. Bul. 460.

Ragsdale, A.C., H.J. Thompson, D.M. Worstell and S. Brody. 1951. Missouri Agr. Expt. Sta. Res. Bul. 471.

Ragsdale, A.C., H.J. Thompson, D.M. Worstell and S. Brody. 1953. Missouri Agr. Expt. Sta. Res. Bul. 521.

Rainwater, F.H. 1962. USGS Hydrol. Invest. Atlas H-61, Washington D.C.

Ray, D.E. and C.B. Roubicek. 1971. J. Animal Sci. 33:72.

Razdan, M.N., D.D. Sharma, P.K. Bhargava and M.S. Chawla. 1971. J. Dairy Sci. 54:1200.

Reid, J.T., G.H. Wellington and H.O. Dunn. 1955. J. Dairy Sci. 38:1344.

Ritzman, E.G. and F.G. Benedict. 1924. N. Hampshire Agr. Expt. Sta. Tech. Bul. 26.

Rosemann, M., and P. Morrison. 1967. Physiol. Zool. 40:134.

Roubicek, C.B. 1969. In: Animal Growth and Nutrition. Lea & Febiger, Pub. Co.

Ruckebush, T., J.P. Laplace and J.P.Perret. 1967. Nutr. Abstr. Rev. 37:138.

Schmidt-Nielsen, K. 1964. Desert Animals, Physiological Problems of Heat and Water. Oxford Univ. Press.

Schoen, A. 1972. E. African Agr. For. J. 37:1, 325.

Seif, S. M., H.D. Johnson and L. Hahn. 1973. J. Dairy Sci. 56:581.

Sekine, J., Y. Asahida and Y. Hirose. 1972. J. Fac. Agr. Hokkaido Univ. 57:51.

Siebert, B.D. and W.V. MacFarlane. 1969. Aust. J. Agr. Res. 20:613.

Siebert, B.D. and W.V. MacFarlane. 1971. Physiol. Zool. 44:225.

Siebert, B.D. and W.V. MacFarlane. 1975. Physiol. Zool. 48:36.

Sims, P.L. and J.E. Butcher. 1966. Proc. West. Sec. Amer. Soc. Animal Sci. 17:211.

Smith, B.S.W. and A.R. Sykes. 1974. J. Agr. Sci. 82:105.

Solovyh, A.G. 1959. Nutr. Abstr. Rev. 29:1369.

Squires, V.R. and A.D. Wilson. 1971. Aust. J. Agr. Res. 22:283.

Stiles, R.P., D.G. Grieve, D.G. Butler and R. A. Willoughby. 1974. Can. J. Animal Sci. 54:73.

Sundstrom, C. 1970. Wyoming Wildlf. 34(2):14.

Taneja, G.C. 1965. Indian J. Expt. Biol. 3:259.

Taneja, G.C. 1966. Indian J. Expt. Biol. 4:167.

Taylor, C.R. 1968. Nature 219:181.

Taylor, C.R. 1969. Physiol. 217:317.

Thomas, T.P. 1971. Animal Prod. 13:399.

Thompson, H.J., D.M. Worstell and S. Brody. 1949. Missouri Agr. Expt. Sta. Res. Bul. 436.

Thornton, R.F. and N.G. Yates. 1968. Aust. J. Agr. Res. 19:665.

Thronton, R.F. and N.G. Yates. 1969. Aust. J. Agr. Res. 20:185.

Thornton, R.F. and N.G. Yates. 1970. J. Agr. Res. 21:145.

Utley, P.R., N.W. Bradley and J.A. Boling. 1970. J. Animal Sci. 31:130; J. Nutr. 100:551.

Wade, L. and L.B. Sasser. 1970. Amer. J. Vet. Res. 31:1375.

Waldo, D.R., R.W. Miller, M. Okamoto and L.A. Moore. 1965. J. Dairy Sci. 48:1473.

Wallace, J.D., D.N. Hyder and K.L. Knox. 1972. Amer. J. Vet. Res. 33:921.

Warner, A.C.I. and B.D. Stacy. 1968. Brit. J. Nutr. 22:389.

Weeth, H.J. and A.L. Lesperance. 1965. Proc. West. Sect. Amer. Soc. Animal Sci. 16:xix.

Weeth, H.J., A.L. Lesperance and V.R. Bohman. 1968. J. Animal Sci. 27:739.

Weeth, H.J., D.S. Sawhey and A.L.Lesperance. 1967. J. Animal Sci. 26:418.

Weeth, H.J., R. Winton, C.F. Speth and R.C. Blincoe. 1970. J. Animal Sci. 30:219.

Wellington, G.H., J.T. Reid, L.J. Bratzler and J.I. Miller. 1956. J. Animal Sci. 15:76.

Williams, C.M. 1959. Proc. West. Sec. Amer. Soc. Animal Sci. 10:XLII.

Wilson, A.D. 1966. Aust. J. Agr. Res. 17:503.

Wilson, A.D. 1970. Aust. J. Agr. Res. 21:273.

Wilson, A.D. 1974. Aust. J. Agr. Res. 25:339.

Winchester, C.F. and M.J. Morris. 1956. J. Animal Sci. 15:722.

Wohlt, J.E. et al. 1976. J. Animal Sci. 42:1280

Wrenn, T.R., et al. 1962. J. Dairy Sci. 45:205.

Wright, D.E. and B.A. Jones. 1974. N.Z. J. Agr. Res. 17:417.

Chapter 3 - Nitrogen Metabolism and Requirements

By D.C. Church and J.P. Fontenot

Quantitatively, protein is required by ruminant animals in amounts second only to energy, thus this topic is of great concern in the nutrition of ruminant animals. Blaxter (1977) has pointed out that the protein requirements of young, rapidly growing animals are on the order of 2-3X those of man, a reflection of the much greater daily rate of protein accretion during growth by young animals. On the other hand the efficiency of converting feed to human food protein is rather low, ranging from about 3% for a sheep flock to about 23% for a dairy herd (Blaxter, 1977). Thus, it is essential to develop and apply more information on protein and N metabolism so that N can be utilized with greater efficiency when possible.

Rumen metabolism of protein, digestion and partial digestion were covered in some detail in Vol. 1 of this series. In this chapter the main emphasis will be on utilization of absorbed N and on protein requirements. The authors regret that the chapter is not more complete; there is a large volume of literature on the topic and it is not possible to do justice to most of it in this chapter.

METABOLISM OF ABSORBED NITROGEN

Absorption

In the rumen a substantial portion of the dietary nitrogenous compounds is degraded to ammonia and organic acids. The amount degraded is dependent upon the chemical nature of the protein or NPN and its solubility, level of feed intake and other dietary and physiological factors. Ammonia which is not incorporated into microbial protein is absorbed through the rumen wall or in the lower GI tract and is transported via the portal vein to the liver. Absorption from the rumen is markedly affected by ruminal pH (and thus by diet), since an acid pH reduces absorption and a basic pH increases absorption (see Vol. 1 for further details). With regard to amino acids, Liebholz (1971) demonstrated that amino acids may be absorbed from the rumen of sheep. However, the ruminal content of free amino acids is quite low, thus there is little reason to believe that the quantity absorbed is a significant amount (Nolan and Leng, 1972).

Protein N in the gut consists of the microbial fraction from the reticulo-rumen, some portion of the dietary protein which escaped ruminal degradation and the normal metabolic sources derived from secretions and sloughed cells. Following digestion (reduction in molecular size and increased solubility) by abomasal, pancreatic and enteric enzymes, amino and nucleic acids are absorbed by the gut wall, primarily the ileum (Ben-Ghendalia et al, 1976; Phillips et al, 1976). The relative order of three amino acids for affinity to absorption sites was lysine>methionine>glycine; the relative rate of transport was methionine>lysine>glycine (Johns and Bergen, 1973). Armstrong and Hutton (1975) have pointed out that amino acids are absorbed by carrier-mediated transport which is sodium dependent, presumably by the same mechanisms as utilized by monogastric species.

Williams (1969) noted differences in rate of absorption of different amino acids in acute studies with sheep, but they did not find differences in overall rate when concentrations were 1.5 or 3mM. When net absorption of amino acids was measured from the portal vein, Hume et al (1972) observed that ratios of individual amino acids to individual amino acids absorbed were similar to those in rumen bacterial protein. Abomasal infusion of leucine depressed net absorption of only lysine, although it depressed the concentration of several other amino acids in portal and/or ventral plasma. When amino acid absorption was measured by portal-jugular venous differences in sheep fed early or late cut alfalfa, sheep fed the early cut alfalfa absorbed ca. 2.8X as much amino acids and essential amino acids as those fed late cut alfalfa (Prewitt et al, 1975).

Normal Blood Levels

The concentration of normal blood components may be variable, depending on age, diet and other factors. With regard to blood ammonia, very little ammonia is found in peripheral blood supplies unless ruminal ammonia levels exceed 50 mM/l. and portal blood exceeds 0.8 mM/l. (Lewis et al, 1957). Normal blood ammonia levels tend to be on the order of 0.10-0.15 mg/100 (Bartley et al, 1976). For other N components in the blood, mean (range) values for lactating cows are: urea, 13.4 mg/100 ml (6.3-25.5); albumin, 3.1 (2.8-3.6) g/100 ml; globulin, 4.3 (3.5-4.9) g/100 ml; hemoglobin, 10.9 (9.1-12.7) g/100 ml. Mean values for plasma urea N in preruminant lambs has been reported to be 12-15 mg of urea N/100 ml (Kirk and Walker, 1976) and ca. 14.5 for preruminant calves (Kitchenham et al, 1975). Normal albumin and globulin levels in calves are 3.2 (2.7-3.7) and 4.4 (3.2-5.6) g/100 ml, respectively (Kitchenham et al, 1975). In milk from cows, urea tends to be about 10-12 mg/100 ml, although it may be quite variable and tends to reflect blood levels of urea (Ide et al, 1966). With regard to plasma amino acids, values in milk-fed calves are on the order of 170 μ M/100 ml as compared to 190 μ M/100 ml in ruminating calves and 188 μ M/100 ml in older steers (Williams and Smith, 1974, 1975; Redd et al, 1975).

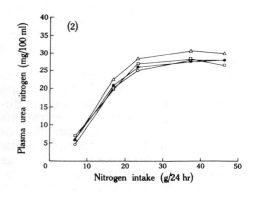

Fig. 3-1. Blood urea levels in sheep consuming increasing amounts of N from wheat straw and/or alfalfa hay From McIntyre (1970).

Blood Urea

There is ample evidence to show that blood urea increases with an increased consumption of protein or NPN (see papers by Polan et al, 1970; Egan and Kellaway, 1971; Cross et al, 1974; or Huber et al, 1976). This is illustrated graphically in Fig. 3-1. In addition, blood urea is related to ruminal ammonia levels (Fig. 3-2). Although blood urea levels tend to increase with an increased consumption of NPN or protein, it may also be high in situations which result in catabolism of body proteins; for example during a period when consumption of food is

not adequate to maintain the animal, in starvation, or severe cases of diarrhea (see Ch. 17) or other debilitating diseases.

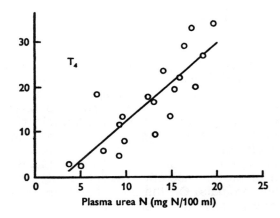

Fig. 3-2. Relationship between ruminal ammonia N and plasma urea N concentrations 4 hr after feeding. Sheep were fed 20 different fresh frozen forages. From Egan and Kellaway (1971).

Plasma Free Amino Acids (PFAA)

In non-ruminants dietary level of protein or of certain amino acids has been shown to affect PFAA and attempts have been made to relate N utilization to PFAA in ruminants. Results were obtained by Theurer et al (1966) indicating that the concentration of PFAA in jugular blood is fairly representative of the portal blood concentration with the possible exception of methionine and lysine. Theurer et al (1968) found that PFAA of sheep fed soybean meal and corn gluten meal was related to the levels in the dietary protein sources. Concentrations of most PFAA increased with feed intake in lambs (Nimrick et al, 1971).

Oltjen and Putnam (1966) found that the plasma levels of glycine and serine were higher and the levels of valine, isoleucine, leucine and phenylalanine were lower for cattle fed purified diets containing urea as the only N source than for cattle fed soy protein as the N source (Table 3-1). They suggested that insufficient quantities of branched chain fatty acids in the rumen may be responsible for the lower levels of valine, leucine and isoleucine. Virtanen (1966) found that the plasma concentration of most of the amino acids, especially the essential ones, was lower in cows fed a purified diet in which essentially all of the N was supplied by urea. In these studies the decrease in histidine was particularly striking. Virtanen also

Table 3-1. Free amino acids in the plasma of steers fed various experimental diets.[a]

Amino acid	Isolated soy		Urea	
	Glucose + starch	Starch	Glucose + starch	Starch
	μM/100 ml			
Lysine	6.8	5.1	5.3	7.2
Histidine	3.0	2.8	3.5	3.1
Tryptophan	0.7	0.7	0.4	0.8
Arginine	5.4	4.7	4.4	5.4
Aspartic acid	0.5	0.5	0.3	0.4
Threonine	2.7	3.1	2.4	3.4
Serine	3.6	4.7	5.9	4.9
Proline	3.4	4.1	3.7	3.5
Glutamic acid	3.7	6.0	5.6	4.1
Glycine	18.2	22.3	30.5	27.0
Alanine	12.5	15.4	14.0	11.5
Valine	14.7	18.9	11.6	12.3
Cystine	1.2	1.3	1.0	1.1
Methionine	1.0	1.0	1.0	1.2
Isoleucine	6.3	7.4	5.3	6.0
Leucine	6.9	8.3	5.5	5.1
Tyrosine	1.5	1.8	1.4	1.4
Phenylalanine	2.4	2.6	2.0	1.0
Total	94.5	110.7	103.8	99.4

[a] From Oltjen and Putnam (1966).

noticed an increase in glycine in plasma. Freitag et al (1968) observed lower levels of plasma valine, isoleucine, lysine, leucine, phenylalanine, alanine, tyrosine and glutamic acid in steers when urea and corn were substituted for soybean meal. Other researchers have reported differences in PFAA in animals fed urea as the supplemental or only source of N, but the significance of these changes has not been elucidated (Ludwick et al, 1972; Young et al, 1973; Burris et al, 1975).

Fate of Absorbed N

The absorbed compounds of major significance are ammonia, the amino acids and the purines and pyrimidines which result from intestinal degradation of nucleic acids. Other components are present, but in extremely small amounts.

Ammonia absorbed from the rumen or from the gut passes through the liver and a large portion of it is removed and synthesized into urea via the Krebs-Henseleit cycle (see any good biochemistry text). Enzymes concerned in the cycle have been shown to be present in ruminant liver tissues. In one instance it was shown that feeding relatively high levels of urea did not appear to result in an increase in liver enzymes concerned with

urea utilization (Boling et al, 1976) and in one report there was a reduced concentration of most liver enzymes in the Krebs-Henseleit cycle of sheep fed urea (Chalupa et al, 1970).

It has been presumed that unless the critical level of ruminal ammonia is exceeded, all of the absorbed ammonia is converted to urea (Lewis, 1961; Blackburn, 1965; Tillman and Sidhu, 1969). This assumption is based on the fact that usually no increase in peripheral blood ammonia occurs in spite of increased levels of ammonia reaching the liver. Alternative pathways of ammonia utilization include incorporation into glutamic acid, glutamine and carbamyl phosphate and subsequently into purines, pyrimidines and non-essential amino acids.

Although some of the earlier work suggests that most of the plasma urea was derived from absorption of ammonia from the rumen, more recent work indicates that a substantial amount of urea is synthesized elsewhere. For example, Nolan and Leng (1972) infused labeled ammonium sulfate and urea into sheep. They calculated that urea was synthesized in the body at a rate of 18.4 g of urea N/day (daily consumption was 22.8 g N) of which 2.0 g N/day was from ammonia absorbed through the rumen wall and 16.4 g N/day apparently arising from deamination of amino acids and ammonia absorbed from the lower GI tract.

Amino acids are the principal nitrogenous compounds absorbed from the intestine. In studies using labeled amino acids with sheep, Wolff et al (1972) have shown that most of the amino acids, including all the essential ones, are added to portal vein plasma in highly significant amounts. However, uptakes of aspartic and glutamic acids were limited, implying extensive metabolism of these amino acids in the gut wall. They also noted an appreciable net production of alanine consistent with the occurence of extensive transamination reactions between glutamate and aspartate or glutamate and pyruvate.

The liver removes most of the absorbed amino acids with the exception of some of the branched chain acids. Large hepatic uptakes of glycine, alanine and glutamine and to a lesser extent serine, tyrosine, arginine and phenylalanine occur (Wolff et al, 1972). Following transport to the liver and transport by way of plasma proteins or free amino acids, it is assumed that extensive metabolism occurs in peripheral tissues, particularly muscle, but this is a topic outside the scope of this chapter.

The catabolic pathways of major significance for amino acids are transamination reactions involving gluctamic acid coupled with oxidative deamination by glutamic acid dehydrogenase. Glutamic dehydrogenase catalyzes the amination of α-keotglutaric acid to glutamic acid. This same enzyme deaminates glutamic acid and the fact that deamination is reversible is of considerable significance in ruminants.

It does not appear likely that amination is of substantial importance in the synthesis of other amino acids since the oxidase activity level is low for the enzymes concerned with other amino acids (West et al, 1968). However, it appears that the reversible glutamic acid oxidative deamination is of utmost importance. Other amino acids can be produced by transamination reactions involving glutamic acid and the corresponding α-keto acids. Although α-ketoglutaric and glutamic acids are most commonly involved, α-keto and α-amino monocarboxylic acids may transaminate. Since transaminase enzymes are found in most animal tissues, especially in liver, kidney and other organs, undoubtedly synthesis of amino acids occurs in various tissues (West et al, 1968).

A relatively large number of studies have been conducted with ruminant animals in which the pathways of labeled carbon or N from amino acids have been evaluated. Most of these papers will not be discussed here. Some of the early work with ^{14}C-labeled acetate indicated that ruminant tissues apparently cannot synthesize the usual essential amino acids with the exception of arginine (Black et al, 1957; Downes, 1961). Later studies (Ford and Reilly, 1969; Heitmann et al, 1973) demonstrated quite clearly that amino acids are utilized in substantial amounts for glucogenesis or directly as a source of energy for the animal (see Ch. 6). Other reports are available giving information on turnover rates and interconversions of amino acids in ruminants (Egan et al, 1970; Wolff et al, 1972) or relating to the uptake of labeled sulfur and incorporation into tissue proteins (see Ch. 4).

A reasonable number of studies have also been done relating to milk production (Mepham, 1971). It is generally believed that the major milk proteins (β-casein, α-lactalbumin and β-lactoglobulin) are synthesized in the mammary gland from free blood amino acids. Some of the minor components

(α-casein, immune globulins and milk serum albumin) probably enter milk preformed from the bloodstream. There is no question that free plasma amino acids are taken up by the mammary gland in quantities large enough to account for milk protein synthesis (Verbeke and Peters, 1965; Mepham and Linzell, 1966).

There is ample evidence to show that purines and pyrimidines are degraded in the rumen by ruminal microorganisms (see Ch. 13, Vol. 1). However, information on absorption and tissue utilization is rather meager. The general pathways of degradation are known. Allantoin is the principal excretory product of purine catabolism in ruminants and there is a linear relationship between the disappearance of nucleic acids from the small intestine and the quantity of allantoin in sheep urine. The pathway of breakdown of the pyrimidines, uracil and cytosine, in sheep and cattle probably involves β-alanine formation and the degradation of thymine involves the production of β-aminoisobutyric acid. It is likely that these products are further metabolized in the tissues (Armstrong and Hutton, 1975).

Based on disappearance from the small intestine, Ellis and Bleichner (1969) calculated that total urinary purines accounted for 14 to 47% of apparently absorbed purines. Kaplan and Pobirskii (1975) demonstrated that rumen, blood and urine concentration of purines decreased very rapidly in fasted cattle and that there were high correlations between the ruminal content of nucleic acids and concentrations of allantoin and uric acid in plasma and urine. In one experiment when ^{14}C-labeled compounds were given via the abomasum, the amount of the label recovered was 3.8% (uracil) to 32% (adenine) in urine; 3.4% (adenine) to 64% (uracil) in expired gases; and combined recoveries in urine and gases ranged from 6.7% (uracil) to 35% (adenine) (Condon et al, 1970). Labeled carbon from adenine, uracil and RNA was incorporated into tissue RNA and DNA. In subsequent work from this laboratory (Condon and Hatfield, 1971), it was calculated that 82% of abomasally infused RNA-N was digested; urinary recovery ranged from 92 to 110% of intake. Based on this and other studies, they calculated that 63% of nucleic acid N would be lost as undigested (20%) or as purine derivatives excreted in the urine (43%). An additional 37% of the N may be of value to the host via N derived from deamination of nucleic acids. Information is not available to show if intact purines or pyrimidines are incorporated into the cellular tissues of the host.

PROTEIN UTILIZATION

The diet of grazing ruminants contains protein ranging from ca. 3% in poor quality roughages to >25% in lush, young vegetation. The natural plant proteins of herbage or that from protein concentrates varies in amino acid composition and solubility. In fresh herbage as much as 30% of the N may be in NPN form. Seeds such as corn grain or soybean seed also contain NPN which may be as high as 30-40% at the immature stage with levels more on the order of 4-5% at maturity. Thus, the amount and chemical nature of nitrogenous compounds in the diet may be extremely variable.

Dietary N is used, first, for nourishment of the rumen microorganisms. Ultimately, however, the function of dietary N is for tissue maintenance or for tissue and milk synthesis; amino acids may also provide a significant amount of the total energy in many situations.

The degree of efficiency of N utilization is of considerable importance in the economical production of animal products. This is particularly true as our planet becomes more crowded with people and as food and feed supplies become more competitive. Since ruminants are able to use dietary NPN, it

appears that increased levels of NPN will be fed to these species in the future.

Measures of protein and N utilization may include yield of useful products such as meat, milk and wool. For more specific and usually more exact measures, nutritionists resort to evaluations based on digestibility, N retention in the tissues of growing animals or production in milk, biological value (% of digested N retained in the body), protein efficiency ratio (weight gain/unit of protein consumed), net protein value (BV x digestion coefficient for protein), or changes in rumen or blood components such as blood urea or amino acids. Some procedures are applicable in certain situations while others may be more useful at times. Many of these methods have been or will be referred to in this chapter.

Protein Quality

Protein quality is generally defined as the ability of a specific protein to provide essential amino acids in the required amounts to a given animal performing a specific function such as growth, milk production, etc. In the case of ruminant animals, it has been assumed in the past that protein quality is of relatively little importance and that proteins of equal digestibility are of equal value. This assumption has been based on the fact that ruminal microorganisms synthesize the essential amino acids.

Table 3-2. Nutritive value of various nitrogen sources.[1]

Biological measure	Nitrogen sources[2]			
	Soybean meal	Casein	Zein	Urea
True digestibility, %	88.90[a]	79.80[a]	68.10[b]	88.70[a]
Biological value	84.80[a]	78.30[bc]	84.30[ab]	76.40[c]
Net protein value	75.39[a]	62.48[b]	57.40[c]	67.77[ab]
Nitrogen balance, g/day[3]	0.04[c]	-0.53[a]	-1.00[b]	-0.66[a]
Nitrogen balance, g/day[4]	0.04	-0.68	-1.23	-0.85

[1]Hembry et al (1975).

[2]Values without common superscripts are different (P<0.10).

[3]Determined.

[4]Calculated from true digestibility of protein requirement = (endogenous urinary nitrogen + 1 + metabolic fecal nitrogen) X 6.25 X 100/biological value where 1 is the daily nitrogen deposition in wool. This rearranges to: nitrogen balance = digestible nitrogen intake - (endogenous urinary nitrogen + 1 + metabolic fecal nitrogen) (100/biological value).

Some older reports in the literature have demonstrated relatively marked differences in animal gain or N retention when relatively pure sources of protein have been fed to ruminants (for example, Lofgreen et al, 1947; Ellis et al, 1956; Oltjen et al, 1962). A more recent example is given in Table 3-2. Numerous other examples could be given for this type of comparison.

There is little doubt that quality of proteins in the gut has an effect on animal performance or that the same comment applies to preruminant animals (see Ch. 10). In ruminants one example worth citing is the paper of Colebrook and Reis (1969). In this experiment whole egg protein, egg albumen, corn gluten and gelatin were given to sheep via the abomasum. Casein increased wool growth rate 140-200% and similar responses were obtained from the egg proteins; corn gluten produced about half this response and gelatin had little effect. Numerous other examples could be cited, particularly where amino acids such as lysine, methionine or cystine have been infused into the abomasum or gut (Downes et al, 1970; Schelling et al, 1973; Boila and Devlin, 1975; Clark, 1975).

In cases where certain proteins have given a markedly better response, data show that more intense ruminal fermentation occurs and there is a high correlation between biological value of the protein and numbers of ruminal bacteria (Williams and Moir, 1951; Tagara, 1969).

Microbial Quality

McNaught et al (1954) found that the biological value of protein from rumen bacteria and protozoa were similar, the values being 81 and 80, respectively. However, the true digestibility was only 74% for bacterial protein as compared to 91% for protozoal protein. Thus, net protein utilization was much higher for the protozoal protein.

The amino acid composition of rumen bacterial protein seems to be rather constant. A comparison of the values between laboratories yielded a correlation of 0.98 (Purser, 1970). Ration does not appear to affect the composition, since correlation coefficients of 0.98 and 0.99 were found in comparing the bacterial protein from animals fed different rations (Purser, 1970). Purser also reported that the composition of bacterial and protozoal protein was highly correlated (r = 0.97). Amino acid composition of acid hydrolysates of ruminal bacteria

in cattle were similar when free of ruminal ciliated protozoa or if ruminal holotrichs or entodiniomorphs were present (Williams and Dinusson, 1973). Thus, one suspects causes other than amino acid content of rumen microbes for differences in performance from feeding different N sources.

Potter et al (1969) found that the quantity of N apparently reaching the abomasum was approximately 80% as high for steers fed a natural ration supplemented with urea as for steers fed a ration supplemented with soybean meal (Table 3-3). Also, a higher proportion of the abomasal N was in the form of protein in the soy-fed steers. Quality of the protein reaching the abomasum was not affected by the ration fed, since the essential amino acid composition of the abomasal protein was similar for the steers supplemented with the two N sources. Tucker and Fontenot (1970), using lambs fed purified diets, found that the protein N reaching the abomasum was lower for lambs fed urea as the only N source than for those fed a similar ration containing soy protein as the only N sources throughout a 50-day period. About 18% more essential amino acids reached the abomasum of lambs fed a high quality forage than for lambs fed a low quality forage (Amos et al, 1976).

Table 3-3. Nitrogen in the abomasum of steers fed soybean meal or urea[a]

| Item | Supplemental N | |
	Soybean meal	Urea
N intake, g/day	94.4	90.4
Abomasal N, g/day	73.7	58.6
Abomasal N, % of N intake	77.6	65.7
Relative N in abomasum, %	100.0	79.5
Protein N, % of abomasal N	50.2	41.2

[a]Adapted from Potter et al (1969).

Differences were recorded in amino acid availability from rumen microbes from cattle fed different protein supplements (Burris et al, 1974), as shown in Table 3-4. Although no difference in bulk amino acid patterns was evident, ruminal bacteria isolated from cattle fed a high concentrate ration had a higher biological value for the laboratory rat than the bacteria fed a high roughage ration (Keyser et al, 1978).

Table 3-4. Liberation of amino acids in rumen bacteria by pepsin-pancreatin digestion.[a]

| | Protein supplement | | | |
| | None[b] | Soybean meal | Fish-meal | Linseed meal |
Amino acid	1	2	3	4
Aspartic acid	5.70	7.03	6.19	6.33
Threonine	15.69	16.28	12.73	13.15
Serine	11.57	17.12	15.00	10.49
Glutamic acid	10.42	16.93	9.45	9.78
Proline[c]	6.53	11.65	N.D.	5.79
Glycine	10.63	15.22	7.51	12.29
Alanine	26.28	47.1	25.91	27.40
Valine	22.74	35.51	21.13	26.72
Cystine	N.D.	12.04	N.D.	N.D.
Methionine	42.77	38.71	59.85	44.86
Isoleucine	28.36	36.34	30.79	30.31
Leucine	44.35	53.35	44.77	45.56
Tyrosine	53.46	52.84	48.25	52.25
Phenylalanine	53.50	58.35	49.30	55.94
Lysine	48.50	57.14	46.98	55.45
Histidine	41.32	45.49	38.30	50.49
Arginine	57.82	66.81	54.14	49.32
Total	25.59	31.46	25.67	27.05

[a] Burris et al (1974)

[b] Percent of each bacterial amino acid released upon in vitro digestion

[c] N.D. = not detectable

Effect of Quantity of Protein Consumed

One major factor affecting protein digestibility is the amount of protein consumed per day. This is illustrated in work by Egan and Kellaway (1971) in which they fed sheep 20 different fresh frozen herbages ranging from 1.5 to 5.2% N. Results of this procedure on apparent protein digestibility are shown in Fig. 3-3. Note that there is a good linear response between N intake and apparent digestibility. One of the reasons is that metabolic fecal N represents a smaller and smaller amount of the N excreted in feces as dietary consumption increases (see section on maintenance in Nitrogen Requirement section). In addition, soluble and digestible protein in a given plant material generally increase as N content increases.

Urinary N also increases as N intake increases as shown in Fig. 3-3, but at a somewhat slower rate. The overall effect of increasing N consumption on urinary excretion and on N retention is illustrated in Fig. 3-4. The response is curvilinear as might be expected; for that matter the curve on apparent digestibility would be curvilinear if consumption increases enough. Urinary N

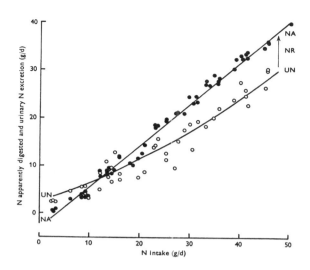

Fig. 3-3. General relationships in sheep between the intake, apparent absorption, urinary excretion and retention of herbage N. Apparently digested N (NA) •; urinary N excretion (UN) o; NR, retained N. Courtesy of Eagan and Kellaway (1971).

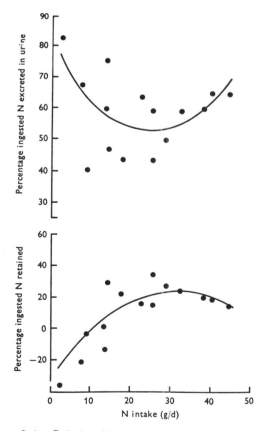

Fig. 3-4. Relationships between percentage of ingested N excreted in urine and percentage of ingested N retained, and N intake. Courtesy of Egan and Kellaway (1971).

Table 3-5. Effect of increasing protein levels on N utilization by growing cattle. [a]

Item	Crude protein in diet, % of DM[b]			
	14.5	19.9	23.7	28.5
Digestibility, %				
Dry matter	63.3	65.0	63.0	64.0
Crude protein	60.5	67.8	72.1	75.0
N utilization, 5/day				
Intake	84.8	109.8	136.0	166.1
Fecal N	33.5	35.2	37.9	41.3
Urinary N	23.7	37.3	55.3	80.0
N retention	27.4	37.3	42.8	44.6
% N retained	32.6	33.8	31.1	26.4
Biological value	53.4	50.0	43.1	35.3

[a] Data from Neville et al (1977)

[b] Increasing levels of protein supplied by soybean and cottonseed meals.

production, as a % of intake, is strongly dependent upon level of N intake. At low levels of N intake the urinary N output is high because of endogenous N components in urine; at high levels of intake, N is utilized with lower efficiency, again resulting in a high percentage of the ingested N appearing in urine. At some intermediate point, N utilization is at highest efficiency and urinary N output as a percentage of N intake is at a minimum (Egan and Kellaway, 1971).

Similar data on the amount of N consumed on efficiency of utilization are shown in Table 3-5 when growing calves were fed complete rations in which the majority of the added protein was supplied by cottonseed and soybean meals. Note that digestibility of protein increased with increasing consumption. Fecal N increased slightly and urinary N increased about 4 fold, but N retention also increased. The percentage retained dropped off at the highest level (28.5%) and the biological value decreased with each increase in dietary protein. Thus, the results with dry, mixed diets are essentially the same as with herbage diets.

It should be pointed out that apparent digestibility of N is always low on a roughage diet that has very low N content. Due to the normal excretion of metabolic fecal N, a dietary crude protein content of 4-5% will often yield just enough digestible protein to balance off the endogenous excretion, resulting in apparent digestibility of about zero.

Protein-Energy Relationships

There is a considerable amount of evidence in the literature to show that energy concentration in the ration affects N utilization. The older literature has been reviewed by writers such as Blaxter (1962) and Mitchell (1964). More recent reviews as related to N requirements have been discussed by Ørskov (1977), Garrett (1977) and Journet and Verite (1977).

In monogastric species, particularly for specific situations such as production of broilers or eggs, it has been demonstrated time and again that there are optimum protein:energy relationships. Broilers and eggs are produced in very specific conditions as compared to the many different feeding situations that are used for ruminant animals. However, as early as 1923, Mollgard (cited by Mitchell, 1964) observed that energy was used most efficiently by dairy cows when protein supplied from 15 to 25% of the net energy. Energy was used less efficiently when protein supplied either less than 15% or more than 25%. In other studies with different animals, it has been shown that utilization of ME does not continuously increase as the protein level increases; rather, it increases for a time, then remains constant throughout a considerable range and then decreases above some critical proportion (Mitchell, 1964).

In preruminant lambs Black and Griffiths (1975) observed that N balance was independent of energy intake when N intake was less than the amount required. Rather, it was linearly related to absorbed N and metabolic weight. When N intake was in excess of the amount required, N balance increased linearly with ME intake at a rate that decreased with increasing live weight. N requirement/MJ decreased with increasing body weight. In calves efficiency of transformation of dietary protein to tissue protein increases with increased energy concentration (Jahn et al, 1976) and in pregnant ewes retention increased as energy concentration of the rations increased although apparent digestibility of N was not affected (Guada et al, 1975).

In the non-lactating animal an increase in energy intake normally leads to an improvement in N balance. The effect is much less than increased consumption of digestible N. In the lactating cow the daily milk production and the utilization of digestible N for milk production are closely related to ME intake (Broster et al, 1969; Gordon and Forbes, 1970, 1971; Paquay et al, 1973). An example of protein-energy interaction is shown in Table 3-6. In this example yield of lactating cows was depressed by either low energy or low protein and N digestibility was depressed by a combination of high energy and low protein, but N retention + milk N was least on the low energy-low protein combination. Another example is shown in Table 3-7 in which cows were given a diet calculated to be isocaloric based on NRC book values for digestibility (Moe and Tyrrell, 1972). Digestibility of both crude protein and energy were depressed in the low protein diet; NE was lower for the low protein diet, but efficiency

Table 3-7. Effect of increasing protein level on efficiency of energy utilization.[a]

Item	Protein level, %	
	15.9	11.6
Protein digestibility, %	69.2	54.5
Predicted DE, Mcal/kg DM	3.25	3.28
Actual DE, %	68.4	63.0
ME, Mcal/kg DM	2.63	2.47
ME/DE, %	83.9	85.8
NE, Mcal/kg DM	1.55	1.44

[a]From More and Tyrrell (1972)

of energy utilization on the low protein diet was primarily caused by lower digestibility. Comparable results were reported in a more recent paper from this laboratory (Moe and Tyrrell, 1977).

Broster et al (1969) observed that N retention was increased by a supplement of readily available energy through a decrease in urinary N loss. N balance was not increased by a supplement of fibrous energy since this resulted in an increase in fecal N loss. In other studies Paquay et al (1973) observed that N secreted in the milk and the daily milk production depended on the ME intake as well as on stage of lactation and these parameters were related to dietary N:energy ratio. The optimal digestible N:ME ratio ranged from about 2.2 g/MJ during the first 3 mo. of lactation to about 1.7 g/MJ in the 6th and 7th mo. and 1.3 g/MJ from the 10th mo.

Table 3-6. Interrelationship between energy and protein on milk production.[a]

	Treatment			
	1	2	3	4
Starch equivalent, % of requirement	82	120	118	80
Digestible protein, % of requirement	122	119	80	77
Milk yield, kg/day	10.8	13.2	11.3	10.4
Milk energy, Mcal/day	7.39	8.89	7.43	7.12
N intake, g/day	230	253	175	177
Digestibility of N, %	73.9	67.5	58.6	67.9
Retained N + milk N, g/day	59.1	86.9	65.3	50.0

[a]Data from Gordon and Forbes (1970)

Unless protein-energy studies involve feeding restricted amounts of feed, changes in energy concentrations are brought about by substituting feedstuffs with more starch or fat and ration alterations of this type usually have a pronounced effect on rumen metabolism, digestibility, and tissue metabolism. One aspect of such a change was demonstrated by Eskeland et al (1973) who found that I.V. administration of propionic acid resulted in higher N retention than administration of an isocaloric amount of acetic acid. Thus, many of the studies on protein-energy have been confounded by various rumen and metabolic factors and it is not possible to partition out the effects strictly due to alteration of energy or N.

At a given energy intake N intake influences metabolism of energy. When the N content of the diet is low, the voluntary intake of dry matter is limited because of reduced microbial activity in the rumen and a reduced rate of degradation of digesta. It has also been demonstrated that intake of protein in excess of the amount required results in a decreased energy balance (Tyrell et al, 1970) and in a decrease in the net efficiency of ME utilization (Walker and Norton, 1971).

Effect of Solubility

Assuming that dietary factors required by rumen microorganisms are present in adequate amounts, one of the major factors related to protein utilization appears to be that of solubility, both in the rumen and in the gut. When evaluating protein sources for monogastric species, pepsin digestibility has been used as one criterion of availability. However, with ruminating animals, it re-

mains to be seen if pepsin solubility is related to overall N utilization in the total GI tract. It has been known for some time that degree of solubility of natural plant or animal proteins is directly correlated to the rate at which ammonia is released in the rumen. For example, casein may be degraded to the extent of 90% whereas zein (from corn grain) may only be degraded to the extent of 30-40% (Chalmers et al, 1954; McDonald and Hall, 1957; Ely et al, 1967; Mangan, 1972) and other proteins may be considerably less soluble when heat-treated or chemically treated to reduce solubility. Thus, proteins vary considerably in the degree to which they are degraded in the rumen. Much less information is available on solubility and digestibility in the gut. One example is given in Table 3-8 from an experiment in which casein or wheat gluten were infused into the gut. Even though casein is considerably more soluble in water or mineral solutions, both proteins were digested to about the same extent and N retention was reasonably similar.

Since ammonia increases in the rumen with increasing solubility of protein or increased consumption, it is reasonable to conclude that more wastage may occur if ammonia levels exceed the need of ruminal microorganisms, particularly since ammonia is readily absorbed from the rumen. Black (1971) calculated that 46% less protein would be absorbed from the intestines of a ruminant lamb if all dietary protein were degraded in the rumen. However, it has not been established that all of the differences in N utilization between different protein sources are due to differential ruminal ammonia production related to solubility.

Table 3-8. Postal ruminal digestion of casein and wheat gluten infused into the small intestine of rams.[a]

Dietary N intake, g/day	Infused N, g/d	N excreted, g/d		Digested N		Retained N	
		feces	urine	g/d	%	g/d	%
Negative control 4.62	---	4.35	2.31	0.27	5.8	-2.04	-46.9
NC + casein 4.62	19.7	4.95	8.09	19.37	79.6	11.28	46.4
NC + wheat gluten 4.62	22.92	5.57	11.16	21.83	79.3	10.68	38.8

[a] Derived from data of Ben-Ghedalia et al (1976)

For example, Little et al (1963) found that feeding regular or heated soybean meal resulted in a higher rate of gain than feeding of corn gluten meal. Both the heat-treated soy and corn gluten meals were low in soluble N and were converted slowly to ammonia in vitro. However, in another example, feeding corn gluten meal to sheep resulted in more total N, protein, essential and non-essential amino acids reaching the abomasum than feeding distillers dried solubles or soybean meal (Amos et al, 1971). In an experiment in which legume-grass hay was shown to result in superior N utilization as compared with soybean meal, it was demonstrated that hay-fed sheep had higher concentrations of soluble N compounds such as soluble α-amino acid N, diffusible N and diffusible peptide N (Dror et al, 1970).

There has been some work designed to develop appropriate means of evaluating protein solubility (Proksova, 1969; Sniffen, 1974; Wohlt et al, 1976; Crawford et al, 1978), either through the use of mineral solutions designed to simulate saliva or with autoclaved rumen fluid. Wohlt et al (1973) demonstrated that protein solubility increased substantially when pH of the buffer was increased from 5.5 to 6.5. Feeds whose major protein fraction was composed mainly of albumins and globulins had a higher solubility than those composed mainly of prolamins and glutelins. A large amount of variation in soluble N was detected among energy feeds (3.9-42.57%) and protein supplements (2.8-93.27%). When lambs were fed rations in which 13 or 35% of the total protein was soluble as determined by the method of Wohlt et al (1976), urinary N, rumen ammonia and butyrate were higher for lambs fed the rations in which 35% of the dietary protein was soluble. In another experiment reported by Sniffen (1974), lambs were fed rations containing 13, 18 or 22% soluble N in concentrates and hay which had

protein which was 24% soluble. He found that % N excreted increased with increasing solubility in the ration and N balance declined. The author pointed out that the concentrate ration was consumed within 15 min. while the hay was consumed over a 24-hr period; the amount of soluble N consumed/unit of time appeared to be a factor. In a study with lactating dairy cows fed diets in which 22 or 42% of the N was soluble, the soluble N did not affect dry matter, protein or energy consumption. However, cows fed the diets with lower N solubility gave more milk (Majdoub et al, 1978). Thus, it is obvious that further information is needed to evaluate the importance of protein solubility on overall utilization.

Rumen By-pass Studies

As pointed out previously, dietary protein and NPN substances are attacked to a variable extent by rumen microorganisms. The conversion of a protein such as zein to microbial protein may improve protein quality and thus be of benefit. However, this is probably not the case for high quality proteins since the amino acid composition of rumen microorganisms does not seem to be altered substantially by kind of ration. Since not all of the ammonia produced in the rumen is incorporated into microbial protein, when soluble N sources are fed high levels of ammonia N are absorbed. Thus, research workers have studied the effect of by-passing the rumen with certain critical amino acids and high quality proteins in order to avoid the wasteful ammonia production by administering them posterior to the rumen or treating them in such a manner that they will not be attacked easily by rumen microbes.

Chalmers et al (1954) studied the effect of administering 50 g of casein to ewes in the later stages of pregnancy by ruminal and duodenal fistulas. Urinary N excretion was lower and N retention was higher when the

Table 3-9. Effect of duodenal administration of casein on N balance.[a]

Method of casein adminstration	N intake, g/day		N excretion, g/day		N balance, g/day
	Basal	Casein	Feces	Urine	
Ruminal fistula	9.20	6.46	4.27	10.64	0.75
Duodenal fistula	9.20	6.46	4.32	9.20	2.14

[a] Adapted from Chalmers et al (1954)

casein was given via the duodenal fistula (Table 3-9). In experiments with sheep, Reis and Schinckel (1961) observed higher N retention from abomasal administration of casein than when the sheep received equivalent levels of N under normal feeding. Also, they reported that efficiency of conversion of dietary N into wool N was much higher where casein was administered into the abomasum than in experiments involving normal feeding. Other reports showing improvement in wool growth with abomasal infusions of casein include those of Reis and Schinckel (1963, 1964) and Reis and Downes (1971).

Little and Mitchell (1967) showed higher N retention in sheep given soybean protein abomasally as compared to orally. Abomasal administration of zein tended to decrease N retention. Rumen by-pass of fishmeal, soybean meal and casein via closure of the esophageal groove increased N retention and rate of gain in lambs (Ørskov et al, 1970). Administering of casein in the abomasum increased milk protein production in dairy cows (Broderick et al, 1970; Derrig et al, 1974; Vik-Mo et al, 1974).

A practical approach for avoiding rumen fermentation would be to process certain protein sources so that they would not be attacked by rumen microbes but would be digested further down the GI tract. It was suggested by Zelter and Leroy (1966) that tannins could be used to decrease rumen degradation. Tannin-treated samples were not degraded in vitro by rumen microorganisms, while untreated samples were degraded rapidly. Rate of ammonia production and average blood urea levels were lower for fistulated sheep fed the treated protein than for those receiving the untreated protein. Delort-Laval and Zelter (1968) reported a 6% increase in N utilization in lactating goats from tannin treatment of peanut and linseed meal. They reported a 16% increase when tannin-treated milk powder was fed to kids. Ferguson et al (1967) studied the effect of formaldehyde treatment of casein. The solubility of the casein at pH 6 was 8% for the treated and 83% for the untreated casein. At the end of 24 hr of in vitro incubation, 4% of the treated and 89% of the untreated casein was degraded. Feeding the treated casein resulted in a 70% increase in wool growth during an 18-week period. There was a decrease in wool growth when the untreated protein was substituted for the treated material.

Treatment of soybean meal with tannic acid has been reported to increase perfor-mance in cattle and sheep (Hatfield, 1970). N retention was increased in one trial. Wright (1974) found that replacement of part of the casein with formaldehyde-treated casein resulted in a 20% increase in gain and an 8% improvement in feed efficiency in lambs fed a fattening-type ration. Feeding formaldehyde-treated casein to lambs increased rate of gain and feed efficiency (Faichney, 1971), N retention (Macrae et al, 1972) and brought about an increase in concentration of some plasma amino acids (Reis and Tunks, 1970).

A trend for improvement in rate of gain and feed efficiency from formaldehyde treatment of peanut meal was observed in ruminating calves fed a 13% protein ration, but not in calves fed a 20% protein ration (Faichney and Davis, 1972). A decreased rate of gain was noted in calves fed a ration supplemented with formaldehyde-treated soybean meal as compared to those fed untreated soybean meal (Schmidt et al, 1973, 1974). Performance of fattening lambs fed untreated and formaldehyde-treated soybean meal was similar (Wachira et al, 1974). Although the results have not been consistent, post ruminal supplementation of casein has increased milk production 1 to 4 kg/day in experiments of short duration (Clark, 1975).

Treatment of hay or silage with formaldehyde depressed apparent digestibility of protein by sheep (Barry, 1973; 1976; Barry and Fennessy, 1973; Amos et al, 1976b). However, Amos et al (1976b) reported an increase in N retention due to a decrease in urinary excretion in lambs fed formaldehyde treated coastal Bermudagrass.

NPN UTILIZATION

Evidence was obtained by Zuntz in 1891 that ruminants could utilize NPN. Since then a voluminous number of experiments have been conducted concerning the use of NPN to replace at least part of the protein in the diet.

One of the milestones in the research on NPN utilization was the work of Loosli et al (1949) showing that all of the amino acids essential for the growth of rats were synthesized in the rumen of sheep. In this work lambs were fed purified diets containing urea or soy protein as the sole N source. As shown in Table 3-10, they reported evidence of extensive amino acid synthesis.

Table 3-10. Daily amino acid balance of sheep and goats fed a urea diet.[a]

| Amino acid | Apparent amino acid, g | | | | |
| | Intake | | Losses | | |
	Diet	Rumen[b]	Feces	Urine	Retention
Arginine	0.19	1.27	0.48	0.09	0.73
Histidine	0.05	0.59	0.18	0.02	0.39
Isoleucine	0.00	1.38	0.52	0.06	0.80
Leucine	0.15	2.04	0.61	0.08	1.35
Lysine	0.24	2.34	0.71	0.12	1.51
Methionine	0.03	0.66	0.21	0.02	0.43
Phenylalanine	0.05	1.01	0.48	0.04	0.49
Threonine	0.07	1.63	0.67	0.06	0.90
Tryptophan	0.01	0.25	0.13	0.01	0.11
Valine	0.14	1.57	0.69	0.08	0.80

[a] From Loosli et al (1949)

[b] Values were calculated by multiplying the daily nitrogen intakes by the amino acid contents of the rumen material.

The amino acid level of rumen contents was 9-20 fold that of the diet. Furthermore, the lambs receiving NPN as the sole N source were in positive N balance.

In many experiments utilization of NPN by ruminants has been less efficient than that of preformed protein. Urea is readily hydrolyzed in the rumen and the ammonia may be used for microbial protein synthesis or it may be absorbed across the rumen wall and may be resynthesized into urea and excreted. Some writers have suggested that if the rate of hydrolysis were slower or if urea were ingested at periodic intervals, efficiency of N utilization would be increased. However, no differences were observed in N balance or protein N reaching the abomasum between sheep infused with equal amounts of urea twice/day or continuously (Streeter et al, 1973). Likewise, Knight and Owens (1973) reported greater N retention in lambs in which urea was infused during a 1 or 3 hr period following each of two daily feedings as compared to continuous infusion. Aceto-hydroxamic acid was effective in inhibiting ruminal fluid urease activity in vitro (Brent et al, 1971) and in vivo (Jones and Milligan, 1975), but no consistent improvement in N retention has been observed (Moore et al, 1968; Streeter et al, 1969). Feeding a slow release extruded urea product containing urea, starch and carboxy resin improved performance and N retention in sheep (Huston et al, 1974).

Feeding 5% tallow with 1.5% urea tends to depress N retention in sheep and rumen protein synthesis in vitro (Phillips and Church, 1975). These results may explain the depressed performance observed when urea was fed to steers in combination with tallow (Bradley et al, 1966). Dehydrated alfalfa meal was shown to improve N utilization in cattle (Horn and Beeson, 1969) but the response has not been consistent (Owen et al, 1971; Van Slyke et al, 1971). Feeding branched-chain volatile fatty acids improved N retention in lambs fed a urea supplemented high roughage ration (Umunna et al, 1975). An acid-resistant hemicellulose from corn cobs increased microbial protein synthesis in vitro and increased N retention of lambs fed a urea-supplemented high roughage ration (McLaren et al, 1976). Sulfur supplementation did not improve N retention in dairy cows fed a corn silage-based urea-supplemented ration (Grieve et al, 1973). Likewise, adding S to urea-containing rations to give N to S ratios of 9.4:1 or 11.4:1 did not improve performance of early weaned calves (Winter, 1976). Performance of steers fed high urea rations was similar for N to S ratios of 15.4 to 6.4 and 4.0 to 1 (Pendlum et al, 1976).

NPN for Growth

NPN sources have been studied as partial or total substitutes for protein in ruminant rations. The use of urea to replace part of the protein has not affected performance consistently. Even at 2 mo. of age calves are able to utilize urea. Research with older dairy calves shows that urea is utilized but the response, compared to conventional protein supplements, has been variable. Age of the animals fed urea may be a factor. Cattle older than 6 mo. achieved daily gain of 1 kg on corn silage and urea, but younger calves needed alfalfa to support a high rate of gain (Thomas et al, 1975). Performance of lambs fed up to 8.5% urea in purified diets was similar or superior to that of lambs fed high protein and whey and 1.71% urea (Price et al, 1972).

In experiments with cattle wintered on dry range grass, the use of a pelleted supplement, in which urea supplied 25% of the protein equivalent, produced performance similar to cottonseed meal (Gallup et al, 1953). Raleigh and Wallace (1963) reported that urea supplementation to hay resulted in similar gains as cottonseed meal supplementation when the ration for growing cattle contained 6% crude protein but gains were lower for the urea-fed cattle when the rations contained 9% crude protein.

Response to feeding urea to cattle fed high roughage rations has not been consistent. Supplementing a mature grass (6% CP) with molasses-urea improved daily gain (275 vs. -15 g/day in cattle; Chicco et al, 1972). Later work with a larger number of cattle yielded similar results (Carnevali et al, 1973). No response was noted in dry cows, yearlings or calves allowed access to a low N (9% crude protein) urea-molasses mixture (Bond and Rumsey, 1973). No difference was observed

from feeding a urea-molasses supplement (31% crude protein) 3 or 6X/week or self-fed to cattle grazing dry winter range (Rush and Totusek, 1975). Performance was poor for all treatments. Apparently, urea-molasses supplements are beneficial to digestibility of low protein roughages (White et al, 1973). Increases in crude fiber and energy digestibility were reported from adding 1% urea to a ration composed of rice straw and molasses. Supplementing 3% protein hay with urea, molasses and a combination of urea and molasses increased dry matter intake 28, 15 and 65% as compared to hay alone (Ernst et al, 1975). Improvements in straw intake were reported from supplementing with urea, sulfur and wheat (Barry and Johnstone, 1976) or urea-molasses (Hadjipanayiotou et al, 1975).

The results of early research indicated that feeding urea to fattening lambs did not allow performance comparable to that from oil meal supplements (Gallup et al, 1953). However, Meiske et al (1955) and Oltjen et al (1963) obtained similar performance from lambs supplemented with urea or soybean meal although Amos et al (1970) found that corn gluten meal improved gain in lambs as compared to urea. With high straw rations, performance tends to be less with urea than soy protein (Bhattacharya and Khan, 1973; Bhattacharya and Pervez, 1973).

Performance in fattening cattle has usually not been altered by replacing up to one-third of the protein N with urea N (Gallup et al, 1953; Oltjen et al, 1965; Perry et al, 1967a; Fontenot et al, 1968; Clark et al, 1970; Boling

Table 3-11. Examples of experimental results comparing urea with plant protein sources in finishing rations for cattle.

Comparison	Daily gain	Feed conversion	Reference
Corn + soybean meal	1.04	5.67	White et al (1975)
+ urea	0.82	6.47	
Corn + soybean meal*	1.13	7.03	Burris et al (1975)
+ urea	1.15	6.91	
Corn + soybean meal	1.48	6.9	Clark et al (1970)
+ urea	1.52	7.1	
Barley + cottonseed meal	1.37	6.6	Church (1972)
+ urea	1.46	6.2	
Barley + soybean meal	1.06	6.57	Kay and Macdearmid
+ urea	1.13	6.41	(1972)

* Ration consumption restricted to 7.95 kg/day.

et al, 1971; Kay and Macdearmid, 1972; White et al, 1975). However, the results are not consistent. For example, performance of the urea-fed cattle was lower than for those fed conventional protein supplement in one of four trials reported by Clark et al (1970) and one of five trials reported by Perry et al (1967a). But in a number of instances, urea supplements have produced equal if not greater gains than plant protein sources (Table 3-11).

In beef cattle nutrition there is a trend toward using greater amounts of urea. However, as pointed out by Chalupa (1968), even if 90% of the supplementary N is from urea, this will represent only about one-third of the protein equivalent in a typical ration. It appears, however, that some amino acids may be limiting for growth on certain diets. Methionine and threonine appeared to be limiting for growth of calves fed urea or soybean meal as a supplement (Liebholz, 1976) and sulfur containing amino acids were the most limiting for sheep fed urea containing diets (Owens et al, 1973).

There have been a number of growth studies in which virtually all of the dietary N was supplied by NPN (Oltjen, 1969). When NPN completely replaces protein in purified diets, rate of growth and feed efficiency are generally lower than when soy protein is used (Meacham et al, 1961; Oltjen et al, 1962; Matrone et al, 1964; Goodrich and Tillman, 1968). However, palatability may be a factor here.

NPN for Milk Production

Urea or other NPN compounds can be used to replace part of the native protein in dairy rations, but divergent results have been obtained concerning the maximum level of urea which can be used successfully. Recent reports on this topic include those of Knott et al (1972), Clark et al (1973), Huber (1975), Jones et al (1975), Kwan et al (1977) and Polan et al (1976) on dairy cows and that of Champredon and Pion (1972) on lactating goats. In actual practice the trend is to feed either no urea or limit the amount to ca. 1% in early lactation. In mid to late lactation feeding as much as 2.5% (of the concentrate) has been used without any detriment to milk production. The amount of natural occurring NPN compounds and solubility of N in other feedstuffs may be a factor in how much urea can be utilized (Kertz and Everett, 1975; Kwan et al, 1977). Utilization of urea

may have a special application in areas where heat stress is a factor since a limited amount of information suggests that its inclusion will reduce the heat increment of feeding (Colovos et al, 1963). The feeding of urea or other NPN has not affected milk composition consistently.

Usually, when a negative response is observed from feeding urea, a decrease in feed consumption occurs. Wilson et al (1975) reported data showing that feed depression with high urea levels was due to a physiological effect other than taste. Depressions in feed consumption occurred when urea level exceeded 2% of the ration but feed consumption was depressed more when urea was administered directly into the rumen.

NPN for Reproduction

Heifers fed on a purified diet with urea as the only source of N reached puberty and reproduced satisfactorily (Bond and Oltjen, 1973). Age at puberty was higher than for heifers fed a natural diet or purified diet with soy protein as the N source but no differences were observed in estrous cycle, conception rate, birth weight of calves or gestation length. Heifers fed the purified urea diet gave less milk at first lactation and averaged 53 days longer between calving and first estrus. Supplying as much as two thirds of the dietary N as urea did not affect reproductive performance of heifers or performance of their calves. Feeding urea did not affect reproductive performance of cow and ewes in some studies or surveys (Ryder et al, 1973; Thompson et al, 1973). Incidence and regularity of estrus and percent calf or lamb crops from service during one estrus period were not altered by feeding urea nor was the concentration of a number of hormones. Mastitis, digestive disorders, ovarian function, services per conception and birth and survival of calves not aborted were affected by feeding urea to dairy cows (Garverick et al, 1971; Erb et al, 1976). However, abortion of first pregnancy, retained placenta at second calving and calving intervals were increased and gestation periods were decreased from feeding urea to supply 45% of total dietary N up to mid-pregnancy and 36% thereafter.

Adaptation to NPN Feeding

Evidence has been accumulating during the last few years that in some manner ruminants adapt to NPN feeding, but there is no easy explanation for the differences in results when an adaptation response has been demonstrated. A number of reports show that N retention is improved on urea or urea and/or biuret rations when animals have been exposed to the diets for periods of up to 50 days (McLaren et al, 1959, 1965, 1976; Smith et al, 1960; Ludwick et al, 1971). In one case DES reduced the time (McLaren et al, 1959) and the presence of readily available carbohydrates may increase the amount of N absorbed but not the adaptation time (McLaren et al, 1965).

Rumen microbes are not capable of hydrolyzing biuret without adaptation (Gilchrist et al, 1968), although adaptation may sometimes occur quite rapidly (Wyatt et al, 1975). Adaptation was lost if biuret was not fed for a few days (Clemens and Johnson, 1973). Feeding diets low to moderate in starch resulted in faster adaptation to biuret but adaptation was not influenced by the presence of urea or soybean meal (Clemens and Johnson, 1973, 1974).

Although Caffrey et al (1967) reported that rate of ammonia assimilation by rumen microorganisms in vitro was greater using inocula from lambs which had been adapted to a urea-rich diet than from lambs on a normal diet, Barth et al (1961) did not find an adaptation response as measured with in vitro protein synthesis over a 49-day period. In another example Ludwick et al (1970) found that in vitro protein synthesis tended to be higher using microbes from lambs which had been fed urea for 100 days than with microbes from lambs fed soy protein; with washed cell suspensions there were no differences in protein synthesis nor were there any differences in urea-^{15}N incorporation in vitro by whole rumen contents from lambs fed urea or soy protein for ca. 7 mo. Feeding lyophilized rumen contents from sheep adapted to urea did not influence N retention in non-adapted sheep (Waymack, 1976).

A number of studies have demonstrated that urinary N decreases and N retention increases with time in steers or lambs fed purified diets containing urea (Oltjen and Putnam, 1966; Clifford and Tillman, 1968). Although Oltjen (1969) suggested that some experimental results showing an adaptation response may be a reflection of animal adjustment to the purified diet components other than NPN or animal adaptation from an adequate to a lower protein diet, Meiske and Goodrich (1966) and Perry et al (1967b)

obtained indirect evidence of adaptation to urea feeding in finishing cattle fed practical rations. Substantial differences in daily gain were observed between cattle fed supplements containing no urea and high levels of urea, particularly during the first 28 days of the trials. In the study by Meiske and Goodrich (Table 3-12) daily gains were identical for cattle fed linseed meal and urea during the last 74 days.

Table 3-12. Feeding of urea supplements to fattening cattle.[a]

	Linseed meal	Urea supplements
Daily gain, kg		
Total, 102 days	1.29	1.16
First 28 days	1.95	1.44
Final 74 days	1.05	1.05

[a]Meiske and Goodrich (1966)

With lactating cows fed purified diets, Virtanen (1966) reported increased labeling of amino acids of milk protein with ^{15}N following 6 mo. of feeding urea compared to a non-adapted cow. He also reported similar labeling from feeding urea 6 or 25 mo.

Although a variety of theories have been proposed, the nature and site of the adaptation response have not been established. Probably some fo the variations in response are due to differences in rations or methods of feeding urea. In many of the papers reviewed information was not given concerning the manner in which urea was introduced into the ration. In some cases it may have been introduced gradually while in others it may have been introduced abruptly.

Sources of NPN

Although urea is the most common source of NPN now in use, several other NPN compounds are potential commercial sources including various organic and inorganic ammonium salts, anhydrous ammonia, amides and purines. This is a topic that is more suited to Vol. 3 of this series, thus only a brief coverage of the topic will be given here.

A product (Starea) was developed by processing starch (grain) and urea together in cooker-extruder equipment (Helmer et al, 1970). Trends for lower ammonia N and higher bacterial protein in vitro were reported when Starea was used as a substrate as compared to ground or expanded corn plus urea. An increase in milk production was reported from feeding Starea (Helmer et al, 1970; Roman-Ponce et al, 1975), but Jones et al (1975) found no effect as compared to corn and urea. Similar performance was noted for feedlot cattle fed urea or Starea (Thompson et al, 1972). Feeding Starea or sulfur-coated urea did not increase N retention in lambs as compared to urea (Umunna and Woods, 1975) nor did feeding heated complexes of urea and high cellulose sources improve N retention in steers as compared to untreated complexes (Daniels et al, 1971).

Meiske et al (1955) concluded that biuret was a satisfactory source of supplemental N for growing-fattening lambs and biuret appeared to be less toxic than urea when administered in large amounts. Similar results were observed by Berry et al (1956) with lambs although lower gains were observed in steers fed biuret than in those fed urea. Biuret was shown to be of similar value as urea for wintering and fattening cattle (Oltjen et al, 1974) and appears to be similar or better than urea for supplementing low protein dry grass for beef cows (Rush and Totusek, 1976; Rush et al, 1976; Martin et al, 1976). Quite a number of additional studies have been carried out in which biuret has been compared either to urea or natural protein sources. Much of the material has been reviewed by Fonnesbeck et al (1975). It should be noted that it is not permitted to feed biuret to lactating dairy cows in most states.

Other NPN sources such as diammonium phosphate, ammonium sulfate, ammonium polyphosphate, ammonium propionate, butyrate or acetate or anhydrous ammonia have been used in various studies in many different laboratories. Most of these compounds are considerably less toxic than urea when given via drench or fed in large amounts. However, most of them are more costly than urea. Diammonium or mono-ammonium phosphates find some use in liquid supplements and, to a lesser extent, in dry supplements. Anhydrous ammonia appears to be satisfactory when added to silage or whey. Other N-containing compounds are only rarely used in practical situations.

NITROGEN REQUIREMENTS

The N requirements of ruminants are listed in various publications such as the NRC bulletins and other similar publications from other countries. However, there is considerable uncertainty about the accuracy for a wide range of conditions because of many different factors. For example, N requirements are affected by age, sex, species, level and type of production, disease and parasites, and other environmental stresses. In addition, efficiency of N utilization is affected by amount of protein consumed and it is interrelated to energy level of the diet as well as the presence of readily available carbohydrates. Furthermore, there is considerable uncertainty regarding the utilization of the total N supply when NPN is introduced into the diet and it is quite obvious that different N sources are used with different efficiencies. Recent and rather thorough reviews on this topic include that of Swanson (1977) and a series of papers by Roy et al, W. Kaufman, Miller et al, Gordon, and Pfeffer which appeared in the 2nd International Symposium on Protein Metabolism and Nutrition, in 1977. In this section of this chapter it is not the intent to review the published literature on the topic. Rather, the discussion will be directed toward some of the methods used to evaluate N requirements and some of the uncertainties on the topic.

Maintenance Requirements

N or protein is required, of course, at lower levels for maintenance than during active growth or when animals are performing some other function such as milk production. Many different experiments have been carried out to evaluate requirements. Most of the requirement tables have been developed from data obtained on N balance studies and with feeding trials. N balance studies are reasonably useful for maintenance studies; however, for evaluating requirements for growing or lactating animals, it is difficult to confine animals for long enough periods to obtain valid data without resulting in reduced production.

Most of the current feeding standards have been developed using the factorial method suggested by H.H. Mitchell in 1929. This method depends on some reasonably accurate method for arriving at values for minimal N excretion. Data are required for metabolic fecal N (MFN), endogenous urinary N (EUN), losses from skin and hair or wool, and some measure of efficiency of protein utilization by the animal.

EUN can be estimated by feeding diets with no N (not practicable for ruminating animals) or by feeding graded N levels and regressing urinary N excretion to a zero level. After evaluating many different experiments on cattle, Swanson (1977) calculated that EUN = .44 $W^{.5}$ where W (body weight) is in kg. The protein equivalent is 2.75 $W^{.5}$. Additional N losses occur via skin, hair, wool, etc. Swanson (1977) found that these losses are estimated with reasonable precision by the value .22$W^{.6}$.

MFN is more variable and affected to a great degree by level of feed intake and the nature of the feed as well as N digestibility. In healthy preruminant calves essentially 100% of milk protein is digested and all fecal N will be MFN which is excreted at a rate of 2 g/kg of dry matter intake (DMI) or, for protein, at a rate of 1.25% of DMI. With ruminating animals, Swanson (1977) points out that some types of feed which resulted in low MFN included certain low-N grasses and straw, especially tropical grasses and wheat straw below 51% digestible dry matter. Some feeds, such as corn husks, stalks, stover and silage produced more fecal N than grass hay of similar protein content. Thus, these variables complicate evaluation of MFN excretion. Based on analyses of many different trials, Swanson calculated that MFN losses are more closely related to fecal output than to DMI; in other words, the amount of indigestible material passing through the gut has a big effect on MFN excretion. Swanson concluded that MFN (in grams) could be estimated by multiplying fecal dry matter by 10.9 or, in terms of protein this is equal to 6.8% of fecal dry matter. This value is for a digestible DMI ranging from 55 to 70%. It would need to be modified somewhat for very low digestible DMI that might be more representative of beef cow or ewe diets.

Example calculations. For the preruminant calf, milk protein may be completely digested but there is some wastage in metabolism, so that maximal efficiency is near 80% (Roy et al, 1970), but a more practical efficiency range is 70-75%. Swanson (1977) uses the lower value (70%) and other factors previously mentioned to calculate crude protein requirements of milk-fed calves:

CP, g/day = [(2.75$W^{.5}$) + (.2$W^{.6}$) + (0.125 g DMI)]/.7; in this case the first value is for EUN, the second for skin and hair loss, and the third for MFN. For an animal weighing 75 kg and fed 750 g milk DM/day (6 kg milk), the formula is:

CP, g/day = [(2.75 x 8.66) + (.2 x 13.34) +

(.0125 x 750)]/.7 = 36 g.

For ruminating animals, the average absorption efficiency has been estimated at 75% (Satter and Roffler, 1975) and average metabolism efficiency at 60% (Swanson, 1977). The daily requirement can be calculated as:

CP, g/day = [(2.75 $W^{.5}$) + (.2$W^{.6}$) + (.068 g FDM)]/.45. For maintenance of a cow weighing 600 kg and fed 7500 g DM which is 55% digestible, the formula is:

CP, g/day = [(2.75 x 24.5) + (.2 x 46.44) +

(.068 x .45 x 7500)]/.45 = 680 g.

Swanson (1977) points out that young animals have somewhat different efficiencies than older animals, at least partly due to feeding of feeds with higher digestibility. Estimates of combined efficiency factors for calves are .56 for small calves fed mainly concentrates, .50 for medium sized calves (100-150 kg) fed more concentrate than roughages, and .47 for large calves (150-200 kg) fed roughages and concentrates in about equal proportions.

If it is desired to express the requirement in terms of apparently digestible protein, crude protein from these equations must be reduced by the amount of MFN plus crude protein of feed origin which is indigestible.

In practice, ruminants are usually not fed at the absolute minimum levels of protein suggested by factorial computed data. One reason for this is that very low levels of protein result in depressed rumen microbial function and a reduced consumption of poor quality roughage or other feed which may be low in protein. In addition, animals are usually producing some product, although the level of production and the requirement may be low. An example of a ruminant fed at a level approaching maintenance would be a beef cow during the early stages of gestation and not nursing a calf. The maintenance requirement for a 500 kg cow (middle third of pregnancy) is 0.2 kg of digestible protein according to NRC (1976). The values for other weights were calculated at the same rate/unit of $W^{0.75}$.

Growth

The protein requirement for growth includes the requirement for maintenance in addition to that needed for growth. Generally the daily protein requirement increases with age (and size) of the animal up to maturity but the requirement, expressed as % of the ration, decreases with age, since the need to replace endogenous losses forms a greater proportion of the total as age increases and the requirement for growth decreases. Protein requirements may be established by the use of N balance, factorialization and feeding trials. Theoretically, the protein level which will give maximum N retention in a growing animal would be the protein requirement for growth for that animal. However, feed intake is usually not at a maximum in animals confined to metabolism stalls. Thus, nutrient levels may be too low for maximum growth and a low energy intake may lead to false conclusions.

The factorial method has been used in most modern feeding standards to estimate protein needs during growth (illustrated in Maintenance section). The difficulty with this method is that of obtaining accurate values for endogenous N excretions of actively growing animals, plus the fact that efficiency of N utilization varies considerably from feed to feed.

The use fo feeding trials alone has limitations for determining the protein requirement for growth since the composition of the gain is not known. The use of slaughter data to supplement feeding trial data would provide additional valuable data concerning the nature of the increase in weight.

Preston (1966) reported that protein requirements of growing-fattening cattle and lambs are a function of body weight, body weight gain, and digestibility of the protein in the ration. He expressed the digestible protein requirements by the following equations:

$$\text{Cattle, DP} = 2.79\, W^{0.75}\, (1 + 1.905\, G)$$

$$\text{Lambs, DP} = 2.79\, W^{0.75}\, (1 + 6.02\, G)$$

where DP refers to kg of digestible protein, W, is body weight in kg and G is daily gain in kg.

Chiou and Jordan (1973) concluded that the protein requirement of young lambs 2 days to 4 weeks of age and consuming a 20 to 25% fat milk replacer was 24 to 26% protein (dry matter basis). The protein requirement is related to energy level of the ration. The relationship between protein and energy requirement of growing lambs was defined as follows (Black et al, 1973): $Y = 13.4 - 0.242X$, where Y refers to g of protein of ideal amino acid pattern/MJ NE and X refers to liveweight in kg. The N requirement of lambs from 3 to 38 kg was found to be constant at 0.9 g/MJ NE (Black and Griffiths, 1975). The digestible protein requirement for calves from 11 to 60 days of age was increased by increasing the level of feeding of the ration (Donnelly and Hutton, 1976). The protein requirement of growing-finishing cattle is also related to the available energy content of the ration (Peterson et al, 1973). Jahn and Chandler (1976) determined that the protein requirements of calves gaining .6 kg/day from 8 to 20 wk of age were 271, 318 and 407 g for rations with 11, 18 and 25% acid detergent fiber.

Since post-ruminal administration of certain proteins or amino acids has resulted in increased N retention, one cannot discount the possibility that levels of certain amino acids may limit growth. Based on studies using the Plasma Amino Acid Score with microbial protein, Purser (1970) suggested that histidine, cystine, leucine, arginine and lysine were potentially limiting in microbial proteins. Preruminant lambs showed similar sensitivity to dietary amino acid balance as non-ruminant animals (Rogers and Egan, 1974). On the basis of data from steers fed high-silage rations, Chandler (1970) calculated an amino acid balance for production of body protein. Although none of the amino acids were calculated to be in negative balance, he suggested the following rank in order of importance in the limitation of growth: isoleucine, lysine, methionine, arginine, threonine, valine, histidine, phenylalanine, tryptophan, and leucine.

Different kinds of procedures were used during the last few years to study amino acid requirement for growth. From studies using the amino acid oxidation technique with abomasal infusion of amino acids, Brookes et al (1973) estimated the abomasal lysine requirement of a wether lamb to be 6.5 to 6.8 g/day. The lysine requirement of calves was estimated at 18.8 g/day, using a technique involving the rise in plasma amino acid from abomasal infusion (Williams and Smith, 1974). Methionine requirement was estimated to be 4.4 to 9.8 g/day. The total absorbable sulfur amino acid requirement for 274 kg steers was estimated at 18.6 g, using a similar procedure (Fenderson and Bergen, 1975). Lysine, threonine and tryptophan requirements were estimated at 22.5, 15.1 and 3.5 g/day, respectively. Using a procedure involving the rise in plasma amino acids from intraperitoneal administration of amino acids, Hall et al (1974) suggested that lysine, methionine and histidine were the first limiting essential amino acids.

Gestation

The protein (N) required for gestation should include replacement for endogenous losses (maintenance), for the protein in the embryo and embryogenic tissue and losses in metabolism. The amount of protein in the embryo is low until the last half of pregnancy. The higher requirement during the latter stages of pregnancy is reflected in the NRC suggested requirements. Evidence was obtained that tryptophan was the most limiting amino acid in the pregnant ewe (Offer et al, 1975).

Lactation

Since milk is high in protein content (dry basis), milk production results in a substantial increase in protein requirement. For dairy cows the NRC (1978) requirements were derived by the factorial method. Jacobson et al (1970) reported that dietary protein levels ranging from about 10 to 20% resulted in small differences in milk production as dietary crude protein level increased. They also reported that, if milk production was increased, feed consumption (net energy) was also generally increased. They suggested that the prime reason for feeding high levels of protein to dairy cows was to encourage greater voluntary consumption of energy, thereby increasing performance and efficiency of feed to milk. They raised the question whether amino acids limit milk production in lactating cows. The protein requirement of lactating cows appears to be at least 13.5% dry basis (Thomas, 1971; Van Horn et al, 1976). Gardner and Park (1973) obtained evidence that the requirement is higher than this for maximum milk yield. On the basis of calculations of amino acid balance and assuming that milk protein production was the only demand for essential amino acids, Chandler (1970) ranked the amino acids in order of limiting milk production as follows: methionine, valine, iso-leucine, tryptophan and lysine. Due to the higher rates of milk production, protein requirement for milk production in dairy cows is much higher than for beef cows of comparable size.

AMINO ACID SUPPLEMENTATION

It was shown several years ago that the usual essential amino acids, except for arginine, were metabolically essential for the ruminant animal (Black et al, 1957; Downes, 1961). It has been suggested that the sub-optimal performance sometimes observed when NPN is fed was due to deficiencies of certain amino acids (McCarthy et al, 1970). Thus, several workers have tested the value of feeding supplementary amino acids.

Some of the older data suggest that methionine supplementation improved performance in lambs fed urea but not in those fed supplemental soybean meal. Feeding methionine hydroxy analog (MHA) to lambs did not affect rate of gain but increased feed efficiency (Wilson et al, 1972). Wool growth and N retention were increased from feeding 3.8 g of dl-methionine (Doyle and Bird, 1975). Although some data suggest that lysine supplementation may improve performance of cattle or sheep, other reports show no effect. Reports showing positive results include those of Gossett et al (1962) with lysine and methionine and that of McLaren et al (1965) with methionine or tryptophan. On the other hand, Oltjen et al (1962) reported no beneficial effects on gain or feed efficiency in sheep from adding 0.2 or 0.4 dl-methionine or 0.2% of dl-alanine to purified diets in which urea was used as the N source. Including 3% glutamic acid in semipurified rations in which urea supplied 97% of the N did not significantly alter N retention in calves (Oltjen et al, 1964). Likewise, Harbers et al (1961) found no benefit from supplementing low urea rations with lysine.

Feeding MHA to lactating dairy cows had not consistently affected milk production (Polan et al, 1970; Hutjens and Schultz, 1971; Holter et al, 1972; Wallenius and Whitechurch, 1975; Chandler et al, 1976), but the analog may be of some benefit for increasing milk fat percentage (Bhargava et al, 1977). Papas et al (1974) reported results indicating that less than one third of MHA was converted to methionine in lambs.

Bunn et al (1968) studied the effect of supplementing a select group of amino acids based on the composition of alfalfa on growth and N retention of lambs fed a purified diet containing urea as the N source. The amino acid supplementation resulted in an improvement in growth rate but had no effect on N retention. Clifford et al (1968) found that addition of leucine, isoleucine, valine and phenylalanine to a purified diet containing urea as the N source had no significant effect on feed intake and rate of gain of lambs.

Oltjen (1969) concluded that, generally, amino acid additions had not improved animal performance. He suggested the following reasons for the poor response: in most of the studies dl mixtures of the amino acids were used instead of the active l form; the amino acid may have been supplied in insufficient amount; the unprotected amino acids may have been too available in the rumen resulting in rapid catabolism instead of being incorporated into a microbial protein, and the amino acids were not limiting for growth. Hogan (1975) has pointed out the high producing dairy cow, early in lactation, is the most likely animal to be deficient in an amino acid, in particular, methionine. Sheep on high fiber forage may also be deficient in cystine.

Administration of 0.5 to 2.0 g of l-cysteine or equimolar levels of dl-methionine increased wool growth (Reis, 1967). Methionine hydroxy analog (MHA) was as effective as dl-methionine. High levels of l-cysteine (6-8 g/day) resulted in a decrease in wool growth. Abomasal infusion of methionine increased wool growth up to 37% (Robards, 1971). Feeding encapsulated methionine increased gains and feed efficiency in ewes fed a urea containing diet, but not when fed soybean meal (Mowat and Deelstra, 1972). Abomasal infusion of methionine in steers fed a high roughage ration tended to improve N retention (Steinacker et al, 1970). Increased N retention resulted from abomasal infusion of methionine to sheep fed a good quality diet (Schelling et al, 1973). Feeding this type of product did not affect milk production or N utilization by dairy cows (Williams et al, 1970) nor did abomasal infusion of methionine affect milk production of cows (Schwab et al, 1976). However, lysine infusion gave a marked response. N retention was increased in steers by abomasal infusion (Burris et al, 1976).

Oltjen et al (1970) studied the effects of abomasal infusion of valine, isoleucine, leucine and phenylalanine in urea-fed steers and of serine and glycine in soy protein-fed steers given purified diets. Amino acid infusions in the urea-fed steers decreased urinary N excretion and increased N retention. Retention was similar to that of the soy-fed animals. Infusion of serine and glycine in soy-fed steers resulted in an increase in urinary N excretion and a decrease in N retention.

PROTEIN DEFICIENCY

In feral ruminant species the diet has surplus protein at times, particularly during lush growth in the spring (or rainy season), it is adequate for some part of the year, and borderline to deficient during winter months or dry seasons. Probably less fluctuation occurs with domestic stock, but it is a well documented fact that protein may be deficient in many situations, although the deficiency may often be complicated with deficiencies of other nutrients such as some of the mineral elements and available energy. Many, many research papers are in the literature which show that inadequate protein results in lowered growth rates, reduced feed efficiency and impaired reproduction. Specific examples of deficiency will be given for some of these items.

One of the first effects of protein deficiency is a reduced feed consumption by ruminant animals. A recent example of research on this is shown in Fig. 3-5 (Santos, 1978). In this example yearling cattle were given ad libitum access to wheat straw and were fed supplementary protein in graded levels ranging from 0 to 4 g/kg $W^{.75}$. Note that there was a substantial increase in straw consumption with the lower levels of supplementary protein. This appears to be a result of an increased microbial activity in the rumen which allows more complete and more rapid fermentation.

Studies with sheep show that low protein diets will result in reduced wool production (Reis, 1969; Egan, 1970; Langlands, 1971). An interaction between protein and energy levels has also been shown by Walker and Norton (1971) and Black et al (1973).

With regard to milk production, Robinson et al (1974) demonstrated that milk production by ewes was 2.4, 2.9 and 3.1 kg for isocaloric diets containing 10.3, 13.6 and

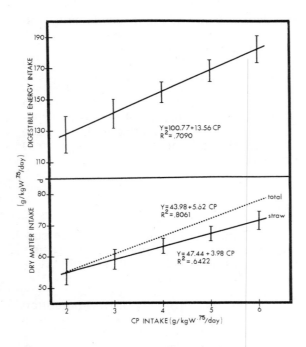

Fig. 3-5. Effect of inadequate protein on dry matter and digestible energy consumption of cattle. Note that as protein consumption increased there was a marked increase in energy consumption as well as dry matter. From Santos (1978).

16.9% crude protein, respectively. In cattle, numerous reports show that reduced protein intake will result in less milk yield and solids (Gordon and Forbes, 1970; Thomas, 1971; Gardner and Park, 1973; Paquay et al, 1973), although another paper suggests that as little as 75% of the estimated requirements did not affect milk yield or quality (Treacher et al, 1976). With regard to reproduction, a number of recent reports show some effect of protein deficiency. In a study with beef heifers, Bedrack et al (1964) found that a protein deficiency resulted in either just maintenance of weight or loss of weight. There were no normal embryos produced (10 animals) and eight of the heifers did not ovulate. With 2-yr-old heifers there were normal embryos in 4 of 7 animals. Some animals ovulated without showing estrus and could not be bred. In other studies Bond and Wiltbank (1970) found that protein level did not affect birth weights of calves but the cows gave less milk. Bull et al (1978) have demonstrated that maternal protein restriction prepartum (beef cows) reduced the ability of the calf to absorb colostral immunoglobulins. Protein restriction during the last 150 days of

gestation did not cause severe loss of body weight of the cow, but calves from restricted cows were more subject to cold stress. In heifers given restricted protein levels, there was a significant correlation between the intake of protein and blood values for hematocrit, hemoblgobin, red blood cell count and prothrombin time and serum values for uric acid, cholesterol and blood urea N.

In an Australian study cows were supplemented with nothing, P or P and protein. Cows that exhibited estrus within 60 days of calving declined from 100% on the P+ protein to 70% on P and 50% on the control diet (Little, 1975). However, in another Australian experiment P did not affect estrus but adequate protein increased estrus activity over no supplemental treatment (Teleni et al, 1977). In studies with ewes, Lamond et al (1973) did not observe any marked effect of low protein diets on fertility, however Christenson and Prior (1976) found that an intake of 149 g of crude protein per day (vs. 213 g) resulted in lower birth weights and lamb survival in lambs from yearling ewes.

In a very severe protein deficiency animals will be anemic. Low hemoglobin and hematocrit values occur and marked declines occur in liver and blood serum protein levels, partly due to a decline in albumin concentration (Bedrak et al, 1964). In sheep fed straw with only 0.5% digestible protein, Masters and Horgan (1962) observed increases in SGOT which was related to centrilobular necrosis observed in the livers. However, total proteins were not affected much and blood urea was constant for five weeks and then declined. Payne and Laws (1978) observed reduced liver DNA and lower activity for a number of enzymes which metabolize amino acids. Comparable changes were not observed in muscle tissue.

There is little question that protein intake influences blood urea levels. Manston et al (1975) observed that more dietary protein increased hemoglobin levels of dairy cows. In another study by Treacher et al (1976), cows on a low protein diet (75% of ARC recommendations) did not show any marked differences from control cows. After 9 weeks of lactation, urea, packed cell volume, hemoglobin and red blood cells begin to rise in the control group but they did not begin to rise in the low protein group until 14 weeks post calving when the cows were transferred to a high-protein concentrate.

Bone disorders have also been related to inadequate protein intake by ruminants. For example, Siebert et al (1975) fed cattle adequate P but low protein. Two steers on this diet developed a disorder which clinicically resembled osteomalacia after 21 weeks of feeding and other animals on the same diet showed varying degrees of lameness. With sheep, Sykes and Field (1972) have demonstrated that low protein resulted in reduced uptake of Ca by the skeleton. A low protein diet (6%) resulted in a skeletal loss of 30 g of Ca while an adequate diet (11.8%) allowed an increase of 42 g in skeletal Ca.

Ruminants apparently have adaptive and compensatory mechanisms which operate during periods of low and high N intakes. When steers were changed from high (15% crude protein) to low (5% crude protein), N retention decreased from 0.95 g to -.17 g $N/kg^{.60}$/day (Biddle and Evans, 1973). The steers were in positive N balance during the third week of the depletion period. Repletion with a high N diet resulted in an immediate improvement in N retention, which reached a maximum value after 2 weeks. The fluctuations in N retention were affected mainly by changes in urinary N. However, the urinary N patterns indicated that conservation mecha-

nisms were operating (Table 3-13). For example the urinary N excretion decreased from 0.46 to 0.33 $g/kg^{.60}$ day between weeks 1 and 3 of depletion. Likewise the urinary excretion was much lower during the first 2 weeks of repletion than during the standardization period prior to depletion. The changes in N retention were mediated mainly through changes in urea N excretion. Similar results were reported by Biddle et al (1975). The changes in urea excretion may mean more of the urea is circulated in the plasma and transferred to the rumen. A negative correlation has been reported between the net increase in ruminal ammonia after injection of urea and the preingestion levels of ruminal ammonia and blood urea in sheep on a diet supplying 11.4 g N/day (Harrop and Phillipson, 1974). No such correlation was recorded in sheep fed a higher dietary N level (20.7 g/day).

Plasma protein and albumin decreased in growing cattle after 5 weeks of depletion and approached predepletion levels only after 6 weeks of depletion (Biddle et al, 1975). Plasma urea N declined from a value of 16 mg/100 ml to 0.8 mg/100 ml during depletion and reached a peak of 18 mg/100 ml after 3 weeks of repletion. These workers

Table 3-13. Effect of level of nitrogen intake on performance of growing steers.[a,b]

Period Protein level	Standard- ization high	Depletion low			Repletion high		
Time, week	4	5	7	8[c]	9	10	12
Body wt, kg$^{.60}$	33.7	33.7	33.8	33.9	33.7	33.8	34.0
Dry matter intake, g/kg$^{.60}$/day	138	132	131	142	150	154	152
Digestibility, %							
Dry matter	70	62	58	59	68	69	77
Nitrogen	73	28	38	72	75	74	80
Retained nitrogen, g/kg$^{.60}$/day							
Ingested	3.25	1.04	1.03	2.57	3.43	3.42	3.39
Fecal	0.84	0.75	0.63	0.72	0.87	0.90	0.69
Urine	1.46	0.46	0.31	0.93	0.99	0.82	1.32
Urea	0.85	0.09	0.03	0.51	0.51	0.26	0.68
Ammonia	0.23	0.11	0.06	0.21	0.19	0.17	0.29
Residual	0.38	0.26	0.22	0.21	0.29	0.39	0.35
Retained	0.95	-.17	0.09	0.92	1.57	1.70	1.38
Retained, % of intake	29	-16	9	36	46	50	41

[a]Biddle and Evans (1973).

[b]Each value is the average of four observations.

[c]On days two and three of this collection repletion diets were fed.

calculated the labile N reserves at 6% of empty body weight N. Paquay et al (1972) concluded that the mature cow is able to store and lose large amounts of protein when N and energy intakes are varied.

EXCESS PROTEIN

For ruminants in their native state, excess protein is not likely to be available except for brief periods of lush plant growth. With domestic stock, there is some possibility that it may be a problem. Urea toxicity is, of course, a well documented fact (see Vol. 1).

In an experiment in which sheep were fed up to 220% of their maintenance requirement, results suggest that various N-containing components were higher in the rumen as was blood urea when the dietary protein content increased (Dror and Bondi, 1969). Fenderson and Bergen (1976) fed diets to steers with 10-40% crude protein. Dry matter intake for the two high levels (32 and 40%) was depressed primarily during days 2 and 3 but they recovered to initial levels between days 5 and 10. Plasma amino acid levels were not markedly influenced, but ruminal ammonia levels and plasma urea levels were increased markedly. Although some steers had ruminal ammonia levels in excess of 100 mg/100 ml, they did not exhibit any signs of ammonia toxicity and the authors concluded that ammonia arising from degradation of preformed protein can be tolerated by ruminants when their amino acid requirements are met. When lactating cows were fed rations with 25% crude protein for 112 days, Hawkins et al (1977) found differences in blood cholesterol and high levels of lymphocytes but blood urea N, hemoglobin, packed cell volume and total white blood cells were not affected. The source and solubility of the proteins had a marked effect on ruminal ammonia.

In a study with goats fed a 45% protein diet, Zucker and Steger (1975) found that feed intake decreased and water intake increased with rising protein intake, but weight remained unaffected. Serum urea increased about 3 fold. They did not observe any histopathological changes in tissues after four weeks of feeding. When cows were given about 1 kg of digestible protein in excess of requirements for several years, Schilling (1965) found some changes in adrenal glands of the cows, but otherwise no pathological or degenerative changes.

In experiments with dairy cows, congestion of the conjunctiva occurred after 2-3 mo. in cows fed excess protein (Yonemura, 1970). Appetite was lost within 1-2 weeks but recovered when fiber was added to the diet. Low protein and low energy resulted in reduced body weight and milk yield and high protein with low energy produced the same results. Ovarian cysts and ovarian dysfunction were frequent in both high and low protein groups. In males semen quality was reduced on low protein and energy and on high protein intake. Sonderegger and Schurch (1977) also observed that excess digestible protein, particularly if it exceeded 250-300 g/cow/day, resulted in lengthened intervals between parturition and first service. Hewett (1971) and Treacher et al (1976) also concluded that high protein levels may interfere with ovarian function in lactating cows, but the mechanism causing the infertility remains obscure.

METABOLIZABLE PROTEIN

Metabolizable protein, a concept introduced by Burroughs et al (1971), is defined as the quantity of protein digested or amino acid(s) absorbed in the post-ruminal portion of the GI tract of ruminants. According to this concept, in non-ruminants it has the same meaning as apparent digestible protein or absorbable amino acids. However, in ruminants the metabolizable protein would include the portion of dietary protein which escaped ruminal degradation and the rumen microbial protein.

The following equation was used to calculate the protein required for maintenance: $P = (0.0125) (70.4W^{.734})$, where P refers to g of maintenance protein and W refers to body weight in kg. They assumed that 40% of absorbed protein was lost in metabolism.

Metabolizable protein values for some feedstuffs were calculated. These values consisted of a summation of undegraded protein reaching the abomasum and the degraded protein converted to microbial protein which reached the abomasum. They estimated 100% conversion of degraded protein into microbial protein, with maximum values of 51.2 g protein/kg of concentrate and 25.6 g/kg of roughage dry matter. Later, Burroughs et al (1975) revised some of the values and calculated the requirement and content of metabolizable protein in feedstuffs. Suggested requirement values are given in Table 3-14 and metabolizable

Table 3-14. Metabolizable protein requirements for lactating cows.[a]

Body wt, kg	Milk fat, %	Dig. feed, kg	Net protein, g	Metaboliz-able protein,[b] g
Maintenance of mature lactating cows				
350		5.0	66	140
450		6.0	78	166
550		7.0	92	196
Maintenance and pregnancy (last 2 mo. gestation)				
350		6.4	116	247
450		7.9	140	298
550		9.3	166	353
Milk production (nutrients required per kg milk)				
		2.5	28	30
		3.0	30	32
		3.5	32	34
		4.0	34	36

[a]Adapted from Burroughs (1975).

[b]Net protein X 2.13, which assumes 53% loss in metabolism for maintenance. For milk production, net protein X 1.05, which assumes 5% loss in metabolism.

protein content of some feedstuffs is shown in Table 3-15.

Burroughs et al (1975) have proposed a urea fermentation potential (UFP), an expression of the amount of urea that can be useful in a given cattle ration. The formula used to assess the UFP of feedstuffs, expressed as g of urea/kg of dry matter consumed was: $UFP = 1.044 (TDN - B)/2.8$. B refers to estimated g of protein in 1 kg of feed consumed and degraded in the rumen, contributing ammonia to the total rumen pool. The 1.044 refers to the estimated potential net g of rumen microbial amino acid protein that results from 10 g of TDN. The 2.8 converts protein to urea N equivalent. The UFP makes use of two well accepted principles in urea utilization, i.e., for good urea utilization the dietary protein level is suboptimal and a supply of readily available carbohydrates is essential, but the values used in the calculations are based on limited data. The development of more experimental data will enable the refinement of the factors used in the calculations of metabolizable protein and UFP.

Satter and Slyter (1974) found that microbial protein yield in vitro increased linearly with supplementary urea until

ammonia started to accumulate in the medium. When ammonia concentration increased above 50 mg/l., higher levels did not

Table 3-15. Metabolizable protein content of some feeds for body purposes.[a]

Feedstuff	Metabolizable protein, g/kg dry matter
Alfalfa hay, 17.3% protein	41.2
Barley grain, 13.0% protein	89.4
Corn, aerial part, ensiled	52.4
Corn cobs, ground	8.1
Corn, ears, ground	62.6
Corn, grain	68.8
Cottonseed hulls, ground	13.1
Cottonseed meal, solvent extracted	150.4
Linseed meal, solvent extracted	135.3
Molasses, sugarcane	19.9
Sorghum grain, milo	90.2
Soybean meal, solvent extracted	168.5
Urea	2225.0

[a]Adapted from Burroughs (1975).

affect microbial protein production. They suggested that NPN supplements would be useful only if the ruminal ammonia concentration is <50 mg NH_3-N/l. of ruminal fluid. Additions of NPN to ruminant rations resulting in predicted ruminal ammonia concentrations greater than 5 mg $NH_3N/100$ ml rumen fluid were of no benefit (Roffler and Satter, 1975). NPN supplementation did not improve milk production if the ration contained $>12.5\%$ crude protein or if the predicted ruminal ammonia concentration was greater than 4 mg NH_3-N/100 ml rumen fluid. The crude protein level at which ruminal ammonia N reached 5 mg/100 ml varied with TDN concentration (Roffler et al, 1976).

References Cited

Amos, H.E., D.G. Ely, C.O. Little and G.E. Mitchell. 1970. J. Animal Sci. 31:767.

Amos, H.E., J. Evans and D. Burdick. 1976a. J. Animal Sci. 42:970.

Amos, H.E., J. Evans, D. Burdick and T. Park. 1976b. J. Animal Sci. 43:1300.

Amos, H.E., C.O. Little, D.G. Ely and G.E. Mitchell, Jr. 1971. Can. J. Animal Sci. 51:51.

Armstrong, D.G. and K. Hutton. 1975. In: Digestion and Metabolism in the Ruminant. Univ. of New England Pub. Unit, Armidale, N.S.W., Australia.

Barry, T.N. 1973. N. Zeal. J. Agr. Res. 16:185.

Barry, T.N. 1976. J. Agr. Sci. 86:379.

Barry, T.N. and P.F. Fennessy. 1973. N. Zeal. J. Agr. Res. 16:59.

Barry, T.N. and P.D. Johnstone. 1976. J. Agr. Sci. 86:163.

Barth, K.M., G.A. McLaren and G.C. Anderson. 1961. J. Animal Sci. 18:1521 (abstr).

Bartley, E.E. et al. 1976. J. Animal Sci. 43:835.

Bedrack, E., A.C. Warnick, J.F. Hentges and T.J. Cunha. 1964. Florida Agr. Expt. Sta. Tech. Bul. 678.

Ben-Ghadalia, D., H. Tagari and A. Bondi. 1976. Brit. J. Nutr. 36:211.

Berry, W.T., J.K. Riggs and H.O. Kunkel. 1956. J. Animal Sci. 15:225.

Bhargava, P.K., D.E. Otterby, J.M. Murphy and J.D. Donker. 1977. J. Dairy Sci. 60:1594.

Bhattacharya, A.N. and A.R. Khan. 1973. J. Animal Sci. 37:136.

Bhattacharya, A.N. and E. Pervez. 1973. J. Animal Sci. 36:976.

Biddle, G.N. and J.L. Evans. 1973. J. Animal Sci. 36:123.

Biddle, G.N., J.L. Evans and J.R. Trout. 1975. J. Nutr. 105:1578,1584.

Black, A.L., M. Kleiber, A.H. Smith and D.N. Stewart. 1957. Biochem. Biophys. Acta. 23:54.

Black, J.L. 1971. Brit. J. Nutr. 25:31.

Black, J.L. and D.A. Griffiths. 1975. Brit. J. Nutr. 33:399.

Black, J.L., G.R. Pearce and D.E. Tribe. 1973. Brit. J. Nutr. 30:45.

Black, J.L., G.E. Robards and R. Thomas. 1973. Aust. J. Agr. Res. 24:399.

Blackburn, T.H. 1965. In: Physiology of Digestion in the Ruminant. Butterworth, Washington, D.C.

Blaxter, K.L., 1962. Energy Metabolism of Ruminants. Hutchinson Pub. Co.

Blaxter, K.L. 1977. In: Proc. Second Int. Symposium on Protein Metabolism and Nutrition Centre for Agr. Publ. and Documentation, Wageningen, The Netherlands.

Boila, R.J. and T.J. Devlin. 1975. Can. J. Animal Sci. 55:297.

Boling, J.A., N.W. Bradley, R.E. Tucker and D.D. Kratzer. 1971. J. Animal Sci. 33:895.

Boling, J.A., P.J. Katanyukul and C.T. Nuzum. 1976. Int. J. Vit. Nutr. Res. 46:395.

Bond, J. and R.R. Oltjen. 1973. J. Animal Sci. 37:141,1040.

Bond, J. and T.S. Rumsey. 1973. J. Animal Sci. 37:593.

Bond, J. and J.N. Wiltbank. 1970. J. Animal Sci. 30:438.

Bradley, N.W., B.M. Jones, G.E. Mitchell and C.O. Little. 1966. J. Animal Sci. 25:480.

Brent, B.E., A. Adepoju and F. Portela. 1971. J. Animal Sci. 32:794.

Broderick, G.A., T. Kowalczyk and L.D. Satter. 1970. J. Dairy Sci. 53:1714.

Brookes, I.M., F.N. Owens, R.E. Brown and U.S. Garrigus. 1973. J. Animal Sci. 36:965.

Broster, W.H., V.J. Tuck, T. Smith and V.W. Johnson. 1969. J. Agr. Sci. 72:13.

Bull, R.C. et al. 1978. Proc. West Sect. Amer. Soc. Animal Sci. 29:339,343.

Bunn, C.R., J.J. McNeill and G. Matrone. 1968. J. Nutr. 94:47.

Burris, W.R., J.A. Boling, N.W. Bradley and A.W. Young. 1976. J. Animal Sci. 42:699.

Burris, W.R., N.W. Bradley and J.A. Boling. 1974. J. Animal Sci. 38:200.

Burris, W.R., N.W. Bradley and J.A. Boling. 1975. J. Animal Sci. 40:714.

Burroughs, W., D.K. Nelson and D.R. Mertens. 1975. J. Dairy Sci. 58:611.

Burroughs, W., A.H. Trenkle and R.L. Vetter. 1971. Vet. Med. Small Anim. Clin. 66:238,598.

Caffrey, P.J., E.E. Hatfield, H.W. Norton and U.S. Garrigus. 1967. J. Animal Sci. 26:595.

Carnevali, A.A., T.A. Shultz, E. Shultz and C.F. Chicco. 1973. Agronomia Tropical 21:565.

Chalmers, M.I., D.P. Cuthbertson and R.L.M. Synge. 1954. J. Agr. Sci. 44:254.

Chalupa, W. 1968. J. Animal Sci. 27:207.

Chalupa, W., J. Clark, P. Opliger and R. Lavker. 1970. J. NUtr. 100:170.

Champredon, C. and R. Pion. 1972. Ann. Biol. Anim. Bioch. Biophys. 12:307.

Chandler, P.T. 1970. Proc. Va. Feed Conven. Nutr. Conf., p. 22.

Chandler, P.T. et al. 1976. J. Dairy Sci. 59:1897.

Chicco, C.F. et al. 1972. J. Animal Sci. 35:859.

Chiou, P.W. and R.M. Jordan. 1973. J. Animal Sci. 37:581.

Christenson, R.K. and R.L. Prior. 1976. J. Animal Sci. 43:1104.

Church, D.C. 1972. Feedstuffs 44(46):40.

Clark, J.H. 1975. J. Dairy Sci. 58:1178.

Clark, J.H., S.L. Spahr and R.G. Derrig. 1973. J. Dairy Sci. 56:763.

Clark, J.L. et al. 1970. J. Animal Sci. 30:297;31:961.

Clemens, E.T. and R.R. Johnson. 1973. J. Animal Sci. 37:1027; J. Nutr. 103:1406.

Clemens, E.T. and R.R. Johnson. 1974. J. Animal Sci. 39:937.

Clifford, A.J. and A.D. Tillman. 1968. J. Animal Sci. 27:484.

Colebrook, W.F. and P.J. Reis. 1969. Aust. J. Biol. Sci. 22:1507.

Colovos, N.F. et al. 1963. J. Dairy Sci. 46:696.

Condon, R.J., G. Hall and E.E. Hatfield. 1970. J. Animal Sci. 31:1037 (abstr).

Condon, R.J. and E.E. Hatfield, 1971. Proc. Fed. Amer. Soc. Expt. Biol. 40:403 (abstr.).

Crawford, R.L., W.H. Hoover, C.J. Sniffen and B.A. Crooker. 1978. J. Animal Sci. 46:1768.

Cross, D.L., R.L. Ludwick, J.A. Boling and N.W. Bradley. 1974. J. Animal Sci. 38:404.

Daniels, L.B., M.E. Muhrer, J.R. Campbell and F.A. Martz. 1971. J. Animal Sci. 32:348.

Delort-Laval, J. and S.Z. Zelter. 1968. Proc. Second World Conf. Animal Prod., p.457.

Derrig, R.G., J.H. Clark and C.L. Davis. 1974. J. Nutr. 104:151.

Donnelly, P.E. and J.B. Hutton. 1976. N. Zeal. J. Agr. Res. 19:289.

Downes, A.M. 1961. J. Biol. Sci. 14:254.

Downes, A.M., P.J. Reis, L.F. Sharry and D.A. Tunks. 1970. Aust. J. Biol. Sci. 23:1077.

Doyle, P.T. and P.R. Bird. 1975. Aust. J. Agr. Res. 26:337.

Dror, Y. and A. Bondi. 1969. J. Agr. Sci. 72:327.

Dror, Y., H. Tagari and A. Bondi. 1970. J. Agr. Sci. 75:381.

Egan, A.R. 1970. Aust. J. Agr. Res. 21:85.

Egan, A.R. and R.C. Kellaway. 1971. Brit. J. Nutr. 26:335.

Egan, A.R., F. Moller and A.L. Black. 1970. J. Nutr. 100:419.

Ellis, W.C. and K.C. Bleichner. 1969. J. Animal Sci. 29:157 (abstr).

Ellis, W.C., G.B. Garner, M.E. Muhrer and W.H. Pfander. 1956. J. Nutr. 60:413.

Ely, D.G., C.O. Little, P.G. Woolfold and G.E. Mitchell. 1967. J. Nutr. 91:314.

Erb, R.E. et al. 1976. J. Dairy Sci. 59:656.

Ernst, A.J., J.F. Limpus and P.K. O'Rourke. 1975. Aust. J. Exp. Agr. Anim. Husb. 15:451.

Eskeland, B., W.H. Pfander and R.L. Preston. 1973. Brit. J. Nutr. 29:347.

Faichney, G.J. 1971. Aust. J. Agr. Res. 22:453.

Faichney, G.J. and H.L. Davies. 1972. Aust. J. Agr. Res. 23:167.

Fenderson, C.L. and W.G. Bergen. 1975. J. Animal Sci. 41:1759.

Fenderson, C.L. and W.G. Bergen. 1976. J. Animal Sci. 42:1323.

Ferguson, K.A., J.A. Henesley and P.J. Reis. 1967. Aust. J. Sci. 30:215.

Fonnesbeck, P.V., L.C. Kearl and L.E. Harris. 1975. J. Animal Sci. 40:1150.

Fontenot, J.P., W.H. McClure and R.C. Carter. 1968. V.P.I. Res. Div. Res. Rpt. 126:22.

Ford, E.J.H. and P.E.B. Reilly. 1969. Res. Vet. Sci. 10:96,409.

Freitag, R.R., W.H. Smith and W.M. Beeson. 1968. J. Animal Sci. 27:478.

Gallup, W.D., L.S. Pope and C.K. Whitehair. 1953. Okla. Agr. Expt. Sta. Bul. B-409.

Gardner, R.W. and R.L. Park. 1973. J. Dairy Sci. 56:390.

Garverick, H.A., R.E. Erb, R.D. Randel and M.D. Cunningham. 1971. J. Dairy Sci. 54:1669.

Garrett, W.N. 1977. In: Proc. 2nd Int. Symposium on Protein Metabolism and Nutrition. Centre for Agr. Pub. and Documentation, Wageningen, The Netherlands.

Gilchrist, F.M., E. Potgieter and J.B.N. Ross. 1968. J. Agr. Sci. 70:157.

Goodrich, R.D. and A.D. Tillman. 1968. J. Animal Sci. 25:484.

Gordon, F.J. and T.J. Forbes. 1970. J. Dairy Res. 37:481.

Gordon, F.J. and T.J. Forbes. 1971. J. Dairy Res. 38:381.

Gossett, W.H. et al. 1962. J. Animal Sci. 21:248.

Grieve, D.G. et al. 1973. J. Dairy Sci. 56:218,224.

Guada, J.A., J.J. Robinson and C. Fraser. 1975. J. Agr. Sci. 85:175.

Hadjipanayiotou, M., A. Louca and M.J. Lawlor. 1975. Animal Prod. 20:429.

Hall, G.A.B., E.E. Hatfield and F.N. Owens. 1974. J. Animal Sci. 38:124.

Harbers, L.H., R.R. Oltjen and A.D. Tillman. 1961. J. Animal Sci. 20:880.

Harrop, C.J.F. and A.T. Phillipson. 1974. J. Agr. Sci. 82:399.

Hatfield, E.E. 1970. Fed. Proc. 29:44.

Hawkins, G.E., T.O. Lindsey and D.R. Strength. 1977. J. Dairy Sci. 60:66 (abstr).

Heitmann, R.N., W.H. Hoover and C.J. Sniffen. 1973. J. Nutr. 103:1587.

Helmer, L.G. et al. 1970. J. Dairy Sci. 53:330,883.

Hembry, F.G., W.H. Pfander, and R.L. Preston. 1975. J. Nutr. 105:267.

Hewett, C.D. 1971. Nord. Vet. Med. 23:65.

Hogan, J.P. 1975. J. Dairy Sci. 58:1164.

Holter, J.B., N.F. Colovos, H.A. Davis and W.E. Urban. 1968. J. Dairy Sci. 51:1243,1403.

Holter, J.B., C.W. Kim and N.F. Colovos. 1972. J. Dairy Sci. 55:460.

Horn, G.W. and W.M. Beeson. 1969. J. Animal Sci. 28:412.

Huber, J.T. 1975. J. Animal Sci. 41:954.

Huber, J.T., R.L. Boman and H.E. Henderson. 1976. J. Dairy Sci. 59:1936.

Hume, I.D., D.R. Jacobson and G.E. Mitchell, Jr. 1972. J. Nutr. 102:495.

Huston, J.E., M. Shelton and L.H. Brever. 1974. J. Animal Sci. 39:618.

Hutjens, M.F. and L.H. Schultz. 1971. J. Dairy Sci. 54:1637.

Ide, Y., K. Shimbayashi and T. Yonemura. 1966. Jap. J. Vet. Sci. 28:321.

Jacobson, D.R., H.H. Van Horn and C.J. Sniffen. 1970. Fed. Proc. 29:35.

Jahn, E. and P.T. Chandler. 1976. J. Animal Sci. 42:724.

Jahn, E., P.T. Chandler and R.F. Kelly. 1976. J. Animal Sci. 42:736.

Johns, J.T. and W.G. Bergen. 1973. J. Nutr. 103:1581.

Jones, G.A. and J.D. Milligan. 1975. Can. J. Animal Sci. 55:39.

Jones, G.M., C. Stephens and B. Kensett. 1975. J. Dairy Sci. 58:689.

Journet, M. and R. Verite. 1977. In: Proc. 2nd Int. Symposium on Protein Metabolism and Nutrition. Centre for Agr. Pub. and Documentation, Wageningen, The Netherlands.

Kaplan, V.A. and N.N. Pobirskii. 1975. Nutr. Abstr. Rev. 45:281.

Kay, M. and A. Macdearmid. 1972. Animal Prod. 14:367.

Kertz, A.F. and J.P. Everett, Jr. 1975. J. Animal Sci. 41:945.

Keyser, R.B., K.E. Webb, Jr. and J.P. Fontenot. 1978. J. Animal Sci. (in press).

Kirk, R.D. and D.M. Walker. 1976. Aust. J. Agr. Res. 27:109.

Kitchenham, B.A. et al. 1975. Brit. Vet. J. 131:436.

Knight, W.M. and F.N. Owens. 1973. J. Animal Sci. 36:145.

Knott, F.N., C.E. Polan and J.T. Huber. 1972. J. Dairy Sci. 55:466.

Kwan, K. et al. 1977. J. Dairy Sci. 60:1706.

Lamond, D.R. et al. 1973. J. Animal Sci. 36:363.

Langlands, J.P. 1971. Aust. J. Exp. Agr. Anim. Hus. 11:9.

Leibholz, J. 1969. J. Animal Sci. 29:628.

Leibholz, J. 1971. Aust. J. Agr. Res. 22:639,647.

Leibholz, J. 1976. Aust. J. Agr. Res. 27:287.

Lewis, D. 1961. In: Digestive Physiology and Nutrition of the Ruminant. Butterworths, London.

Lewis, D., K.J. Hill and E.F. Annison. 1957. Biochem. J. 66:587.

Little, C.O., W. Burroughs and W. Woods. 1963. J. Animal Sci. 22:358.

Little, C.O. and G.E. Mitchell. 1967. J. Animal Sci. 26:411.

Little, D.A. 1975. Aust. J. Expt. Agr. Animal Hus. 15:25.

Lofgreen, G.P., J.K. Loosli and L.A. Maynard. 1947. J. Animal Sci. 6:343.

Loosli, J.K. et al. 1949. Science 110:144.

Ludwick, R.L., J.P. Fontenot and R.E. Tucker. 1970. J. Animal Sci. 31:248 (abstr).

Ludwick, R.L., J.P. Fontenot and R.E. Tucker. 1971. J. Animal Sci. 33:1298.

Ludwick, R.L., J.P. Fontenot and R.E. Tucker. 1972. J. Animal Sci. 35:1036.

Macrae, J.C., M.J. Ulyatt, P.D. Pearce and J. Hendtlass. 1972. Brit. J. Nutr. 27:39.

Majdoub, A., G.T. Lane and T.E. Aitchison. 1978. J. Dairy Sci. 61:59.

Mangan, J.L. 1972. Brit. J. Nutr. 27:261.

Manston, R., A.M. Russell, S.M. Dew and J.M. Payne. 1975. Vet. Rec. 96:497.

Martin, L.C., C.B. Ammerman, W.C. Burns and M. Koger. 1976. J. Animal Sci. 42:21.

Masters, C.J. and D.J. Horgan. 1962. Aust. J. Agr. Res. 13:1082.

Matrone, G., C.R. Bunn and J.J. McNeill. 1964. J. Nutr. 84:215.

McCarthy, R.D., R.A. Patton and L.C. Griel, Jr. 1970. Fed. Proc. 29:41.

McDonald, I.W. 1954. Biochem. J. 56:120.

McDonald, I.W. and R.J. Hall. 1957. Biochem. J. 67:400.

McIntyre, K.H. 1970. Aust. J. Agr. Res. 21:501.

McLaren, G.A. et al. 1959. J. Animal Sci. 18:1319.

McLaren, G.A. et al. 1965. J. Animal Sci. 24:231; J. Nutr. 87:331.

McLaren, G.A. et al. 1976. J. Animal Sci. 43:1072; Nutr. Rept. Internat. 14:497.

McNaught, M.L., E.C. Owens, K.M. Henry and S.K. Kon. 1954. Biochem. J. 56:151.

Meacham, T.N. et al. 1961. J. Animal Sci. 20:387 (abstr).

Meiske, J.C. and R.D. Goodrich. 1966. Univ. Minn. Res. Rpt. B-68.

Meiske, J.C., W.J. Van Arsdell, R.W. Luecke and A. Hoefer. 1955. J. Animal Sci. 14:941.

Mepham, T.B. 1971. In: Lactation. Butterworths, London.

Mepham, T.B. and J.L. Linzell. 1966. Biochem. J. 101:76.

Mitchell, H.H. 1964. Comparative Nutrition of Man and Domestic Animals. Academic Press

Moe, P.W. and H.F. Tyrell. 1972. J. Dairy Sci. 55:318.

Moe, P.W. and H.F. Tyrell. 1977. J. Dairy Sci. 60:69 (abstr).

Moore, M.J., W.R. Woodsend and T.J. Klopfenstein. 1968. J. Animal Sci. 27:1172.

Mowat, D.N. and K. Deelstra. 1972. J. Animal Sci. 34:332.

Neville, W.E., R.E. Hellwig, R.J. Ritter and W.C. McCormick. 1977. J. Animal Sci. 44:687.

Nimrick, K., F.N. Owens, E.E. Hatfield and J. Kaminski. 1971. J. Dairy Sci. 54:1496.

Nolan, J.V. and R.A. Leng. 1972. Brit. J. Nutr. 27:177.

NRC. 1976. Nutrient Requirements of Beef Cattle. Nat. Acad. Sci., Washington, D.C.

NRC. 1978. Nutrient Requirements of Dairy Cattle. Nat. Acad. Sci. Washington, D.C.

Offer, N.W., M.V. Tas, R.F.E. Axford and R.A. Evans. 1975. Brit. J. Nutr. 34:375.

Oltjen, R.R. 1969. J. Animal Sci. 28:673.

Oltjen, R.R., J. Bond and G.V. Richardson. 1969. J. Animal Sci. 28:717.

Oltjen, R.R., W.C. Burns and C.B. Ammerman. 1974. J. Animal Sci. 38:975.

Oltjen, R.R., W. Chalupa and L.L. Slyter. 1970. J. Animal Sci. 31:250.

Oltjen, R.R., R.E. Davis and R.L. Hiner. 1965. J. Animal Sci. 24:192.

Oltjen, R.R. and P.A. Putnam. 1966. J. Nutr. 89:385.

Oltjen, R.R., J.D. Robbins and R.E. Davis. 1964. J. Animal Sci. 23:767.

Oltjen, R.R., R.J. Sirny and A.D. Tillman. 1962. J. Animal Sci. 21:277; J. Nutr. 77:269.

Oltjen, R.R., L.L. Slyter, A.S. Kozak and E.E. Williams. 1968. J. Nutr. 94:193.

Oltjen, R.R., L.L. Slyter and R.L. Wilson. 1972. J. Nutr. 102:479.

Oltjen, R.R., G.R. Waller, A.B. Nelson and A.D. Tillman. 1963. J. Animal Sci. 22:36.

Ørskov, E.R. 1977. In: Proc. 2nd Int. Symposium on Protein Metabolism and Nutrition. Centre for Agr. Publ. and Documentation. Wageningen. The Netherlands.

Ørskov, E.R., C. Fraser and E.L. Corse. 1970. Brit. J. Nutr. 24:803.

Ørskov, E.R., R. Smart and A.Z. Mehrez. 1974. J. Agr. Sci. 83:299.

Owen, F.G., E.L. Fisher and P.J. Cunningham. 1971. J. Dairy Sci. 54:52.

Owens, F.N., W.M. Knight and K.O. Nimrick. 1973. J. Animal Sci. 37:1000.

Papas, A., G.A.B. Hall, E.E. Hatfield and F.N. Owens. 1974. J. Nutr. 104:653.

Paquay, R., R. DeBaere and A. Lousse. 1972. Brit. J. Nutr. 27:27.

Paquay, R., J.M. Godeau, R. De Baere and A. Lousse. 1973. J. Dairy Res. 40:93;329.

Payne, E. and L. Laws. 1978. Brit. J. Nutr. 39:441.

Pendlum, L.C., J.A. Boling and N.W. Bradley. 1976. J. Animal Sci. 43:1307.

54

Perry, T.W., W.M. Beeson and M.T. Mohler. 1967a. J. Animal Sci. 26:1434.
Perry, T.W., W.M. Beeson, D.M. Robinson and M.T. Mohler. 1967b. Purdue Agr. Expt. Sta. Res. Prog. Rpt. 303.
Peterson, L.A., E.E. Hatfield and U.S. Garrigus. 1973. J. Animal Sci. 36:772.
Phillips, R.L. and D.C. Church. 1975. J. Animal Sci. 41:588.
Phillips, W.A., K.E. Webb, Jr. and J.P. Fontenot. 1976. J. Animal Sci. 42:201.
Polan, C.E. et al. 1970. J. Dairy Sci. 53:607,1578.
Polan, C.E., C.N. Miller and M.L. McGilliard. 1976. J. Dairy Sci. 59:1910.
Potter, G.D., O. Little and G.E. Mitchell. 1969. J. Animal Sci. 28:711.
Preston, R.L. 1966. J. Nutr. 90:157.
Prewitt, L.R. et al. 1975. J. Animal Sci. 41:1722.
Price, W.D., J.A. Brown, E.E. Menvielle and W.H. Smith. 1972. J. Animal Sci. 35:848.
Proksova, M. 1969. Nutr. Abstr. Rev. 39:442.
Purser, D.B. 1970. J. Animal Sci. 30:988.
Raleigh, R.J. and J.D. Wallace. 1963. J. Animal Sci. 22:330.
Razzaque, M.A. and J.H. Topps. 1973. Proc. Nutr. Soc. 32:59 (abstr).
Redd, T.L. et al. 1975. J. Animal Sci. 40:567.
Reis, P.J. 1967. Aust. J. Biol. Sci. 20:809.
Reis, P.J. 1969. Aust. J. Biol. Sci. 22:745.
Reis, P.J. and A.M. Downes. 1971. J. Agr. Sci. 76:173.
Reis, P.J. and P.G. Schinckel. 1961. Aust. J. Agr. Res. 12:335.
Reis, P.J. and P.G. Schinckel. 1963. Aust. J. Biol. Sci. 16:218.
Reis, P.J. and P.G. Schinckel. 1964. Aust. J. Biol. Sci. 17:532.
Reis, P.J. and D.A. Tunks. 1970. Aust. J. Biol. Sci. 23:673.
Robards, G.E. 1971. Aust. J. Agr. Res. 22:261.
Robinson, J.J., C. Fraser, J.C. Gill and I. McHattie. 1974. Animal Prod. 19:331.
Roffler, R.E. and L.D. Satter. 1975. J. Dairy Sci. 58:1889.
Roffler, R.E. and C.G. Schuab and L.D. Satter. 1976. J. Dairy Sci. 59:80.
Rogers, Q.R. and A.R. Egan. 1974. Aust. J. Biol. Sci. 28:169.
Roman-Ponce, H. et al. 1975. J. Dairy Sci. 58:1320.
Rowlands, G.J., W. Little and B.A. Kitchenham. 1977. J. Dairy Res. 44:1.
Roy, J.H.B. et al. 1970. Brit. J. Nutr. 18:467.
Rush, I.G., R.R. Johnson and R. Totusek. 1976. J. Animal Sci. 42:1297.
Rush, I.G. and R.Totusek. 1975. J. Animal Sci. 41:1141.
Rush, I.G. and R. Totusek. 1976. J. Animal Sci. 42:497.
Ryder, W.L., D. Hillman and J.T. Huber. 1972. J. Dairy Sci. 55:1290.
Santos, A. 1978. M.S. Thesis. Oregon State University, Corvallis, OR.
Satter, L.D. and R.E. Roffler. 1975. J. Dairy Sci. 58:1219.
Satter, L.D. and L.L. Slyter. 1974. Brit. J. Nutr. 32:199.
Schelling, G.T., J.E. Chandler and G.C. Scott. 1973. J. Animal Sci. 37:1034.
Schelling, G.T. and E.E. Hatfield. 1969. J. Nutr. 96:319.
Schilling, E. 1965. Nutr. Abstr. Rev. 33:391.
Schmidt, S.P., N.J. Benevenga and N.A. Jorgensen. 1974. J. Animal Sci. 38:646.
Schmidt, S.P., N.A. Jorgensen, N.J. Benevenga and V.H. Brungardt. 1973. J. Animal Sci. 37:1233.
Schwab, C.G., L.D. Satter and A.B. Caly. 1976. J. Dairy Sci. 59:1254.
Siebert, B.D., D.M.R. Newman, B. Hart and G.L. Mitchell. 1975. Aust. J. Expt. Agr. Animal Hus. 15:321.
Smith, G.S. et al. 1960. J. Nutr. 71:20.
Sniffen, C.J. 1974. Proc. Cornel Nutr. Conf., p. 12.
Sonderegger, H. and A. Schurch. 1977. Livestock Prod. Sci. 4:327.
Steinacker, G., T.J. Devlin and J.R. Ingalls. 1970. Can. J. Animal Sci. 50:319.
Streeter, C.L., C.O. Little, G.E. Mitchell, Jr. and R.A. Scott. 1973. J. Animal Sci. 37:796.
Streeter, C.L., R.R. Oltjen, L.L. Slyter and W.M. Fishbein. 1969. J. Animal Sci. 29:88.
Swanson, E.W. 1977. J. Dairy Sci. 60:1583.
Sykes, A.R. and A.C. Field. 1972. J. Agr. Sci. 78:109.
Tagari, H. 1969. Brit. J. Nutr. 23:455.
Tagari, H., D. Ben-Ghedalia and S. Zamwel. 1976. Animal Prod. 23:81.
Teleni, E., B.D. Siebert, R.M. Murray and C.D. Nancarrow. 1977. Aust. J. Expt. Agr. Animal Hus. 17:207.

Theurer, B., W. Woods and G.E. Poley. 1966. J. Animal Sci. 25:175.

Theurer, B., W. Woods and G.E. Poley. 1968. J. Animal Sci. 27:1059.

Thomas, C., J.M. Wilkinson and J.C. Taylor. 1975. J. Agr. Sci. 84:353.

Thomas, J.W. 1971. J. Dairy Sci. 54:1629.

Thompson, L.H. et al. 1973. J. Animal Sci. 37:399.

Thompson, L.H., M.B. Wise, R.W. Harvey and E.R. Barrick. 1972. J. Animal Sci. 35:474.

Tillman, A.D. and K.S. Sidhu. 1969. J. Animal Sci. 28:689.

Tiwari, A.D., F.N. Owens and U.S. Garrigus. 1973. J. Animal Sci. 37:1396.

Treacher, R.J., W. Little, K.A. Collis and A.J. Starck. 1976. J. Dairy Res. 43:357.

Tucker, R.E. and J.P. Fontenot. 1970. J. Animal Sci. 30:330 (abstr).

Tyrrell, H.F., P.W. Moe and W.P. Flatt. 1970. In: Energy Metabolism of Farm Animals. 5th Symposium, Juris Druck & Verlag, Zurich.

Umunna, N.N., T. Klopfenstein and W. Woods. 1975. J. Animal Sci. 40:523.

Umunna, N.N. and W.R. Woods. 1975. J. Sci. Fd. Agr. 26:413.

Van Horn, H.H. et al. 1976. J. Dairy Sci. 59:902.

Van Slyke, G.G., W.M. Beeson and T.W. Perry. 1971. J. Animal Sci. 33:671.

Verbeke, R. and G. Peeters. 1965. Biochem. J. 94:183.

Vik-Mo, L., R.S. Emery and J.T. Huber. 1974. J. Dairy Sci. 57:869.

Virtanen, A.I. 1966. Science 153:1603.

Wachira, J.D., L.D. Satter, G.P. Brooke and A.L. Pope. 1974. J. Animal Sci. 39:796.

Walker, D.M. and B.W. Norton. 1971. J. Agr. Sci. 77:363.

Wallenius, R.W. and R.E. Whitechurch. 1975. J. Dairy Sci. 58:1314.

Waynack, L.B. 1976. J. Animal Sci. 43:712.

Webb, D.W., E.E. Bartley and R.M. Meyer. 1972. J. Animal Sci. 35:1263.

West, E.S., W.R. Todd, H.S. Mason and J.T. Van Brugger. 1968. Textbook of Biochemistry (4th ed.). The McMillan Co., New York.

White, T.W., W.L. Reynolds and F.G. Hembry. 1973. J. Animal Sci. 37:1428.

White, T.W., W.L. Reynolds and F.G. Hembry. 1975. J. Animal Sci. 40:1.

Williams, A.P. and R.H. Smith. 1974. J. Nutr. 32:421.

Williams, A.P. and R.H. Smith. 1974. Proc. Nutr. Soc. 33:35 (abstr).

Williams, A.P. and R.H. Smith. 1975. Brit. J. Nutr. 33:149.

Williams, L.R., F.A. Martz and E.S. Hilderbrand. 1970. J. Dairy Sci. 53:1709.

Williams, P.P. and W.E. Dinusson. 1973. J. Animal Sci. 36:151.

Williams, V.J. 1969. Comp. Biochem. Physiol. 29:865.

Williams, V.J. and R.J. Moir. 1951. Aust. J. Sci. Res. 4:377.

Wilson, G., F.A. Martz, J.R. Campbell and B.A. Becker. 1975. J. Animal Sci. 41:1431.

Wilson, L.L. et al. 1972. J. Animal Sci. 35:128.

Winter, K.A. 1976. Can. J. Animal Sci. 56:567.

Wohlt, J.E., C.J. Sniffen and W.H. Hoover. 1973. J. Dairy Sci. 56:1052.

Wohlt, J.E. et al. 1976. J. Animal Sci. 42:1280.

Wolff, J.E. et al. 1972. Amer. J. Physiol. 223:438,447.

Wright, P.L. 1974. J. Animal Sci. 33:137.

Wyatt, R.D., R.R. Johnson and E.T. Clemens. 1975. J. Animal Sci. 40:126.

Yonemura, T. 1970. JARQ. 5:50.

Young, A.W., J.A. Boling and N.W. Bradley. 1973. J. Animal Sci. 36:803.

Zelter, S.Z. and F. Leroy. 1966. Z. Teirphysiol. Tierernaehr. Fiittermittelk 22:39.

Zucker, H. and A. Steger. 1975. Wiener Tierarztliche Monatsschrift 62:338.

Chapter 4 - The Macro (Major) Minerals

By J.P. Fontenot and D.C. Church

The macro minerals have been recognized to be dietary essentials for many years. These include calcium, chlorine, magnesium, phosphorus, potassium, sodium and sulfur. They are present in the animal body and are required at relatively high levels as compared to the micro or trace minerals. The approximate concentrations of the macro minerals in the animal body are (%): Ca, 1.33; Cl, .11; K, .19; Mg, .04; Na, .16; P, .74; S, .15 g.

In addition to many specific functions, the macro minerals perform certain general physiological functions which are critical for support of animal life. These include osmotic pressure, buffering activity which stabilizes pH in tissues, maintenance of irritability of nerves and muscles, catalytic functions and as components of certain organic substances. Not only is the presence of a given mineral important for normal health and production, but the ratio of some minerals has to be optimized.

Research with macro minerals continues at a rather rapid pace in spite of the fact that they have been recognized to be essential for many years. Continued research has been essential because of changing production systems to more concentrated livestock operations and use of more highly refined by-product feedstuffs which may be low in minerals or, for some by-products, contain excessive amounts of mineral elements.

Information on specific functions of the various minerals has been deleted from the second edition of this volume. This type of information is available in most introductory nutrition or biochemistry text books.

Data have been presented in Ch. 5, Vol. 1 for mineral levels in saliva, in Ch. 9, Vol. 1, concerning absorption from different parts of the gastro-intestinal tract (GI tract), and Ch. 15, Vol. 1 relating macro minerals to rumen fermentation. These items will not be discussed further in this chapter. For further information, the reader is referred to a standard biochemistry text such as Leninger (1975), Comar and Bronner (1962, 1964), ARC (1965), Underwood (1966), Dyer (1969), or Church and Pond (1974).

CALCIUM

Tissue Distribution

Calcium is found in the body in larger amounts than any other mineral. It is the main element in bone, accounting for 8% of bone, on a wet basis. The Ca:P ratio in bone is rather constant at 2:1. Approximately 99% of the Ca in the body is found in bone and teeth, with the other 1% distributed in various soft tissues. Ca content of the total body is not a constant value. For example, in cattle it may be expected to decline from about 1.6% in young animals to about 1% in adult animals (ARC, 1965), although the Ca content of bone will increase with age up to a point. Ca in bone ash was shown to increase from 3 mo. to 1 yr but remained constant thereafter (Blincoe et al, 1973). Various bones of cattle contain similar concentrations of Ca (Bohman et al, 1962).

The normal blood plasma of serum Ca is 10 mg/100 ml with a range between 9 and 12. Levels of plasma Ca in beef cows were not affected by intake of feed or supplemental minerals (Fisher et al, 1972), but the levels were shown to vary with season in sheep (Grace and Scott, 1974). Fifty to 70% of the Ca is in ionic form of salts such as phosphates and bicarbonates, and the remainder is bound to serum proteins, particularly albumin and γ-globulin, which is non-diffusible. The forms are in equilibrium and redistribution between them is a relatively rapid process. The level of blood Ca is a reflection of the balance between that which enters and that which leaves the blood and represents a balance between absorption, withdrawal or deposition in the skeleton, and excretion via urine or feces. The animal uses a number of homeostatic control routes to adapt to variable intakes of minerals, including Ca (Miller, 1975).

The animal is able to maintain a normal plasma level for short periods by mobilization from the bone. Feeding dairy cows a ration with 0.25% Ca for 9 wk did not cause a lowering of plasma Ca, compared to feeding a ration with 0.75% Ca (Belyea et al, 1976). Intracellular Ca is about 20 mg/100 g of tissue (White et al, 1973).

In experiments in which radio Ca was recovered from various parts of the GI tract 30 hr following injections, 1.2% was found in the rumen contents, 0.33% in omasal contents, 0.07% in abomasal contents, 0.37% in the small intestine and 1.4% in the large intestine (Hansard et al, 1952). The specific activity was rather uniform in soft tissues. In the bone, highest activity was in the sternal end of the rib, followed by the vertebra and mandible. The lowest amount was found in incisor teeth. In the soft tissues examined (oral dose), the order of activity was: plasma >kidney > spleen > liver = muscle.

It appears that Ca in fetal tissues is not in equilibrium with that of the dam's tissues. Virtually all of the radio Ca injected in fetal tissue was present 5-6 hr later, with little or no transfer to the mother or twin fetuses (Braithwaite et al, 1972). Thus, movement of Ca across the placenta is a one way process. Rate of transfer of minerals appears to be important in the growth of multiple fetuses in sheep. Maximum rate of transfer of Ca, regardless of the number of fetuses, was ca. 2.8 g/day (Twardock et al, 1973). The rate was attained by 112 days when quadruplets were carried, 126 days for triplets and 140 days for twins.

Absorption and Excretion

Sites of Absorption and Excretion. Early work with cattle by Hansard et al (1952) indicated that radio Ca could be recovered in substantial amounts in the small intestine only a few minutes after I.V. dosage, thus indicating secretion into the small intestine. In the young calf (2-5 wk of age). Smith (1962) found that Ca and other mineral elements were temporarily held up in the abomasum due to association with coagulated milk. He observed that net absorption up to the end of the small intestine was about 86% of intake, although absorption apparently decreased with age. Net exchange of Ca in the large intestine was negligible at all times. In subsequent work with older calves (Smith and McAllan, 1966), it was shown that about 60-90% of the Ca in the ileum was nonfilterable, although this form was in partial equilibrium with soluble forms of Ca.

Van't Klooster (1969) also observed that the solubility of Ca decreased from the duodenum to the terminal ileum. Subsequent work was reported with calves by Chandler and Cragle (1962) in which ^{144}Ce was used as a marker. They were studying calves 7-15 wk of age which were fed on skim milk and/or a starter ration. They found little exchange of Ca in the rumen, but a net secretion in the omasum, a large absorption by the abomasum, secretion between the abomasum and the proximal third of the small intestine and the greatest net absorption in the middle portion of the small intestine. Net exchange in the remainder of the tract was small, but data indicated slight secretion between the distal third of the intestine and the cecum and in the colon.

In research with sheep, Jones and Mackie (1959) used ^{45}Ca to study sites of secretion or absorption and the sheep were sacrificed 1 hr after they were given I.V. doses. Their data indicated that 15% of the total radioactivity recovered in the GI tract was in the rumen contents, 36.9% was in the 3rd of 4 equal segments of the small intestine, 14% in the 4th segment, and lesser amounts in other areas. These data would seem to show that Ca is excreted farther down the small intestine in sheep than in cattle. Phillipson and Storry (1965) have also investigated sites of absorption in sheep with the use of intestinal loops. Their data indicated that Ca absorption occurred from the upper jejunum and ileum, the amount being related to the Ca concentration. Absorption was apparently complete by the end of the ileum. In experiments with calves, Perry et al (1967) reported a net secretion of Ca in the upper small intestine although net absorption was high in the total small intestine. Van't Klooster (1969) observed a slight net secretion in the large intestine. Pfeffer et al (1970) reported net secretions of Ca during passage through the reticulo-rumen, omasum, abomasum and small intestine and a trend for net losses during passage through the cecum and colon and Liebholz (1974) reported that 38.8 to 50.1% of ingested Ca disappeared by the time the ingesta reached the duodenum of sheep equipped with a re-entrant duodenal cannula, indicating absorption before reaching the small intestine.

Studies with animals which have had I.V. doses of ^{45}Ca (Shroder and Hansard, 1958; Tillman and Brethour, 1958; Thompson et al, 1959) show that a substantial amount of fecal Ca may be of endogenous origin and that true digestibility may be on the order of 20-60%. The endogenous Ca in feces thus may account for 50% or more of fecal Ca in some situations (Tillman and Brethour, ibid). It may be that fecal endogenous Ca is excreted in the upper GI tract (bile, intestinal juices) and not reabsorbed and that little excretion takes place in the large intestine.

Adequate information is not available to resolve this question.

Effect of Age. Hansard et al (1954), using isotopic techniques, reported that net Ca absorption in cattle decreased with age, from 99% in the young calf to 23% in cattle 12-15 yr of age. Absorption dropped from 95% at 1 mo. of age to 41% at 6 mo. of age and was gradually reduced thereafter. The effect of age on apparent absorption was confimed by Garces and Evans (1971) (Fig. 4-1). Of course, part of this early drop would be due to a changeover from a highly absorbable form of Ca in milk to less soluble forms in other feedstuffs (Lengemann et al, 1957), although Smith (1962) observed an apparent decrease in absorption in calves from 2 to 5 wk of age. Ca absorption was studied in wethers varying in age from 2 to 70 mo. (Braithwaite and Risguddin, 1971). The greatest effect was a large decrease in absorption during the period from a young growing animal to a mature adult, but slight changes occurred in young and old animals. True digestibility of Ca in 2-5 day, milk-fed lambs was 88% (Walker, 1972). Cowan et al (1968) found that yearling deer retained more ^{45}Ca and ^{89}Sr than 2-yr olds. The younger deer also transferred more to their growing antlers. Bronner (1964) states that there is some evidence that the actual amount of Ca absorbed stays about the same as an animal grows older, but with an increasing intake of feed (and Ca), the percentage of absorbed Ca declines.

Effect of Stage of Production. Rate of absorption from the intestine of ewes increased steadily during pregnancy (Braithwaite et al, 1970). Absorption was less in ewes with single than those with twin fetuses. During lactation, ewes which had been depleted of Ca during pregnancy absorbed about twice as much Ca as previous estimates for lactating ewes (Sykes and Dingwall, 1975). The authors suggested that this was due mainly to an enhanced active absorption.

Absorption from Ca Sources. Ca in feedstuffs is present as a variety of different salts (carbonates, phosphates, phytates and oxalates) and the solubility in the GI tract is believed to be related to the prevailing pH; however, there is very little direct evidence that pH is a factor in the ruminant GI tract (Smith and McAllan, 1966). Matsushima et al (1955) demonstrated that particle size of limestone or bone meal did not appear to be a factor in absorption, thus these sources must be readily soluble in the intestines. Hansard and others (1957) found that Ca in various inorganic sources appeared to be utilized slightly more efficiently by cattle than that from alfalfa, lespedeza or orchardgrass hay, but differences were small and not statistically different. The biological availability of Ca in ruminants is highest from bone meal, monocalcium phosphate and dicalcium phosphate, intermediate from limestone and defluorinated phosphate and lowest from hay (Peeler, 1972). The true digestibility of Ca varies greatly with a range from about 20 to 60%. Apparent digestibility, however, will usually be very low, more on the order of 5-10% or less in mature animals on maintenance rations.

Organic Dietary Factors. Fats were shown to have a depressing effect on Ca utilization by ruminants (Tillman and Brethour, 1958), presumably due to the formation of insoluble Ca soaps (Roberts and McKirdy, 1965) (see Ch. 7). However, no interrelationship was observed between added fat and Ca levels indicating that steers fed added fat did not have a higher Ca requirement than those fed rations without added fat (Hatch et al, 1972). Lactose and other sugars stimulate Ca absorption in other species although the mechanism is not specific for Ca, and some amino acids, particularly lysine, are known to be stimulatory in the young rat. Stillings

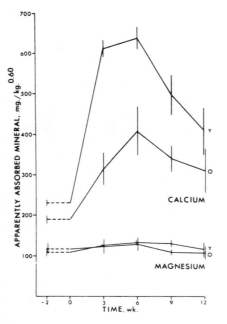

Fig. 4-1. Apparent Ca and Mg absorption for animals which were 15 mo. (Y) and 44 mo. (O) of age. From Garces and Evans (1971).

et al (1964) have shown that Ca retention was greater in animals consuming high N forages as compared to low N forages even though Ca intake was less. Supplemental vitamin D improved Ca absorption and retention on the low N forage. Grains are generally believed to facilitate Ca absorption (Brochart, 1965; Paquay et al, 1968) in dairy cattle although there is contradictory evidence.

It is interesting to note that feed ingestion and accompanying metabolic changes has been reported to increase urinary excretion of Ca (Stacy, 1969). Stacy concluded that this may have been due to a reduced blood pH, probably resulting, in turn, from an increased absorption of the VFA and lowered plasma bicarbonate.

Vitamin D, of course, is considered to have a most important function in regulating Ca absorption (see Ch. 9 and 12), evidence on this subject having been available for some time in ruminants.

Effect of Other Minerals on Absorption. Numerous experiments have demonstrated that Ca utilization is affected by the amount of P in the diet. Dowe et al (1957) fed beef calves Ca:P ratios varying from 1.3:1 to 13.7:1 in which the P intake was considered to be adequate. Liveweight gain was decreased as Ca intake increased and the authors suggested that a critical ratio may exist between 4.3:1 and 9.1:1. The excess Ca was not reflected in blood Ca levels. In one trial blood P was depressed. Wise et al (1963) studied Ca:P ratios varying from 0.4:1 to 14.3:1 in calves fed semipurified diets. They observed that performance and nutrient conversion were markedly decreased with Ca:P ratios lower than 1:1. Ratios between 1:1 and 7:1 gave similar and satisfactory results. Ratios above 7:1 resulted in decreased performance, but adverse effects were not as marked as with ratios below 1:1 (see Table 4-1).

Luick and others (1957) found that dairy cows were unable to maintain positive Ca balance when the dietary Ca:P ratio was less than 1:1. Cows responded to changes in Ca or P in the diet by adjusting absorption and excretion, and cows on low Ca and high P diets utilized dietary Ca less efficiently than cows on higher Ca diets. In work with lambs, Fontenot and others (1964) have observed that high ratios of Ca:P (4:1 and 8:1) depressed rate of gain and feed efficiency. In growing Holstein steers, feeding a ration with an 8:1 ratio of Ca:P reduced daily gain, compared to a 1:1 ratio, but feeding a 4:1 ratio had no effect (Ricketts et al, 1970). Manston (1967) indicated that increasing the Ca and P intake increased absorption for a few days, but absorption then returned to near its initial level. Long term experiments with pregnant heifers showed better absorption of both elements when given a 2:1 than when given a 1:1 ratio (Steevens et al, 1971). Absorption, retention and efficiency of utilization of Ca was greatest in steers receiving a Ca:P ratio of 1:1, compared to 4:1 and 8:1 (Ricketts et al, 1970). Lomba et al (1978) observed that P + chloride and sulfate tended to stimulate Ca digestibility under some circumstances.

Data obtained with isotopic techniques (Young and others, 1966) showed that wide ratios of Ca:P had little effect on P utilization; however, an inadequate supply of P

Table 4-1. Effect of various Ca:P ratios when fed to calves.[a]

Ca, %	0.27	0.27	0.27	0.81	0.81	0.81	2.43	2.43	2.43
P, %	0.17	0.34	0.68	0.17	0.34	0.68	0.17	0.34	0.68
Ca:P ratio	1.6	0.8	0.44	4.8	2.4	1.2	14.33	7.2	3.6
Daily gain, g	669	503	281	712	694	631	494	664	503
Daily feed intake, g	3.6	3.4	2.7	3.4	3.5	3.5	3.2	3.6	3.4
Feed efficiency	5.6	6.7	14.6	4.8	5.1	5.9	6.5	5.5	6.9
Serum Ca, mg % terminal	15.3	15.0	13.3	16.6	14.8	14.0	16.1	14.9	14.6
Serum P, mg % terminal	9.4	9.7	10.2	7.7	10.2	10.3	7.2	9.8	11.3

[a] From Wise et al (1963)

reduced Ca deposition in and removal from bone and decreased Ca absorption. Urinary Ca was higher in animals given inadequate P in the diet.

There is evidence to show that the feeding of high levels of Zn will either depress the effects of a high Ca:P ratio on rate of gain and feed efficiency (Fontenot et al, 1964) or the net retention and true digestibility of dietary Ca (Thompson et al, 1959). However, the beneficial effects have not been observed consistently. Supplementing a diet with a high Ca:P ration with Zn did not improve rate of gain in young calves (Cobic et al, 1971). Information on other mineral elements is sparse and incomplete.

There is little reason to believe that Ca absorption or retention is related to the Mg status of the animal (Care and Van't Klooster, 1965; Hjerpe, 1968), even though these elements are similar in many respects, both chemically and physiologically. There is some evidence in monogastric species that Mg may replace some Ca when it is lost from bone (White et al 1973). Adding 100 ppm F in drinking water depressed Ca absorption in calves (Ramberg et al, 1970). Supplementing of calves with NH_4CL increased absorption and urinary excretion of Ca and decreased urinary pH (Braithwaite, 1972). Oral administration of NH_4Cl in goats increased exchangeable Ca (Vagg and Payne, 1970) and acidosis increased urinary excretion of Ca in sheep (Stacy and Wilson, 1970).

Miscellaneous Factors. Diethylstilbestrol, a synthetic estrogen, has been shown to result in increased retention of Ca (Whitehair et al, 1953), apparently by reduction of fecal excretion (Shroder and Hansard, 1958). In other species, cortisone or ACTH, estrogens, or progesterone have been implicated in Ca metabolism. Implanting of hexestrol increased absorption and urinary excretion of Ca (Braithwaite et al, 1972). They suggested that the increased retention was due to stimulating the production of growth hormone. Braithwaite (1975) found that SQ administration of bovine growth hormone increased absorption rate of Ca in mature wethers. Some of the variation in mineral metabolism may be related to genetics (Wiener and Field, 1971). Gastrointestinal irridiation reduced plasma Ca, but the effect appeared to be due to lowered intake (Sasser et al, 1974).

Route of Excretion

Hansard et al (1952) have studied the metabolism of Ca in older cattle (7-32 mo. of age) which were in a slightly positive Ca balance. They found that 85% of the dietary Ca intake was excreted via feces. When ^{45}Ca was administered I.V., about 2% of the total excretion was via urine and 98% via feces, although only 15% of the total dose was excreted. Elam and Autry (1961) also found that only about 23% of total Ca excretion was via urine in steers. Gueguen and Mathieu (1965) found that Ca urinary concentration varied little in calves given from 8 to 16 g/day, although apparent absorption of Ca varied from about 60% on the low level to 35% at the higher level. Jones and Mackie (1959) compared the absorption of ^{45}Ca and ^{89}Sr in sheep. Almost 4X as much Ca as Sr was absorbed and deposited in the skeleton. The kidney was able to excrete more Sr, but both Ca and Sr were excreted primarily in the intestines. Other Ca balance studies with sheep (Shroder and Hansard, 1958; Tillman and Brethour, 1958; Thompson et al, 1959) show that only 25% of excreted Ca was recovered in urine.

Regulation of Blood Ca

Blood Ca is believed to be largely regulated by action of hormones which control absorption to some extent or which influence bone deposition and withdrawal. There may also be some effect on fecal excretion due to hormones. Parathormone from the parathyroid gland has been shown to have a controlling effect on Ca absorption in the presence of vitamin D, and thyrocalcitonin from cells in the thyroid gland has a depressing effect on blood Ca by decreasing absorption or reducing bone mobilization (see Ch. 12 for further details). Indirectly, Luick et al (1957) have shown the effect of hormones in dairy cows. In their research they found that lactating cows utilized dietary Ca more efficiently than non-lactating cows, and pregnant cows were more efficient than open cows. Similar results were observed in sheep (Braithwaite et al, 1970). Ca clearance and parathormone declined with age in cows 4.5 to 7.8 yr of age (Ramburg et al, 1976). The authors suggested that a decrease in Ca clearance tended to increase plasma Ca, which led to a decreased rate of parathormone secretion. Feeding Ca deficient diets prepartum has been used successfully to prevent parturient paresis, presumably by inducing increased

PTH secretion (Goings et al, 1974; Wiggers et al, 1975). Reductions in blood Ca were noted at parturition in cows and goats, but not in ewes (Barlet et al, 1971).

Ca Deficiency

It is generally assumed that Ca can be withdrawn readily from the skeleton during periods of inadequate dietary intake or insufficient absorption since the bone salts are said to be readily available in time of need. As an example, Benzie et al (1956) studied the deposition and withdrawal of Ca in pregnant and lactating ewes when fed 2 or 5 g of Ca daily. Ewes were sacrificed at various stages so that bone ash could be measured. When fed the low level of Ca, they found 18% less bone ash at mid-lactation than during early gestation and 6.5% less on the high level of Ca. Ewes that were continued on the low Ca diet had not replaced losses in bone by the middle of the dry period. Loss of bone ash was greater in the skull, mandible and cervical vertebra than in most other bones (end of radius and meta-carpel). Serum Ca fell after early lactation on the low Ca diet and did not return to the level found in early gestation although there was an increase after weaning of the lambs. Serum P tended to vary inversely with Ca. McRoberts and others (1965) found that a diet low in Ca caused a moderately large depression in serum Ca when fed to growing lambs. The low Ca intake also resulted in reduced bone ash but did not produce clinical defects of the skeleton. The teeth of these animals erupted slowly, had slight hypoplasia of the enamel and eventually became severely worn. Annenkov et al (1969) have published some interesting data on experiments in which ^{45}Ca and ^{32}P were used with sheep. They reported that plasma Ca administered I.V. had a half life of less than 1 hr and that the half life of that exchanging with the skeleton was 8.6 hr. Of interest, however, is the observation that the half life of Ca in the skeleton was 275 days, about half that of rabbits. Very little of the labeled Ca recovered in fetuses was derived from the skeleton, although they observed that pregnant ewes had much larger ex-changeable Ca pool (6.2 g) than after parturi-tion (2.6 g). These data indicate that the skeleton may be relatively resistant to depletion.

Some of the papers mentioned indicate that sheep may respond to low Ca diets with a reduction in serum Ca and a gradual deple-tion of skeletal reserves. However, there is evidence to indicate that cattle are relatively resistant to depletion in serum Ca, (Wise et al, 1963). Feeding a low Ca ration for 5 mo. prior to parturition increased plasma Ca during the subsequent lactation (Dunham and Ward, 1971).

Older animals, particularly lactating adults, may develop osteomalacia (osteo-porosis), a condition in which the bones become thin, brittle, and low in total ash. Such symptoms have been reported in dairy cattle. An affected cow is shown in Fig. 4-2. This condition results in a stiff gait, moderate lameness and fractures of the bones.

In addition to the skeletal changes that may occur with long term Ca deficiency, other symptoms of a deficiency may include depressed feed intake, reduced rate of gain, or reduced milk production in lactating cows (Underwood, 1966). Data showing involve-ment in reproductive problems are scanty and incomplete.

Rickets is a disorder of the bone in which there is inadequate mineralization of the bone and a resultant malformation of the bone in young rapidly growing animals. Although low Ca diets apparently may result in rickets in humans and other species

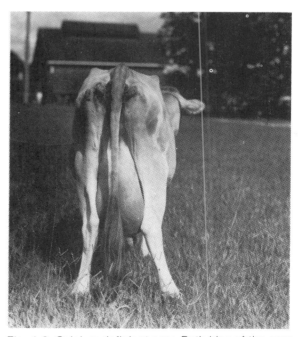

Fig. 4-2. Calcium deficient cow. Both hips of the cow have been broken (knocked down) as a result of demineralization of the bones. Courtesy of R.B. Becker, Florida Agr. Expt. Sta.

(Thomas and Howard, 1964), ruminants seem to be resistant to low Ca rickets (McRoberts et al, 1965). However, rickets has been reported in lambs fed a low Ca-low P ration (Field et al, 1975).

Osteodystrophy (osteodystrophia fibrosa) is a condition known to occur in horses fed diets with excessive P or a low Ca:P ratio. Curtis et al (1969) have diagnosed a condition in sheep believed to be osteodystrophy. In this disease there is a demineralization of the bones accompanied by a fibrous dysplasia. The bones are very weak and there may be a separation of muscular and tendinous attachments in horses. Articular erosions occur and there may be a displacement of the bone marrow (Blood and Henderson, 1968). Some of the symptoms are believed to be a result of hyperparathyroidism. In these particular sheep the lambs were weaned at 10 wk of age and put on a high grain ration. The condition first appeared 3 wk after weaning and about 10% of the lambs died, 20% being affected. No particular symptoms were observed except osteodystrophy which was believed to be a combination of rickets and hyperparathyroidism. Calculated Ca:P ratios of the diet were 1:2. Aas Hansen et al (1968) have observed similar findings when goats were fed rations low in Ca. Extra vitamin D had a protective effect. Serum Ca was depressed to 3-4 mg/100 ml and serum glutamic pyruvic transaminase values were elevated. Osteodystrophia has been described in a goat, apparently due to an abnormal Ca:P ratio (Saha and Deb, 1973).

A calcinosis was described in sheep in which mineralization of the aorta, arteries, lungs and kidneys occurred (Gill et al, 1976). It was suggested that it was due to complex mineral imbalance. Excessive dietary Ca resulted in hypercalcitoninism in bulls (Krook et al, 1971).

Milk fever (parturient paresis) is a metabolic problem associated with abnormal metabolism of Ca and perhaps other minerals during the early stages of lactation (see Ch. 12); it might be considered to be a short-term deficiency, but it is not, as such, related to Ca stores in the bones.

Dietary Requirements

The Ca requirements of sheep and cattle have been discussed at length by ARC (1965) and it is not the intent of this discussion to go into this subject for the many different situations that may affect Ca requirements.

Ca needs are related to P and vitamin D status. Other factors that must be taken into consideration include density of the ration (if Ca need is expressed in terms of % of ration), level of performance (rate of gain, amount of milk produced), age of the animal, solubility and digestibility of the Ca source (milk vs. mineral supplements vs. plant sources), amount of fat in the diet and species of animal in question.

Examples of recommendations, in terms of percentage of the diet, dry basis, are shown. These are taken from NRC publications. The reader is referred to these publications or to ARC (1965) for further details on Ca requirements of ruminants.

Beef cattle:
growing-finishing cattle, 1.04-0.18%
pregnant females, 0.23-0.18%
early lactation, 0.42-0.25%

Dairy cattle:
growing cattle, 0.70-0.40%
mature bulls, 0.24%
maintenance plus reproduction, 0.37%
milk production, 0.60-0.43%

Sheep:
fattening lambs, 0.37-0.26%
non-lactating ewes, 0.30-0.21%
lactating ewes, 0.52-0.48%

The large variation among growing-finishing ruminants is due to age and rate of gain. The requirement during lactation is related to the level of milk production. Recent work in lambs from 5 to 70 days of age has defined the Ca requirement in these young animals (Hodge et al, 1973). It was concluded that a Ca intake of 250 mg/kg body weight/day is adequate for young lambs slaughtered for meat production at an early age. Hodge (1973) estimated Ca requirements for young lambs by the factorial method. The values for lambs gaining at the rate of 100, 200, 300 and 400 g/day were 1.0, 1.9, 2.9 and 3.9 g/day for 10 kg lambs, and 1.2, 2.4, 3.6 and 4.8 g/day for 18 kg lambs.

Feeding limestone increased fecal pH and feed efficiency and decreased starch losses in feces of dairy cattle (Wheeler and Noller, 1976). Data were obtained indicating that the optimum level of Ca in high concentrate diets may be higher than the level recommended by NRC for fattening cattle (Varner and Woods, 1972).

PHOSPHORUS

Tissue Distribution

Phosphorus is widely distributed in both plant and animal tissues. The P content of bone ash is 16-17% or about 4-4.5% of wet bone tissue, and is found in a rather constant Ca:P ratio of 2:1. The amount of P in the bones of young animals will be less than that in adults since their bones are not completely mineralized. About 75-80% of the total body P is found in the skeleton and teeth. Whole blood contains about 35-45 mg/100 ml of P, much of which is found in the red cells. The inorganic P level of serum or plasma in ruminants is 3-6 mg/100 ml but may range from 4-9 mg/100 ml. The range may be partly due to the fact that hydrolysis of organo-P complexes occurs if blood is allowed to stand outside the body, resulting in analytical errors. Much of the plasma P is ionized, but part of it is complexed with proteins, lipids or carbohydrates. P is found at a level of about 0.08% in smooth muscle and 0.21% in skeletal muscle. Brain tissue may have 0.24-0.44% (cattle), and liver about 0.28%. The order of uptake of ^{32}P in various tissues of sheep has been reported to be: bile, liver, kidney, heart, spleen, lung, muscle and brain (Smith et al, 1952).

Absorption and Excretion

Sites of Absorption and Excretion. The absorption and utilization of P has been studied extensively in ruminant species, probably because P is usually more apt to be a limiting nutrient than Ca or some of the other mineral nutrients. One of the earliest reports dealing with the use of ^{32}P was that of Shirley et al (1951). In this case a steer was fed grass hay fertilized with radio P, and the contents of the GI tract and tissues were counted for radioactivity. Approximately 45% of the activity was found in the GI tract, of which 36% was in the reticulo-rumen (animals were slaughtered about 40 hr after feed first presented). Feces contained 1.34% and urine 1.54% of the activity. No activity was found in feces during the first 12 hr, but 0.92% of the dose was present in 24 hr. Values were given on various soft and skeletal tissues.

The question of where P is absorbed or secreted into the GI tract has been examined by Smith et al (1955) in sheep and cattle by sacrificing animals at intervals after administration of an I.V. dose of ^{32}P. Examination of their data on young (1 mo. of age) lambs indicated probable secretion in the rumen (saliva or through the rumen wall), the abomasum and the small intestine with little change in the large intestine. In older lambs (4 mo. of age), there was some indication of secretion into the abomasum, small intes-

tine and rectum; in lambs 10 mo. of age there was apparent secretion in the omasum in addition to the other sites. Based on changes with time, data indicated apparent absorption in the small intestine or cecum. With respect to calves, there was an apparent secretion in the omasum and the small intestine, but little into the rumen. Adult cows secreted large amounts into the rumen and lesser amounts in the small intestine and colon. Apparent absorption occurred in the abomasum and the small intestine or cecum in calves. Van't Klooster (1969) also found a small net excretion in the large intestine of cows.

Chandler and Cragle (1962) studied this aspect with the use of ^{144}Ce as a marker with calves 1 and 15 wk of age. Their data indicated a net secretion in the reticulo-rumen, omasum and small intestine (1st of 6 segments); data also indicated a slight secretion in the colon. There was substantial absorption in the abomasum and the lower half of the small intestine. Older calves (15 wks vs 1 wk of age) showed greater secretion in the omasum and absorption in the abomasum.

The true digestibility of P is usually quite high for most inorganic sources, being on the order of 70-80%. Since this is the case and since most of the excreted P is fecal P (see section on route of excretion), a very substantial amount of net excretion must occur in the GI tract. The experiments mentioned above do not show this, however. Of course, it may be that most of the endogenous P is excreted in the upper small intestine and that it is not reabsorbed to the same extent as dietary P. This could occur if insoluble complexes were formed in bile, for example.

Effect of Other Nutrients on P Utilization. As noted in the section on Ca, excess Ca may interfere with the utilization of P. A report of Hansard and Barth (1962) adds further information on this subject. The source of P (as phytin or tricalcium phosphate) or level of Ca had no significant effect upon total blood P (or Ca) nor upon P excretion. True digestibility of P was not affected by source or levels of Ca, although data indicated that Ca absorption augmented metabolic excretion of P. Compere et al (1965) have reported similar data, indicating that the Ca:P ratio did not affect urinary excretion of P nor its true digestibility, but increased fecal excretion. Manston (1967) found that absorption

Table 4-2. Phosphorus metabolism of lambs fed different levels of calcium.[a]

Ca intake[b]	P intake, mg/kg/d	Apparent absorption, %	Fecal P, mg/kg/d	Urinary P, mg/kg/d
50 mg/kg/d				
Period 1	292	96	12	203
2	206	90	25	121
250 mg/kg/d				
Period 1	315	93	22	150
2	224	80	45	90
450 mg/kg/d				
Period 1	311	87	41	90
2	222	67	74	51
650 mg/kg/d				
Period 1	319	86	44	84
2	219	64	79	38

[a]Adapted from Hodge (1973).
[b]Period one from 5-37 days and period 2 from 37 to 69 days of age.

of P (and Ca) increased when the dietary intake of the element increased, but only for a few days. Absorption of both elements were near optimum when cows were given a Ca:P ratio of 2:1. Ca and P were retained in a constant ratio of 1.25 to 1 in sheep; it has been suggested that P retention is controlled by the rate of Ca retention (Braithwaite, 1975). Hodge (1973) reported that Ca levels did not markedly affect apparent digestibility of P in lambs between 5 and 37 days. However, apparent absorption of P was depressed in the calves from 37 to 69 days of age by each increase in Ca level (Table 4-2). Westerlund (1956), working with milking cows, found that fecal P rose with increasing loss of Ca (in negative balance). Fecal P decreased with increasing P in milk and urine and with increasing N retention; milk P was inversely related to fecal and urinary P and N balance. Reduction of P in the feed led to an increased loss of Ca. His results indicated that, if reserves were withdrawn from the bone, the mineral in excess would be excreted. Ca:P ratio and supplemental vitamin D did not affect plasma inorganic P in lactating cows (Dunham and Ward, 1971) and different supplemental levels of Mg apparently have no effect on serum P (Dutton and Fontenot, 1967).

Thompson et al (1959) have reported that added zinc sulfate interfered with P absorption from the GI tract of lambs. Since Zn did not change the metabolic fecal P, they concluded that there was a reduction in absorption. Aluminum sulfate did not change P absorption or excretion (see Table 4-3). Shirley et al (1950) studied the effect of sodium molybdate or copper sulfate on P utilization by steers. When high Cu levels were fed, there was a big increase in labeled P found in the rectum, particularly. High Mo resulted in a comparable increase in the GI tract with a particularly large increase of labeled P in the jejunum. The addition of either of these minerals (Cu or Mo) resulted in a very marked decrease in excretion of urinary P and high Mo resulted in at least a two-fold increase in total excretion of P (see Table 4-3). In view of the scanty information on the site of P absorption and excretion in the GI tract, it is difficult to determine if Cu or Mo was interfering with absorption or increasing excretion. The latter was deemed likely since tissue concentration of ^{32}P was not markedly reduced by Cu or Mo. A high Fe level (1000 ppm) depressed plasma P and tended to decrease apparent absorption of P in cattle (Standish et al, 1971).

Although vegetable oils have been shown to decrease absorption of Ca, corn oil has no apparent effect on true digestibility or retention of P (Tillman and Brethour, 1958). Sudden dietary changes have been shown to result in reduced blood P levels with no apparent effect on milk concentration (L'Estrange and Axford, 1966) although an increased water intake may be expected to increase urinary P excretion (Suttle and Field, 1966). High N forages have been

Table 4-3. Effect of some other mineral elements on P balance and digestibility.

Item	Sheep[a]			Cattle[b]			
	Basal diet	Basal + 1% Al	Basal + 1% Zn	Basal diet	Basal + high Mo	Basal + high Cu	Basal + high Mo + high Cu
Fecal P, g	2.06	2.07	1.92	5.16	15.60	4.7	4.68
Urinary P							
g	0.05	0.04	0.07	2.30	0.03	0.04	0.54
% of excreted							
Net retention, g	-.10	-.17	-.50				
True digestibility, %	88.3	76.6	81.6				

[a] From Thompson et al (1959)

[b] From Shirley et al (1950)

indicated as causing an improved retention of P and higher serum levels (Stillings et al, 1964) as compared to low N forage. Also a reduction in the amount of protein in the diet may result in increased urinary P and reduced P retention in calves (Mudgel and Kay, 1967). Van't Klooster (1969) has shown that a substantial amount of intestinal P is insoluble, the percentage increasing from duodenum to ileum.

Ewer (1951) reported that a single massive dose of the vitamin D would result in a temporary cure of rickets and improve the P retention of sheep maintained on a low P diet. Conrad et al (1956) have also shown that massive doses of vitamin D increased the absorption of ^{32}P in cattle, although net retention was not affected much since excretion also increased, particularly via the urine.

Effect of Miscellaneous Factors. A number of factors have been reported to influence P serum levels or P utilization by ruminants. Seasonal trends have been observed in serum P, the high values tending to be during the winter and spring (Vaskov et al, 1969). Daily trends have also been noted (Unsheim and Rappen, 1969). The concentration of blood P has been shown to be related to pregnancy and lactation, values generally being lower during lactation and pregnancy than for dry animals (Kirchegessner, 1958; Vaskov et al, 1969). Urinary excretion of P apparently diminishes following the cessation of lactation (Gueguen and Mathieu, 1965). The concentration of P increases with fetal age (Field and Suttle, 1967), but some data indicate that most of the fetal P is derived from dietary P rather than from body stores (Annenkov et al, 1969). The maximum rate of placental transfer of P was approxi-

mately 1.4 g/day, regardless of the number of fetuses (Twardock et al, 1973). There is also an effect of age on serum P (Lane et al, 1968; Unshelm and Rappen, 1969), one paper indicating a decline of 0.44 mg/100 ml per year in cattle.

Synthetic hormones such as diethylstilbestrol have been shown to increase P retention, probably by way of reduced urinary excretion (Whitehair et al, 1953; Shroder and Hansard, 1958). Thyroidectomy apparently results in reduced accumulation of P in the bones of goats (Symonds, 1969), and other hormones such as oxytocin may result in reduced serum P while vasopressin temporarily increases blood P in sheep (Moodie, 1968).

Route of Excretion

There is ample evidence in the literature to show that relatively small amounts of total P excretion occur via the urine. Typical literature on sheep (Shroder and Hansard, 1958; Tillman and Brethour, 1958) indicates that about 95% of total P excretion is via the feces, although there is some evidence that urinary excretion may represent a relatively higher percentage (16%) in the case of lambs in negative P balance (Ellis and Tillman, 1961). In the case of cattle, Kleiber et al (1951) reported that urinary P was less than 1% of fecal P, values in agreement with reports by Ammerman et al (1957) and O'Donovan et al (1965). Tillman et al (1959) found urinary P to be 4.5% of total excreted by steers. Mayer et al (1968) have presented graphical data on cows which indicated relatively low urinary P, although the values showed quite a range (see Fig. 4-3). Two extreme variations from these papers might be of interest. Shirley and others (1950) found that fecal P represented 69% and urinary P about 31% of total P excreted by steers. When ^{32}P was injected intramuscularly, 19% was excreted via feces and 81% via urine (one steer). In another example, Reed et al (1965) found that urinary P ranged from 26 to 53% of total excreted by steers fed diets "mainly of maize." Perhaps some of these differences are due to the influence of parathyroid hormone (see section on regulation of blood P).

Urinary P excretion was in excess of normal in 10% of dairy cows in confinement (Manston and Vagg, 1970). This occurred only in cows which were permanently housed. Fine grinding of oat hulls increased urinary P excretion in sheep, which was ameliorated by addition of polyethylene flakes (Tomas, 1974). However, fecal P excretion was lower and balance was higher for the sheep fed the ground oat hulls. The authors indicated that the decreased endogenous fecal excretion of P appeared to be compensated by an increase in urinary excretion. Tomas (1974) found that diversion of parotid saliva from the rumen to the blood increased urinary P excretion, and P balance was not changed.

Most of the studies with radio P indicate that a very substantial amount of the total fecal P is of endogenous origin (i.e., excreted into the GI tract). The values in the literature vary considerably, depending upon the amount of P in the diet, the nature of the P source, and other factors. Nevertheless, published values indicate that about 40-90% may be of metabolic origin (Kleiber et al, 1951; Lofgreen and Kleiber, 1953; Luick and Lofgreen, 1957; Tillman et al, 1959).

Since the available data on excretion of P into the GI tract indicates that a substantial amount of P is excreted in the small intestine or in areas anterior to the small intestine, it would be interesting to know how much of this might be recycled in the body. One would think that P secreted into the upper small intestine might be reabsorbed unless it was present in insoluble complexes with other minerals or organic chelates. Recycling, of course, should result in a lower dietary requirement.

Regulation of Blood Phosphorus

The maintenance of blood P, like that of many other minerals, is presumed to be a reflection of the combined values of absorption, excretion and withdrawal from or deposition in the bones or other tissues. Information reviewed by White et al (1973) and Irving (1964) on species other than ruminants

indicates that a major mechanism of controlling blood P is via control over excretion through the kidney by the parathyroid hormone. The reduction in P excretion that occurs when I.V. Ca infusions are given can be reduced by parathormone and the hormone, when administered to hypoparathyroid patients, causes a marked phosphate diuresis. In cases of renal insufficiency the serum P is elevated. The feeding of excess Ca, Fe or Al has no effect on fasting serum P in normal individuals, but causes an abrupt fall in serum P in patients with renal insufficiency. Furthermore, I.V. injection of parathormone into one renal artery will lead to phosphaturia of that kidney, but not by the other. The only conclusive evidence in ruminants is that published by Mayer et al (1966, 1968). Their research has shown that a bovine parathyroid extract, when administered to dry cows, resulted in a marked increase in urinary excretion of P, the peak occurring 3-5 days after treatment of intact cows. Parathyroidectomy was followed by a decline in urinary P and a rise in fecal P. Fecal P was reduced in intact cows treated with the PHE or in parathyroidectomized cows treated with the extract (see Fig. 4-3). The effect of some other hormones has been mentioned previously. Vitamin D may also have some effect since data of Conrad et al (1956) indicated an increase in serum P following treatment with massive doses of the vitamin; the dose also increased urinary P.

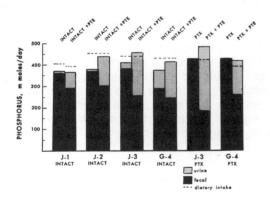

Fig. 4-3. Changes in fecal and urinary P excretion of cows associated with parathyroid extract administration and parathyroidectomy. Note that the parathyroid extract administration was always accompanied by an increase of urinary P with an offsetting decrease in fecal P so that changes in total P excretion were small. Parathyroidectomy was followed by a decline in urinary P and an increase in fecal P. From Mayer et al (1968).

Phosphorus Deficiency

Phosphorus deficiency appears to be a wide-spread problem throughout the world. Most of the forage that ruminants consume is little more than adequate in P content and weathered, leached forage is nearly always borderline or deficient in P. Consequently, P is usually one of the most limiting of the mineral nutrients for ruminants in many situations.

Usually, the first evidence of P deficiency is a drop in plasma inorganic P below the normal levels (4-6 $\pm$ mg/100 ml for adults; 6-8 $\pm$ mg/100 ml for young animals). Plasma phosphatase values increase. The mineral content of the bones becomes depleted and the bones become fragile. Another result of a P deficiency is that the joints become stiff (see Fig. 4-4), lameness may develop and fractures may occur. Upon postmortem, the articulating cartilages in the joints appear to be eroded (NRC publications). Field et al (1975) reported twisting of the forelegs in lambs fed low Ca (0.07%) and low P (0.13%).

Anorexia (reduced appetite) is the first clinical symptom of P deficiency, but it is not specific for a P deficiency, of course. Most animals develop pica (a depraved appetite) in which case they will chew and ingest material not usually considered to be food—articles such as rocks, dirt, wood, bones or hair (see Fig. 4-5). Pica is not specific for P, either, since it may occur with a Na or K deficiency. As a result of pica,

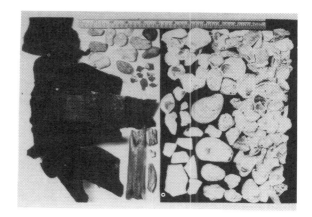

Fig. 4-5. Pica or depraved appetite in P-deficient cattle Picture illustrates material recovered from the stomach of a deficient cow. It includes oyster shells, 6 pieces of porcelain, 3 teeth, a 4.5 in. section of cannon bone, inner tube, tire casing, pieces of metal and pebbles. Courtesy of R.B. Becker, Florida Agr. Expt. Sta.

cattle may consume carcass debris when available and may, at times, be poisoned by *Clostridium botulinum*, an organism that produces a toxin which causes paralysis.

Less drastic deficiencies result in an appearance typical of the animal shown in Fig. 4-6, which is characterized by a listless appearance with a dull, dry hair coat; the appearance of the hair coat is not specific for P deficiency and is, very likely, simply a reflection of the fact that sick animals do not lick and care for their hair as do normal healthy animals. A P deficiency may also interfere with the utilization of vitamin A stores in the liver since a deficiency results in a reduced output of vitamin A in the milk without depleting liver stores (Thomas et al, 1953). In young, growing animals, teeth as well as bones will be less dense and less completely mineralized (Benzie et al, 1959).

Gain or milk production will be reduced in P-deficient animals; the older literature indicates that fertility is apt to be reduced in females. Morrow (1969) and Jakovac et al (1968) have presented data which indicate that fertility of dairy cows was markedly reduced when deficient in P. Supplementation with P resulted in prompt recovery of blood P levels and a restoration of normal fertility. It is of interest to note that, in each case, these problems occurred in areas where intensive agricultural practices were carried out, apparently resulting in depletion of soil P and, inevitably, producing plant tissues with insufficient P to adequately

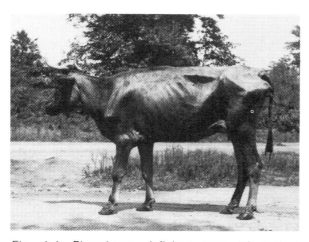

Fig. 4-4. Phosphorus deficient cow. "A typical advanced case of sweeny or stiffs in a cow on a P-deficient range. Note the stiffness and thin condition. Her bones were depleted to such an extent that the 13th rib was broken in a casual examination." Courtesy of R.B. Becker, Florida Agr. Expt. Sta.

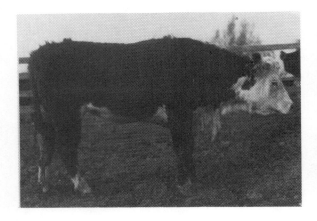

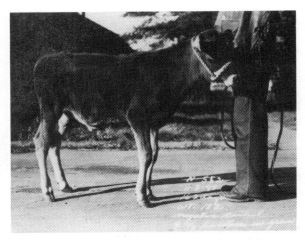

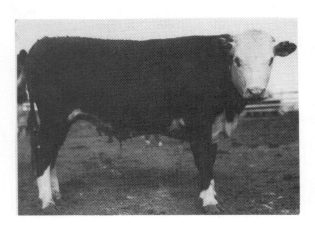

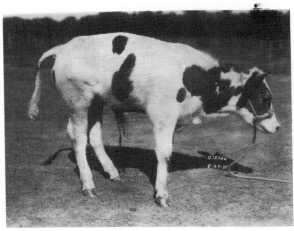

Fig. 4-6. P deficient (top) and adequately fed steer. The deficient steer received a ration with 0.12% P as compared to 0.18% for the other steer. Idaho Agr. Expt. Sta. photo. Courtesy of W.M. Beeson, Purdue Univ.

Fig. 4-7. Rickets in the calf. The upper picture shows a Jersey heifer with a moderate case of rickets. Note the foreward position of the knees. The lower picture shows a more severe case in which the legs are more deformed and the animal assumes a kypotic stance. Courtesy of J.W. Thomas, Michigan State Univ.

supply the amounts needed for high producing animals. Stevens et al (1971) found that ovarian dysfunction and a number of services per conception were higher in cows fed 0.4% P as compared to 0.6%. P supplementation of cows grazing native winter pastures in a P deficient area of Queensland, Australia, increased the percentage of cows exhibiting estrus 3 mo. after calving, but was not as effective as a combination of supplemental protein and P (Little, 1975).

In the young ruminant a deficiency of P and/or vitamin D will result in rickets. Typical symptoms of rickets are described in the NRC publication on dairy cattle. The condition is first manifested with a thickening and swelling in the metacarpal (pastern or ankle) or metatarsal bones or both. As the

case becomes more severe, the forelegs may bend forward or sideways, or both. The joints, especially the knee and hock, become swollen and stiff, the pastern straight, and the back humped. The animal assumes what is termed a kypotic stance (Fig. 4-7). In more severe cases synovial fluid accumulates in the joints. Posterior paralysis may occur as a result of fractured vertebra (Fig. 4-8). The advanced stages of the disease are marked by a stiffness of the gait, dragging of the hind feet, hyperirritability, tetany, labored and fast breathing, anorexia except for milk, weakness and retardation of growth. On autopsy the gall bladder is frequently distended by accumulation of viscous, ropy orange-yellow bile. Enteritis occasionally occurs.

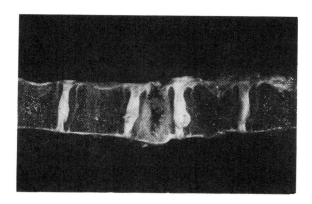

Fig. 4-8. Rickets in the calf. An isolated section of the spinal column showing a compressed fracture of the 1st lumbar vertebra as a result of incomplete mineralization of the bone. Courtesy of L.E. Krook, Cornell Univ.

Osteomalacia or osteofibrosis, a disease which may be caused by insufficient Ca, may also develop as a result of insufficient P in older animals. This disease (discussed in section of Ca) is characterized by a low bone ash and difficulty in movement, sore joints, fractures, etc. Inadequate protein intake has also resulted in a bone disorder resembling osteomalacia (Siebert et al, 1975).

Phosphorus Requirements

The ARC (1965) has done a detailed job of calculating the deposition of P in the tissues as related to body weight, rate of gain, the added increment due to pregnancy or lactation of sheep and cattle. They have expressed estimated requirements in terms of these various factors along with changing estimates of P retention, and have presented graphs showing how their recommendations compare to the NRC recommendations. Generally speaking, the suggested levels put forth by ARC are higher than NRC recommendations, particularly at heavier body weights. Sykes and Dingwall (1976) suggested that the P requirement for a 50 lb ewe carrying twins increases at the rate of 1.1 g/day during the first month and 2.5 g/day during the last month of gestation.

The type of recommendations put forth by the NRC are shown below:

Dairy cattle (% of dry matter)
    growing cattle, 0.50-0.26%
    dry pregnant cows, 0.26%
    lactation, 0.40-0.26%
    mature bulls, 0.18%

Beef Cattle (% of dry matter)
    growing-fattening cattle, 0.70-0.18%
    pregnant females, 0.23-0.18%
    lactating cows, 0.38-0.25%
    bulls, 0.26-0.18%
Sheep (% of diet)
    finishing lambs, 0.23-0.16%
    nonlactating ewes, 0.28-0.20%
    ewes, lactation, 0.37-0.34%
    rams, 0.19-0.16%

The adequacy of the recommendations put forth will, of course, depend upon the Ca:P ratio, the availability of the P sources, the presence of factors in the diet which may interfere with the P utilization, the performance of the animal and the amount of feed consumed by the individual.

Excess Phosphorus

There are no data, as such, which show that naturally occurring P compounds are toxic, with the possible exception of phosphates found in saline waters. There are, however, several situations in which a relative excess of P in relation to Ca may result in very detrimental situations. One of these is the effect of a relative excess of P in milk fever situations (Ch. 12) with the resultant inability of the animal to mobilize Ca at a sufficiently rapid rate. A second is the problem of urinary calculi (Ch. 13) which results in the deposition of phosphatic stones in the bladder. The third is the possibility of osteodystrophy in sheep which was mentioned in the section on Ca.

Other more concentrated chemicals may be toxic. For example, feeding 3 g of phosphoric acid resulted in decreased bodyweight and in death in Merino sheep (McMeniman, 1973). Supplementing with monosodium phosphate or bone flour had no effect, nor did increasing P intake from 1.5 to 2.3 g/day (cattle) by supplementing with Christmas Island rock phosphate (Siebert et al, 1975). Whether P, as such, is toxic or the result is from an imbalance of Ca and P, it behooves the nutritionist to be concerned with the dietary concentrations of these two elements and to take into consideration the various factors that influence their utilization by the body.

Supplemental Phosphorus Sources

A rather large amount of P in plant material is present as phytin or phytic acid (a hexaphosphoric acid ester or inositol). Utilization of this complex by non-ruminant animals is rather low, but in ruminants, the rumen microorganisms can hydrolyze phytin and utilize the P (Raun et al, 1956). Tillman and Brethour (1958) found that Ca phytate and monocalcium phosphate were utilized with about equal efficiency by sheep. True digestibility was 63% from the phytate and 70% from the inorganic source. Ellis and Tillman (1961) however, found that the true digestibility of phytin P from wheat bran was only 25% when fed to young sheep (4 mo. of age). Hansard and Barth (1962) have also shown that P from phytin was well utilized, although absorption of Ca was lower from the phytate. Approximately 100% of natural phytate phosphorus was hydrolyzed in 56 day old calves or 9 mo old steers (Nelson et al, 1976).

Various inorganic sources of P are the primary supplementary sources available for ruminant rations, although oil seed meals and middlings or bran from grain processing are important sources. Some of the research relating to utilization of P sources is reviewed briefly.

Ammerman et al (1957) compared various sources of inorganic P in steer and lamb balance trials. Based on P retention and maintenance of blood P, dicalcium phosphate, calcined defluorinated phosphate, bone meal, soft phosphate with colloidal clay, and Curacao Island phosphate were of equal value for steers. With lambs, dicalcium phosphate and Curacao phosphate were well utilized, but soft phosphate and defluorinated phosphate were poorly utilized. Gamma Ca phosphate was essentially unavailable. Vitreous Ca metaphosphate was utilized to some extent, but significantly less so than the orthophosphate (monocalcium phosphate). In an experiment with depleted calves, Arrington et al (1962) found the true digestibility of dicalcium phosphate, Curacao phosphate and defluorinated phosphate to be 98.2, 85.7 and 82.7%, respectively. Improvement in plasma P was 2.9. 2.6 and 2.6 mg/100 ml. Chicco et al (1965) used absorption and tissue deposition data of labeled P and celluloytic activity of rumen microorganisms to evaluate a variety of P sources. Based on both in vivo and in vitro data, Ca orthophosphate, Na ortho- and metaphosphate appeared to be equally available as sources of P. Na pyrophosphate was equal to these sources when solubility, cellulose digestion and tissue deposition were considered, but apparent absorption was lower. Ca pyrophosphate was essentially unavailable to rumen microorganisms and was the least available for absorption and tissue deposition. Ca metaphosphate was intermediate in absorption, tissue deposition and cellulose digestion. Long et al (1957) found that steamed bone meal, Curacao Island phosphate and dicalcium phosphate were of equal availability to growing heifers. O'Donovan et al (1965) found that dicalcium phosphate had higher apparent digestibility than defluorinated phosphate for steers. True digestibility was not different, although data indicated somewhat higher serum P for steers fed dicalcium phosphate. Hemingway and Fishwick (1975) reported that defluorinated rock phosphate was equal in value as a P supplement to dicalcium phosphate for sheep. In other work, Tillman and Brethour (1958) found phosphoric acid to be equal to dicalcium phosphate for steers and that Na pyrophosphate was equally available as monosodium phosphate. Vitreous Na metaphosphate caused an increased fecal excretion, but true digestibility of these sources was not different (Tillman and Brethour, 1958).

Two rock phosphate materials from Christmas Island were inferior to dicalcium and tricalcium sources for growing sheep (Fishwick, 1976). P retentions were 0.26 and 0.27 g/day for the naturally occurring rock phosphate materials, compared to 0.61 and 0.83 g/day for the dicalcium and tricalcium phosphate products, respectively. Blood P was lower for lambs fed the Christmas Island products, than for those fed the other two supplemental sources. The Christmas Island materials were low in F, but contained high levels of Fe and Al. Superphosphate is not a satisfactory P supplement for animals due to its high F content. Supplementation of lambs with superphosphate decreased daily gain and retention of Ca and P, compared to a standard P supplement (Agarwala et al, 1971). Calcination of superphosphate at 600° C for 2 hr lowered the F content from 23,500 to 1,600 ppm. Feeding this supplement did not result in the effects noted when untreated superphosphate was fed (Fig. 4-9). Low F Mexican rock phosphate was found to be equal in value to other P sources such as defluorinated phosphate and monosodium phosphate (Webb et al, 1975). A chemical mixture of 87% mono- and 13% dicalcium phosphate tended to be lower in value than other P supplements.

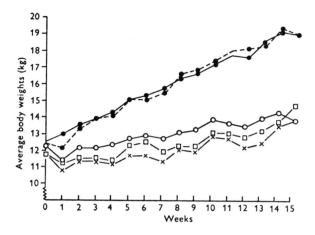

Fig. 4-9. Growth response of lambs fed 'different P supplements. •—•, fed "Supermindiff" mineral mixture; • - - •, fed calcined superphosphate; °—°, superphosphate; x—x, superphosphate + oral Co; □—□ superphosphate + parenteral B₁₂ . From Agawala et al (1971).

MAGNESIUM

Mg is an element that is very similar to Ca, both in terms of its chemical reactions and its functions in biological systems. In contrast to Ca, on which information has been available for many years, there is much more recent information dealing with Mg. The relatively large amount of research that has been done on Mg metabolism in ruminants is related to the involvement of Mg in the grass tetany syndrome (see Ch. 13).

Distribution in Tissues

Mg is widely distributed in plant and animal tissues, representing about 0.5-0.7% of bone ash. About 70% of total body Mg is present in the skeleton of ruminants in a Ca:Mg ratio of about 55:1. Serum Mg in adequately fed ruminants is usually on the order of 1.8 to 3 mg/100 ml. Pregnancy caused an increase in plasma Mg up to 3-4 wk before parturition and lactation caused a decrease in plasma level 3-4 wk after parturition in mature dairy cattle grazing ryegrass clover pasture in New Zealand (Grace, 1972). Pregnancy or lactation had no effect in sheep or young dairy cattle. About 33% of serum Mg appears to be bound to proteins such as albumin and globulin. Mg tends to be concentrated in the intracellular spaces of soft tissues and liver (16-26 mg/100 g). Striated

muscle contains relatively high concentrations, in cattle about 190 mg of Mg/kg of tissue as compared to about 100 mg in nervous tissue. The distribution of ^{28}Mg in the tissues of sheep following I.V. administration has been reported (Field, 1961; McAllese et al, 1961). There were marked variations in the specific activity between soft tissues, between bones and between parts of the same bone. The order of decreasing specific activity was bile, kidney, plasma, liver, spleen, skeletal muscle and bone (Field, ibid). Bovine and ovine milk contain about 125 and 175 mg/kg (ARC, 1965).

Absorption and Excretion

Sites of Absorption and Excretion. Field (1961) has reported on the specific activity of ^{28}Mg in the GI tract of sheep following I.V. administration. The percent of specific activity in various areas was: rumen, 4.4; abomasum, 7.2; 1st of 6 segments of the small intestine, 24.8; 2nd and 3rd segments, 22.0; 4th segment, 11.3; 5th segment, 9.25; 6th segment, 6.3; cecum, 8.1; colon, 6.4; and rectum, 0.6. The activity in the rumen might very well have been from Mg secreted in saliva. Other workers have shown that appreciable excretion of Mg in other species occurs in bile, gastric juices and pancreatic juice, so excretion (or secretion) at these sites may account for the high values noted by Field. Other studies (McAllese et al, 1961) in which ^{28}Mg has been used with lambs indicated maximum plasma isotope levels 12-14 hr after oral dosing. When the isotope was administered I.V., most of the ^{28}Mg was cleared in 8-10 hr. Absorption of Mg from the oral dose was considerably higher by Mg-deficient lambs than by those not deficient.

Smith (1962) has studied ion exchange in the GI tract of the milk-fed calf by using fistulas at various points with PEG (polyethylene glycol) as a marker. In calves 2-5 wk of age he found that net absorption of Mg up to the distal end of the small intestine was about 25% and that through the large intestine was 35% of intake. He concluded that the true percentage absorption of Mg up to the end of the small intestine decreased with increasing intake. Other work from that laboratory (Smith and McAllan, 1966) indicated that 34-74% of Mg in the intestine was non-ultrafilterable, although this form was in partial equilibrium with soluble forms. A reduction of pH in the ileum indicated that some precipitation of Mg occurred, partly dependent upon phosphate although other factors such as ammonium were implicated. Van't Klooster (1969) found that solubility of Mg decreased from the duodenum to the ileum.

Perry et al (1967) have also used markers (Cr_2O_3 or ^{144}Ce) to determine changes in Mg concentration throughout the GI tract of calves. Their data indicated a net secretion of Mg in the proximal small intestine when fed three different diets. However, there was little change indicated in the cecum and small intestines. When studying absorption in a loop of the upper ileum (Care and Van't Klooster, 1965), it was shown that Mg absorption occurred only when absorption was favored by concentration gradients. Similar information was shown for a loop in the mid-ileum. However, in a loop of the terminal ileum, no net absorption occurred, although it was shown that absorption could take place when ^{28}Mg was used. Phillipson and Storry (1965) have used similar procedures with somewhat similar results.

Recent research indicates that the stomach is the primary site for net Mg absorption in ruminating animals. Grace and MacRae (1972) reported net absorption of Mg from the stomach region of all sheep. They also found that endogenous Mg entering the small intestine exceeded the amount absorbed (Table 4-4). Marongiu (1971), Grace et al (1974) and Tomas and Potter (1976) confirmed the stomach to be the major site for Mg absorption, however net absorption occurred from the large intestine at high dietary intakes of Mg (Grace et al, 1974). Axford et al (1975) found that 34% of dietary Mg was absorbed in the stomach in sheep with no net absorption in the small intestine. It has been found that the principal site of Mg absorption from the ruminant stomach is the reticulo-rumen and that no significant absorption of Mg occurs from the omasum or abomasum of sheep (Tomas and Potter, 1976). They reported that post-ruminal absorption of Mg is not sufficient to maintain normal Mg status. Although no net absorption occurred from the small intestine, there was some absorption from the large intestine (Tomas and Potter, 1976).

These papers on Mg absorption from the ruminant GI tract, particularly that of Field, indicate that a substantial amount of Mg is either secreted into the proximal part of the intestine, probably by way of bile and perhaps through pancreatic juice or through the wall of the small intestine. Studies on uptake of Mg would indicate that most of the Mg had been absorbed by the end of the small intestine, although it seems likely that some further absorption may occur in the large intestine. The fact that Mg is secreted or excreted prior to an area where absorption occurs means that some of it should be recycled and utilized again. This should make for very efficient utilization of the element and would markedly reduce the amount likely to be needed in the diet.

With respect to fetal absorption of labeled Mg, Rogers et al (1964) presented data which indicate that fetal uptake was slow as compared to the dam or calves.

Effect of Other Nutrients on Mg Utilization. There are several pieces of evidence (see Ch. 13) indicating that high K rations may result in reduced apparent absorption of dietary Mg. Wise et al (1963) found that serum Mg was reduced when high levels of dietary P and low Ca were fed. It has also been reported that Mg absorption was not altered when organic P replaced inorganic P supplements (Dutton and Fontenot, 1967). Care and Van't Klooster (1965) suggested that Mg absorption in ileal loops was depressed by high concentrations of Ca in perfusion fluids; however, Wise et al did not notice any depression in serum Mg when high levels of Ca or high Ca and P were fed to calves. Lomba et al (1968) suggest that Mg absorption is enhanced by increasing Mg and Ca intake, while N and, to a lesser extent, fat, result in reduced absorption. High levels of Ca and P appear to lower Mg

Table 4-4. Quantities of Mg flowing through the GI tract of sheep fed dried grass.[a]

Consumed, g/day	1.67
Duodenum, g/day	
Observed	.90
Cr adjusted	1.09
Ileum, g/day	
Observed	1.01
Cr adjusted	1.17
Feces	1.04
Apparent absorption, %	38
Net absorption	
Stomach, % of total	89
Intestine, % of total	11

[a] From Grace and MacRae (1972)

absorption (Chicco et al, 1973; Pless et al, 1975; Nel, 1976), but the effect does not appear to be as severe as high levels of dietary K. Although fertilization of pastures with high levels of N appears to lower Mg utilization, high levels of dietary N per se do not appear to reduce absorption of Mg (Moore et al, 1972).

There is little evidence (Smith, 1958, 1962) to suggest that vitamin D has any influence on Mg absorption in ruminants except in one instance (Stillings et al, 1964) in which vitamin D improved the utilization of Mg in low N forages. Excessive water intake may be a factor in Mg retention since Suttle and Field (1960) found that water infused intra-ruminally increased urinary Mg by about 31% in sheep, although fecal losses were not affected.

Effect of Age and Hormones. Smith (1962) found that in young calves (2-5 wk of age) absorption of Mg in the large intestine decreased with age. In previous work (Smith, 1958) it was observed that fecal Mg excretion increased from 32% of dietary Mg at about 3 wk of age to 86% at about 16 wk of age after which it did not change appreciably. Net Mg absorption from forages by adult animals is usually on the order of 10-20%. Differences in age from 10 to 88 mo. did not affect apparent absorption or retention of Mg (Garces and Evans, 1971). Chicco et al (1973) found that plasma Mg and voluntary feed intake were reduced sooner in mature than younger sheep fed a low Mg diet. Field and Suttle (1967) have shown that the Mg content of the fetus increased with age.

There is little evidence to suggest that a variety of different hormone preparations have had any marked effect. Scott and Dobson (1965) found that I.V. infusions of aldosterone resulted in some reduction in serum Mg, but Moodie (1968) found no effect on blood levels or on absorption when several hormones from the posterior pituitary gland were administered to sheep. Care et al (1965) have shown that adrenalectomized sheep maintained with cortisone and deoxycortisone has little change in Mg status. Madsen et al (1975) reported data indicating higher absorption and retention of Mg in hypothyroid sheep.

It has been pointed out previously that a considerable amount of Mg is given off into the intestinal tract of ruminant species. Therefore, we might anticipate that the majority of the element excreted would be by way of the fecal route. In the case of young calves, Blaxter et al (1954) found that urinary Mg did not vary greatly and represented only a small percentage (usually < 5%) of combined fecal and urinary excretion even when some calves were in a negative Mg balance. Hutton et al (1965) have carried out Mg balance studies with milking cows consuming Mg at the rate of 0.1 g/kg of live weight. In this trial they found that 80% was excreted via feces, 12% was found in urine and 8% either in milk or retained in the body. In lactating beef cows it has been shown that urinary Mg was highly related to the amount of Mg fed, but no data were given on fecal Mg (O'Kelley and Fontenot, 1969). This is in contrast to the conclusions of Lomba et al (1968) who suggested that urinary losses of Mg were not related to Mg intake and digestibility.

In the case of studies with sheep, Stillings et al (1964) found that Mg excretion on low N forages resulted in 82% excreted via feces and 13% via urine. Comparable values on high N forage were 88% and 10.7%, respectively. In this case total Mg excretion varied from 133 to 166 mg/day, not much different to be sure. When sheep were fed semi-purified diets, Dutton and Fontenot (1967) found that 36 to 42% of total Mg was excreted via urine. Perhaps the difference here may be partly related to availability of Mg salts in the purified diet. McAllese et al (1961) have published data on lambs given ^{28}Mg both orally and I.V. When control lambs were given an I.V. dose (adequate intake of Mg), 60% of the isotope was recovered in urine as compared to 9% when given an oral dose. Mg deficient lambs secreted < 5% in urine and < 4% when given an oral dose. Decreased absorption of Mg from feeding a high K level was accompanied by lower urinary excretion of Mg (Newton et al, 1972) and a high correlation was observed between absorbed and urinary Mg (Chicco et al, 1972). It seems likely that the relative amount of Mg that is excreted in urine must be related to solubility and absorption as well as the total intake.

Utilization of Different Mg Sources

There is little doubt that Mg may be utilized less efficiently from some vegetative sources than from hays, other dry feeds or inorganic sources. As an example Care et al (1965) demonstrated that changing sheep from a hay diet to lush grass resulted in reduced serum Mg and a slower Mg turnover. Likewise, Stillings et al (1964) found that

Table 4-5. Effect of different Mg sources on mineral retention.[a]

Item	Magnesium supplement		
	None	Dolomitic limestone	Magnesium oxide
Mg intake, g/day	4.85	14.4	13.5
Mg excretion, g/day			
Fecal	2.28	10.5	6.50
Urinary	1.56	0.97	24.92
Mg absorption, % of intake	52.9	27.3	51.5
Mg availability from supplement, %		14.3	51.1
Ca intake, g/day	19.7	19.3	19.7
Ca retention, g/day	4.5	2.4	5.4
P intake, g/day	12.5	12.5	12.5
P retention, g/day	4.1	3.5	4.9
Dry matter digestibility, %	69.0	60.0	70.0

[a] From Gerken and Fontenot (1967)

utilization of Mg was less in high N forage than in low N forages. Other examples of this type are discussed in Ch. 13.

With respect to inorganic sources of Mg, Stewart and Moodie (1956) found that sheep absorbed Mg from the nitrate salt more quickly than from Mg sulfate. Gerken and Fontenot (1967) have compared utilization of Mg from dolomitic limestone vs that from Mg oxide when fed to steers. The availability of Mg was estimated to be 14% from the dolomitic limestone vs 52% from Mg oxide, thus indicating a marked difference (see Table 4-5). Feeding dolomitic limestone also resulted in a marked depression in digestibility of energy. Subsequent work from that same laboratory (Moore et al, 1971) indicated that the lower availability of Mg from dolomitic limestone, as compared to Mg oxide or Mg carbonate, was associated with an increase in passage rate through the GI tract. When working with sheep, Ammerman et al (1972) calculated the true absorption from Mg carbonate, Mg oxide, Mg sulfate and mangesite to be 72, 73, 78 and 14%, respectively. Net retention followed the same trends as the data on absorption. Apparent absorption of Mg from magnesium oxide and magnesium phosphate was similar, when these were fed to growing sheep (Fishwick and Hemingway, 1973); however, apparent absorption was lower from a calcium magnesium phosphate than from magnesium oxide. Hemingway and Ritchie (1969) have reported that Mg "bullets"

composed of Mg, Al and Cu were utilized by suckling calves; the bullets were dissolved in the rumen over a 3 wk period.

Magnesium Deficiency

Acute Mg deficiencies in the rat results in vasodilation manifested by erythema and hyperemia, accompanied by increasing neuromuscular hyperirritability culminating in generalized seizures. Chronic deficiency results in alopecia, skin lesions, hematomas of the ear and swollen hyperemic gums. Inflammatory necrotic foci develop in the small blood vessels and these foci become fibrotic and are widely distributed in body tissues. Calcium casts may be seen in the convoluted tubules in the kidneys.

In ruminants a deficiency in young animals may develop in animals restricted to a milk diet. Blaxter et al (1954) and Blaxter and Rook (1954) have described such deficiencies. The symptoms observed did not resemble those in the rat. No hyperemia, vasodilation or hair or skin changes were observed. The first unequivocal sign was a retracted head (opisthotonus) which resembles that seen in thiamin deficiency (Fig. 4-10), although thiamin treatment did not alleviate it. The gait was ataxic and the calves frequently carried their ears backward and slightly downwards. The calves were hypersensitive to tactile or sound stimuli. Later, muscle tremors were observed which finally gave way to convulsions. Stamping of the feet and violent head retraction were observed prior to convulsions.

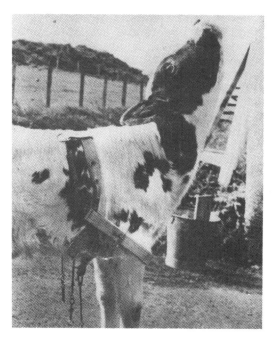

Fig. 4-10. Mg-deficient calf fed a liquid diet containing 0.5 mg of Mg/100 ml. Note the retracted position of the head which resembles a thiamin deficiency. From Blaxter et al (1954).

Animals that died usually did so during convulsions. No marked postmortem findings were observed except extensive hemorrhaging. They found that it was necessary to deplete calves of ca. one third of body Mg in order to cause convulsions. Subsequent data (Blaxter and Rook, 1955) indicated that Mg deficiency in calves resulted in an increased heat production and a fall in energy retention. The increased heat production was apparently due to tonic muscular activity and not to an increased heat increment. Increased levels of blood pyruvic acid were observed.

Martin et al (1964) found that Mg deficiency resulted in a reduced appetite, changes in the rumen flora, and a marked reduction in digestibility in vivo and cellulose digestion in vitro. Similar results were reported in sheep (Ammerman et al, 1971). Larvor et al (1965) observed that deficient calves were slightly anemic and had jaundice, with an increase of bilirubin and decreased glucose-6-phosphate dehydrogenase in the red blood cells. Kiesel and Alexander (1966) have also observed jaundice in sheep with some degree of impaired clotting of the blood. Liver damage was seen in some sheep and there was a reduced amount of serum albumin and globulins. Kiesel et al (1969) reported other changes in serum enzymes. Hjerpe (1968) found that serum Ca and P levels were increased in Mg deficient sheep although net retention was not changed. Other biochemical changes observed in the grass tetany syndrome are discussed in Ch. 13.

Magnesium Requirements

The Mg requirements of different classes of ruminant animals have not been well defined and experimental results differ, partly because different types of diets have been utilized in research studies. In some of the older literature (Blaxter et al, 1954) requirements suggested for calves were on the order of 20-30 mg/kg of body weight, or 0.07-0.08% of the diet (Hawkins, 1954).

The ARC (1965) have discussed the requirements of Mg by ruminants in some detail. Their estimated requirements for some classes of ruminants are shown:

Cattle: growing animals, 50-400 kg
0.33 kg gain/day, 0.4-6.6 g
0.50 kg gain/day, 0.5-7.0 g
1.0 kg gain/day, 0.8-8 g
during pregnancy
young cattle, 6.5-8.0 g/day
mature cattle, 7.8-9.4 g/day
added lactation requirement
10 kg milk/day, 13.8 g/day
20 kg milk/day, 20.1 g/day
30 kg milk/day, 26.4 g/day

Sheep: lambs (values given for different rates of gain at different weights)
14-47 mg/kg live weight/day
pregnant ewes
12-20 mg/kg live weight

O'Kelley and Fontenot (1969) have suggested that beef cows need about 21, 22 and 18 g/day during early, mid and late lactation, respectively. These latter values would be comparable to 0.18, 0.19 and 0.16% of Mg in the dry matter of the ration. These requirements are considerably higher than those suggested by Blaxter and McGill (1956) and higher than suggested by Rook et al (1964) who found that 9.1 g of Mg/day maintained normal serum Mg in lactating dairy cows. Other dietary factors such as K, N, chelating factors in forage, and relative solubility of the Mg sources may have a considerable effect on the amount of Mg required in the diet. O'Kelley and Fontenot (1973) reported that the Mg requirement for pregnant beef cows was considerably lower than the values given previously for lactating beef cows. The requirement appears to be 8.5, 7.0 and 9.0 g Mg/day at 155, 200 and 255 days gestation, respectively.

Toxicity. With respect to Mg toxicity, there is little information available in the literature. In monogastric species it is known that a high intake of Mg salts will result in diarrhea. With respect to ruminants, Pierce (1959) has shown that a $MgCl_2$ concentration of 0.1% along with 1.2% NaCl in water had no adverse effect on sheep. When 0.2 or 0.5% $MgCl_2$ was given with 1.05 or 0.7% NaCl, there was a reduction in feed intake and occasional diarrhea, particularly with the 0.5% $MgCl_2$ solutions.

SODIUM

Sodium in the Tissues

Na is generally considered to be primarily confined to the extracellular fluids (plasma, cerebrospinal and interstitial fluids); however, an appreciable amount of the body store is found in bone or cartilage (Forbes, 1962). Data indicate that 30-45% of the body Na is found in the skeleton in man, 40-45% in the dog, monkey and rabbit, and 21% in the rat. Bone Na appears to be firmly bound to the inorganic crystals and appears to be present in the extracellular phase of bone and cartilage. Na is found in muscle at levels of 20-45 meq/kg of fat-free muscle of which 30-35% is intracellular Na. In red blood cells of cattle and sheep, 70-80 meq/kg is found, whereas plasma may have 120-140 meq/l. (ca. 300 mg/100 ml. The Na in erythrocytes of ruminants is considerably higher than that found in species such as man (4-17 meq/kg), rabbits and rats, but less than that found in some carnivores such as dogs and cats (104-106 meq/kg). Na ions in plasma make up 90% or more of the bases found. Ruminants also produce saliva with considerably more Na than some species; mixed ruminant saliva averages about 180 meq/kg. Low dietary intake of Na is not consistently reflected in low plasma Na. Hagsten and Perry (1975) reported a trend for higher plasma Na in lambs during Na depletion. Na content of the dura mater tended to be lower in calves fed a low vitamin A level (Mikkilineni et al, 1973).

Absorption and Excretion

Sites of Absorption and Excretion. Data on absorption and excretion of Na in ruminant species are less extensive than for some of the other mineral elements; nevertheless, a fair number of papers are available. Smith (1962), using PEG as a marker, found that the net exchange of Na in young calves was about 40% of intake up to the end of the small intestine, but absorption was almost complete in the large intestine. There was no marked effect of age in these studies. Perry et al (1967), using markers, found a net secretion in the upper small intestine. They estimated that an average of 133 g of Na were secreted in the upper small intestine daily. During passage through the lower gut, 87% of the Na was absorbed from the small intestine and, essentially, the other 13% from the cecum and large intestine. Mylrea (1966) calculated that 53% of the Na in the small intestine was absorbed, considerable amounts being secreted into the upper part of the small intestine of calves. Van't Klooster (1969) found that there was a net absorption of 500 g of Na in the small intestine of cows. Of that which passed into the large intestine, about 88% was absorbed there. Goodal and Kay (1965) have studied absorption in the cecum and large intestine by means of sheep fitted with a re-entrant cannula in the terminal ileum of sheep. They found that the Na concentration varied as much as 29 fold in the ileal samples. By comparing ileal and fecal samples, however, they estimated that 96% of the ileal Na was absorbed in the large intestine. Thus, these experiments, although of a limited nature, indicate rather complete reabsorption of Na in the large intestine, a mechanism which provides a means of drastically reducing the dietary N requirement.

Route of Excretion. The papers that have just been cited indicate that Na absorption in the gut is relatively complete. However, it might be of interest to look at some other work that shows the relative excretion of Na via urine or feces.

Perry et al (1966) have used [28]Na in studies with dairy heifers. Four-day excretions of oral [28]Na averaged 2.3% of the dose in urine and 1.8% in feces, or 56% via urine and 44% via feces. The average 4-day fecal excretion of I.V. [28]Na was 1.3%. Administration of K bicarbonate did not influence excretion of oral Na, but it did increase urinary excretion of I.V. doses, resulting in 4.4% urinary vs. 1.5% for controls. Kemp (1964) reported that the availability of Na from fresh herbage was 85% of which 15% was excreted in feces. Feeding 400 g of KCl/day caused an increase in the Na excretion via urine and less via feces with no net change in excretion. Renkema et al (1962) have shown that fecal excretion of Na was greatly increased as the intake increased and that there was a reciprocal change in fecal Na and K.

Nelson et al (1955) studied the effect of high salt intake (6% of the diet) on Na excretion and on digestibility of nutrients by cattle and sheep. When steers consumed 3.5 g of Na, 1.42 g were excreted via feces and 1.90 via urine. When Na intake increased to 94.4 g, fecal excretion was 3.5 and urinary excretion was 82.2 g, indicating that most of the excess Na was absorbed and excreted via the urine. About the same situation was found for sheep, except that urinary excretion was a much larger percentage of the total on a basal ration, being 0.22 g via feces and 3.04 g via urine. Devlin and Roberts (1965) fed sheep purified rations which contained 4, 44 or 129 meq. of Na. Urinary excretion averaged 61.6, 68.3 and 76.2% of total excretion, values which were generally less than those reported by Nelson et al. Renkema et al (1962) fed cattle either 3 or 40 g of Na daily. Concentration of Na in feces was about 10X as great with the high Na intake as with the low intake. In a second experiment with a cow, excretion of Na in feces increased about 4-fold when supplemental Na was given; however, almost as much additional Na was excreted in feces as in urine. Elam and Autry (1961) found that 74.9% of Na was excreted via the urine when 1.8% NaCl was fed in the diet of steers. Some of their data are shown in Table 4-6. Notice the effect of NaCl intake on retention of K, particularly. Wilson and Dudzinski (1973) showed that addition of 1.5 or 2.0% Na to drinking water did not affect Na excretion by sheep. The increased Na intake was excreted via the urine. Tomas et al (1973)

Table 4-6. Effect of NaCl intake on excretion of various minerals by steers.[a]

Item	NaCl intake		
	1%	4%	8%
Sodium			
fecal, g	5.9	7.1	10.2
urinary, g	17.1	47.5	126.2
% retained	11.9	36.8	7.9
Chloride			
fecal, g	3.2	3.6	6.8
urinary, g	46.0	94.3	217.2
% retained	0.9	24.5	8.1
Calcium			
fecal, g	16.9	14.7	13.1
urinary, g	0.2	0.1	1.0
% retained	-4.4	19.1	21.2
Phosphorus			
fecal, g	14.0	11.1	10.9
urinary, g	4.8	4.9	9.2
% retained	6.2	20.0	-1.1
Potassium			
fecal, g	7.0	4.2	5.2
urinary, g	35.2	62.7	63.8
% retained	25.9	-30.7	-22.9
Magnesium			
fecal, g	8.9	7.7	7.6
urinary, g	1.0	1.4	1.5
% retained	24.9	28.3	23.8

[a] From Elam and Autry (1961)

showed that adding 0.8 or 1.3% NaCl increased fecal excretion of Na in sheep, but most of the increased Na excretion was via the urine (Table 4-7).

Table 4-7. Excretion of Na in sheep given water with 0, 0.8 or 1.3% NaCl.[a]

Item	Na in water, %		
	0	0.8	1.3
Fecal excretion, mM/day	24.2	42.5	60.1
Urinary excretion, mM/day	52.6	488.5	977.3
Balance, mM/day	-2.6	12.1	14.3
Urinary, % of total excretion	67.6	92.1	94.3

[a] From Tomas et al (1973)

These experiments, then, would indicate that Na excretion via the feces may be quite variable. The data show that the Na:K ratio has a marked influence on the relative route of excretion as it does on saliva. We could also conclude that probably a bigger percentage of Na will be excreted via feces when the intake of Na is low, reflecting the irreducible amount that is to be expected in fecal excretions. On the other hand, when large amounts of Na are administered, most of the increased excretion is via the urine.

Other Factors Influencing Excretion

Although Na may be very efficiently absorbed from the small and large intestines, some excretion via urine occurs even on diets containing very small quantities of Na. Data in the paper of Devlin and Roberts (1965) show an excretion of about 18 meq/day (30 day average) when the intake by sheep was only 4 meq/day. Consequently, we must conclude that even ruminant animals cannot control excretion completely. The half-life of radiosodium in humans appears to be about 11 days (Forbes, 1962). In the kidney of man, about 99.5% of Na in the glomerular filtrate may be reabsorbed. Kidney excretion is limited, however, as evidenced by the fact that many mammals cannot exist on saline waters such as sea water. The problem appears to be that they cannot concentrate the Na in urine sufficiently to remove it from the blood at a rapid enough rate. In other words, the osmolarity of urine will be less than that of sea water. In ruminants it has been shown that an increase in water intake will result in an increased urinary excretion of Na (Suttle and Field, 1966). Dobson and others (1966) have studied the effect of some dietary changes on Na balance, the results generally indicating that Na retention on frozen grass was essentially equal to intake even though intake was low. When changed to a ration of meal and hay, Na retention increased although urinary levels were reduced. When changed back to the frozen grass, Na excretion via the urine increased. It is not possible to explain these facts with the information at hand, but it may be partly due to the likely increase in water intake and its effect on Na excretion observed by Suttle and Field. Protein and/or energy intake may be a factor since Horrocks (1964) reported data indicating an improvement in Na retention by steers when a low quality roughage was supplemented with a protein-grain pellet.

The adrenal hormones are known to have a very important effect on Na (and K) excretion. Aldosterone is particularly potent. The administration of adrenocortical hormones such as aldosterone usually leads to Na retention (and K loss) which is reflected in decreased excretion of Na in the urine. Removal of the adrenal glands produces the opposite effect, and it has been demonstrated that adrenalectomized animals require much larger amounts of Na in their diet. The adrenal hormones stimulate kidney resorption of Na as well as intestinal absorption and reduce excretion in sweat (Forbes, 1962; Blair-West et al, 1965). Widths of cortex and zona glomerulosa were greater in steers fed a diet with .003% Na than those given supplementary Na at a level of 3.1 g/day (Morris and Gartner, 1971). Histological studies of adrenal cortices of lambs fed low Na diets (.01%) showed wider zona glomerulosa (Hagsten and Perry, 1975).

Sodium Deficiency

Na deficiency may develop as a result of inadequate intake, from excessive losses from the GI tract during diarrhea or vomiting, in cases of renal insufficiency, adrenocortical failure, or due to excessive sweating. In the ruminant animal inadequate intake is presumed to be the most important factor, although diarrhea is probably a big factor in young animals. Na deficiency can be a serious problem in ruminants, although the likelihood is recognized and NaCl is usually fed to domestic animals. Its importance in wild species is not known at this time.

As a Na deficiency develops, the Na content of plasma, saliva and other fluids is decreased and the K content generally is increased. This has been demonstrated to be under the control of aldosterone and is, presumably, a mechanism for conserving the body supply of Na (Blair-West et al, 1965).

Of the relatively recent papers on Na deficiency in ruminants, one of the better ones is the report of Smith and Aines (1959) dealing with dairy cows. The first clinical deficiency symptom noted was a craving for salt as evidenced by reactions when cows were teased with salt. This developed within a 2-wk period after the start of an experiment. After approximately 2 mo., cows showed signs of pica which was evidenced by licking of the hands and clothing of herdsmen, consumption of soil soaked with urine or the runoff from a manure pile, and licking of barn walls. Deficient cows were observed drinking urine from NaCl supplemented cows. A decrease in body weight was noted after 10-11 mo. and was correlated with a loss of appetite. Roughage consumption—first silage and then hay—declined before concentrate consumption and, eventually, there was complete anorexia. Deficient cows assumed a gaunt, "tucked-up" appearance and developed a dry, harsh skin (particularly on the neck), the hair became unkempt, and they were listless (Fig. 4-1). In some cows tetany and a staggered gait in the hind legs was evident. Some cows collapsed and died and in others irregular heart action was detected. In one cow, blood values on the day of collapse were 208 mg/100 ml Na (vs normal of 250) and 275 mg/100 ml Cl (vs normal of ca. 360). Enlarged adrenals were noted in some cows, indicating hyperactivity.

Hawkins et al (1965) did not mention depraved appetites in a study with dairy steers and papers by Devlin and Roberts (1965) or McClymont et al (1957) did not mention pica, nor did Denton and Sabine (1961, 1963) other than for a craving for Na salts. In the latter reports the authors found that sheep made deficient with parotid salivary fistulas showed a marked craving for Na salts and would usually take NaHCO$_3$ in preference to NaCl. They found that Na deficient sheep have the ability to consume enough Na in solutions to replete the deficiency and that they did not usually over consume. Their sheep would quit drinking a Na solution after consuming enough Na to replete body stores—much sooner than it could possibly have been absorbed.

Many animal experiments dealing with Na have utilized NaCl in the studies, thus it is possible that some of the deficiency symptoms reported may be a combination of Na and Cl deficiencies. Aines and Smith (1957) have investigated this problem in lactating cows. In the experiment reported, salt deficient cows were fed NaCl, NaHCO$_3$, or MgCl$_2$. When NaCl was fed, increases in milk production, body weight and roughage consumption occurred. Sodium bicarbonate feeding resulted in increases in production, although less than with NaCl. MgCl$_2$ failed to elicit a response. These data along with those of Smith and Aines (1959) would indicate that Na was more limiting than Cl.

In a short term experiment with calves made deficient with parotid fistulas (Whipp et al, 1966), it was found that the Na:K ratio in saliva decreased from 27.6 to <0.5 within a 2 wk period. Plasma Na concentration decreased from an initial value of 141 to 125 meq/l. during the same time, although no changes in plasma K were detected. Feeding a Na deficient diet decreased Na concentration and increased K concentration in saliva (Morris and Gartner, 1971). Na:K ratio in saliva of Na deficient cattle was < 1, compared to values between 11 and 21 for those fed 3.1 g Na/day. European work with identical twin dairy cows (Helfferich et al, 1966; Bertzback et al, 1966; Pfeffer et al, 1966) has shown that cows on a low Na intake (3.2 and 5.5 g/day) lost a total of 190 g of body Na during the first 7 wk of lactation, but then milk production fell rapidly and Na equilibrium was established. Loss of Na in urine and feces was low although milk concentration was almost normal as was serum. There was some indication that the low Na diet resulted in a negative Ca balance. Plasma volume was low and hematocrit values increased. Body losses of Cl in the 1st 50 days of lactation amounted to about 280 g and weight fell rapidly. Serum Cl declined from 100 to <90 meq/l. Skydsgaard (1968) suggests that analyses of salivary Na and K can be used to diagnose Na deficiency in cattle. He found the normal Na:K ratio to be from 17:1 to 25:1 and suggests, if it is between 10:1 and 15:1 that Na deficiency can be suspected.

Available data indicate that sheep are more resistant to Na deficiency than cattle, although comparisons between wether sheep and lactating cows are hardly to be expected to give good interspecies comparisons since it is known that salt requirements of lactating cows are greater than for dry cows. Devlin and Roberts (1965) found that Na deficiency resulted in reduced feed intake and increased N excretion, but no other

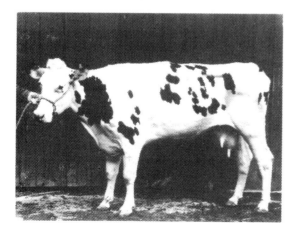

Fig. 4-11. Salt deficient cow. Note the dehydrated appearance of the animal. From Smith and Aines (1959).

symptoms were observed. As noted previously, Denton and Sabine observed a craving for Na-containing salts. Phillips and Sundaram (1966) have studied Na depletion in pregnant ewes with parotid fistulas. They found that the Na content of saliva declined from 173 to 38 meq/l. and that of K rose from 5 to 96 meq/l. Plasma volume fell, its Na content fell from 150 to 135 meq/l. and the K fell from 4.6 to 4.2 meq/l. Some decline was observed in fetal plasma and amniotic fluid, but there was no apparent change in K. Morris and Peterson (1975) found that a constant Na:K in parotid saliva in lactating ewes was reached when the ewes received 820 mg Na/kg diet which represents about 38% of the NRC requirement. Cows fed low Na levels showed physiological adaptation manifested in decreases of Na in urine, feces, milk, plasma, saliva and rumen fluid (Van Leeuwen, 1970). Na depletion by acute cannulation of a parotid duct in sheep resulted in decreases in salivary, urinary and plasma Na (Abraham et al, 1976).

Sodium Requirements

Smith and Aines (1959) calculated that lactating cows need about 30 g of supplemental NaCl for the production of 20 kg of milk. In their experiments they fed 15 or 60 g of NaCl/day. Their analytical data indicated a Na intake in feed of 8-15 g/day, so those cows getting 15 g of NaCl were apparently getting from 14-21 g of Na and those receiving 60 g of NaCl were receiving 31.6-36.8 g of Na. Production responses indicated that the lower intake was not adequate. Horrocks (1964) calculated 0.5 g of Na was the minimum amount that could be excreted via urine and feces when steers were fed maintenance rations of hay. Diets with 0.2 g of Na/day were shown to be inadequate as compared to diets with approximately 10 g of supplemental Na/day. Morris and Gartner (1971) suggested that the Na requirement for steers fed a 50% roughage ration was 31 g/day, based on Na:K ratio in saliva and ruminal fluid, width of adrenal cortex zona glomerulosa, daily feed intake and rate of gain. A level of up to 168 g K/day did not affect the Na requirement of growing steers (Morris and Gartner, 1975).

The NRC recommends 0.10% salt in the diet dry matter for beef cattle. Morris and Murphy (1972) reported results indicating that 80 to 110 kg beef calves gaining 0.6 kg/day require 1.2 to 3.4 g Na/day. According to NRC the salt requirement of growing lambs approximates 0.4% of diet dry matter. Morris and Peterson (1975) concluded that the NRC values for lactating ewes was excessive and suggested an allowance of 870 mg/kg diet for maintaining normal Na:K ratio in parotid saliva. McClymont et al (1957) got a response in gain on rations of oats and alfalfa chaff when 0.25% NaCl was added to diets containing 0.009-0.62% Na and 0.05-0.42% Cl. Devlin and Roberts (1965) suggested that Na requirements for lambs were on the order of 1.0 g/day or 2.6 g of NaCl. Hagsten et al (1975) reported that the total salt requirement for fattening lambs was approximately 0.4%. They indicated that since typical diets would supply the equivalent of 0.2% salt, the recommended supplemental level is approximately 0.2%. NRC estimated the Na requirement of milk cows at 0.18% (0.46% salt) of dry matter. Salt requirements of beef cattle appear to be higher on high roughage rations (Cunha, 1976).

Salt Toxicity

Na deficiencies in ruminants may frequently be a problem, probably more so for wild species in the USA than for domestic animals. Excess Na, however, may also be a serious problem, particularly when water supplies are saline. According to Forbes (1962) an acute excess of Na results in a gain in body water and an increase in body fluid volume. Large excesses, such as may occur when sea water is consumed, result in hypertonicity of extracellular fluid, intracellular dehydration, and eventually in death due to the fact that the maximal concentration of Na that the kidney can achieve is below that of the fluid ingested.

Salt mixed with protein supplements has been used as a means of limiting intake of protein supplements for wintering animals. Data reported by Nelson et al (1955) indicated that rations containing up to 6% NaCl were not detrimental to cattle or sheep; however, Sandals (1978) reported total toxicity in 2 of 6 animals following sudden access to a protein supplement containing 5% salt. Elam (1961) and Elam and Autry (1961) found that 8% NaCl decreased digestibility of organic nutrients when fed to cattle; there was a variable effect on other mineral elements. The lower level of NaCl (1 or 2%) increased Ca retention. P retention was higher on intermediate NaCl levels; Mg retention was not affected, although there was a substantial increase in urinary K excretion. Meyer et al (1955) fed NaCl at levels of 0.66-12.8% of the ration to growing lambs and found no detrimental effect on digestibility or growth. Carcass grades were depressed somewhat at the highest level of salt intake. The kidneys were larger in lambs receiving 9.4 or 12.8% NaCl, but there was no effect on adrenal weight, blood albumin, or hematocrit. Steers also tolerated a level of 9.3% NaCl without adverse effects.

Feeding a barley-NaCl mixture containing 30% NaCl at such a level (260 g/day) to supply 3.1 g Na/day reduced dry matter and organic matter intake and organic matter digestibility in sheep (Moseley and Jones, 1974). Liveweight gain and efficiency of utilization of organic matter were also lowered, but self feeding steers grazing tropical forages a supplement containing 30% salt did not alter gains or apparent digestibility of dry matter, cellulose or protein (Chicco et al, 1971).

Cardon (1953) and Johnson et al (1959) found no effect on in vitro cellulose digestion by high additions of salt or on in vivo digestion by steers (Cardon, ibid). However, Wilson (1967) found that water with 2% NaCl reduced in vitro rumen digestion by sheep. Concentration of protozoa and selenomonods in the rumen were decreased from feeding 150 g NaCl/day to sheep (Hemsley et al, 1975). Based on measurements of DNA and polysaccharide it appeared there was a trend for a reduction of total microbial population in the rumen of sheep drinking a 1.3% NaCl solution (Potter et al, 1972). However, the rumen microflora adapted to high concentrations of NaCl in rumen of animals drinking the high NaCl solution.

When studying the salt tolerance of sheep, Pierce (1957, 1959) provided water with 1 to 2% NaCl. NaCl at 1% had no adverse effects; 1.5% was detrimental to some sheep; and 2% was detrimental to all. There was a decrease in food consumption and body weight of affected animals. Several sheep on 2% became very emaciated and weak, and some died. Occasional diarrhea was noted. There was no effect on plasma K, Na, Ca or Mg but Cl concentration was significantly higher in the 2% group. In another experiment 0.20 or 0.50% Mg chloride was given with 1.05 or 0.69% NaCl in water; these combinations were detrimental to some sheep. The principal effect was a reduced feed intake and occasional diarrhea. Wilson (1966) noted similar results in an experiment in which 10-20% NaCl was given in feed or 1.2-2.0% in water. Feed intake de-

creased as salt concentration increased and water intake increased in relation to the amount of NaCl ingested, irrespective of diet or means of ingestion (food or water). When sheep were introduced suddenly to 2% NaCl in water (Wilson, 1967), intake of feed fell sharply for 3 days and then increased again and within 5 to 7 days reached a stable value about 160 g below the intake when given fresh water. In another experiment sheep were fed diets containing from 7.5 to 15% added NaCl (Wilson and Hindley, 1968). When access to water was restricted to once daily, there was a reduction in feed intake, the reduction being more severe with the more salty diets. Merino sheep drank less (5 l./day) than Border Leicester sheep (7.6 l./day).

Potter (1963) found that sheep responded to saline water (1.3% NaCl) by a slight increase in plasma K and Cl and increased urinary excretion of Na and Cl and somewhat more K. Urinary pH was increased and osmolarity reduced. No change in kidney function was detected. In subsequent research (Potter, 1968) sheep adapted to water with 1.3% NaCl were infused with 10% NaCl solutions and compared with those given rain water to drink. The sheep which drank rain water were often affected by the infusion and exhibited signs resembling K deficit. The diuresis produced by infusions was more prolonged in rain water sheep, and the excretion of Na and Cl was greater in those maintained on saline water. Plasma K was reduced in all sheep and urinary excretion of K increased. Hemsley (1975) reported large increases in wool growth of sheep from feeding 130 g NaCl/day to sheep fed a 37% crude protein diet. They suggested that the effects of salt were due to reduced rumen degradation of protein.

Weeth et al (1960, 1961, 1962, 1968) have studied the effect of excess salt consumption by cattle in various situations. In one experiment with heifers they found that 1% NaCl in water was tolerated very well, whereas 2% was definitely toxic and caused severe anorexia, weight loss, and dehydration. Animals were lethargic and rectal temperatures were lowered. Blood serum Na was elevated, as was K (winter time). In another experiment heifers just maintained their weight on 1.5% NaCl and 1.75% was detrimental during the winter. In the summer, 1.2% salt water was toxic. Water consumption was increased 47 to 69%, respectively, by the addition of 1 and 1.2%

Table 4-8. Effect of watering when consuming tap or saline water.[a]

Item	Tap water			0.5% NaCl water		
	Ad lib	Once/day	Once/ 2 days	Ad lib	Once/day	Once/ 2 days
Hay consumption, kg/day	6.3	6.4	5.2	6.4	6.3	5.3
Water consumption						
kg/day	30.4	27.2	20.9	35.8	29.9	22.2
kg/kg of hay intake	4.82	4.25	4.02	5.59	4.75	4.19
Urine produced, kg/day	5.7	5.9	4.7	16.1	13.2	8.9
Urinary urea N, g/day	12.8	19.3	20.7	30.2	25.9	27.1
Urine osmolality, mOsmol/kg	780	871	863	680	781	926

[a] From Weeth et al (1968)

NaCl to the drinking water. Blood hematocrits increased and pulse and respiration rates were increased except during the hot part of the day. Further work (Weeth and Lesperance, 1965) showed that water with 1.5% NaCl resulted in increased urinary excretion of urea N by 37% over animals receiving tap water. Plasma osmolality increased from control values of 291 to 332 mOsmol/kg. The effect of intermittent watering with saline water has also been studied (Weeth et al, 1968). They found that watering once/day decreased water consumption when compared with ad libitum intake, and that watering every 2 days further decreased consumption of saline water. Some of the data presented in this paper are shown in Table 4-8. Note the effect of salt consumption on urine volume and urinary urea-N excretion. Requiring sheep to drink water with 2% salt for up to 4 years did not cause hypertension (Potter, 1972).

CHLORINE

Chlorine in the Tissues

The animal body contains about 0.10-0.11% Cl, and it has been estimated that less than 16% of body Cl is intracellular (Cotlove and Hogben, 1962; White et al, 1973). Normal plasma or serum values in ruminants are about 360-370 mg/100 ml (ca. 103 meq/l.) and about 220-260 mg/100 ml in whole blood. Values of 104 and 98 meq Cl/l. of plasma were obtained from 144 cattle and 20 sheep, respectively (Phillips, 1970). Muscle contains about 60 mg/100 ml and mixed ruminant saliva about 100 meq/l. Red

blood cells are estimated to have 55-64 meq/kg (humans); skin about 10-50 meq/kg and nervous tissues about 18 meq/kg. Chlorides are also found in large concentrations (80-125+ meq/l.) in gastric juices, gastric mucas, bile, pancreatic juice, intestinal secretions, synovial fluid, cerebrospinal fluid, and sweat.

Absorption and Excretion of Cl

Data published by Smith (1962) indicate that calves absorbed 80-95% of the dietary intake of Cl in the small intestine and that some further net absorption occurred in the large intestine. Goodall and Kay (1965) have studied absorption in the large intestine of sheep with the use of re-entrant cannulae in the terminal ileum. They found that there was a considerable variation in the concentration of Cl in the ileal effluent. Of the Cl that entered the large intestine, they calculated that 98% of it was absorbed. Care and Van't Klooster (1965) have studied absorption in sheep with the use of re-entrant cannula in various sites. Not much information was given on Cl, but they did conclude that there was little change in Cl concentration in the sites studied. Mylrea (1966) calculated that net absorption occurred in calves in the lower small intestine to the extent of about 80%. Other studies indicate that the digestion and utilization of chloride is not influenced by the amount of injected chloride at the time of the trial, but the most important fate of dietary chloride appears to be the necessity for cows to eliminate large amounts of K in the urine (Paquay et al, 1969).

Nelson et al (1955) found that steers and lambs excreted very little Cl in feces, average values showing that 98% of the Cl was excreted in urine. Elam and Autry (1961) found, however, that somewhat larger percentages of Cl were excreted in feces, the amount depending on the amount of Cl in the diet. With 1% added NaCl in the diet, 6.5% of the Cl was excreted via the feces. This value declined to 3% when the diet contained 8% NaCl. Tomas et al (1973) observed a small increase in Cl excretion in feces in sheep allowed access to a 1.3% NaCl solution (20.4 vs 38.8 mM/day), but a large increase in urinary excretion (271.3 vs 1184.5 mM/day). Adding salt at concentrations of 1.0 and 1.3% to drinking water caused distress at parturition to some of the ewes and neonatal mortality in the lambs (Potter and McIntosh, 1974). Adding salt to the water increased plasma levels of Na and K and lowered the levels of Ca and Mg.

Chloride Deficiency

Deficiency symptoms that can be attributed to Cl alone have not been described in ruminants since most feeds contain appreciable amounts. For example, the Cl content of cereal grains is 0.04 to 0.15%, that of protein supplements is about 0.10%, and dry forage on the order of 0.3 to 0.7%. Thus, most diets probably contain an abundant amount of Cl.

Early work suggests that, on a very low Cl intake, growth is retarded or lacking and animals are stunted. Whether the differences described for Na deficiency in sheep and those for NaCl in cattle may be ascribed to Cl remains a debatable question at the present time. The general opinion of most nutritionists seems to be that Na is a more limiting nutrient than Cl for ruminant animals. Data reported by Smith and Aines (1959) on urinary excretion of Cl indicate this since urinary Na reached minimal values long before Cl did.

Not much information is available concerning Cl requirement. The NRC bulletin on beef cattle states that the Na and the Cl requirement can be met by including 0.10% salt in dry diet matter. The data of Smith and Aines (1959) indicated that lactating dairy cows maintained normal blood Cl levels when fed 60 g of NaCl/day (36+ g of supplemental Cl) and had subnormal values when fed 15 g of NaCl (9.1 g of supplemental Cl). Intake of Cl from the feed ranged from about 70-125 g/day (plus supplemental Cl), thus an intake of about 80-125 g/day of Cl was indicated to be inadequate and a level of about 105-160 g/day was adequate.

POTASSIUM

There has been a renewed interest in the place of K in ruminant nutrition in recent years, partly because of the increased use of low forage rations for fattening cattle. These rations are borderline or deficient in K. A review of K as related to the nutrition and digestive physiology of ruminants is available (Ward, 1966).

Potassium in the Tissues

The majority of K in the body is found in the cells. White et al (1973) state that total K content of a 70 kg human adult is about 4,000 meq, of which only 70 meq is found in extracellular fluids. Data on the rat show that plasma has about 4-5 meq/l. and about 106 meq/kg for erythrocytes. The spleen of the rat is very high in K, being about 265 meq/kg (Wilde, 1962). In the ruminant animal normal values for serum K are about 3.4-4.5 meq/l. (ca. 14-18 mg/100 ml). Mixed ruminant saliva contains 16-46 mg/100 ml. Lohman and Norton (1968) have presented detailed analyses of tissues from cattle, the data showing that muscle (3.32 g/kg) contains more K than other tissues, although bone (3.07 g/kg) and the GI tract and its contents (2.71 g/kg) were relatively high. Adipose tissues contained less K (0.77 g/kg) than the other tissues with the exception of a group lumped together (blood, mesenteric fat and feet). Other workers have reported no difference in K of the carcass of different liveweights, when expressed on a fat-free basis (Clark et al, 1972). ^{40}K has been used to estimate body composition of live animals. The use of this method depends on the constancy of K relative to other body components (Clark et al, 1972). Johnson et al (1972) found that K level in the diet affected whole body ^{40}K counts in cattle, but it appeared that the main influence was due to K content in GI tract contents. Use of a combination of K in live animals and liveweight was effective in predicting N, ether extract, water and GE of the carcass (Clark et al, 1976). The R^2 values were 0.87, 0.87, 0.84 and 0.84, respectively.

Absorption and Excretion

Smith (1962) found that K was very well absorbed by the milk fed calf and that most of the absorption occurred in the small intestine, although some occurred in the large intestine. Perry et al (1967) reported a net secretion in the upper small intestine and absorption in the lower small intestine in calves, with minimal values in the large intestine. They estimated that 36 g of K were secreted into the upper small intestine and that absorption from the small intestine accounted for 90% of the K absorbed from the gut. Goodall and Kay (1965) estimated that 53% of the K entering the large intestine was absorbed there, and Care and Van't Klooster (1965) found that K was absorbed in the duodenum and in the upper and mid ileum but not in the terminal ileum of sheep. Mylrea (1966) estimated that K in the small intestine was nearly completely absorbed (90-97%) in calves. In cows (Van't Klooster, 1969) it has been shown that there was a relatively high absorption of K in the small intestine (200-300 g). Of the K that entered the large intestine, about 54% of it was absorbed.

Perry et al (1966) carried out experiments with older heifers concerning excretion of K. They found that about 49% of oral ^{42}K was excreted in urine by 4 days and 2.3% in feces. When additional $KHCO_3$ was fed (132 g), the 4-day urinary excretion was increased to 57%. Intravenous ^{42}K was increased to 68% in the urine by the dose of K bicarbonate as compared to 46% for controls. In balance trials with lambs, Devlin and Roberts (1963) found that 62-63% of K excretion was via urine (30.5 meq fed) when medium and high levels of Na were fed. When a low level of Na was fed (4 meq), fecal excretion of K increased to about 53% of the total and total K excretion was increased from 20 to 30 meq. Moseley and Jones (1974) also noted increased K excretion via the urine when 3% Na was supplemented to sheep. Newton et al (1972) found that K excretion in urine (% of total) was higher for lambs fed a high K level. Elam and Autry (1961) reported that urinary K (83-94% of total) increased as NaCl intake increased in cattle; however, St. Omer and Roberts (1967) found that dietary K did not influence urinary or fecal Na excretion of heifers. Dewhurst et al (1968) noted that about 90% of K was excreted in urine by sheep. When KCl or K acetate was infused, the amount excreted in the urine was 82 and 64%, respectively. In most experiments the administration of K salts produced a marked kaliuresis (K urinary excretion) as well as natriuresis even with a low Na intake. Scott (1969) found that I.V. or intraruminal infusions of HCl did not change K excretion. L'Estrange and Axford (1966) noted that K excretion was little changed by diets of fresh herbage and hay plus supplement nor was

there a change in milk concentration. Suttle and Field (1966) and Scott (1969) both found that there was no effect on the amount of K excreted when changes in urine volume were caused by intraruminal water infusions.

Whole blood concentration of K has been shown to be positively related to Mg and Ca and negatively correlated to Na. Month of pregnancy of cows was related to K, and milk production was negatively related to K, and a significant age effect was found, highest values being at intermediate ages (Lane et al, 1968). Fetal concentration of K appears to decrease with age in sheep (Field and Suttle, 1967).

Potassium Deficiency

K deficiency is not believed to be a problem in ruminants with rare exceptions nor, for that matter, in most other species since the K content of most grains is 0.5% or greater and in most forages it is >1% of the dry matter.

In studies on rats with purified diets it was reported that K deficiency resulted in a reduced appetite and growth rate. The animals became lethargic and comatose and they often died after 3 wk on deficient diets. They had an untidy appearance, cyanotic skin, short fur-like hair, diarrhea and distended abdomens. Postmortem examination revealed ascites (edema of the peritoneal cavity) and, frequently, hydrothorax. Pathological lesions were widespread. Humans, apparently may frequently be K-deficient following surgery; the condition is characterized by extreme muscular weakness, lethargy, anorexia, myocardial degenerative changes, pulmonary edema, and peripheral paralysis. Histological and functional lesions are observed in the kidneys. The convoluted tubules appear engorged and the cells develop vacuoles. Concomitantly, there is a striking diminution in concentrating ability of the kidney, with a conservation of K and excretion of an alkaline urine containing large amounts of ammonia. Na reabsorption may be excessive, resulting in its accumulation with consequent edema (White et al, 1973).

There have been several papers describing some details of K deficiency in ruminants. Devlin et al (1969) found that deficient steers had a poor appetite, the daily gain was negligible and some lost weight. Other symptoms included partial to near complete inanition and pica which involved hair licking and pulling and eating of wooden fences.

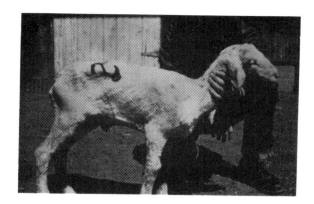

Fig. 4-12. A K-deficient lamb fed a semi-purified diet with 0.1%K. Note the listless and emaciated appearance. University of Missouri photo. Courtesy of R.L. Preston.

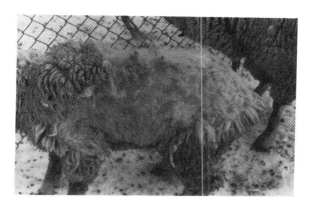

Fig. 4-13. K deficient lamb. This photo illustrates the wool biting and pulling that may occur in deficient animals. University of Manitoba photo. Courtesy of W.K. Roberts.

The hair coats were rough, giving the animals a haggard appearance. During the late stages of the experiment a general weakness was observed in 2 steers and, when forced to move quickly, these individuals showed incoordination and wobbling of the hind quarters. Serum K values were low (3.7 meq/l.), but Mg and Cl were increased in deficient animals and there was an apparent increase in serum P. In vitro rumen fermentation was depressed in deficient animals. In other work from that laboratory (St. Omer and Roberts, 1967), it was shown that K-deficient rations had no effect on N balance or on apparent digestibility. Urinary ammonia excretion was increased, however, and plasma P was higher in deficient animals. Pradhan and Hemken (1968) have reported similar deficiency symptoms in lactating dairy cows. They found, in addition, that blood hematocrit readings were increased and a relatively greater decrease in milk K than blood plasma K. Na content of milk increased in deficient cows. Examples of deficient animals are shown in Fig. 4-12, 13,14.

Telle et al (1964) reported that lambs on low-K rations showed a marked decrease in feed intake after 10 days on deficient diets. They soon showed signs of listlessness and impaired response to sudden disturbances. Stiffness in the hind legs was observed which progressed to the forelegs, the neck and into the back. Deficient lambs were emaciated (Fig. 4-12). No mention was made of pica. Deficient lambs had high hematocrits (42%), and low K in whole blood, plasma and red cells. Red cell Na was increased and there was an apparent decrease

in red cell Ca. The kidneys of lambs fed 0.1% K had cortex cells which were swollen and had a cloudy appearance and there were small focal areas of connective tissue replacement in the cortex of one of the lambs. Some histological changes in muscle were noted. They also observed that rumen papillae were short. During K depletion urinary K excretion decreased during the initial stages, and continued to decrease up to 40 hr, but fecal K decreased only moderately (Cowa and Phillips, 1973). Campbell and Roberts (1965) have observed wool biting and pulling in deficient sheep (Fig. 4-13).

Potassium Requirements

There have been several research reports dealing with the K requirements of ruminants that are of interest. In the case of lambs,

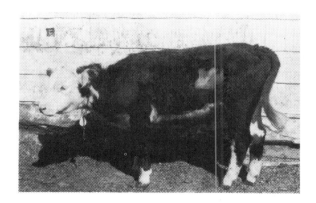

Fig. 4-14. A K-deficient steer. This steer was fed a ration containing 0.27% K. During a period of 110 days this steer lost 57 kg of body weight. University of Manitoba photo. Courtesy of W.K. Roberts.

Table 4-9. Effect of feeding different potassium levels to dairy cows.[a]

Item	Potassium level, %		
	0.45	0.55	0.66
Daily milk production, kg			
Pre-experimental,[b] 15 days	27.2	27.6	26.3
Experimental period			
0-4 wk	23.7	23.3	25.0
5-8 wk	22.0	24.2	23.1
9-12 wk	20.0	22.7	20.2
Post trial[c], 19 days	19.2	21.2	18.5
Body weight gain, kg	15.7	54.5	92.9
Daily feed intake, kg			
Pre-experimental[b], 15 days	16.8	13.2	14.0
Experimental period			
0-4 wk	16.6	14.8	18.0
5-8 wk	16.2	16.8	21.0
9-12 wk	14.6	17.5	20.6
Post-trial, 19 days	18.2	18.8	20.8

[a] Adapted from Dennis et al (1976)
[b] All cows fed 0.45% K
[c] All cows fed 0.66% K

Telle et al (1964) used semipurified rations varying from 0.1 to 0.81% K. After 49 days, lambs on 0.1 and 0.2% K were transferred to 0.62% K and others to 0.81% K. Results of this feedlot trial indicated that lambs receiving diets with 0.42 or 0.62% K gained more than lambs receiving 0.38% K. Blood K values were essentially the same for lambs on 0.42 or 0.62% K. Lambs switched from the low levels to 0.62 or 0.81% K did slightly better on the 0.62% diet. The authors calculated that the optimal level was about 0.55% of dry matter or about 65 mg/kg of body weight. Blood values below 12 mg/100 ml would be indicative of a K deficiency. Campbell and Roberts (1965) also used semipurified diets with 0.3, 0.5 and 0.7% K. Lambs given 0.7% K gained significantly more than those getting 0.3% in an equalized feeding trial. Balance studies indicated a daily requirement of <56 meq or about 64 mg/kg of body weight, thus agreeing with the data of Telle et al.

St. Omer and Roberts (1967) carried out balance trials with heifers fed diets with 157, 439 or 1089 meq of K. The low level resulted in a negative K retention while the other rations resulted in positive balances. N balance was not affected by treatment, but urinary ammonia excretion was higher on the low-K diet. They calculated that the K re-

quirement for maintenance was about 133 meq/kg of body weight daily. In work with steers Devlin et al (1969) fed diets ranging from 0.27 to 0.85% in one experiment and from 0.36 to 0.77% in the second. Data from the first trial (gains, feed intake, blood values, in vitro digestion) indicated that the requirement was greater than 0.51% but not more than 0.72% K. In the second trial, data indicated a requirement between 0.67 and 0.77% K, values considerably higher than indicated for sheep. With respect to dairy cows, it has been reported that milk production was similar for cows fed rations with 0.45, 0.55 and 0.66% K (Dennis et al, 1976). However, weight gain was highest for the cows fed 0.66% K (Table 4-9). Later research from this laboratory (Dennis and Hemken, 1978) indicated that 0.7% K was adequate for cows in mid to late lactations, but the requirement may be higher than 0.7% for high-producing cows in early lactation.

Potassium Toxicity

A number of papers indicate that ruminants may ingest rather large quantities of K without any detrimental effects of an immediate nature. Rook and Balch (1962) calculated that dairy cows consuming lush grass may consume more than 300 g/day without producing any major differences in the metabolism of Na, K, or water. Ward (1966) pointed out that cows consuming alfalfa hay may be expected to consume more than 500 g of K/day, also without apparent ill effect. Pearson et al (1949) found that ewes could consume 5% K bicarbonate without effect on the amount of serum Ca, Mg or K. Likewise, Fontenot et al (1960) fed rations containing 4.7% K in combination with high protein to sheep in balance trials. Apparent absorption of Mg was lower for the lambs fed the high K, high protein ration; Newton et al (1972) also observed a 46% reduction in Mg absorption in lambs resulting from feeding a 5.5% K ration.

The toxicity of K when administered I.V. can be demonstrated. Anderson and Pickering (1962) found that 2 l. of 1 N KCl could be administered slowly without ill effects to cows. However, in calves, Bergman and Sellers (1954) found that K began to be toxic when plasma reached a concentration of 8 meq/l. At this concentration calves were irritable and urinated frequently. Dennis and Harbaugh (1948) found that a dose of 648 g killed one of 2 cows, the other recovering after a dose of Ca gluconate. Two cows receiving 300 and 400 g showed no clinical symptoms; a third cow receiving 350 g showed symptoms typical of milk fever and recovered after treatment with Ca gluconate. Feeding 227 KCl increased udder edema in Holstein heifers (Randall et al, 1974).

White et al (1973) state that electrocardiographic changes in humans are easily detected at serum K concentrations greater than 5 meq/l. At progressively higher concentrations the alterations become more severe and above 10 meq/l. the heart may stop in diastole. These changes are referable solely to the extracellular accumulation of K. In calves with severe diarrhea it seems likely that excessive serum K may be a problem (Roy et al, 1959; Fisher, 1965) since K is not excreted as rapidly as Na in such situations. The high serum K in calves with diarrhea suggests that cardiac arrest may be a contributing cause of death.

The depressing effect of high K on Mg absorption is well documented (Newton et al, 1972). Feeding lambs increased levels of K from 0.7 to 3% decreased weight and energy gain (Jackson et al, 1971).

SULFUR

Sulfur in the Tissues

Only a very small amount of S is found in the animal body in the form of sulfates. Practically all of the S is present in proteins in the form of the S-containing amino acids (cystine, cysteine, methionine and cystathionine) or in the tissues as metabolic derivatives of these amino acids. The total S content of most proteins varies from 0.3 to 1.6%, averaging about 1%. Wool and hair contain large amounts of cystine and may have as much as 4 and 5% S, respectively. S is also found in the vitamins, biotin and thiamin; in peptides such as glutathionine, in esters or phenols, in carbohydrates and lipids, and numerous other compounds present in small amounts. Muscle has about 0.25% S, and brain tissue about 0.5%. In human plasma about 0.7-1.5 meq/l. of sulfate is found. Normal sulfate in sheep are probably about 2-5 mg/100 ml of sulfate S. Hansard and Mohammed (1968, 1969) have presented information on the S content of various tissues of sheep and cattle. The S content of sheep (pregnant females) was generally between 2.2 and 3.6 mg/g of fresh tissue and that of cattle (pregnant females) from 2.0 to 4.0 mg/g of fresh tissue. Liver and heart tissues usually had the highest concentration. Following an I.V. dose of ^{35}S as Na sulfate, the radio S was particularly high in liver, kidney, spleen and adrenal glands. In the fetal tissues, high concentrations were shown in liver, brain and pituitary tissues as well as some bones in the sheep. Trends were similar in cattle.

Absorption, Metabolism and Excretion of S

There is very little information concerning absorption of various forms of S by ruminants. Some time ago, Weir and Rendig (1954) found that there was a rapid increase in blood sulfate S when animals were given doses of Na sulfate. Bray (1969) has studied the absorption and excretion of ^{35}S as the sulfate or sulfide when administered I.V., intraruminally and via the duodenum. His results show that sulfide S was excreted very rapidly in urine, with 51-55% being excreted within 6 hr. He found that 80-84% of the dose was excreted via urine within 24 hr. Negligible amounts were found in feces. With respect to the sulfate, intraruminal administration resulted in 23% being excreted via urine within 6 hr and 34-51% within 24 hr. About 15% was excreted via feces. Duodenal administration resulted in urinary excretion of 18-20% in 6 hr and 38-39% in 24 hr and substantially higher amounts (34-51%) were excreted via feces; thus, his results indicate clearly that ruminal administration resulted in a much greater absorption from the GI tract than did duodenal administration. However, I.V. administration of sulfate resulted in fecal excretion of 12-19% of the dose, indicating that a substantial amount of fecal S may be of endogenous origin. Bray suggests that some of the sulfate entering the lower gut may have been reduced to sulfide which may have been absorbed. If this takes place (no evidence), it would further complicate estimates of absorption and excretion. Other work of Bray's (1969) shows that substantial amounts of S may be absorbed through the rumen wall, but little returns from the blood through the rumen wall.

Apparent absorption of S when sodium sulfate was infused continuously into the rumen of sheep was 93, 95 and 96%, respectively, when the amounts infused were 1.5, 3.0 and 6.0 g/day (Bird and Moir, 1971). The values when the sodium sulfate was infused into the duodenum were 93, 92 and 82%, respectively. When the salt was infused intraruminally, 87-94% of the fecal S was in the neutral S fraction, 4.1 to 5.4% was ester sulfate S, and 0.5 to 4.0% was inorganic sulfate S (Bird, 1971).

When ^{35}S from taurine was administered by a single intraduodenal infusion in sheep, 41 to 51% was recovered in bile and pancreatic secretions, less than 1% in feces and less than 4% in the urine in 3 days (Bird, 1972). On the other hand, when labeled sodium sulfate was administered, 63 to 76% of the ^{35}S was recovered in urine in 4-5 days. The results showed that taurine is conserved, contributing to the S economy of the animal.

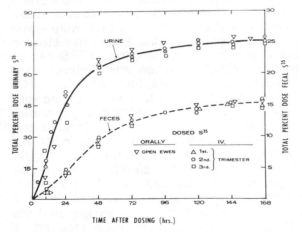

Fig. 4-15. Graph showing the accumulative fecal and urinary excretion of orally and I.V. administered ^{35}S by open and gravid ewes at 3 trimesters of pregnancy. From Hansard and Mohammed (1968).

Hansard and Mohammed have studied the excretion of Na sulfate administered I.V. or orally to sheep (1968) and cattle (1969). The results with sheep (Fig. 4-15) show that about 75% of the dose was excreted via urine and about 15% via feces within a period of 168 hr; thus, about 80% of the excretion was via the urine. Data presented on cattle were similar except that a slightly larger percentage was excreted via urine and slightly less via feces. Route of administration had little effect on route of excretion. Older data published by Thomas et al (1951) on sheep fed purified diets showed that 66 to 93% of S was excreted via urine, the percentage increasing as the S content in the diet decreased.

With elemental S, Starks et al (1953) found that fecal examination accounted for about two thirds of total excretion. Results reported by Jacobson et al (1967, 1969) with dairy cows fed practical type diets, however, did not show this trend since urinary S excretion decreased, percentage wise, from 28% of excretion on adequate diets to 13% on moderately low S diets. There have been some reports indicating that the N:S ratio in urine is relatively constant (Barrow and Lambourne, 1962), however, the results of Thomas et al (1951) do not show this, since N:S ratios were 5.6:1 on adequate diets and 3:1 on deficient diets. Neither do the results of Jacobson et al show a constant N:S ratio in urinary S. In the latter report fecal N:S ratios were similar for cows on an adequate or a low S diet. Bray and Hemsley (1969), working with sheep, found that fecal S increased as dietary S levels increased and the fecal N:S ratio decreased; likewise, the percentage of S excreted via urine increased from 23% on a low S diet to 72% on one with excess S, most of which was represented by urinary sulfates. Excretion of fecal S was shown to be related to intake of S, organic matter and digestible organic matter, and urinary S excretion varied with intake of S and organic matter (Kennedy, 1974).

The mean recovery of ^{35}S in ileal digesta 48 hr after a single I.V. infusion was 24.5% (Bird and Thornton, 1972). The distribution of the S was protein, 49.4%; soluble organic S, 10.1%; reducible S, 40.5%. They estimated that 40% of the infused ^{35}S was cycled to the rumen and incorporated into microbial protein. Of the ^{35}S labeled methionine infused intraruminally, 74% of the ^{35}S flowed to the omasum (Bird and Moir, 1972). The distribution of ^{35}S in feces, urine, and wool after ruminal and abomasal infusions was 30 vs 11%, 39 vs 30% and 5.6 vs 22.8%, respectively.

The organic sulfates normally found in urine consist of compounds such as phenol and indole conjugated with sulfate. Compounds such as phenol and indole are quite toxic; they most probably originate from bacterial action in the gut and conjugation with sulfate is a mechanism utilized to render such compounds less toxic (White et al, 1973).

Concerning retention of S in the tissues, Hansard and Mohammed (1969) found that pregnant cows excreted 73% of total S and retained 9.2% of a single oral dose of radiosulfur. Substantial amounts were transferred to fetal tissues. With sheep, they (Hansard and Mohammed, 1968) estimated that third trimester ewes absorbed and retained about 56% of the dose and that 44% was transferred to fetal tissues (fetus, 77%; placenta, 16%; placental fluids, 7%).

Sulfur Deficiency

S in some form is a required nutrient for ruminants. One of the earliest pieces of research to demonstrate this in ruminants was the report of Thomas et al (1951). In this research purified diets were fed to sheep. Low S diets resulted in a gradual failure of appetite, loss in body weight, emaciation, wool pulling and death. Depraved appetites evidenced by chewing on wooden pens and pulling and consumption of wool were observed in all deficient animals. The N in the diet (urea) was apparently not utilized, since deficient lambs were consistently in negative N and S balance. The rate of wool growth was reduced, but apparently the amino acid composition did not change. Animals fed the same diet with supplemental Na sulfate gained weight, had positive N and S balances, and exhibited none of the deficiency symptoms. Likewise, when deficient animals were transferred to the S-supplemented diets, their performance rapidly improved. Starks et al (1953) have reported similar symptoms in sheep, noting that lambs began losing wool after about 1 mo. on the deficient diet. Other symptoms noted included excessive lacrimation, profuse salivation, dullness, weakness, and cloudy eyes. In some of the animals histological lesions were observed in liver (vacuolated cells), heart (degeneration of muscle fibers and proliferation of fibroblasts), skeletal muscle (proliferation of lymphocytes and degeneration of fibers), and spleen. A deficient animal is shown in Fig. 4-16.

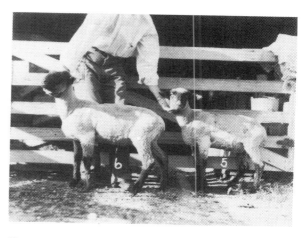

Fig. 4-16. Sulfur deficient lamb (no. 5). The deficient lamb received a low-S basal ration while the other lamb received the basal + 3 g of elemental S per day. Note the patches where wool has been lost. Courtesy of U.S. Garrigus, Univ. of Illinois.

Martin et al (1964) carried out short-term experiments with steers transferred to S-deficient diets. They reported that digestibility of cellulose by steers was reduced by 95%. Whanger and Matrone (1966) have studied the in vitro production of VFA from sheep fed purified diets. They found that deficient diets resulted in large quantities of lactate from substrates such as glucose, the lactate apparently not being converted to VFA in the usual manner. An appreciable amount of the lactate produced was the d form, which could be detected in the blood of deficient animals. Blood sugar levels of deficient animals were higher than S-supplemented animals. Bray and Hemsley (1969) found that blood sulfate levels were reduced and both salivary and blood urea were increased in deficient lambs. In addition, rumen VFA were reduced and propionic and n-valeric acids were lower. No lactate analyses were reported. Rumen ammonia N and TCA N were also reduced in deficient animals. Rumen sulfide levels were very low, also.

Supplementing S to increase the intake from 135 mg to 494 mg/day increased flow of protein to the omasum, N retention, organic matter digestibility and energy intake (Bird, 1972). For example, organic matter digestibility was increased from 44 to 66%. The S to N ratio was 13.5 in the supplemented ration.

Utilization and Requirements of S

It is apparent from some of the research reports which have been reviewed that sulfide and sulfate S can be absorbed by the

Table 4-10. Cumulative radiosulfur excretions and retentions through day 11 after administration to lambs. [a]

	Form of ^{35}S administered		
Item	Elemental sulfur	Sodium sulfate	l-methionine
^{35}S excretion, % of dose			
Feces	64.0	22.2	22.2
Urine	9.2	21.8	7.8
Total	73.2	44.0	30.0
True digestibility of ^{35}S, % of dose[b]	36.0[b]	77.8[c]	77.8[c]
True retention of ^{35}S, % of dose[f]	26.8[d]	56.0[e]	70.0[e]
Absorbed ^{35}S retained, %	73.8	72.0	90.0

[a]From Johnson et al (1971)

[bc]Means with different superscript letters differ (P<.01)

[de]Means with different superscript letters differ (P<.05)

[f]Assuming that radioactive fecal and urinary losses through day 11 represented all of the exogenous loss and an insignificant amount of endogenous radioactive sulfur.

ruminant GI tract, although these two forms may be utilized to different degrees. Much of the research with S in ruminant rations has been directed toward the study of metabolism of inorganic S. More S from sodium sulfate was incorporated into casein than from calcium sulfate (Bouchard and Conrad, 1973). Also, more ^{35}S was excreted in the urine of cows when the Ca salt was used.

A number of papers indicating utilization by rumen microorganisms have been discussed in Vol. 1 (Ch. 15). These generally indicate a more efficient utilization of organic forms of S or sulfide S than for sulfates or elemental S. Further proof that S in various forms can be utilized by the ruminant has been obtained by feeding with ^{35}S and by recovering label in various body tissues or milk. For example, Hale and Garrigus (1953) recovered ^{35}S in blood proteins and wool of sheep fed inorganic S and sulfate S. Other papers reporting isolation of labeled S from host tissues include those of Kulwish et al (1957), Hansard and Mohammed (1968, 1969) and Johnson et al (1971).

True digestibility of S was 65 to 67% from molasses; 77 to 87% from sodium sulfate and 42 to 53% from lignon sulfonate (Bouchard and Conrad, 1973). In research using ^{35}S from elemental S, sodium sulfate and l-methionine, Johnson et al (1971) found that true digestibility of S from these three sources in sheep was 36.0, 77.8 and 77.8%, respectively. True retention values were 26.8, 56.0 and 70.0% for the three respective S sources (Table 4-10). In sheep on forage diets, apparent digestibility of S decreased linearly with the reciprocal of dietary S content and was predicted to be zero when dietary S was 0.81 g S/kg organic matter (Langlands et al, 1973). The availability of S from white clover and perennial ryegrass is about 56% (Joyce and Rattray, 1970).

Some time ago Whiting et al (1954) concluded that the S requirement for sheep did not exceed 0.1% of the ration. When working with lambs, Starks et al (1953) fed a basal ration containing 0.06% S. When this was increased to 0.705% S, N retention and wool growth were increased and weight loss reduced. Lofgreen et al (1953) fed 0.02% supplemental Na sulfate to sheep receiving partially purified diets containing 40% of the dietary N as urea. The basal ration contained 0.23% total S and 0.15% inorganic S. The additional S had no effect on weight gain, N retention or wool growth in this experiment. Albert and co-workers (1956) fed supplemental S as Na sulfate, methionine or elemental S to growing lambs receiving a purified ration containing 4% urea. On the basis of curves fitted to their data, these authors calculated the requirements to be 0.64% methionine, 1.27% Na sulfate, or 0.47% elemental S for maximum daily gain. This would be equivalent to 0.138, 0.29 and 0.47% S from the three sources, respectively; it is obvious that their data indicated much more efficient utilization of S from the methionine and sulfate than from elemental S. Weir and Rendig (1954) calculated that lambs needed 1.7 g or more S/day based on feeding trials with low S alfalfa hay and added methionine.

The work of Bray and Hemsley (1969) with sheep indicated no improvement in performance of sheep fed diets with 0.143% total S as compared to rations with 0.318%. Moir et al (1968) have suggested that the N:S ratio should be approximately 10:1 and Bray and Hemsley (1969) agreed with this conclusion, although their range of diets were not sufficient to confirm their suggestion with conclusive evidence. Maintenance requirement for S, calculated from metabolic urinary and fecal losses and S content of wool growth showed that 0.48 g of retainable S was required daily in sheep (Johnson et al, 1971). Langlands and Southerland (1973) reported that approximately 70 g S were secreted to produce 2 kg clean wool, 50 g S in a lactation yielding 100 l. of milk and 8 g S in birth of a single lamb. Joyce and Rattray (1970) calculated the daily maintenance S requirement of 20 to 40 kg growing sheep to be 0.54 g/day.

In work with dairy cows (Jacobson et al, 1967, 1969), it was concluded that rations with about 0.09% S (dry basis) were inadequate and that rations with about 0.13% S were adequate. Supplementing S to a semi-purified diet containing 0.1% S with increased dry matter intake and digestibility by dairy cows (Bouchard and Conrad, 1973). Regression analysis indicated that an S level of 0.12% would approximate S balance and 0.18% would allow for a positive S balance of 4 g/day in cows producing 8 to 37 kg milk/day. Supplementing a diet composed of hay containing 0.13% S and a grain mixture with 0.28% S did not increase performance of dairy cows (Burgess and Nicholson, 1971). Supplementation of diets containing 0.11 or 0.13% S did not affect feed intake or milk production in dairy cows (Grieve et al, 1973).

Goodrich et al (1967) indicated a response from supplementation when rations contained appreciable amounts of urea. Chalupa et al (1973) reported that 0.13% S appeared adequate for performance in beef steers. Chalupa et al (1971) observed that the S needs of bull calves were satisfied with 0.3% S from elemental S. The parameters included performance, N balance, plasma amino acids and tissue S levels.

Toxicity

There is some information which indicates that high S supplements may result in reduced performance of lambs (Johnson et al, 1968) or beef steers (Shively et al, 1966). However, this subject requires further study in order to determine the level that might be detrimental and the physiological response resulting from a toxic level.

Lower dry matter intakes were recorded in dairy cows when the level of S was 0.35% or above (Bouchard and Conrad, 1974), but feeding up to 0.62% S to beef steers did not cause any deleterious effects (Chalupa et al, 1973). No overt toxicity was reported in heifers allowed access to drinking water with up to 2,500 ppm sulfate (Digesti and Weeth, 1973).

Sulfur toxicity was reported in a group of 20 yearling heifers which had consumed S mixed with corn (Julian and Harrison, 1975). The animals showed respiratory disease and abdominal pain. Vasculites and necrosis of the rumen and abomasal wall were recorded upon examination of one of the animals. Lower feed and water consumption, weight loss and diuresis were reported in growing heifers offered water containing 5,000 ppm sulfate (Weeth and Hunter, 1971). Water intake was not affected by adding 1,462 or 2,814 ppm sulfate to the drinking water, but hay intake was depressed at the higher level (Weeth and Capps, 1972). Rate of gain was decreased by both sulfate levels. In a later study Digesti and Weeth (1976) concluded that 2,500 ppm sulfate in drinking water represents a safe tolerance concentration. Bird (1972) observed temporary respiratory distress and collapse in sheep given single ruminal or ileal infusion of sulfide (0.95 g S). Continuous ruminal infusion of 2.93 g S/day or sulfide decreased dry matter intake. He suggested that addition of a maximum of 4 g S/day to ruminant diets of 0.2% S should meet the requirement without adversely affecting feed intake.

The minimum lethal dose of sodium metabisulfite in sheep was 2.25 g/kg bodyweight (Nikolaev and Dzhidzheva, 1973). The LD_{50} was 2.25 mg/kg. Signs of toxicity were restlessness, feed refusal, ruminal atony, rapid pulse and respiration, cyanosis and death. Kaemmerer et al (1972) reported no harmful effects in sheep fed dried beet pulp containing 1% SO_2 as sodium disulfite in a ration of 500 g hay, 500 g dried beet pulp and 200 g ground oats.

GENERAL OBSERVATIONS ON MINERALS

Shown in Table 4-11 is a summary showing typical blood values and relative amounts of absorption and excretion of the major minerals in various areas of the ruminant GI tract. These relative estimates are not very precise, but are included to give the reader a summary based on available information. Data are also shown for the approximate percentage of excretion via urine for each of these elements. These values too, will vary considerably, depending upon the amount of the element in the diet, its chemical form, the presence of other elements, and the relative over supply of the element in the diet. However, the data in the table should provide a convenient summary for "typical" values.

The reader will be aware that there has been a vast amount of research effort expended on investigations dealing with the various elements over the past 50 to 60 years. Even so, it is apparent when summing up the findings that much remains to be learned with respect to absorption and excretion—the sites, factors affecting, interactions with other nutrients—as well as needed information on the amount of a given element required in the diet under different situations and for different species and other items of interest such as toxicity. The lack of some of this information is, no doubt, not a critical factor with respect to present day feeding and management practices. However, it can be said with a high degree of certainty that the better the understanding of a nutrient's metabolism and its relationship to other nutrients or to physiological functions, the more nearly we should be able to formulate diets with optimum nutrient content or to supplement forage with limiting nutrients. Much remains to be done in the area of mineral nutrition.

Table 4-11. Typical blood values for the major minerals and sites in the ruminant gastro-intestinal tract where net secretion (+) or absorption (-) has been shown to occur.[a]

Element	Concentration in plasma or serum, mg %	Rumen	Omasum	Abomasum	Small intestine Upper	Mid	Lower	Large intestine	Urinary excretion, % of total
Ca	9-12	+ *	+	--	+ + +	---	-	+	1-5
Mg	1.8-3	+ + +	---	--	+ +	-	-	--	10-40
K	14-18	+ or -	-		+ + +	---	--	-	60-90
Na	300	+ + + *	-		+ + +	---	--	--	60-80
P	4-9	+ + *	+	-	+ + +	---	--	+ +	1-5
Cl	360	+ *		+ + +	+ + +	--	--	--	95-98
S[b]	2-5	-				--	--	+	75-80

[a] More than one + or - indicates relative amount

[b] As sulfate S

* Salivary contribution.

References Cited

Macro Minerals, General References

ARC. 1965. The Nutrient Requirements of Farm Livestock. No. 2 Ruminants. Agr. Research Council, London.

Church, D.C. and W.G. Pond. 1974. Basic Animal Nutrition and Feeding. O&B Books, Corvallis, Oregon.

Comar, C.L. and F. Bronner (ed.). 1962, 1964. Mineral Metabolism. Vol. 2, part A & B. Academic Press.

Dyer, I.A. 1969. In: Animal Growth and Nutrition. Lea & Febiger Pub. Co.

Leninger, A.L. 1975. Biochemistry. Worth Publ. Inc., N.Y.

NRC. 1975. Nutrient Requirements of Sheep. Nat. Acad. Sci., Washington, D.C.

NRC. 1976. Nutrient Requirements of Beef Cattle. Nat. Acad. Sci. Washington, D.C.

NRC. 1978. Nutrient Requirements of Dairy Cattle. Nat. Acad. Sci., Washington, D.C.

Underwood, E.J. 1966. The Mineral Nutrition of Livestock. Commonwealth Agricultural Bureaux.

White, A., P. Handler, E.L. Smith. 1973. Principles of Biochemistry. 5th Edition. McGraw-Hill Book Co.

Calcium

Aas Hansen, M., J.L. Flatla and T. Mikkelsen. 1968. Nutr. Abstr. Rev. 38:1403.

Annenkov, B.N., J.P.Fomicev, V.E. Madison and I.I. Cepel. 1969. Nutr. Abstr. Abstr. Rev. 39:520.

Barlet, J.P., M.C. Michel, P. Lowar and M. Theriez. 1971. Ann. Biol. Anim. Bioch. Biophys (Fr.) 11:415.

Belyea, R.L., C.E. Coppock and G.B. Lake. 1976. J. Dairy Sci. 59:1068.

Benzie, D. et al. 1956. J. Agr. Sci. 48:175.

Blincoe, C., A.L. Lesperance and V.R. Bohman. 1973. J. Animal Sci. 36:971.

Blood, D.C. and J.A. Henderson. 1968. Veterinary Medicine. Williams & Wilkins Co.

Bohman, V.R., M.A. Wade and C. Blincoe. 1962. Science 136:1120.

Braithwaite, G.D. 1972. Brit. J. Nutr. 27:201.

Braithwaite, G.D. 1975. Brit. J. Nutr. 33:309.

Braithwaite, G.D., R.F. Glascock and S.H. Riazuddin. 1970. Brit. J. Nutr. 24:661.

Braithwaite, G.C., R.F. Glascock and S.H. Riazuddin. 1972. Brit. J. Nutr. 27:417; 28:269.

Braithwaite, G.C. and S.H. Riazuddin. 1971. Brit. J. Nutr. 26:215.

Brochart, M. 1965. Nutr. Abstr. Rev. 35:257.

Bronner, F. 1964. In: Mineral Metabolism. Vol. 2, part A. Academic Press.

Care, A.D. and A.T. Van't Klooster. 1965. J. Physiol. 177:174.

Chandler, P.T. and R.G. Cragle. 1962. Proc. Soc. Expt. Biol. Med. 111:431.

Cobic, S., S. Vucetic and S. Bacvanski. 1971. J. Sci. Agr. Res. (Yugoslavia) 24:109.

Cowan, R.L., E.W. Hartsook and J.B. Whelan. 1968. Proc. Soc. Expt. Biol. Med. 129:733.

Curtis, R.A., R.G. Thomson and L. Weirenga. 1969. Can. Vet. J. 10:20.

Dunham, J.R. and G. Ward. 1971. J. Dairy Sci. 54:833.

Dowe, T.W., J. Matsushima and V.H. Arthaud. 1957. J. Animal Sci. 16:811.

Elam, C.J. and I.K. Autry. 1961. Proc. West. Sec. Amer. Soc. Animal Sci. 12:LXIX.

Field, A.C., N.F. Suttle and D.O. Nisbet. 1975. J. Agr. Sci. 85:435.

Fisher, L.J. et al. 1975. Can. J. Animal Sci. 52:693.

Fontenot, J.P., R.F. Miller and N.O. Price. 1964. J. Animal Sci. 23:875 (abstr).

Garces, M.A. and J.L. Evans. 1971. J. Animal Sci. 32:789.

Gill, B.S., M. Singh and A.K. Chopra. 1976. Amer. J. Vet. Res. 37:545.

Goings, R.L. et al. 1974. J. Dairy Sci. 57:1184.

Grace, N.D. and D. Scott. 1974. New Zealand J. Agr. Res. 17:165.

Gueguen, L. and C.M. Mathieu. 1965. Ann. Zootech. 14:231.

Hansard, S.L., C.L. Comar and G.K. Davis. 1954. Amer. J. Physiol. 177:383.

Hansard, S.L., C.L. Comar and M.P. Plumlee. 1952. J. Animal Sci. 11:524.

Hansard, S.L., H.M. Crowder and W.A. Lyke. 1957. J. Animal Sci. 16:437.

Hatch, C.F., T.W. Perry, M.T. Mohler and W.M. Beeson. 1972. J. Animal Sci. 34:483.
Hjerpe, C.A. 1968. Amer. J. Vet. Res. 29:143.
Hodge, R.W. 1973. Aust. J. Agr. Res. 24:237.
Hodge, R.W., G.R. Pearce and D.E. Tribe. 1973. Aust. J. Agr. Res. 24:229.
Jones, H.G. and W.S. Mackie. 1959. Brit. J. Nutr. 13:335.
Krook, L. et al. 1971. Cornell Vet. 61:625.
Leibholz, Jane. 1974. Aust. J. Agr. Res. 25:147.
Lengemann, F.W., C.L. Comar and R.H. Wasserman. 1957. J. Nutr. 61:571.
Lomba, F. et al. 1978. Brit. J. Nutr. 39:425.
Luick, R.R., J.M. Boda and M. Kleiber. 1957. J. Nutr. 61:597.
Manston, R. 1967. J. Agr. Sci. 68:263.
Matsushima, J. et al. 1955. J. Animal Sci. 14:1042.
McRoberts, M.R., R. Hill and A.C. Dalgarno. 1965. J. Agr. Sci. 65:1.
Miller, W.J. 1975. J. Dairy Sci. 58:1549.
Paquay, R., F. Lomba, A. Lousse and V. Bienfet. 1968. J. Agr. Sci. 71:173.
Peeler, H.T. 1972. J. Animal Sci. 35:695.
Pfeffer, E., A. Thompson and D.G. Armstrong. 1970. Brit. J. Nutr. 24:197.
Phillipson, A.T. and J.E. Storry. 1965. J. Physiol. 181:130.
Perry, S.C., R.G. Cragle and J.K. Miller. 1967. J. Nutr. 93:283.
Ramberg, C.F., Jr., G.P. Mayer, D.S. Kronfeld and J.T. Potts, Jr. 1976. J. Nutr. 106:671.
Ramberg, C.R. et al. 1970. J. Nutr. 100:981.
Ricketts, R.E. et al. 1970. J. Dairy Sci. 53:898; Amer. J. Vet. Res. 31:1023.
Roberts, W.K. and J.A. McKirdy. 1965. J. Animal Sci. 23:682.
Saba, A.C. and S.K. Deb. 1973. Indian Vet. J. 50:14.
Sasser, L.B., L. Wade, Jr. and M.C. Bell. 1974. J. Animal Sci. 38:178.
Shroder, J.D. and S.L. Hansard. 1958. J. Animal Sci. 17:343.
Smith, R.H. 1962. Biochem. J. 83:151.
Smith, R.H. and A.B. McAllan. 1966. Brit. J. Nutr. 20:703.
Stacy, B.D. 1969. Quart. J. Expt. Physiol. 54:1.
Stacy, R.D. and B.W. Wilson. 1970. J. Physiol. 210:549.
Steevens, B.J., L.J. Bush, J.D. Stout and E.I. Williams. 1971. J. Dairy Sci. 54:655.
Stillings, B.R., J.W. Bratzler, L.F. Marriott and R.C. Miller. 1964. J. Animal Sci. 23:1148.
Sykes, A.R. and R.A. Dingwall. 1975. J. Agr. Sci. 84:245.
Thomas, W.C. and J.E. Howard. 1964. In: Mineral Metabolism. Vol. 2, part A. Academic Press.
Thompson, A., S.L. Hansard and M.C. Bell. 1959. J. Animal Sci. 18:187.
Tillman, A.D. and J.R. Brethour. 1958. J. Animal Sci. 17:782.
Twardock, A.R., H.W. Symonds, B.F. Sansom and G.J. Rowlands. 1973. Brit. J. Nutr. 29:437.
Vagg, M.J. and J.M. Payne. 1970. Brit. Vet. J. 126:531.
Van't Klooster, A.T. 1969. Nutr. Abstr. Rev. 39:129.
Varner, L.W. and W. Woods. 1972. J. Animal Sci. 35:415.
Walker, D.M. 1972. J. Agr. Sci. 79:121.
Wheeler, W.E. and C.H. Noller. 1976. J. Dairy Sci. 59:1788.
Whitehair, C.K., W.D. Gallup and M.C. Bell. 1953. J. Animal Sci. 12:331.
Wiener, G. and A.C. Field. 1971. Proc. Nutr. Soc. 30:91.
Wiggers, K.D., D.K. Nelson and N.L. Jacobson. 1975. J. Dairy Sci. 58:430.
Wise, M.B., A.L. Ordozeva and E.R. Barrick. 1963. J. Nutr. 79:79.
Young, V.R., et al. 1966. Brit. J. Nutr. 20:727, 783, 795.

Phosphorus

Agarwala, O.N., K. Nath and V. Mahadevan. 1971. J. Agr. Sci. 77:467.
Ammerman, C.B. et al. 1957. J. Animal Sci. 16:796.
Annenkov, B.N., J.P. Fomicev, V.L. Madison and I.I. Cepel. 1969. Nutr. Abstr. Rev. 39:520.
Arrington, L.R. et al. 1962. J. Animal Sci. 21:987 (abstr).
Benzie, D. et al. 1959. J. Agr. Sci. 52:1.
Braithwaite, G.D. 1975. Brit. J. Nutr. 34:311.
Chandler, P.T. and R.G. Cragle. 1962. Proc. Soc. Expt. Biol. Med. 111:431.
Chicco, C.F. et al. 1965. J. Animal Sci. 24:355.
Compere, R., S. Vanuytrecht and J. Fabry. 1965. C.R. Soc. Biol. 159:1258.
Conrad, H.R., S.L. Hansard and J.W. Hibbs. 1956. J. Dairy Sci. 39:1697.

Dunham, J.R. and G. Ward. 1971. J. Dairy Sci. 54:863.

Dutton, J.E. and J. P. Fontenot. 1967. J. Animal Sci. 26:1409.

Ellis, L.C. and A.D. Tillman. 1961. J. Animal Sci. 20:606.

Ewer, T.K. 1951. Brit. J. Nutr. 5:298;305.

Field, A.C. and N.F. Suttle. 1967. J. Agr. Sci. 69:417.

Field, A.C., N.F. Suttle and D.F. Nisbet. 1975. J. Agr. Sci. 85:435.

Fishwick, G. 1976. New Zealand J. Agr. Res. 19:307.

Gueguen, L. and C.M. Mathieu. 1965. Ann. Zootech. 14:231.

Hansard, S.L. and J. Barth. 1962. J. Animal Sci. 21:384 (abstr).

Hemingway, R.G. and G. Fishwick. 1975. J. Agr. Sci. 84:381.

Hodge, R.W. 1973. Aust. J. Agr. Res. 24:921.

Irving, J.T. 1964. In: Mineral Metabolism. Vol. 2, part A. Academic Press.

Jakovac, M., D. Supe and K. Mikulec. 1968. Nutr. Abstr. Rev. 38:694.

Kirchgessner, M. 1958. Nutr. Abstr. Rev. 28:1114.

Kleiber, M., A.H. Smith, N.P. Ralston and A.L. Black. 1951. J. Nutr. 45:253.

Lane, A.G., J.R. Campbell and G.F. Krause. 1968. J. Animal Sci. 27:766.

L'Estrange, J.L. and R.E. Axford. 1966. J. Agr. Sci. 67:295.

Little, D.A. 1975. Aust. J. Exp. Agr. Animal Husb. 15:25.

Lofgreen, G.P. and M. Kleiber. 1953. J. Animal Sci. 12:366.

Long, T.A. et al. 1957. J. Animal Sci. 16:444.

Luick, J.R. and G.P. Lofgreen. 1957. J. Animal Sci. 16:201.

Manston, R. 1967. J. Agr. Sci. 68:263.

Manston, R. and M.J. Vagg. 1970. J. Agr. Sci. 74:161.

Mayer, G.P., R.R. Marshak and D.S. Kronfeld. 1966. Amer. J. Physiol. 211:1366.

Mayer, G.P., C.F. Ramberg and D.S. Kronfeld. 1968. J. Nutr. 95:202.

McRoberts, M.R., R. Hill and A.C. Dalgarno. 1965. J. Agr. Sci. 65:1,11,15.

McMeniman, N.P. 1973. Aust. Vet. J. 49:150.

Moodie, E.W. 1968. Quart. J. Expt. Physiol. 53:250.

Morrow, D.A. 1969. J. Amer. Vet. Med. Assoc. 154:761.

Mudgal, V.D. and S.N. Kay. 1967. Indian J. Dairy Sci. 20:5.

Nelson, T.S., L.B. Daniels, J.R. Hall and L.G. Shields. 1976. J. Animal Sci. 42:1509.

O'Donovan, J.P., M.P. Plumlee, W.H. Smith and W.M. Beeson. 1965. J. Animal Sci. 24:981.

Raun, A., E. Cheng and W. Burroughs. 1956. J. Agr. Food Chem. 4:869.

Reed, W.D.C., R.C. Elliott and J.H. Topps. 1965. Nature 208:953.

Shirley, R.L., G.K. Davis and J.R. Neller. 1951. J. Animal Sci. 10:335.

Shirley, R.L., R.D. Owens and G.K. Davis. 1950. J. Animal Sci. 9:552.

Shroder, J.D. and S.L. Hansard. 1958. J. Animal Sci. 17:343.

Siebert, B.D., D.M.R. Newman, B. Hart and G.L. Michell. 1975. Aust. J. Exp. Agr. Animal Husb. 15:321.

Smith, A.H. et al. 1952. J. Animal Sci. 11:638.

Smith, A.H. et al. 1955. J. Nutr. 57:507;58:95.

Standish, J.F., C.B. Ammerman, A.Z. Palmer and C.F. Simpson. 1971. J. Animal Sci. 33:171.

Steevens, B.J., L.J. Bush, J.D. Stout and E.I. Williams. 1971. J. Dairy Sci. 54:655.

Stillings, B.R., J.W. Bratzler, L.F. Marriott and R.C. Miller. 1964. J. Animal Sci. 23:1148.

Suttle, N.F. and A.C. Field. 1966. Brit. J. Nutr. 20:609.

Sykes, A.R. and R.A. Dingwall. 1975. J. Agr. Sci. 84:245.

Symonds, H.W. 1969. Res. Vet. Sci. 10:218.

Thomas, O.O., W.D. Gallup and C.K. Whitehair. 1953. J. Animal Sci. 12:372.

Thompson, A. S.L. Hansard and M.C. Bell. 1959. J. Animal Sci. 18:187.

Tillman, A.D. and J.R. Brethour. 1958. J. Animal Sci. 17:100,104,782,792.

Tillman, A.D., J.R. Brethour and S.L. Hansard. 1959. J. Animal Sci. 18:249.

Tomas, F.M. 1974. Aust. J. Agric. Res. 25:485,495.

Twardock, A.R., H.W. Symonds, B.F. Sansom and G.J. Rowlands. 1973. Brit. J. Nutr. 29:437.

Unshelm, J. and W.H. Rappen. 1969. Nutr. Abstr. Rev. 39:449.

Van't Klooster, A.T. 1969. Nutr. Abstr. Rev. 39:129.

Vaskov, B. et al. 1969. Nutr. Abstr. Rev. 39:450.

Webb, K.E., Jr., J.P. Fontenot and M.B. Wise. 1975. J. Animal Sci. 40:760.

Westerlund, A. 1956. Nutr. Abstr. Rev. 27:470.

Whitehair, C.K., W.D. Gallup and M.C. Bell. 1953. J. Animal Sci. 12:331.
Wise, M.B., S.E. Smith and L.L. Barnes. 1958. J. Animal Sci. 17:89.

Magnesium

Ammerman, C.B., C.F. Chicco, P.E. Loggins and L.R. Arrington. 1972. J. Animal Sci. 34:122.
Ammerman, C.B. et al. 1971. J. Dairy Sci. 54:1288.
Axford, R.F.E., M.V. Tas, R.A. Evans and N.W. Ofter. 1975. Res. Vet. Sci. 19:333.
Blaxter, K.L. and R.F. McGill. 1956. Vet. Rev. Anot. 2:35.
Blaxter, K.L. and J.A.F. Rook. 1954. J. Comp. Path. Therap. 64:176.
Blaxter, K.L. and J.A.F. Rook. 1955. Brit. J. Nutr. 9:121.
Blaxter, K.L., J.A.F. Rook and A.M. MacDonald. 1954. J. Comp. Pathol. Therap. 64:157.
Care, A.D., D.B. Ross and A.A. Wilson. 1965. J. Physiol. 176:284.
Care, A.D. and A.T. Van't Klooster. 1965. J. Physiol. 177:174.
Chicco, C.F., C.B. Ammerman, W.G. Hillis and L.R. Arrington. 1972. Amer. J. Physiol. 222:1469.
Chicco, C.F., C.B. Ammerman and P.E. Loggins. 1973. J. Dairy Sci. 56:822.
Dutton, J.E. and J.P. Fontenot. 1967. J. Animal Sci. 26:1409.
Field, A.C. 1961. Brit. J. Nutr. 15:349.
Field, A.C. and N.F. Suttle. 1967. J. Agr. Sci. 69:417.
Fishwick, G. and R.G. Hemingway. 1973. J. Agr. Sci. 81:441.
Garces, M.A. and J.L. Evans. 1971. J. Animal Sci. 32:789.
Gerken, H.J. and J.P. Fontenot. 1967. J. Animal Sci. 26:1404.
Grace, N.D. 1972. N.Z. J. Agr. Res. 15:79.
Grace, N.D. and J.C. Macrae. 1972. Brit. J. Nutr. 27:51.
Grace, N.D., M.J. Ulyatt and J.C. Macrae. 1974. J. Agr. Sci. 82:321.
Hawkins, G.E. 1954. J. Dairy Sci. 37:656.
Hemingway, R.G. and N.S. Ritchie. 1969. Vet. Rec. 3:465.
Hjerpe, C.A. 1968. Amer. J. Vet. Res. 29:143.
Hutton, J.B., K.E. Jury and E.B. Davies. 1965. N.Z. J. Agr. Res. 8:479.
Kiesel, G.K. and H.D. Alexander. 1966. Amer. J. Vet. Res. 30:381.
Kiesel, G.K., H.D. Alexander and G. Brooks. 1969. Amer. J. Vet. Res. 30:381.
Larvor, P., T. Kwiatowski and M. Lamand. 1965. Ann. Biol. Animale Biochim. Biophys. 5:389.
Lomba, F., R. Paquay, V. Bienfet and A. Lousse. 1968. J. Agr. Sci. 71:181.
Martin, J.E. et al. 1964. J. Nutr. 83:60.
Madsen, F.C. et al. 1975. Proc. Soc. Expt. Biol. Med. 149:207.
Marongiu, A. 1971. Bolletino della Societa' Italiana di Biologia Sperimentale. 47:768.
McAllese, D.M., M.C. Bell and R.M. Forbes. 1961. J. Nutr. 74:505.
Moodie, E.W. 1968. Quart. J. Expt. Physiol. 53:250.
Moore, W.F., J.P. Fontenot and R.E. Tucker. 1971. J. Animal Sci. 33:502.
Moore, W.F., J.P. Fontenot and K.E. Webb, Jr. 1972. J. Animal Sci. 35:1046.
Nel, J.W. 1976. S. Afr. J. Animal Sci. 6(11-16):2.
Newton, G.L., J.P. Fontenot, R.E. Tucker and C.E. Polan. 1972. J. Animal Sci. 35:440.
O'Kelley, R.E. and J.P. Fontenot. 1969. J. Animal Sci. 29:959.
O'Kelley, R.E. and J.P. Fontenot. 1973. J. Animal Sci. 36:994.
Perry, S.C., R.G. Cragle and J.K. Miller. 1967. J. Nutr. 93:283.
Phillipson, A.T. and J.E. Storry. 1965. J. Physiol. 181:130.
Pierce, A.W. 1959. Aust. J. Agr. Res. 10:725.
Pless, C.D., J.P. Fontenot and K.E. Webb, Jr. 1975. V.P.I. & S.U. Res. Div. Rep. 153:104.
Rogers, T.A., M.B. Simesen, T. Lunaas and J.R. Luick. 1964. Acta. Vet. Scand. 5:209.
Rook, J.A.F., R.C. Campling and V.M. Johnson. 1964. J. Agr. Sci. 62:273.
Scott, D. and A. Dobson. 1965. Quart. J. Expt. Physiol. 50:42.
Smith, R.H. 1958. Biochem. J. 70:201.
Smith, R.H. 1962. Biochem. J. 83:151.
Smith, R.H. and A.B. McAllan. 1966. Brit. J. Nutr. 20:703.
Stewart, J. and E.W. Moodie. 1956. J. Comp. Path. Therap. 66:10.
Stillings, E.R., J.W. Bratzler, L.F. Marriott and R.C. Miller. 1964. J. Animal Sci. 23:1148.
Suttle, N.F. and A.C. Field. 1966. Brit. J. Nutr. 20:609.
Tomas, F.M. and B.J. Potter. 1976. Brit. J. Nutr. 36:37; Aust. J. Agr. Res. 27:437.
Van't Klooster, A.T. 1969. Nutr. Abstr. Rev. 39:129.
Wise, M.B., A.L. Ordoveza and E.R. Barrick. 1963. J. Nutr. 79:79.

Sodium

Abraham, S.F. et al. 1976. Quart. J. Exp. Physiol. 61:185.

Aines, P.D. and S.E. Smith. 1957. J. Dairy Sci. 40:682.

Bertzbach, J., B. Helfferich, E. Pfeffer and W. Lendeit. 1966. Nutr. Abstr. Rev. 36:872.

Blair-West, J.R. et al. 1965. In: Physiology of Digestion in the Ruminant. Butterworths Pub. Co.

Cardon, B.P. 1953. J. Animal Sci. 12:536.

Chicco, C.F. et al. 1971. J. Animal Sci. 33:142.

Cunha, T.J. 1976. Feedstuffs 48(20):18.

Denton, D.A. and J.R. Sabine. 1961. J. Physiology. 157:97.

Denton, D.A. and J.R. Sabine. 1963. Behaviour. 20:364.

Devlin, T.H. and W.K. Roberts. 1965. J. Animal Sci. 22:648.

Dobson, A., D. Scott and J.B. Bruce. 1966. Quart. J. Expt. Physiol. 51:311.

Elam, C.J. 1961. J. Animal Sci. 20:931 (abstr).

Elam, C.J. and L.K. Autry. 1961. Proc. West. Sec. Amer. Soc. Animal Sci. 12:LXIX.

Forbes, G.B. 1962. In: Mineral Metabolism. Vol. 2, part B. Academic Press.

Goodall, E.D. and R.N.B. Kay. 1965. J. Physiol. 176:12.

Hagsten, I. and T.W. Perry. 1975. J. Animal Sci. 40:1205.

Hagsten, I., T.W. Perry and J. B. Outhouse. 1975. J. Animal Sci. 40:329.

Hawkins, G.E., K.M. Autrey and J.W. Huff. 1965. J. Dairy Sci. 48:790 (abstr).

Helfferich, B., J. Bertzbach, E. Pfeffer and W. Lenkeit. 1966. Nutr. Abstr. Rev. 36:872.

Hemsley, J.A. 1975. Aust. J. Agr. Res. 26:709.

Hemsley, J.A., J.P. Hogan and R.H. Weston. 1975. Aust. J. Agr. Res. 26:715.

Horrocks, D. 1964. J. Agr. Sci. 63:369;373.

Johnson, D.E., L.H. Harbers and J.M. Prescott. 1959. J. Animal Sci. 18:599.

Kemp, A. 1964. Netherlands J. Agr. Sci. 12:263.

McClymont, G.L., K.N. Wynne, P.K. Briggs and M.C. Frankling. 1957. Aust. J. Agr. Res. 8:83.

Meyer, J.H., W.C. Weir, N.R. Ittner and J.D. Smith. 1955. J. Animal Sci. 14:412.

Mikkilineni, S.R. et al. 1973. J. Dairy Sci. 56:395.

Morris, J.G. and R.J.W. Gartner. 1971. Brit. J. Nutr. 25:191.

Morris, J.G. and R.J.W. Gartner. 1975. Brit. J. Nutr. 34:1.

Morris, J.G. and G.W. Murphy. 1972. J. Agr. Sci. 78:105.

Morris, J.G. and R.G. Peterson. 1975. J. Nutr. 105:595.

Moseley, G. and D.I.H. Jones. 1974. J. Agr. Sci. 83:37.

Mylrea, P.J. 1966. Res. Vet. Sci. 7:394.

Nelson, A.B., R.W. MacVicar, W. Archer and J.C. Meiske. 1955. J. Animal Sci. 14:825.

Pierce, A.W. 1957. Aust. J. Agr. Res. 8:711.

Pierce, A.W. 1959. Aust. J. Agr. Res. 10:725.

Perry, S.C., R.G. Cragle and J.K. Miller. 1967. J. Nutr. 93:283.

Perry, S.C., J.H. Schaffer, R.G. Cragle and J.K. Miller. 1966. J. Animal Sci. 25:907 (abstr).

Pfeffer, E., B. Helfferich, J. Bertzbach and W. Lenkeit. 1966. Nutr. Abstr. Rev. 36:872.

Phillips, G.D. and S.K. Sundaram. 1966. J. Physiol. 184:889.

Potter, B.J. 1963. Aust. J. Agr. Res. 14:518.

Potter, B.J. 1968. J. Physiol. 194:435.

Potter, B.J. 1972. Aust. J. Exp. Biol. Med. Sci. 50:387.

Potter, B.J., D.J. Walker and W.W. Forrest. 1972. Brit. J. Nutr. 27:75.

Renkema, J.A., T. Senshu, B.D.E. Gaillard and E. Brauwer. 1962. Netherlands J. Agr. Sci. 10:52.

Sandals, W.C.D. 1978. Can. Vet. J. 19:136.

Skydsgaard, J.M. 1968. Nutr. Abstr. Rev. 38:411.

Smith, R.H. 1962. Biochem. J. 83:151.

Smith, S.E. and P.D. Aines. 1959. Cornell Agr. Expt. Sta. Bul. 938.

Suttle, N.F. and A.C. Field. 1966. Brit. J. Nutr. 20:609.

Tomas, F.M., G.B. Jones, B.J. Potter and G.L. Langsford. 1973. Aust. J. Agr. Res. 24:377.

Van't Klooster, A.T. 1969. Nutr. Abstr. Rev. 39:129.

Van Leeuwen, J.M. 1970. Versl. landbouok. Onderzoek. 737:218.

Weeth, H.J. and L.H. Haverland. 1961. J. Animal Sci. 20:518.

Weeth, H.J., L.H. Haverland and D.W. Cassard. 1960. J. Animal Sci. 19:845.

Weeth, H.J., J.E. Hunter and E.L. Piper. 1962. J. Animal Sci. 21:688.

Weeth, H.J. and A.L. Lesperance. 1965. J. Animal Sci. 24:441.

Weeth, H.J., A.L. Lesperance and V.R. Bohman. 1968. J. Animal Sci. 27:739.

Whipp, S.C., E.A. Usenik, A.F. Weber and A.L. Good. 1966. Amer. J. Vet. Res. 27:1229.
Wilson, A.D. 1967. Aust. J. Expt. Agr. 7:321.
Wilson, A.D. and M.L. Dudzinski. 1973. Aust. J. Agr. Res. 24:245.
Wilson, A.D. and N.L. Hindley. 1968. Aust. J. Agr. Res. 19:597.
Wilson, G.W. 1966. Aust. J. Agr. Res. 17:503.

Chlorine
Care, A.D. and A.T. Van't Klooster. 1965. J. Physiol. 177:174.
Cotlove, E. and C.A.M. Hogben. 1962. In: Mineral Metabolism. Vol. 2, part B. Academic Press.
Elam, C.J. and L.K. Autry. 1961. Proc. West. Sec. Amer. Soc. Animal Sci. 12:LXIX.
Goodall, E.D. and R.N.B. Kay. 1965. J. Physiol. 176:12.
Mylrea, P.J. 1966. Res. Vet. Sci. 7:394.
Nelson, A.B., R.W. MacVicar, W. Archer and J.C. Meiske. 1955. J. Animal Sci. 14:825.
Paquay, R., F. Lomba, A. Lousse and V. Bienfet. 1969. J. Agr. Sci. 73:223.
Phillips, G.D. 1970. Brit. Vet. J. 126:409.
Potter, B.J. and G.H. McIntosh. 1974. Aust. J. Agr. Res. 25:909.
Smith, R.H. 1962. Biochem J. 83:151.
Smith, S.E. and P.D. Aines. 1959. Cornell Agr. Expt. Sta. Bul. 938.
Tomas, F.M., G.B. Jenes, B.J. Potter and G.L. Langsford. 1973. Aust. J. Agr. Res. 24:377.

Potassium
Anderson, R.S. and E.C. Pickering. 1962. J. Physiol. 164:180.
Bergman, E.N. and A.F. Sellers. 1954. Amer. J. Vet. Res. 15:25.
Campbell, L.D. and W.K. Roberts. 1965. Can. J. Animal Sci. 45:147.
Care, A.D. and A.T. Van't Klooster. 1965. J. Physiol. 177:174.
Clark, J.L., H.B. Hedrick and G.B. Thompson. 1976. J. Animal Sci. 42:352.
Clark, J.L. et al. 1972. J. Animal Sci. 35:542.
Cowa, T.J.J. and G.D. Phillips. 1973. Can. J. Animal Sci. 53:653.
Dennis, J. and F.G. Harbaugh. 1948. Amer. J. Vet. Res. 9:20.
Dennis, R.L. and R.W. Hemken. 1978. J. Dairy Sci. 61:757.
Dennis, R.J., R.W. Hemken and D.R. Jacobson. 1976. J. Dairy Sci. 59:324.
Devlin, T.J. and W.K. Roberts. 1963. J. Animal Sci. 22:648.
Devlin, T.J., W.K. Roberts and V.V. St. Omer. 1969. J. Animal Sci. 28:557.
Dewhurst, J.K., F.A. Harrison and R.D. Keynes. 1968. J. Physiol. 195:609.
Elam, C.J. and L.K. Autry. 1961. Proc. West. Sec. Amer. Soc. Animal Sci. 12:LXIX.
Field, A.C. and N.F. Suttle. 1967. J. Agr. Sci. 69:417.
Fisher, E.W. 1965. Brit. Vet. J. 121:132.
Fontenot, J.P., R.W. Miller, C.K. Whitehair and R. MacVicar. 1960. J. Animal Sci. 19:127.
Goodall, E.D. and R.N.B. Kay. 1965. J. Physiol. 176:12.
Jackson, H.M., R.P. Kromann and F.E. Ray. 1971. J. Animal Sci. 33:872.
Johnson, R.R., L.E. Walters and J.V. Whiteman. 1972. J. Animal Sci. 35:931.
Lane, A.G., J.R. Campbell and G.F. Krause. 1968. J. Animal Sci. 27:766.
L'Estrange, J.L. and R.F.E. Axford. 1966. J. Agr. Sci. 67:295.
Lohman, T.G. and H.W. Norton. 1968. J. Animal Sci. 27:1266.
Moseley, G. and D.I.H. Jones. 1974. J. Agr. Sci. 83:37.
Mylrea, P.J. 1966. Res. Vet. Sci. 7:394.
Newton, G.L., J.P. Fontenot, R.E. Tucker and C.E. Polan. 1972. J. Animal Sci. 35:440.
Perry, S.C., R.G. Cragle and J.K. Miller. 1967. J. Nutr. 93:283.
Perry, S.C., J.H. Schaffer, R.G. Cragle and J.K. Miller. 1966. J. Animal Sci. 26:907 (abstr).
Pradhan, K. and R.W. Hemken. 1968. J. Dairy Sci. 51:1377.
Randall, W.E., R.W. Hemken, L.S. Bull and L.W. Douglas. 1974. J. Dairy Sci. 57:472.
Rook, J.A.F. and C.C. Balch. 1962. J. Agr. Sci. 59:103.
Roy, J.H.B. et al. 1959. Brit. J. Nutr. 13:219.
Scott, D. 1969. Quart. J. Expt. Physiol. 54:16,25.
Smith, R.H. 1962. Biochem. J. 83:151.
St. Omer, V.V. and W.K. Roberts. 1967. Can. J. Animal Sci. 47:39.
Suttle, N.F. and A.C. Field. 1966. Brit. J. Nutr. 20:609.
Telle, P.P., R.Preston, L.C. Kintner and W.H. Pfander. 1964. J. Animal Sci. 23:59.

Van't Klooster, A.T. 1969. Nutr. Abstr. Rev. 39:129.

Ward, G.M. 1966. J. Dairy Sci. 49:268.

Wilde, W.S. 1962. In: Mineral Metabolism. Vol. 2, part B. Academic Press.

Sulfur

Albert, W.W., U.S. Garrigus, R.M. Forbes and H.W. Norton. 1956. J. Animal Sci. 15:559.

Barrow, N.J. and L.J. Lambourne. 1962. Aust. J. Agr. Res. 13:461.

Bird, P.R. 1971. Aust. J. Biol. Sci. 24:1329.

Bird, P.R. 1972. Aust. J. Biol. Sci. 25:817,1073,1087.

Bird, P.R. and R.J. Moir. 1971. Aust. J. Biol. Sci. 24:1319.

Bird, P.R. and R.J. Moir. 1972. Aust. J. Biol. Sci. 25:835.

Bird, P.R. and R.F. Thornton. 1972. Aust. J. Biol. Sci. 25:1299.

Burgess, P.L. and J.W.G. Nicholson. 1971. Can. J. Animal Sci. 51:711.

Bouchard, R. and H.R. Conrad. 1973. J. Dairy Sci. 56:1276,1429,1435.

Bouchard, R. and H.R. Conrad. 1974. Can. J. Animal Sci. 54:587.

Bray, A.C. 1969. Aust. J. Agr. Res. 20:725,739,749.

Bray, A.C. and J.A. Hemsley. 1969. Aust. J. Agr. Res. 20:759.

Chalupa, W., R.R. Oltjen, L.L. Slyter and D.A. Dinius. 1971. J. Animal Sci. 33:278.

Chalupa, W., R.R. Oltjen and D.A. Dinius. 1973. J. Animal Sci. 37:340.

Digesti, R.D. and H.J. Weeth. 1973. Proc. West. Sec. ASAS 24:259.

Digesti, R.D. and H.J. Weeth. 1976. J. Animal Sci. 42:1498.

Goodrich, R.D., J.H. Johnson and J.C. Meiske. 1967. J. Animal Sci. 26:1490 (abstr).

Grieve, D.G., W.G. Merrill and C.E. Coppock. 1973. J. Dairy Sci. 56:224.

Hale, W.H. and U.S. Garrigus. 1953. J. Animal Sci. 12:492.

Hansard, S.L. and A.S. Mohammed. 1968. J. Nutr. 96:247.

Hansard, S.L. and A.S. Mohammed. 1969. J. Animal Sci. 28:283.

Jacobson, D.R., J.W. Barnett, S.B. Carr and R.H. Hatton. 1967. J. Dairy Sci. 50:1248.

Jacobson, D.R. et al. 1969. J. Dairy Sci. 52:472.

Johnson, W.H., R.D. Goodrich and J.C. Meiske. 1971. J. Animal Sci. 32:778.

Johnson, W.H., J.C. Meiske and R.D. Goodrich. 1968. J. Animal Sci. 27:1166 (abstr).

Joyce, J.P. and P.V. Rattray. 1970. N.Z. J. Agr. Res. 13:792.

Julian, R.J. and K.B. Harrison. 1975. Can. Vet. J. 16:28.

Kaemmerer, K., E. Barke and M.J. Seidler. 1973. Nutr. Abstr. Rev. 43:177.

Kennedy, P.M. 1974. Aust. J. Agr. Res. 25:1015.

Kulwish, R., L. Strugglia and P.B. Pearson. 1957. J. Nutr. 61:113.

Langlands, J.R. and H.A.M. Sutherland. 1973. Brit. J. Nutr. 30:529.

Langlands, J.P., H.A.M. Sutherland and M.J. Playce. 1973. Brit. J. Nutr. 30:538.

Lofgreen, G.P., W.C. Weir and J.F. Wilson. 1953. J. Animal Sci. 12:347.

Martin, J.E. et al. 1964. J. Nutr. 83:60.

Moir, R.J., M. Sommers and A.C. Bray. 1968. Sulphur Inst. J. 3:15.

Nikolaev, K. and V. Dzhedzheva. 1973. Veterinarnomeditsinski Nauki. 10:61.

Shively, J., D. Wolf, A. Trenkle and W. Burroughs. 1966. J. Animal Sci. 25:1256 (abstr).

Starks, P.B., W.H. Hale, U.S. Garrigus and R.M. Forbes. 1953. J. Animal Sci. 12:480.

Thomas, W.E., J.K. Loosli, H.H. Williams and L.A. Maynard. 1951. J. Nutr. 43:515.

Weeth, H.J. and D.L. Capps. 1972. J. Animal Sci. 34:256.

Weeth, H.J. and J.E. Hunter. 1971. J. Animal Sci. 32:277.

Weir, W.C. and V.V. Rendig. 1954. J. Nutr. 54:87.

Whanger, P.D. and G. Matrone. 1966. Biochem. Biophys. Acta. 124:273.

Whiting, F., S.B. Slen, L.M. Bezeau and R.D. Clark. 1954. J. Animal Sci. 12:936.

Chapter 5 - The Trace Elements

by D.C. Church, S.L. Hansard, J.K. Miller
and P.D. Whanger

Although traces of certain minerals were recognized in plant and animal tissues early in the 19th century, it was nearly 6 decades before significant biological importance was attached to some of them (Nicholas and Ega, 1973). More than 60 inorganic elements have been identified in tissues of man, animals, fungi, bacteria and dietary components and the importance of many of them in biochemical and physiological processes has been established. The microminerals comprising <1% of the total ash in the animal body have been so designated primarily on the basis of mass occurrence.

Underwood (1977) has arbitrarily divided the microminerals into three groups:

Dietary essential—cobalt, copper, iodine, iron, manganese, molybdenum, nickel, selenium and zinc.

Possible essential—arsenic, cadmium, chromium, fluorine, silicon, tin and vanadium

Contaminants—aluminum, barium, boron, bromine, cesium, lithium, rubidium, strontium and titanium.

Definite proof that a mineral element is required is not always easy to come by. Natural foods and feeds, soil, and water supplies may have sufficient quantities of the elements to satisfy requirements. Purified diets have been most helpful in this respect. Even here, however, many laboratory reagent grade chemicals have traces of a variety of different elements other than the chemical compounds specified on the label. Consequently, a "pure" diet may be difficult to achieve. The senior author well remembers a story told to him by an agronomic student who was trying to show that wheat required boron. The student was carrying out a study using a hydroponic technique and, in the course of the work, mixed his mineral solutions in a stone crock. The solutions were transferred to the hydroponic tank with a glass beaker. Using this procedure he could not show any results by adding boron. Eventually, he found that the glass beakers used had boron in the glass which was soluble enough in the mineral solution so that no requirement could be shown.

F has been recognized in the prevention of dental cavities and has shown other possibilities in animal metabolism. Studies with purified diets have indicated that V, Sn, Cr and As may be essential for specific physiological functions. However, other elements, such as Al, Cs, Sr, Br and B, which appear to be required by plants, have not been identified as being essential for animals.

With the exception of Fe in hemoglobin, myoglobin, and some storage compounds, most trace minerals seem to function as biological catalysts. Their roles may range from weak ionic effects to specific combinations with proteins to form metallo-enzymes (Underwood, 1977). A great volume of in vitro data on trace element-enzyme associations has been accumulated during the last 20 years. Underwood (1977) has pointed out, however, that several pathological disorders cannot yet be explained in biochemical or enzyme terms, strongly suggesting either undiscovered metalloenzymes or other vital roles yet unknown for the micro-elements (i.e. nonenzymic functionally active compounds). I and Co are two examples of this thesis. Wacker and Valee (1959) suggest that some trace elements play a role in the configuration of the RNA molecule, perhaps linking purine or pyrmidine bases or both through covalent bonds and hence, bearing a functional relationship to protein synthesis and the transmission of genetic information.

For additional reading the authors would suggest the classic book by Underwood, now in its 4th edition (1977). Other relatively recent compilations include that edited by Mills (1970), Hoekstra et al (1974), and Mortvedt et al (1972). Additional references are listed under the General Reference list at the end of the chapter.

COBALT

Experimental data on Co date back a good many years, and a substantial amount of information on its distribution in plants has been available for more than 40 years. With respect to animals, Co was first shown to be beneficial to sheep in 1935 (see Underwood, 1977). Since that time there have been many,

many papers dealing with the distribution of Co in the tissues, its function in animal metabolism, deficiency symptoms, and methods of supplementing animals with Co in deficient areas. For further details on the subject refer to Smith (1962) or Underwood (1977).

Distribution of Tissue Co

Data from a variety of sources show that Co is found in highest concentrations in the kidney, adrenals, spleen and pancreas. Lesser amounts may be found in other organs or tissues. Typical concentrations in the liver of ruminants on adequate diets are on the order of 0.15 ppm or more of Co, although normal animals may be found with lower levels than this (Andrews et al, 1959). Only small quantities of Co are found in blood or milk. In the rumen contents of adequately fed animals, Co may be found in amounts on the order of 0.4-0.7 mcg/100 g. The rumen microorganisms take up substantial quantities of dietary Co.

Plant tissues vary tremendously, and there are species as well as seasonal differences. Andrews (1956) points out that the Co content of pastures (in New Zealand) tends to increase in the late autumn and winter and to decrease in spring and summer. The grasses are generally lower than legumes in Co content.

Metabolism of Co

Absorption and Excretion. Comar et al (1946) and Comar and Davis (1946) have studied the excretion of radiocobalt when administered orally or I.V. to cattle. After an oral dose, about 80% appeared in the feces but only 0.5 in the urine. The liver was the main site of tissue storage, but contained only 0.4% of the dose by five days after dosing. After an I.V. dose, about 65% of the dose was recovered in the urine, with 7% and 30% in the feces in different experiments. Co in the blood disappeared relatively quickly and none was detected in the rumen. Distribution in the tissues was general, although high concentrations were found in the kidney, liver, bone marrow, lymph glands and bile. They calculated that 5-15% of the I.V. dose was excreted via bile. Small amounts were found in abomasal contents. Very limited amounts were transferred across the placenta of a pregnant animal. With respect to sheep, Monroe et al (1952) found that 85% of an oral dose of radiocobalt was recovered in feces and ca. 11% in urine. After an I.V. dose, 8% was recovered in feces and 78% in urine.

Rothery et al (1953) found that liver and kidney of sheep concentrated labeled Co more than any other tissues. When sheep were killed at intervals after an oral dose, the highest concentration was found in the rectal contents (330-2,300 mcg/kg of wet tissue). Co passed out of the rumen rapidly, but was still recovered in substantial amounts in the rectum 24 hr after the last oral intake.

Co and Vitamin B$_{12}$ Metabolism. Information available at this time indicates that Co occupies a unique position for one of the trace elements in that it is an integral part of the molecule of cyanocobalamin, or vitamin B$_{12}$. Information on this subject became available in 1948, and it provided a much better understanding of the role of Co in the nutrition of animals. Although Co may be present in the tissues in bound forms other than B$_{12}$, no other physiological function has been demonstrated. In blood plasma studies with B$_{12}$ labeled with ^{60}Co show that B$_{12}$ is bound to the α-2 fraction of serum globulins (Gille et al, 1971). Infusion studies with isolated jejunal sections of sheep gut suggest that Co reduced motor activity of the gut. In addition, when infused with other salts or organic compounds, Co reduced absorption of Na, K, P, glucose, glycine and water but increased excretion into the intestinal lumen of Na and Ca absorption (Li and Abdrakhamanov, 1975). Oral CoCl$_2$ apparently reduces Mo retention, particularly when combined with KI (Odynets et al, 1972).

With respect to ruminant species, there are a number of studies which show that Co, per se, is apparently not required by the animal, whereas B$_{12}$ is, without question, required by the tissues. The rumen microorganisms, then, provide the link between Co and B$_{12}$ by synthesizing the vitamin which is required by the host's tissues.

The need for oral intake of Co has been shown in many different studies. Although some (Smith et al, 1950; Lee and Marston, 1969) research indicated that I.V. administration of Co resulted in no improvement of Co-deficient lambs, others (Ray et al, 1958; Keener et al, 1951; Monroe et al, 1952) have shown that I.V. dosage of Co resulted in some improvement in the performance of deficient animals and improved B$_{12}$ synthesis in the rumen, indicating recycling of Co to the rumen, either through the saliva or through the rumen wall. Administration of Co via the duodenum or abomasum has been shown to improve growth in one experiment (Phillipson and Mitchell, 1952) but not in others (Lee and Marston, 1969; Kercher and Smith, 1956) although there may be a greater concentration of B_{12} in the cecum and large intestine as a result (Kercher and Smith, 1956). Monroe et al (1952) found that about 10X as much ^{60}Co was recovered in the liver as B_{12} after ingestion as after I.V. dosing. They calculated that 10% of oral Co was recovered as B_{12} in the feces as compared to 0.2% after I.V. dosing.

Numerous experiments have shown that I.V. or oral dosing with Co will increase liver concentration of Co, but the correlation between Co and liver B_{12} is not high when large doses of Co are given (Andrews et al, 1959). The liver, itself, has been reported to take up only 14% of labeled B_{12} administered I.V. (Marston et al, 1961).

The amount of B_{12} synthesis in the rumen is very substantial, since rumen contents may contain up to 10 mcg of B_{12} activity/g of dry matter. Apparent synthesis in the GI tract of sheep on natural rations has been estimated at ca. 2,000-3,000 mcg/day (Pearson et al, 1953). However, only a fraction of this is true vitamin B_{12}. Rumen microorganisms synthesize a variety of Co-containing B_{12}-like molecules (Hine and Dawbarn, 1954) that are believed to have no physiological function for the host (Monroe et al, 1952; Hopper and Johnson, 1955; Smith, 1962). Hine and Dawbarn pointed out that total B_{12} activity in rumen contents was 10-20X greater than true B_{12} activity. It has been estimated that the absorption of B_{12} is very low (Kercher and Smith, 1955) since an oral dose of B_{12} required about 35X as much as a parenteral dose. Marston (1970) calculated that absorption efficiency was <3% in sheep.

It is also possible that rumen microorganisms might metabolize dietary or rumen B_{12}, possibly producing some of the pseudo vitamins. At any rate, data available indicate that only a small portion of Co synthesized into B_{12} may be of use to the host. This, then, offers a possible explanation of why the Co requirement of ruminants is greater than that of species such as the horse, rabbit or quokka. It is assumed that these species derive their B_{12} requirement from absorption of B_{12} produced in the cecum or large intestine. In the case of the rabbit, some of the dietary B_{12} may be obtained by coprophagy. It has been shown that the pseudo B_{12} compounds do appear in the liver of calves (Hopper and Johnson, 1955). Their function in the rumen is unknown also, but it is known that some of these compounds are growth-promoting factors for some types of bacteria.

Cobalt Deficiency

Underwood (1977) has summarized the older literature dealing with ruminants. For the purposes of this discussion, it will suffice to briefly recapitulate some of his discussion without documenting much of the original research. Evidence indicates that cattle, sheep and goats are affected. Presumably, wild ruminants are affected also, but information is lacking on this subject.

The time required to develop deficiency symptoms depends on the dietary intake as well as tissue reserves of B_{12}. For example, when lambs were put on a diet with 0.042 ppm of Co, it required 7 mo. for low hemoglobin to show up but plasma B_{12} was not depressed until 258 days (Jones and Anthony, 1970). In another case lambs were grazed on pasture where the soil had 0.17 ppm of Co. By the end of 8 wk, at least 50% of the lambs had a clinical deficiency (Russel et al, 1975).

The severity of Co deficiency may vary from a mild deficiency to an acute stage. In the latter, the appearance of the animal (see Fig. 5-1,2) resembles that of starvation, the animal being listless and emaciated. In addition, the animal appears anemic, since the mucous membranes are blanched and the skin is pale. The eyes may water excessively, also. A characteristic finding is that a depressed appetite accompanies or precedes the symptoms that develop. Plasma glucose is also said to be quite low in affected sheep as well as plasma alkaline phosphatase (MacPherson et al, 1973; MacPherson and Moon, 1974).

Young animals are generally said to be more susceptible to a Co deficiency than adults, probably because of a higher requirement due to their more rapid growth rate and higher metabolic rate than adults. Likewise, yearlings are generally more susceptible than adults.

The liver of severely affected animals shows fatty degeneration and the spleen shows hemosiderosis. There may be hypoplasia of the bone marrow and other bone marrow abnormalities (Ibbotson et al, 1970). Red blood cells and hemoglobin levels are low, although there is no apparent agreement on what specific type of anemia is present. Although animals are anemic, plasma proteins do not appear to be affected (Jones and Anthony, 1970). Some data

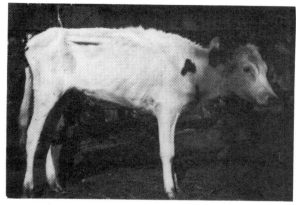

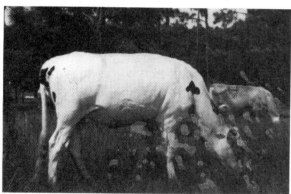

Fig. 5-1. Co deficient animal (top). Note the severe emaciation. Bottom. The same animal several weeks after Co administration. Courtesy of R.B. Becker, Florida Agr. Expt. Sta.

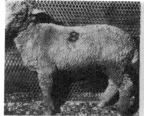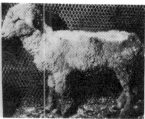

Fig. 5-2. Co-deficient sheep. Note the severe emaciation and wool chewing that has occurred (right). The lamb on the left received an adequate diet. Courtesy of S.E. Smith, Cornell Univ.

indicate that treatment with folic acid will restore normal erythropoiesis, but has no effect otherwise (Marston et al, 1961); thus, it is often said that the anemia that develops is secondary.

A normal liver Co level is on the order of 0.2-0.3 ppm, whereas Co-deficient animals may have levels of 0.04-0.06 ppm or less. In normal sheep, a typical value for B_{12} in the blood is 1-3 mcg/l. Andrews et al (1959) suggest that sheep show the first clinical symptoms when the blood of ewes reaches a value of 0.26 mcg/l. and, for lambs, a value of 0.30 mcg/l. They further suggest that liver B_{12} should be at least 0.30 ppm of fresh tissue to be considered adequate.

Co-deficient animals generally have very little body fat remaining. Deficient sheep are less efficient in absorbing N. Animals on a Co-deficient diet but with adequate tissue reserves of B_{12} apparently do not have altered metabolism of N or energy and production of methane or digestibility of roughage were not altered (Smith and Marston, 1970). Wool with low breaking strength has been observed in deficient sheep (Jones and Anthony, 1970). Holmes (1965) has reported data showing tissue changes in water, collagen, lipids and nitrogenous compounds. Rozybakiev (1967) indicated that addition of a Co supplement to a deficient diet increased the volume of combined secretions from the bile and pancreatic ducts. The Cl content of these secretions was increased, but urea and dry matter were reduced. Proteolytic activity rose and lipolytic and diastatic activity fell.

As was noted previously, a decreased appetite is a noticeable symptom of a Co deficiency. Supplementation with Co will stimulate the appetite within a matter of a few days. This rapid response may be partly due to changes in the rumen microflora, since there is one paper which indicates a change in rumen bacteria on Co-deficient rations. Marston et al (1961, 1972) have presented data which show that Co-deficient sheep could not remove propionic acid from the blood as rapidly as normal sheep, although there was no effect on formic or acetic acids. In vitro studies with liver showed that deficient animals could metabolize malate and succinate normally, but could not handle propionate conversion to succinate. This led to an accumulation of the intermediate, methylmalonyl CoA. When the B_{12}-containing enzyme, methylmalonyl co-isomerase, was added, the conversion of methylmalonyl Co A to succinyl Co A was restored. Metabolism of glutamate was normal. Since it has been shown (Ch. 11) that high blood levels of propionate may depress the appetite, these authors suggest that this may be the explanation for the depressed appetite in Co-deficient animals.

Data published by Gawthorne (1968) showed that urinary excretion of methylmalonic acid in deficient sheep was 5-12X that of normals, and that of formimino-glutamic acid was increased more than 30X.

The latter acid increased in the early stages more so than the former. The significance of this latter change remains to be determined. Serum B_{12} concentration is inversely related to urinary formimino glutamic acid concentration (Russel et al, 1975).

Hine and Dawbarn (1954) point out that withdrawal of Co from a diet, otherwise adequate, resulted in a marked fall in B_{12} activity in rumen contents to a value only 4-12% of the previous level. Marston et al (1961) suggest that a normal level of Co in the rumen is about 40 mcg/l. When this falls below 20, synthesis of B_{12} falls from a normal level (said to be 600-1,000 mcg/day) to less than 50 mcg/day. They further suggest that there is no obvious impairment of physiological function until liver B_{12} falls below 0.15 ppm.

With respect to synthesis of B_{12} in the rumen, Tribe et al (1954) reported that administration of penicillin was effective in curing sheep while they remained on a Co-deficient diet. They suggested that this might be accounted for by a change in the rumen microorganisms to a population that favored the utilization of the limited dietary Co more efficiently.

A conditioned B_{12} deficiency in cattle has been reported from Japan (Shashi et al, 1953). It is believed to be caused by the presence in the drinking water of silico-fluoride which is toxic to some rumen organisms shown to be responsible for some B_{12} synthesis. The disease can be induced in healthy animals by giving silicofluoride and responds to treatment with vitamin B_{12}.

Lee and Marston (1969) pointed out that the degree of Co deficiency may differ greatly from season to season and from year to year. Andrews (1956) suggested that some of the seasonal and yearly changes may be due to changes in the composition of pastures, since it was shown that the Co content of grasses was less than that of legumes and that seasonal changes occurred in Co content of forage, also. Lee (1950) has also pointed out that Co deficiency occurs in areas (in Australia) where the soils have largely been derived from shells of marine origin. Andrews et al (1958) found that Co deficiency was more apt to develop on lightly grazed pastures than on heavily grazed pastures; they suggested that animals on the heavily grazed pastures might be picking up more Co from the soil.

Cobalt Requirements

Andrews (1956) states that young, growing sheep have the highest Co requirement, followed by mature sheep, calves of 6-18 mo. of age, and mature cattle. Field data indicate that severe Co deficiency results in cattle and sheep maintained on forage containing 0.02-0.05 ppm Co (dry basis). Andrews et al (1958) suggest that lambs require about 0.11 ppm under New Zealand conditions. Although lower levels than this have been proposed based on research from other countries (see Underwood, 1977), Lee and Marston (1969) calculated that ewes required about 0.08 mg/day and that lambs may require as much as 0.2 mg/day of Co. Somer and Gawthorne (1969) found that plasma vitamin B_{12} concentration progressively increased as the dietary Co level was raised from 0.04 ppm to 0.34 ppm. Their data, based on plasma B_{12}, indicated a requirement of at least 0.10 ppm of Co.

The Co requirement of bovines has not been as well defined as that for sheep. The limited data indicate that the requirement may be on the order of 1 mg/day or more (Underwood, 1977).

Limited data on B_{12} supplementation indicate a high requirement if this vitamin is to replace Co in the diet, but the data are not sufficiently precise to establish a dietary requirement. For that matter, there would be no point in this except for preruminants.

Other Nutrient Factors

Davis et al (1956) reported that high Mo in the diet of cattle (200-400 ppm) changed the distribution of B_{12} in liver and heart tissues, probably due to the fact that the high Mo diets appeared to reduce the synthesis of B_{12}. Addition of Co to such rations increased the synthesis of B_{12}. Data from Florida (Ammerman, 1970) showed that Co additions to the diet of heifers improved the utilization of Cu and Fe in animals on a low Mo diet, and that Co also improved the utilization of Fe for blood hemoglobin formation in heifers receiving Mo in the diet. Co did not appear to modify the reduced liver Cu seen with the addition of Mo. MacPherson et al (1973) also concluded that injected B_{12} or oral Co helped to prevent a Cu deficiency in cattle.

Phalaris staggers is a disease of cattle and sheep that occurs when these animals graze the perennial grass, *Phalaris tuberosa*. This disease has been observed in Australia, New Zealand, South Africa and the USA. Lee and Kuchel (1953) found that there was no incidence of staggers amongst 10 ewes which were dosed each wk with 7 mg of Co, while

11 of 15 untreated ewes were affected, six of them fatally. However, Lanigan and Whittem (1970) observed that prior treatment with Co did not reduce morbidity or mortality of sheep which ingested toxic alkaloids from *Heliotropium europaeum*.

Prevention of Co Deficiency

Co deficiency can readily be prevented provided a regular intake of the element can be obtained. Fertilization of pastures has been used successfully, data from New Zealand (Andrews, 1956) showing that Co sulfate applied at the rate of about 140 g/acre this level would usually suffice up to 3 yr. Spraying of plant foliage (Andrews, 1956; Griffiths et al, 1970) has also been used successfully. Inclusion in supplemental feed at the rate of 2 g/ton was found to be adequate in an area of marginal deficiency (Keener et al, 1954), or the addition to salt licks may be successfully used.

Drenching of animals is one sure way of getting Co into animals where it may not be feasible to fertilize. However, data of Lee and Marston (1969) showed that animals should be drenched at least once per week in order to obtain maximum gain. Previous information reviewed shows that the B$_{12}$ and Co concentration in the rumen drop rapidly when the dietary intake is stopped. Irving (1959) presented data which showed that liver Co levels are also depleted in 10-30 days after drenching.

One means of eliminating the tedious task of drenching is to use the Co "bullets" which were devised by Dewey et al (1958). These products are prepared of cobaltic oxide and clay and compressed to provide a dense, long-lasting source of Co. Other data (Andrews et al, 1958; Andrews and Stephenson, 1966) show that this method can be used quite successfully, provided the animal does not regurgitate and lose the pellet. In young animals, some information (Owen et al, 1960) indicates that the bullets may become encrusted with phosphatic salts, thus reducing the release of Co. This may be partially alleviated by inclusion of steel screws which serve to abrade off any coatings (see Underwood, 1977).

Cobalt Toxicity

Co toxicity can be produced in sheep and cattle by administration of large doses, Becker and Smith (1951) finding that doses of 4.4-11 mg/kg of weight resulted in severely depressed appetite, weight losses

and anemia at the higher levels, although levels up to 3.5 mg/kg could be tolerated for as long as 8 weeks. I.V. doses of 75 mg resulted in death of several animals. Postmortem studies showed liver degeneration, lung congestion and hemorrhaging in the small intestine.

In studies with calves (Dunn et al, 1952; Ely et al, 1948, 1952), it was shown that I.V. doses of 0.66 mg/kg of weight were toxic, resulting in symptoms such as increased lacrimation and salivation, dyspnea, incoordination, defecation and urination. Oral doses of 0.9 mg/kg of weight were toxic. I.V. injections of methionine reduced the severity of the symptoms. Keener et al (1954) state that Holstein calves could tolerate up to 100X the amount of Co usually fed. These data indicate that calves are much more susceptible than sheep to Co toxicity. Dickson and Bond (1974) suggest that Co toxicity in cattle may occur rather frequently in Australia, particularly when Co has been used in salt licks, in mixed rations and when applied to pastures. Neathery and Miller (1977) concluded that the maximum safe level for cattle is 20 ppm and for sheep, 50 ppm.

Gardiner and Nairn (1969) have shown that ewes develop some of the signs of clover disease when grazed on pastures primarily of subterranean clover (*Trifolium subterraneum*) which have been heavily fertilized with Co. The symptoms observed involved such things as depressed fertility and cystic degeneration of the cervix and uterus. The administration of Se appeared to reverse, to some extent, the adverse effects of the Co.

COPPER AND MOLYBDENUM

The essentiality of Cu for animals has been recognized for over 45 years. Since that time a vast amount of literature has been accumulated on Cu requirements, deficiency and toxicity. Mo was first recognized for its toxicity, but abnormalities may also result in both ruminant and monogastric animals when dietary Mo is very low (Poitevint and Nelson, 1978). Because of the close interrelationship between the two elements, Cu and Mo will be discussed together. Recent reviews of Cu and Mo requirements, toxicities and interactions in ruminants include those of Suttle (1975a), Pitt (1976), Roberts (1976), Underwood (1977), Poitevint and Nelson (1978), and Ward (1978).

Tissue Cu and Mo

Underwood (1977) has summarized literature from a variety of sources on Cu

Table 5-1. Distribution of blood Cu of sheep of different ages.[a]

Item	Whole blood Cu, mcg%	Plasma Cu, mcg%	Direct reading Cu, mcg%[*]	Indirect reading Cu, mcg%[**]	Red blood cell Cu, mcg%
Adults	98	102	20	81	95
Fetus	45	26	17	11	78
Lambs, new-born	83	63	47	16	104

[a] From McCosker (1968)

[*] Equivalent to albumin-bound Cu

[**] Equivalent to ceruloplasmin Cu

concentration in various tissues of different species of animals. In the blood, Cu is found in the red cells in a nearly colorless protein complex called erythrocuprein, with a molecular weight of about 35,000 and containing ca. 0.34% Cu. In the plasma, Cu is found in ceruloplasmin, an α-globulin complex containing 8 atoms of Cu. Plasma also contains another Cu-containing fraction called direct reading (or direct-reacting) Cu, a fraction which reacts with diethyldithiocarbamate. The Cu in this fraction, which is high after I.V. injection of Cu, is loosely bound to albumin, nondialyzable, and involved in Cu transport. Cu in the plasma or whole blood is typically near 100 μg/100 ml for sheep (Lorenz and Gibb, 1975; Bremner, 1976) and cattle (Huber et al, 1971). With high dietary Mo (25 ppm) and sulfate (0.5%), plasma Cu of sheep increased to 145 μg/100 ml (Bremner, 1976).

McCosker (1968) has examined these blood fractions in sheep of various ages and in various other situations (Table 5-1). These data show that plasma Cu is low in the young lamb, but red cell Cu is more similar to adults. Even lower plasma Cu levels of 38 μg/100 ml (Barlow et al, 1976) and 11 μg/100 ml (Suttle et al, 1970) have been reported for lambs born to ewes with normal plasma Cu levels. McCosker also reported data on sheep afflicted with a variety of diseases. His data indicated that plasma Cu (ceruloplasmin) was increased by acute arthritis, infected wounds, meningitis and abscessed feet. An infection of trichostrongylus increased plasma Cu, but hemonchosis infection reduced it. Increases were noted in animals with hypocalcemia, hypomagnesemia and pregnancy toxemia—probably because of degenerative changes of the liver known to occur in these situations.

Bingley and Dufty (1973) measured Cu in whole blood, plasma and erythrocytes of Hereford cattle throughout pregnancy.

Whole blood Cu remained relatively constant at 83 to 91 μg/100 ml from 32 days before insemination through day 284 of gestation. Plasma Cu increased from 83 μg/100 ml at insemination to 102 μg/100 ml between days 90-119, then declined to 88 μg/100 ml by day 284. Conversely, erythrocyte Cu decreased from initial levels of 79-89 μg/100 ml to 61 μg/100 ml between days 123 and 151 then returned to 95 μg/100 ml by day 284.

Of ruminant tissues analyzed, the liver has by far the greatest concentration of Cu. Claypool et al (1975) measured Cu levels in 540 paired blood and liver samples from cattle. They concluded that plasma Cu was of little value in predicting liver Cu but plasma Cu levels of 50 μg/100 ml or less were indicative of low liver Cu levels. Liver Cu levels may range from 100 to 600 ppm, dry weight basis, in normal adult ruminants (Huber et al, 1971; Suttle et al, 1970; Underwood, 1977) although in the western parts of the USA, liver Cu is typically lower than this, more on the order of 30-100 ppm (Lesperance and Bohman, 1963; Cook et al, 1966). Liver Cu (dry matter basis) may fall below 10 ppm during Cu deficiency or Mo excess (Suttle et al, 1970; Smith and Coup, 1973; Idris and Tartour, 1975; Smith, 1975; Smith et al, 1975; Rogers and Pool, 1978) or exceed 1300 ppm when dietary Cu is excessive (Tait et al, 1971).

The tissue uptake of ^{64}Cu after oral or I.V. administration has been reported for the bovine (Comar et al, 1948) and ovine (Moss et al, 1974). In the case of one bovine sacrificed 19 hr after I.V. administration, ^{64}Cu recoveries were 9.4% of the dose in blood and 33% in the liver. Nearly all other tissues contained <1% of the dose. Some values given for tissues with the higher concentrations were (% of dose): kidney, 0.72; lung, 0.96; rumen tissue, 1.2; large intestine tissue, 1.8; large intestine contents, 0.6; and bile, 0.1. Of the total ^{64}Cu retained in ovine tissues after I.V. administration, percentages in liver increased from 60% at 2 hr to 95% at 24 hr.

Moss et al (1974) also measured accumulation of ^{64}Cu byproducts of conception in 136-day pregnant ewes. At 2 hr after dosing fetal liver contained almost all of the fetal ^{64}Cu, but this dropped to 32% after 24 hr. Other organs contained only trace amounts. The placenta accumulated much more ^{64}Cu than did the fetus, indicating a concentration barrier for Cu between the ewe and fetus. At 2 hr post dosing the placenta contained approximately 99% of the ^{64}Cu in the total products of conception and still maintained at least 63% of the dose at 24 hr. Williams et al (1978) found the instantaneous rate of Cu deposition in the fetus increased exponentially between the 80th and 144th day of gestation. The proportion of total fetal Cu in the liver was always above 50%.

Cu concentrations in milk of ewes fed a 1 ppm Cu ration averaged 26 μg/100 ml; when 11 ppm Cu was fed, milk Cu averaged 116 μg/100 ml on the first day of lactation and 52 μg/100 ml on the 52nd day (Suttle et al, 1970). Several investigators have reported Cu concentrations near 10 μg/100 ml in bovine milk (Vanderveen and Keener, 1964; Huber et al, 1971; Hankinson, 1975; Ho et al, 1977). Feeding high levels of Mo increased milk Cu 10-fold in one study (Huber et al, 1971) but was without effect in another (Vanderveen and Keener, 1964).

Blood levels of Mo vary sharply with Mo intake, increasing from 1-5 μg/100 ml in ruminants receiving normal rations to 160-280 μg/100 ml in sheep fed diets containing 4.5 ppm (Suttle, 1975b) and to 700 μg/100 ml in cows fed 173-300 ppm Mo (Huber et al, 1971). Mo concentrations in other tissues were also increased markedly when cows were fed high Mo levels. Mo concentrations in cows' milk ranged from 0.02 to 0.10 ppm (Vanderveen and Keener, 1964; Huber et al, 1974). Anke et al (1971) dosed 4 lactating goats orally with [99]Mo and 96 hr later found 6.9% of the dose was incorporated into the body exclusive of the GI tract. Of the total retained [99]Mo, 27.4% was in the skeleton, 19.9 in liver, 14.3 in skin, 11.6 in muscles and 0.1 in hair. Relative [99]Mo concentrations in tissue dry matter were kidney, 100; liver, 60; ovaries, 28; blood, 18; skin and bones, 12 each; hair, 3 and muscle, 3.

Functions of Cu and Mo

Cu is a constituent of several enzymes or is essential for their activity. Its involvement in a broad range of biochemical functions in the animal body has been reviewed by Evans (1973) and Underwood (1977). Evidence has also been presented for the involvement of Cu in prostaglandin synthesis (Maddox, 1973) and its role in formation of aortic elastin (Hill et al, 1967). Gallagher and Reeve (1976) suggested Cu is a component of the adenine nucleotide binding sites of mitochondrial membranes because ADP binding was depressed by Cu-complexing agents and increased when mitochondrial membrane Cu content was increased. Erythrocuprein functions as a superoxide dismutase (McCord and Fridovich, 1969), catalyzing the dismutation of monovalent superoxide anion radicals into hydrogen peroxide and oxygen and scavenging of singlet oxygen in metabolism (Arneson, 1970). Sharoyan et al (1977) reported cerebrocuprein, a water soluble protein containing 0.33% Cu isolated from bovine brain, also had superoxide dismutase activity. Ceruloplasmin is a ferroxidase involved in Fe utilization and in promoting the rate of Fe saturation of transferrin in plasma (Osaki et al, 1966). Ceruloplasmin also oxidizes epinephrine, norepinephrine, serotonin and melatonin and may function in controlling the plasma level of certain amines (Osaki et al, 1964). The albumin-bound direct reacting Cu, rather than ceruloplasmin, is considered to be the transport Cu (Gubler et al, 1953).

Monoamine oxidase, an enzyme with a molecular weight of 195,000 daltons, contains 4 atoms of Cu/molecule. It catalyzes the oxidative deamination of a variety of monoamines to the corresponding aldehydes and is involved in maintaining the structural integrity of both vascular and bone tissue. According to Ishizoki and Yasurobu (1976), bovine plasma amine oxidase has a molecular weight of about 170,000 and contains 2 atoms of Cu per mole of protein. Tyrosinase, which also requires Cu, is essential in the pigmentation process since it catalyzes the first two steps in the synthesis of melanin from tyrosine.

Dietary Mo has been associated with development of Cu toxicity when at the lower extreme of intake (Suttle, 1975a). Apart from its reactions with Cu, other biochemical functions of Mo are related to the formation and activities of xanthine oxidase, aldehyde oxidase and sulfite oxidase (Underwood, 1977). Mo participates in the reaction of xanthine oxidase with cytochrome c and the reduction of cytochrome c by aldehyde oxidase.

Absorption and Excretion of Cu

Urinary excretion of Cu is low in most species, amounting to only 1 to 2% of total Cu excreted by sheep fed purified diets (Smith et al, 1968) or cattle fed grass or alfalfa hay (Lesperance and Bohman, 1963). The excretion of ^{64}Cu following oral or I.V. dosage has been reported by several investigators. Comar et al (1948) found that young bulls excreted 75% of an oral dose in feces and 3% via urine during a 5-day period. When the dose was given I.V., about 3% of the dose was excreted via each route. In research with sheep, Lassiter and Bell (1960) also found that excretion of an I.V. dose was about equally divided between feces and urine—about 3% in each case. With sheep fed purified diets, Smith et al (1968) recovered about 5% of an I.V. dose of radio Cu in feces and 1% in urine over a 5-day period. Excretion of ^{64}Cu by two non-pregnant ewes during 5 days after oral dosing averaged 92% of the dose in feces and 0.4% in the urine (Moss et al, 1974).

Suttle (1973a) measured ^{64}Cu absorption by lambs using [103]Ru as a non-absorbed reference. Cu absorption decreased linearly from 71% at 28 days before weaning and 47% 14 days later to 11% at 15 days after weaning. True availability of Cu, estimated from relative responses in blood of hypocupremic ewes to Cu given orally or intravenously, ranged from 4 to 11% (Suttle 1974b).

Effect of Cu Source. There is little evidence to indicate quantitatively how well forage sources of Cu are utilized, although there is evidence that water-soluble complexes of Cu in herbage are used by the rat more efficiently than some inorganic sources (Mills, 1954). There is also evidence to show that rumen microorganisms readily take up plant sources of Cu (Mills, 1958). In the case of various inorganic sources of Cu, Lassiter and Bell (1960) have studied uptake in blood and excretion by sheep of Cu from a variety of cupric salts as well as cupric oxide powder and needles, and Cu wire. In one experiment cupric chloride resulted in higher blood concentrations than the sulfate or nitrate salts, but fecal excretion was little different. In another experiment, data indicated that carbonate and the various oxides were poorly utilized. Dick (1954) found that Cu sulfide, when fed to sheep, resulted in less liver storage than Cu sulfate. MacPherson and Hemmingway (1968) have observed that oral supplementation of sheep with Cu as the sulfate, glycinate or EDTA salt resulted in

similar blood and liver values. When studying Cu poisoning, it has been observed (Todd et al, 1962) that the acetate was more toxic than the sulfate, thus one would assume a greater absorption.

GI Sites of Cu Absorption. Ivan and Grieve (1976) investigated absorption of Cu from various GI tract sections of Holstein bull calves by the Cr_2O_3 ratio technique. Absorption along the tract, measured by comparing each segment with the preceding segment, indicated net secretion of Cu in the abomasum but no absorption from the intestines. Net secretion of Cu into the reticulo-rumen was also associated with low dietary Cu. In experiments with cows equipped with rumen fistula and intestinal re-entrant cannulae, Bertoni et al (1976) also found net secretion of Cu anterior to the small intestine and net absorption in the rest of the tract. Grace (1975) also reported net absorption of Cu from the large intestine of rumen-fistulated, intestinal-cannulated sheep, but found no significant differences in quantities of Cu entering and leaving the forestomachs or small intestine.

Absorption and Excretion of Mo

Urinary excretion of Mo, unlike Cu, can be substantial, exceeding 80% of an I.V. [99]Mo dose in sheep (Bell et al, 1966). During 7 days following an oral [99]Mo dose, steers fed a roughage ration excreted 92% in feces and only 4.5% in urine (Bell et al, 1964). When dosed I.V., excretions were 30% in feces and 9.5% in urine. Blood [99]Mo reached a peak 96 hr after an oral dose, indicating a very low absorption. Excretion of [99]Mo by sheep was markedly influenced by both ration and GI site of dose deposition (Bell et al, 1966). With a concentrate ration, 7-day urinary [99]Mo excretion totalled 45% of abomasal compared to only about 10% of ruminal doses. Corresponding fecal [99]Mo excretions were 20% of the abomasal dose and over 80% of the ruminal dose. When sheep were fed the same roughage ration fed to steers above, excretions were 5% of abomasal and 2% of ruminal doses in urine and 75% of abomasal and 95% of ruminal doses in feces. Work with sheep (Dick, 1953; Scaife, 1956) indicates that the relative amount of Mo excreted via urine is a function of the Mo intake. As the Mo intake increases, a relatively higher percentage of the total excretion will be via urine. In contrast, added stable Mo had little influence on [99]Mo metabolism in cattle (Bell et al, 1964; Fisher et al, 1976).

Robinson et al (1964) calculated that the biological half-life of [99]Mo was about 19-20 hr in lactating cows. Of the total [99]Mo recovered, they found 52% in urine, 22% in feces and 26% in milk. During 9 days following I.V. administration of [99]Mo to lactating cows, Cragle et al (1965) reported 5% was recovered in milk, 6.7% in feces and 31.7% in urine. Percentages of the [99]Mo dose recovered in 96 hr after oral administration to lactating goats averaged 51 in feces, 25.4 in urine, 2.4 in milk and 14.3 in GI tract contents (Anke et al, 1971). [99]Mo absorption, calculated as 100% minus percentages in feces and GI tract contents, was 34.7%. Different rations in the above experiments perhaps account for the relative differences in urinary and fecal excretions.

GI sites of Mo absorption, calculated by ratio to a non-absorbed reference material, indicated [99]Mo was absorbed from each section from the abomasum through the small intestine (Miller et al, 1972). There was net secretion of [99]Mo into the rumen but no appreciable absorption from the rumen or omasum. In vitro studies with ovine small intestine showed that the rate of Mo uptake was highest in the distal ileum, lower in the mid small intestine and even lower in the proximal duodenum (Mason and Cardin, 1977).

Factors Modifying Cu and Mo Metabolism

The effects of Mo and sulfate on Cu metabolism have been described in many research reports. In order to present these in a rational manner, it is considered preferable to discuss the effects of Mo and sulfate separately with a following discussion of Mo-sulfate interactions. This will result in more repetition but, hopefully, it will result in greater clarity for those unfamiliar with the subject.

Effect of Mo on Cu. Suttle (1975a) considers the Cu-Mo antagonism to be of practical nutritional significance where Mo in feed is either exceptionally low (<0.2 ppm) or high (> 7 ppm). The antagonism may be associated with the development of Cu toxicity at the lower and Cu deficiency at the upper extreme. Cu deficiency in cattle has also been associated with higher available soil and herbage Mo and lower Cu:Mo ratio in herbage (Rogers and Pool, 1978).

Sheep have frequently been used in Cu-Mo studies although they are less sensitive than cattle to Mo excess. Liver Cu storage was reduced in sheep receiving 9 mg Cu/day when Mo intake was raised from 5 to 20 mg/day (Dick, 1954). Fattening lambs fed rations containing 24 ppm Cu, a near toxic level, had liver Cu contents near the upper limit of the normal range, 59% higher than that of lambs also fed 7.7 ppm Mo (Harker, 1976). Liver Cu storage was also reduced when dietary Mo level was increased from 2 to 8 ppm (Goodrich and Tillman, 1966) or in sheep fed rations containing 5.2 ppm Cu and 0.04% sulfate when Mo was raised from 0.8 to 5.1 ppm (Wynne and McClymont, 1956). Cunningham and Hogan (1959) have studied the response of young sheep grazing pastures containing about 7 ppm Cu, 0.2 to 0.4% sulfate, and <1 ppm compared to 8 ppm Mo. The high-Mo pasture had no adverse effects on growth or hematology although there was an accumulation of Mo in bones, kidney and spleen. The effect on liver storage depended on sulfate content of the pasture (see succeeding section).

Blood Cu of sheep may be unaffected (Goodrich and Tillman, 1966) or increased (Dick, 1954) by increasing Mo intake. Plasma Cu distribution in sheep was not changed by rations containing up to 8 ppm Mo, but 16 ppm Mo and above increased total plasma Cu by 41% and direct reacting Cu by over 3X (Smith and Wright, 1975). Although absolute concentration of ceruloplasmin Cu was not changed, it was decreased as a proportion of total plasma Cu.

With respect to cattle, Smith et al (1975a) reported induced Cu deficiency in a dairy herd in New Zealand. Average Cu levels were 0.33 mg/l. of plasma and 5.3 mg/kg of dry liver; pasture samples had mean levels of 6.7 ppm Cu and 2.5 ppm Mo. Cunningham et al (1959) found that supplemental Mo increased blood and liver Mo and depressed blood and liver Cu when the ration contained 0.1% sulfate. Lesperance and Bohman (1963) also reported increased plasma Mo and storage in skeletal tissues and liver when beef heifers were fed 100 ppm Mo, but animals on a grass hay and cottonseed meal diet retained more than those on alfalfa hay. Plasma Cu was increased initially on both diets but later changes indicated complex interactions not readily explained. Digestion and balance trials did not show any specific effect of Mo.

Cook et al (1966) found no difference between treatments in plasma and liver Cu in cattle dosed orally with 0, 1.5, or 3.0 mg Mo/kg body weight but values were low at the start. However, plasma Mo and liver Fe were increased and hematocrit values were reduced. Toxicity symptoms were evident within 25 days in some cattle. Huber et al

(1971) fed lactating dairy cows a basal ration containing 6 ppm Cu to which from 53 to 300 ppm Mo was added. Overt symptoms of Mo toxicity were observed in cows receiving 173-200 ppm Mo but in none of the cows on the 53-100 ppm level. The higher Mo levels decreased liver Cu, increased milk Cu but had no effect on blood Cu.

Effects of Sulfates on Cu. The direct antagonism interaction between Cu and sulfate appears to be due to the formation of cupric sulfide (Huisingh et al, 1973). Suttle (1974c) found that the effectiveness of Cu supplements in repleting initially hypocupremic ewes was reduced 39-56% when dietary S was increased from 0.1 to 0.3 or 0.4%. Work with sheep by Dick (1954) suggests a linear decrease in liver Cu retention with increasing sulfate intake. Since supplementation with ferrous sulfide also markedly reduced liver Cu, the assumption was that Cu compounds might have been converted to Cu sulfide which is relatively insoluble. Wynne and McClymont (1956) fed a diet containing 5 ppm Cu and 0.8 ppm Mo to sheep. When this was supplemented with S to give an inorganic sulfate content of 0.4%, liver Cu concentrations fell but not to a level associated with Cu deficiency.

In other work with sheep, Cunningham and Hogan (1959) found that pastures containing about 0.2% sulfate allowed Cu storage even though forage Mo was high, whereas, pastures with 0.4% sulfate resulted in loss of liver Cu. Goodrich and Tillman (1966) also found that, compared to 0.1% sulfate, the 0.4% level decreased Cu and increased Fe in sheep livers. When Cu and Mo intakes were low, the higher level of sulfate reduced gain and feed efficiency, blood hematocrit and plasma P.

Effects of Sulfates on Mo. Early work by Dick (1953) showed that sulfate affected Mo excretion. When the sulfate intake was low, very little Mo was excreted in the urine and blood Mo levels increased to high values. When the sulfate intake increased, large amounts of Mo were excreted, particularly in the urine, and the blood Mo level dropped. Scaife (1956) observed that methionine supplementation also resulted in an immediate increase in Mo excretion and a reduced level of blood Mo, and Cook et al (1966) found that methionine, Na sulfate or Na sulfite all had the ability to reduce plasma Mo levels of heifers given inorganic sources of Mo. Conversely, Scaife (1956) reported that increasing Mo intake from 10 to 50 mg

increased urinary excretion of sulfates from 2-5 to 30-40 mg/100 ml.

Interactions between sulfate and Mo appear to occur at several sites with different effects (Huisingh et al, 1973). Since Mo can inhibit sulfate reduction (Huisingh et al, 1975), it may decrease the amount of sulfide formed in the rumen, thereby increasing Cu availability to the animal. However, results of an in vitro microbial system suggested the inhibitory effect of Mo on sulfide production could be decreased by formation of a non-available complex of Mo with Cu (Bremner, 1975). Initial studies also suggested sulfate and Mo may interact antagonistically at the membrane transport level (Huisingh et al, 1973). Mason and Cardin (1977) found a similar pattern for in vitro uptake of Mo and sulfate by sheep small intestine segments and suggested sulfate inhibits uptake of Mo by competition for sites on a common transport system.

Cu-Mo-Sulfate Interactions

Whitelaw et al (1977) observed evidence of hypocupremia in sheep grazing improved pasture but not in those on adjacent indigenous vegetation. Herbage concentrations of Mo and S were 4 and 2 times, respectively, higher in the improved pasture. Suttle (1974d) has suggested that the Cu-Mo-sulfate antagonism is widely involved in the etiology of both toxicity and deficiency of Cu in sheep and that it might be usefully applied in the treatment and prevention of Cu toxicity. It was shown 25 years ago that Mo limited Cu storage in the liver of sheep only when adequate inorganic sulfate was present. The effect of sulfate was consistent in preventing storage of liver Cu in the presence of Mo. In a subsequent paper, Dick (1956) showed that intakes of 7.5 and 25 mg of Mo allowed liver storage of 308 and 193 mg Cu, but when 3.8 g of sulfate was added, liver Cu storage was reduced to 65 and 2 mg, respectively. Wynne and McClymont (1956) found that sheep maintained on Mo plus sulfate showed a progressive fall in liver and blood Cu levels and developed dystrophic wool and achromatrichia, whereas sulfate or Mo supplements given separately did not result in wool lesions although liver Cu storage was reduced. Cunningham and Hogan (1959) also observed that high sulfate (0.4%) and high Mo (8 ppm) reduced liver Cu storage in sheep.

Work with cattle (Cunningham et al, 1959) indicated that Mo plus sulfate supplements prevented accumulation of Mo but did not increase loss of Cu in blood or liver.

Table 5-2. Effect of Mo + sulfate supplements on blood Cu components.[a]

Diet	Whole blood Cu	Plasma Cu	TCA soluble Cu	Direct reading Cu	Ceruloplasmin Cu	Red blood cell Cu
			---- µg/100 ml ----			
Normal	96	96	96	14	78	95
Mo supplement	118	122	76	20	90	108
Mo + sulfate	152	164	70	58	56	87

[a] Data from McCosker (1968), Bremner (1976), Smith and Wright (1975), Huber et al (1971), Barlow et al (1976), Suttle et al (1970), Bingley and Dufty (1973).

Lesperance and Bohman (1963) found 0.5% added sulfate limited both Mo and Cu storage, and appeared to increase Mo toxicity in cattle.

It was also observed that an increase in Mo intake resulted in increased blood Cu if the diet contained appreciable amounts of sulfate (Dick, 1954). Smith et al (1968) and Bremner (1976) also reported that Mo plus sulfate supplements resulted in higher total and direct-reacting plasma Cu but lower ceruloplasmin (Table 5-2). Bremner (1976) fed three groups of sheep a semi-purified diet containing 10 ppm Cu and 0.08% sulfate alone or supplemented with 25 ppm Mo or 25 ppm Mo plus 0.5% sulfate. His results suggested that Cu and Mo were closely associated in a novel plasma protein fraction which bound Cu firmly only when oxidation was prevented and whose formation was dependent on increased dietary S. Marcilese et al (1969) found that addition of both 0.4% sulfate and 50 ppm Mo to a ration containing 12-14 ppm Cu and 0.03% sulfate inhibited transfer of ^{64}Cu from plasma to tissues in sheep. An interference with Cu entry into liver cells and/or a primary intracellular disturbance in the synthesis of Cu protein compounds including ceruloplasmin was suggested. Addition of 0.4% sulfate plus 50 ppm Mo to the diet also increased accumulation of Cu by the kidney and excretion of Cu in urine but sulfate alone had no effect (Marcilese et al, 1970).

Suttle and McLauchlan (1976) used multiple regression techniques to examine relationships among effects of S and Mo within normal ranges for herbage (0.1-0.4% S and 0.5-4.5 ppm Mo, dry basis) on Cu availability to sheep. The calculations implied that S exerts a predominant and independent effect on Cu availability, whereas Mo has a lesser and S-dependent effect. Results further indicated that increments at the lower end of the normal range of S and Mo concentrations have relatively large depressing effects on Cu availability.

Effects of S and Mo on Cu availability were investigated further by feeding initially hypocupremic ewes basal diets supplemented with 6 to 8 ppm Cu and containing 0.1 or 0.4% S and 0.5 or 4.5 ppm Mo (Suttle, 1973; 1975b). Repletion of plasma Cu was unaffected by Mo alone, only slightly reduced by S alone, and totally inhibited by Mo plus S. Plasma Mo was greatly increased by Mo, slightly decreased by S and unaffected by Mo and S given together. Sulfate, methionine or cysteine were equally as effective as sources of S.

Effects of Mo plus sulfate given to pregnant ewes have been evident in their lambs as stiffness and incoordination of hind legs (Butler et al, 1964), low brain Cu and cytochrome oxidase values (Fell et al, 1965) and brain, liver and blood Cu levels typical of delayed cases of swayback (Suttle and Field, 1968).

Dowdy and Matrone (1968) observed that anemia developed in sheep fed a purified diet containing Mo plus sulfate, but not in those without Mo. They found that Cu sulfate and Na molybdate formed a complex in near neutral solutions. When sheep were given the

112

complex prepared from radio Cu and Mo, removal from the blood of both elements was equal, and the rate was more rapid than removal of Mo when injected I.V. alone. The rate of urinary excretion of Mo from the Cu-Mo complex was also slower than from Mo alone. They concluded that Cu bound in this complex was biologically unavailable and that such a complex could exist in vivo.

Contrasting responses of ruminants and non-ruminants to the Cu-Mo antagonism are probably related to the influence of the rumen (Suttle, 1974d). Neethling et al (1968) found that fecal excretion of ^{64}Cu by sheep was only 35% of the dose when given intra-abomasally compared to 62% when given intraruminally. Similar results have been obtained with Mo which is metabolized differently by ruminants and swine (Bell et al, 1964). During 5 days following oral administration of [99]Mo, percentages of the dose excreted were 15 by swine compared to 75 by cattle in feces and 85 by swine compared to 4 by cattle in urine. Delivery of [99]Mo directly into the abomasum of sheep resulted in urinary and fecal [99]Mo excretions more closely resembling that of swine (Bell et al, 1966). Similar results were obtained with calves (Miller et al, 1972). Although neither Cu (Ivan and Grieve, 1976; Bertoni et al, 1976) nor Mo (Miller et al, 1972) appeared to be absorbed from the rumen, formation in the rumen of an insoluble complex which remained intact on passage through the GI tract could inhibit absorption of both Cu and Mo from the intestines.

The site of the Cu-Mo-S interaction has been shown to be the rumen by several procedures. Dietary S did not prevent repletion of hypocupremic ewes when supplemental Cu was administered by continuous I.V. infusion (Suttle, 1975a). Administration of Mo in the diet and Cu by subcutaneous injection (Suttle and Field, 1974), or by continuous I.V. infusion (Suttle, 1975a) largely circumvented the antagonism. Inhibition of Cu repletion by Mo was also prevented when Cu was given in the diet and Mo was administered by continuous abomasal infusion to bypass the rumen (Fig. 5-3).

Effect of Other Dietary Components. Dick (1954) has published data showing that Ca carbonate supplementation (90 g/day) reduced liver Cu storage in sheep whereas dicalcium phosphate did not. MacPherson and Hemingway (1968) found that liming pasture resulted in lower liver and blood Cu in sheep but did not affect herbage Cu. In

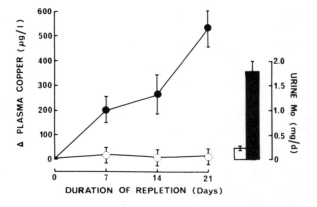

Fig. 5-3. Effects of administering Mo (3.2 mg/day) in the diet (o) or by continuous abomasal infusion (•) on the responses in plasma Cu (μg/l) of initially hypocupraemic ewes given a Cu-supplemented diet (8 mg/kg) and also on urinary Mo excretion between 18 and 21 days. The diet was relatively rich in inorganic sulfate (3 g/kg). From Suttle (1974a).

contrast, after feeding young lambs liquid diets containing 10 ppm Cu and supplemented to provide 50, 250, 450 or 630 mg Ca/kg body weight/day for 2 mo., Hodge and Palmer (1973) found the lowest liver Cu level in lambs fed the lowest Ca level. Liver Cu concentrations in lambs fed the 3 highest Ca levels were well in the region where Cu toxicity symptoms could be expected.

Se may have a favorable interaction with Cu (Hill et al, 1969; Awad et al, 1973; Amer et al, 1973). Oral administration of small Se doses resulted in more gain, heavier wool clip, a higher incidence of twin lambs and increased Cu levels in various organs, blood serum and wool. Dick (1956) reported that Mn improved liver Cu storage by sheep also supplemented with Mo and sulfate. Supplemental Mn may also improve Cu absorption by calves (Ivan and Grieve, 1976). Several studies indicate a Cu-Zn interaction. Corrigall et al (1976) measured alterations in plasma Cu and Zn concentrations associated with the onset and course of several diseases in sheep and cattle and found that plasma Cu rose as Zn declined. They reported that lambs fed rations containing 420 ppm Zn developed a slight anemia.

Dick (1956) has shown that supplementation of sheep with Mo + gluten (100 g/day) reduced liver Cu storage as compared to Mo alone. The addition of Mn to the Mo and gluten further reduced liver Cu. He suggested that sulfide derived in the rumen from the gluten may have accounted for this depression in Cu storage. Goodrich and Tillman (1966) have shown that urea resulted

Table 5-3. Effect of N and S source on Cu liver stores and Cu retention.[a]

Nitrogen source	Urea		Purified Soy Protein	
Sulfur source	Sulfate	Elemental S	Sulfate	Elemental S
Liver Cu, ppm, dry basis				
initial	382	388	383	378
Final	685	1902	630	1003
Cu retention, %	7.8	11.4	-11.9	2.6

[a] From Goodrich and Tillman (1966). Data on liver stores and Cu retention are not on the same animals.

in greater Cu storage as compared to diets supplemented with purified soybean protein (Table 5-3).

Copper Deficiency

Copper deficiency in ruminants results in a number of well described symptoms, but the symptoms depend upon a variety of factors, only some of which are known. Underwood (1977) points out that the manifestations of Cu deficiency depend on the species of animal and its age and sex; on the severity and duration of the deficiency state; and on the particular environment in which the animal is being maintained. Cattle may be unable to maintain normal Cu status under conditions where sheep can (Suttle, 1975c). However, at birth calves generally have high liver Cu levels even when the cows are depleted, so except in extreme deficiency the calf is protected in utero and for up to 2 mo. after birth (Roberts, 1976). In contrast, fetal status parallels that of the ewe in sheep. Todd (1978) reported that symptoms of Cu deficiency in lambs and calves have become more prevalent in Northern Ireland in recent years. He attributed the increase to reduction

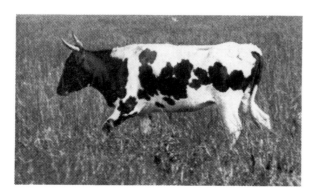

Fig. 5-4. A pacing heifer. This condition is believed to be due to a Cu deficiency. Courtesy of R.B. Becker, Florida Agr. Expt. Sta.

in potato growing and replacement of Cu-based fungicides with non-Cu preparations as well as replacement of Cu sulfate by other antihelmintics.

Typical symptoms that occur in a simple or induced (high Mo and sulfate) Cu deficiency include reduced levels of tissue Cu, which may decline below 10 ppm in liver and 20 μg/100 ml in blood. Brain Cu is reduced as is cytochrome oxidase in brain and liver tissue. Increased liver Fe deposition, with values as high as 4,000 ppm (Cook et al, 1966) may indicate a reduced utilization of Fe in Cu-deficient animals. A high incidence of hemoglobinurea has been reported in hypocupremic cows (Goold and Smith, 1975; Smith, 1975). Suttle (1975c) and Suttle and Angus (1976) listed Cu deficiency symptoms in order of appearance in calves as hypocupremia, growth retardation, impaired feed conversion, rough hair coat, diarrhea, and leg abnormalities. First generation Cu-deficient sheep developed low plasma and tissue Cu and a temporary loss of wool crimp between 6 and 12 mo. but appetite, growth and feed conversion efficiency were not impaired (Suttle et al. 1970).

Blood Changes. A Cu deficiency has been reported to cause a hypochromic anemia in sheep (Howell, 1968) although there are numerous exceptions to this (for example, Suttle and Field, 1968). Smith and Coup (1973) found a Heinz body anemia in many dairy herds where Cu levels were low. Diets with high levels of Mo or sulfate may result in reduced hemoglobin and hematocrit levels in cattle (Cook et al, 1966) and one report indicates a similar situation in sheep (Suttle and Field, 1968), although there are also various exceptions. Serum ceruplasmin activity may also drop in Cu deficiency (Flynn et al, 1977) and has been used as an indicator of Cu status of cattle (Thompson and Todd, 1976a).

Biochemical changes. Decreases in plasma ferroxidase I, plasma monoamine oxidase and liver cytochrome oxidase activities have been detected before the first overt clinical signs of Cu deficiency in cattle (Mills et al, 1976). Lambs from Cu-deficient ewes had extremely low brain cytochrome oxidase and plasma monoamine oxidase activity (Suttle et al, 1970). In Cu-deficient calves, cytochrome oxidase activity was reduced markedly in intestinal mucosa (Suttle, 1975c; Fell et al, 1975) and moderately in cardiac muscle (Suttle and Angus, 1976). Changes in the anterior brain stems of ataxic, Cu-deficient lambs included decreased dopamine and norepinephrine but not seratonin concentrations (O'Dell et al, 1976).

Regardless of clinical appearance, Cu-depleted cattle showed gross or microscopic lesions of the skeleton and cardiovascular system (Mills et al, 1976). In cattle a disease known as falling disease occurs in some areas (particularly Australia) with very low Cu levels in forage. It is characterized by sudden cardiac failure due, apparently, to

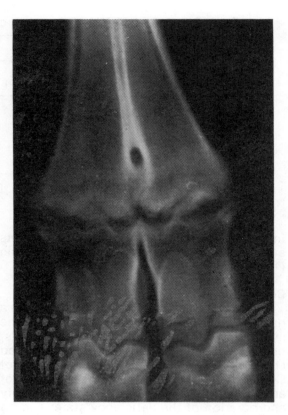

Fig. 5-6. Secondary Cu deficiency. Anteroposterior radiograph of distal metacarpal growth plate of severely affected calf, showing widened zone of cartilage and lipping of the medial and lateral areas of the growth plate. Courtesy of B.P. Smith, Univ. of California, Davis.

fibrosis of myocardial muscles. Leigh (1975) suggested that ultra-structural changes in the myocardium of young steers were specifically attributable to Cu deficiency and that loss of cytochrome oxidase activity was the most likely underlying biochemical defect.

Bone Changes. Lesions associated with lameness in cattle suffering from Cu deficiency associated with high dietary Mo and sulfate included abnormal development of the distal growth plates of the metacarpus and metatarsus (Irwin et al, 1974; Smith et al, 1975b) (Fig. 5-5, 6). Faulty hoof keratinization accompanied decreased hoof Cu and S content and incomplete S cross-linking in the hoof keratin of Alaskan moose subsisting on browse averaging 5.7 ppm Cu (Flynn et al, 1977). Histological changes observed in Cu-deficient sheep (Suttle et al, 1972) but not cattle (Irwin et al, 1974) included decreased osteoblast activity and osteoporosis. Marked bowing of the forelegs may occur (Fig. 5-7).

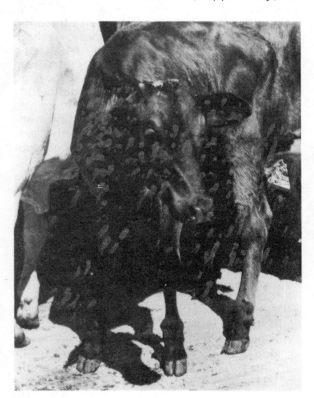

Fig. 5-5. Copper deficiency caused by normal Cu and high S and Mo. The back is arched, pasterns are straight, and the distal metacarpal physeal region is enlarged. Courtesy of B.P. Smith, Univ. of California, Davis.

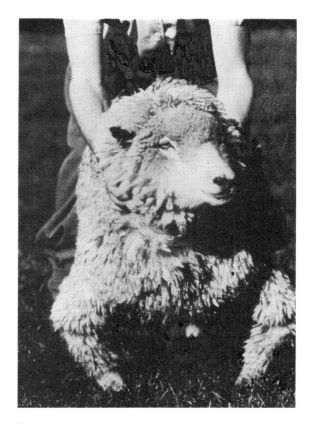

Fig. 5-7. Osteoporosis in sheep. Note the marked outward bowing of the front legs of this lamb. This condition is apparently the result of too little Cu or too much Mo. Courtesy of W.J. Hartley, Univ. of Sidney.

Neonatal Ataxia or Swayback. This is a nervous disorder of lambs and, less frequently, of cattle which is characterized by incoordination and partial paralysis of hind quarters (Fig. 5-8). Some of the lambs are paralyzed at birth and soon die; others develop the condition at a later date. Wiener et al (1969) found that ewes which had produced lambs affected by swayback had lower levels of blood Cu than ewes which produced normal lambs, particularly in winter months. Cu in the brain is low (Butler et al, 1964; Fell et al, 1965; Roberts et al, 1966). Roberts et al described what they believed to be an acute form of swayback. It affected lambs 2-4 weeks of age and resulted in incoordination, muscular tremors, grinding of the teeth and dilation of the pupils of the eyes. Lambs usually died within 24-48 hr. In addition to low blood and brain levels of Cu, they found lesions in the cerebrum which were characterized by edema with cellular degeneration. Idris and Tartour(1975) found demyelination of the nerve fibers in the cerebrum and spinal cord in ataxic

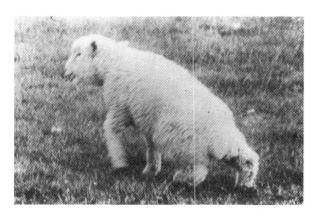

Fig. 5-8. Cu-deficient lamb showing the ataxia that sometimes occurs. Courtesy of W.J. Hartley, Univ. of Sidney.

lambs. Spinal cords of 5 to 8-week old lambs affected with the delayed form of swayback were deficient in myelin lipid components such as cholesterol, cerebrosides and phospholipids (Patterson et al, 1974). Myelin isolated from ataxic lambs was also deficient in Cu.

Suttle and Field (1968) found that liver and brain Cu concentrations of new-born lambs were reduced by feeding their dams low Cu or Mo + sulfate supplemented semi-purified diets. When the two treatments were combined, liver, brain and blood Cu concentrations and brain cytochrome oxidase activities were reduced to levels found in delayed cases of swayback. However, subclinical evidence of swayback was found in only one lamb at birth and there were no clinical cases in the new-born lambs. Thus, the data at this time indicate that there are other factors involved or that ewes which produce affected lambs are, themselves, more subject to Cu depletion than other similar animals. It is possible that the time that a critical deficiency occurs during pregnancy may be important. Petterson and Sweasey (1975) suggested that neonatal swayback arose through a deficiency in the supply of Cu from the ewe to the fetus during the first phase of myelination.

Diarrhea. A very severe diarrhea or scouring of cattle (Fig. 5-9) has been associated with Cu deficiency or Mo excess. Scouring has been only infrequently reported in sheep; however, Suttle and Field (1968) observed severe diarrhea in ewes given semi-purified diets supplemented with Mo and sulfate. The diarrhea ceased after about 12 days, possibly due to a decreased feed intake of about 50%. No diarrhea was

116

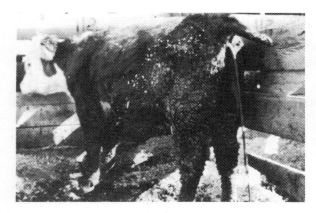

Fig. 5-9. Severe diarrhea produced by feeding 100 ppm of Mo to a heifer on an alfalfa ration. Courtesy of A.L. Lesperance, Univ. of Nevada.

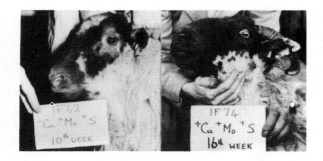

Fig. 5-11. Cu deficiency (on the left) induced by a low level of Cu and high levels of Mo and S. Note achromatricha (bleaching of hair) around eye and muzzle. Courtesy of N.F. Suttle, Moredun Institute, Edinburgh.

observed in sheep not supplemented with Mo + sulfate but given low-Cu diets. Underwood (1977) points out that scouring has, in all cases, been associated with low Cu content of blood and tissues and that it is prevented or cured with supplemental Cu.

Fell et al (1975) correlated diarrhea in Cu-deficient steers with mucosal atrophy in the small intestine, partial villus atrophy, elongation of crypts and goblet cell hyperplasia. These changes together with diminished cytochrome oxidase activity in the small intestine may have produced a malabsorption syndrome resulting in decreased food conversion and diarrhea (Fell et al, 1975; Suttle, 1975c).

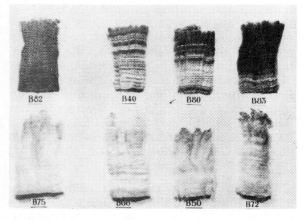

Fig. 5-10. Wool from normal and Cu-deficient sheep. On the left are typical normal black and white wools from a sheep fed a basal diet. The other samples are from sheep on sulfate-Mo supplemented diets, showing banding of black wool, loss of definition of crimp and, in some, occurrence of secondary waves. From Wynne and McClymont (1956).

Depigmentation of Hair or Wool. It has been shown in many instances that hair of cattle or wool of black sheep (see Fig. 5-10, 11) fed diets low in Cu or high in Mo and sulfate will not develop its normal quota of pigment (achromatrichia). Dick (1954) found that it was possible to block pigment formation in black-fleeced sheep within 2 days by raising the Mo and sulfate in the diet. By changing the diet frequently it is possible to produce alternating bands of dark and light wool (see Fig. 5-10). Cattle also show severe bleaching of hair, although there is a great deal of variation between individual animals subjected to the same diet. Suttle and Field (1968) found sheep developed achromatrichia of wool on the head when fed semi-purified diets containing Mo + sulfate supplements, but not without Mo + sulfate, even when supplemental Cu was omitted.

Defective Keratinization of Wool. In sheep it has been shown that a Cu deficiency results in a reduction in both quantity and quality of wool, although there are marked differences in geographical areas (Underwood, 1977). The wool gradually loses its characteristic crimp until the fibers resemble hair more than wool.

Effect on Fertility. Some of the older literature indicates fertility is apt to be reduced in Cu-deficient cattle. Howell (1968) has confirmed this information with sheep. In a group of Cu-deficient sheep, 5 died between the 23 and 34th week and none were pregnant; of the remaining 4, 2 aborted immature fetuses and the others were apparently barren. In a Cu-supplemented group, 1 ewe died in pregnancy and the remaining 5 produced lambs. Wiener et al

(1976) found no apparent association between libido and plasma Cu concentration in rams, but rams which induced pregnancy with the first service had higher Cu levels than those which were less successful.

Requirements for Cu

Cu requirements of ruminant species cannot clearly be defined when various interfering factors are present in the diet. Beck (1962) has classified the pastures of Western Australia on the basis of Cu, Mo and sulfate. He concluded that pastures containing <3 ppm of Cu in the dry matter during the growing period were generally deficient. Values between 3 and 6 ppm were classified as marginal and, in those >6 ppm, deficiency diseases such as enzootic ataxia in sheep and falling disease in cattle were rarely encountered. He pointed out that the Mo and sulfate contents of the various pastures were generally within the same range (0.1 to 4 ppm Mo with <1 ppm; sulfate was from 0.1 to 0.9% with most between 0.2 and 0.4%). MacPherson and Hemmingway (1968) suggest that herbage Cu of 8-9 ppm is inadequate for sheep where the fields have been limed.

Several investigators have used semi-purified diets to study Cu requirements of ruminants. Dowdy and Matrone (1968) found 1 ppm of Cu was insufficient to maintain blood Cu levels of sheep, even with a low level of Mo (0 ppm) or sulfate (0.03%). Wynne and McClymont (1956) observed no marked changes in liver and blood Cu of sheep fed a basal diet with 5.2 ppm Cu, 0.8 ppm Mo and 0.04% sulfate. Suttle and Field (1968) fed semi-purified diets containing 1 or 11 ppm of Cu and/or 50 ppm of Mo and 1% sulfate. The 1 ppm of Cu was not sufficient to prevent a marked decline in plasma Cu and a lower than normal level of blood Cu in the lambs. The 11 ppm of Cu was apparently adequate to maintain normal blood levels, but not in the presence of supplemental Mo + sulfate.

Mills et al (1976) found that addition of 8 ppm Cu to a semi-synthetic diet containing <1 ppm prevented pathological lesions attributable to Cu deficiency in calves. However, this level did not adequately meet their requirement for Cu because, compared to calves fed 15 ppm Cu, there was a marked reduction in liver Cu, a decrease in plasma ferroxidase I activity, and development of diarrhea. Suttle (1978) estimated the components of the Cu requirements of calves by a technique involving the alleviation of hypo-cupremia. The values derived were 3.4 μg Cu/kg liveweight for maintenance and 0.47 mg/kg of weight gain. Dietary requirements of approximately 7 and 15 ppm Cu were predicted for diets containing 2 and 7 ppm Mo, respectively, with growth having little effect. However, somewhat higher Cu intakes were required to maintain initial liver Cu reserves.

Prevention of Cu Deficiency. In areas where Cu deficiency, either simple or induced, is a problem, there are several possibilities for relief. Use of Cu in fertilizer has been successful in many areas in Australia and New Zealand, but only on soils with a low pH. Topdressing a pasture with 5.6 kg Cu sulfate/ha raised Cu from 5.4 to 7.8 ppm and reduced Mo from 5.4 to 3.0 in forage which resulted in increases of Cu from 24 to 68 μg/100 ml in plasma and from 4.4 to 28.6 ppm DM in liver of dairy cows (Smith, 1975). On alkaline soil in the western USA, such practices are not effective and use of Cu may even increase the Mo content of forage. A second method is to provide added Cu in supplemental feeds. The biggest problem of Cu supplementation lies in range areas where it is difficult to supply Cu in either mineral mixes or supplemental concentrates. In areas where waters are naturally saline, it is difficult to obtain adequate Cu intake because the animal may not take supplemental salt or minerals or may take it too irregularly to provide satisfactory performance. If mineral supplementation can be used, a mix with 0.5-1% Cu sulfate will be readily consumed by cattle and sheep.

Where the Mo intake is high, Cu must be provided in relatively high and frequent amounts to obtain satisfactory animal production. As a result many livestock producers have used injectible Cu glycinate or Cu-EDTA complexes which are absorbed slowly (Harvey, 1953; Camargo et al, 1962). Doses of 30-40 mg for sheep and 120-240 mg for cattle can be administered subcutaneously or intramuscularly without undue hazard. The frequency of required dosing is greatly reduced with this method as compared to oral supplementation. Whitelaw (1977) found that plasma Cu of otherwise hypocupremic sheep could be maintained within the normal range of 60 to 160 μg/100 ml by injection at intervals with 12.5 mg CuCa edetate. Improved weight gains and wool quality were also noted. With cows grazing pasture with mean levels of 6.7 ppm Cu and 2.5 ppm Mo, subcutaneous injection with 240 mg Cu as Cu glycinate raised blood Cu from 33 to 97 μg/100 ml, reduced incidence of post parturient hemoglobinuria and maintained higher levels of hemoglobin in the post parturient period (Smith et al, 1975a).

Requirements for Mo

Minimum dietary requirements of Mo for satisfactory growth and health have not been determined nor has Mo deficiency been observed under natural conditions in any species according to Underwood (1977). Ellis et al (1958) found that addition of 2 ppm Mo to a 0.36 ppm Mo basal diet for sheep resulted in faster gains and improved cellulose digestion. Subsequent work from this station did not show any response of sheep when Mo was added to the diet. Sheriha et al (1962) have also looked at Mo supplements. They added 2 or 2.2 ppm supplemental Mo to 3 semi-purified or purified diets which initially contained from 0.01 to 0.45 ppm Mo without response, so they concluded the Mo requirement was <0.01 ppm. Askew (1958) has reported that sheep pastured in areas of New Zealand with low Mo were subject to development of xanthine calculi.

Cu Toxicity

The range between inadequate and excessive dietary Cu levels for ruminants can be relatively narrow, although cattle are less susceptible than sheep to Cu toxicity. Roberts (1976) considers it dangerous to exceed 10 ppm Cu for sheep for any extended period but the Cu requirement of calves appears to be near this level (Mills et al, 1976; Suttle, 1978). Cu-containing insecticides and fungicides have also been implicated in many cases of Cu poisoning. The subject has been reviewed by Todd (1969).

The susceptibility of ruminants to Cu poisoning is at least partly due to the fact that the liver will continue to store Cu when the intake is above that required in a given situation, no control mechanism being operative to restrict absorption and liver uptake. The result is that liver Cu concentration may reach values well in excess of 2,000 ppm on a dry weight basis. Some values in excess of 4,000 ppm have been reported.

Symptoms Observed. Chronic Cu poisoning has three relatively distinct stages (McCosker, 1968). During the first stage there is a gradual accumulation of Cu in the tissues, primarily the liver. No clinical symptoms are observed and blood Cu values are normal. This may occur over an extended period. During stage 2, whole blood Cu may rise to about twice normal levels accompanied by increased plasma billirubin, decreased liver function and a reduced hematocrit. There may also be increases in a variety of blood enzymes and metabolites. The third stage is usually referred to as the hemolytic crisis. Clinical symptoms include dullness, anorexia, dehydration, acute thirst, evidence of abdominal pain, jaundice and hemoglobinuria (Tulloch, 1973; Mylrea and Byrne, 1974; Wasfi and Adam, 1976).

The hemolytic crisis may be accompanied by an increased oxidative state of the blood (Thompson and Todd, 1976b), erythrocyte distortion (Soli and Nafstad, 1976), and a sudden rise in serum creatine phosphokinase (Thompson and Todd, 1974). Methemoglobin content of blood increases and may account for as much as 60% of the hemoglobin of calves. Total hemoglobin level may drop as much as 10 g/100 ml in 48 hr (Todd and Thompson, 1963) to very low levels (1 g/100 ml or less, see Fig. 5-12). Blood glutathione concentration falls drastically and whole blood Cu increases to values 5-8 times normal. Kidney function may be impaired as indicated by rising blood urea but changes in renal function and histology were not detected prior to the hemolytic crisis (Gopinath et al, 1974). These metabolic changes which occur during the hemolytic crisis appear to result from the degeneration of liver cells and the sudden release of Cu into the blood. Animals generally die within 2-4 days after the onset

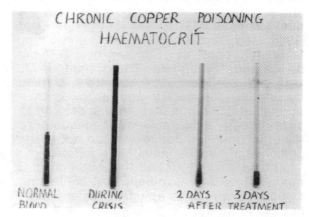

Fig. 5-12. Hematocrits from sheep before, during and after the hemolytic crisis of acute Cu toxicity. Note in the second sample from the left (obtained during the crisis) that it is almost impossible to differentiate between plasma and cells. The amount of hemolysis that has occurred is shown by the two tubes on the right. Courtesy of J.R. Todd, Vet. Res. Labs, Stormont, N. Ireland.

of clinical symptoms. Some breeds of sheep (Merino) are more resistant than others and may survive more than one crisis.

Postmortem findings indicate a generalized icterus (jaundice), including the adipose tissues which may be a dirty-yellow color. The kidney has a distinctive black metallic sheen, the urinary bladder and gall bladder are apt to be distended with dark-colored fluids, and the spleen is enlarged, soft and dark. Outstanding histological changes include necrosis and fatty changes in the liver, dilation and necrosis of renal tubules, petechial hemorrhages on the heart and splenic hemosiderosis (Tullock, 1973; Mylrea and Byrne, 1974; Soli and Nafstad, 1976; and Wasfi and Adam, 1976). Lesions have also been found in the brains of affected animals (Doherty et al, 1969; Morgan, 1973). Observations of many people indicate that added stress, change of environment, transportation, handling of animals, etc. are apt to trigger a hemolytic crisis.

Cu Toxicity in Cattle. Cunningham (1946) reported that yearling heifers and adult cows could tolerate repeated doses of 20-40 g and single doses of up to 100 g Cu sulfate. The lethal amount for a single dose was between 200 and 300 g. However, he fed from 200 to 300 mg of Cu daily for as long as 16 mo. without ill effects. Todd and Gracey (1959) reported a field case in which a heifer died of Cu toxicity after receiving an estimated Cu intake of 454 mg/day or about 68 g over a 5-mo. period. In another report (Todd and Gribben, 1965) a cow with high blood Cu and low hemoglobin (0.75 g/100 ml) had been fed pig feed with 200 ppm of Cu resulting in a calculated Cu intake of 3.3 g/day. Chapman et al (1962) found that daily administration to steers of Cu sulfate in amounts up to 8 g for 12 mo. and then up to 12 g for an additional 4 mo. caused no problem. However, when 12 g of Cu sulfate was given as a drench, 2 or 3 steers died in about 2 mo., which raises some interesting questions on what happens to the Cu in the rumen.

Weiss and Baur (1968) have studied Cu toxicity in young calves given a milk replacer with 50 to 300 ppm. The calf given 50 ppm survived until killed at 116 days, but all others died. Mylrea and Byrne (1974) described acute poisoning in calves following subcutaneous injection of 72 to 144 mg Cu as an EDTA complex. All calves died over a period of 12 days. The liver Cu levels found in these two studies (560-2,100 ppm in dry matter) were lower than those typically found in toxemic sheep. The general opinion (Todd, 1969) seems to be that adult bovines are more resistant to Cu poisoning than sheep and that young bovines are about as susceptible as sheep. Todd (1969) stated that chronic Cu toxicity can be considered as being almost entirely confined to sheep from the point of view of a nutritional disorder.

Cu Toxicity in Sheep. Numerous clinical reports deal with Cu toxicity in sheep. For example, Pearson (1956) mentioned a field case in which ewes died after consuming 1 to 2 lb/day of a feed mix intended for pigs. In other examples Cu poisoning occurred in farm flocks consuming rations with 27 ppm (Tait et al, 1971), 40 ppm (Ross, 1964) or 50 ppm (Pierson and Aanes, 1958) of Cu. A field case (Clegg, 1956) occurred when rams which were given a mineral mix (1,300 ppm Cu) were drenched for worm control with a Cu-containing medicine. Other cases were reported when sheep were put on pasture 2 days following fertilization with a Cu-containing fertilizer (Pryor, 1959) or were pasturing herbage sprayed with Cu sulfate to control liver flukes (Gracey and Todd, 1960). In the latter case, herbage contained up to 200 ppm of Cu and these high levels persisted throughout the dormant winter period in spite of heavy rain and, in some cases, flooding. Tulloch (1973) reported an outbreak in which 40 out of 120 sheep died over 6 weeks when grazed in an orchard 10 weeks after it was sprayed with Cu oxychloride. Sudden cold, dry weather had caused premature fall of autumn leaves which were eaten readily by the sheep.

With respect to experimental studies, clinical symptoms developed in 8 weeks in sheep given 250 mg of Cu/day (Sutter et al, 1958) but not until 13-15 weeks in other sheep supplemented with 1 g of Cu sulfate/day (Barden and Robertson, 1962). Todd et al (1962) have compared the toxicity of Cu sulfate and Cu acetate which were fed at the rate of 0.25 g of Cu/day for 6 weeks and at double this rate thereafter. Cu was found to be more toxic in the acetate than in the sulfate form since animals died earlier and after receiving a smaller dose of Cu. Cu sulfate as a drench was found to be equivalent in toxicity to that fed in meal. Ross (1966) found that 100 mg of Cu as the sulfate given 3/week for 7 weeks to lambs fed a basal ration containing 12-14 ppm of Cu was quite toxic. McCleod and Watt (1970) reported that I.V. injection of the equivalent of 50 mg Cu in solution resulted in the death of 3 out of 4 sheep. Time of death and lesions produced were similar to those occurring on occasion in the field following prophylactic subcutaneous injections.

Adamson et al (1969) has cautioned that 20 ppm Cu in concentrates given to lambs indoors can be dangerous if Mo and sulfate are not present in sufficient quantities to interfere with Cu utilization. Hogan et al (1968) mention that Cu poisoning may occur frequently in penned sheep fed alfalfa hay and pelleted concentrates. In one experiment ewes were fed hay ad lib with about 113 or 454 g/day of 21% crude protein pellets. Liver biopsy samples indicated an increase in liver Cu over a 15-mo. period of from 118 to 887 ppm (dry basis) in those fed the low level of pellets compared to from 116 to 1,326 ppm in the other group. Cu contents were 7 ppm in hay and 11-12 ppm in pellets, but these feeds contained <1ppm Mo and <0.14% sulfate.

In contrast to the paper of Hogan et al, Hemmingway and MacPherson (1967) concluded that Cu toxicity was unlikely to be a problem in lambs fed concentrates in pens. They collected data from animals where Cu intake ranged from 4 to 20 mg/day and calculated a dietary intake of 38 mg/day for 16-20 weeks would be required to raise liver Cu from about 100 to 1,000 ppm. Information was not given on Mo or sulfate intakes. In other work MacPherson and Hemmingway (1965) concluded that additional protein (10% vs 20% diets) might have some protective effect when high levels of Cu were given to sheep.

Bull et al (1956) published some interesting data showing that Cu toxicity may frequently occur in sheep grazing subterranean clover (*Trifolium subterraneum* L.). They found that the early, rapid growth of herbage was apt to have normal amounts of Cu (up to 20 ppm), but negligible amounts of Mo (0.1-0.2 ppm). It has also been suggested that subclinical poisoning with alkaloids by plants such as the heliotrope plant (*Heliotropium europaeum*) may damage the liver and make it more susceptible to accumulation of Cu (Pierson and Aanes, 1958; Bull et al, 1956; Todd, 1969).

Treatment or Prevention of Cu Poisoning. There are several reports (Pierson and Aanes, 1958; Todd et al, 1962; Ross, 1964, 1966) which give evidence that supplementary Mo or Mo + sulfate will stop death losses in sheep that have high and potentially lethal Cu levels. An appropriate level of Mo intake is indicated to be about 100 mg/day. In the long-term feeding experiments carried out by Hogan et al (1968), it was found that the

addition of Ca carbonate to the pelleted part of the ration had no protective effect. The addition of Mo (38 mg/day) and Ca sulfate (5 g/day) did reduce liver Cu storage but did not prevent it. Zn may also have a protective effect. Corrigall et al (1976) observed signs of Cu toxicosis in 3 of 8 lambs fed a ration containing 29 ppm Cu and 143 ppm Zn, only possibly in one of 8 fed 220 ppm Zn and in none fed 420 ppm Zn.

Mo Toxicity

The relationship between a chronic high Mo intake and Cu metabolism has been discussed previously. Individuals who have researched these problems indicate that the symptoms seen are essentially the same whether due to low Cu or high Mo. It seems likely, however, that the great variety of problems that develop (i.e., swayback, falling disease, osteoporosis, achromatrichia, and severe diarrhea) may depend to some extent on the relative deficiency of Cu and the relative over-abundance of Mo.

There are several papers dealing with Mo toxicity that have not been discussed previously. One of these (Thomas and Moss, 1951) dealt with young bull calves given Mo supplements of ca. 300-350 ppm in the diet. Diarrhea was seen early in the experiment but not in later stages. Other typical symptoms included achromatrichia, low blood hematocrit, stiffness of movement, and a total lack of libido. On autopsy marked cartilagenous erosion of the metatarsal joints and deterioration of interstitial cells and germinal epithelium of the testicles were found. Tolgyesi and Elmotz (1967) reported effects of large single Mo doses on cows. A single oral dose of 40 g Mo as ammonium molybdate caused anorexia, weak rumen contractions and diarrhea for 6 to 10 days. The addition of 5-10 g of Mo to the feed caused moderate loss of appetite and mild enteritis, both normalizing in one week. Mo concentrations in the feces, urine, blood and milk were 4 to 60-fold above normal by 5 days after dosage. They concluded that occurrence of severe acute Mo poisoning can be practically excluded due to refusal of the poisoned feed. Mo in inorganic salts or as part of cured forage is less toxic than similar levels in grazed forages (Miller et al, 1970).

IODINE(I)

Goiter has been recognized since ancient times but it was not until the 19th century that its cause was linked to a deficiency of I.

The metabolism of I has since been investigated intensively. These investigations have established much of the general knowledge of I metabolism in mammals and have suggested the most fruitful areas of study with ruminant animals. Numerous reviews have been published on I utilization and its relationship to thyroid function and body metabolism. Investigations dealing more specifically with ruminants have also been reported or summarized in reviews by Daburon et al (1968), Hemken (1970) and Miller et al (1975). Underwood (1977) has his usual good coverage on domestic animals and man.

Absorption and Excretion

Results of many investigations have suggested the I metabolism model shown in Fig. 5-13. Absorption and excretion of radio-iodine in different sections of the bovine digestive tract has been investigated using ^{144}Ce as a non-absorbed reference material (Barua et al, 1964; Miller et al, 1975). These studies indicate that between 70 and 80% of the daily I intake is absorbed directly from the rumen and an additional 10% from the omasum. Although some I is absorbed directly from the abomasum (Miller et al, 1971), re-entry of circulating I into the digestive tract predominates here. Net absorption subsequently occurs from the small and large intestines, including the cecum, at a rate similar to that of other dry matter.

I is secreted by the chief and mucosal cells of the gastric mucosa (Meier-Ruge and Fridrich, 1969). Gastric concentration of iodide from plasma exceeds that of chloride by over 15X in calves dosed daily with both ^{131}I and ^{36}Cl (Miller, 1966). More radio-iodine was recovered from the abomasum than from the entire remaining digestive tract 30 min following intravenous administration of labeled NaI (Barua et al, 1964). During the first 6 hr after intravenous administration to mature cows, >65% of the dose was found in material draining from cannulae placed in ligated abomasa (Miller et al, 1975). Apparently, only iodide is secreted into the abomasum since <5% of ^{131}I given as labeled thyroxine was recovered in abomasal drainage during the first 6 hr.

High dietary I (10-100X normal intake) which effectively blocked thyroid uptake, did not reduce abomasal radioiodine secretion (Miller et al, 1975), but the goitrogen thiocyanate reduced radioiodine uptake by both the thyroid and abomasum (Moss et al, 1968). Gross (1962) has pointed out that the kidney essentially has no threshold for I. Thus, the I concentration action of the abomasum may promote conservation of I by transferring it from vascular to extravascular tissues.

Some of the thyroxine from plasma is constantly being degraded or conjugated in the liver and secreted via bile. Consequently, 30 min after intravenous injection of labeled thyroxine, the highest ^{131}I concentration in

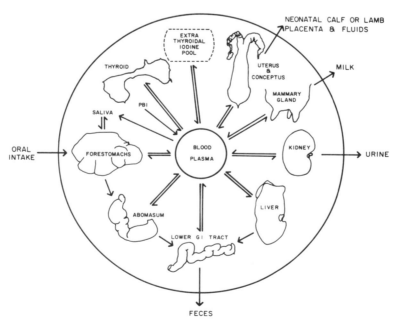

Fig. 5-13. A model for the suggested metabolism of I.

bovine GI tract contents was in the anterior one-sixth of the small intestine (Barua et al, 1964). Some of this I is reabsorbed and recycled since only 74% as much ^{131}I from labeled thyroxine injected intravenously was recovered in feces of intact calves as from cannulated bile ducts of comparable calves (Yatvin et al, 1965). Independent measurements using different techniques indicate about 10% of that thyroxine secreted into the bovine digestive tract is reabsorbed (Mixner and Lennon, 1960; Pipes et al, 1962; Bauman and Turner, 1965).

Major irreversible I losses from the body include urine, feces, and milk (Fig. 5-13). Total radioiodine recoveries in milk, urine and feces during 7 or more days after a single dose compared well with average steady state excretions during daily administration (Lengemann and Swanson, 1957; Binnerts et al, 1962; Cline et al, 1969). Radioiodine excretions following administration to cows as iodide averaged 25% in feces and 40% in urine in 10 reports summarized by Miller et al (1965) in which dietary I intakes were normal (<10 µg/kg body weight per day). Urinary radioiodine excretion can be increased by 50% at daily I intakes above 2 mg/kg body weight (Miller et al, 1965) and more than doubled at much higher intakes (Lengemann and Swanson, 1957), even exceeding the daily dose for short periods. Elevated dietary I had little effect on fecal radioiodine excretion (Miller et al, 1965) and total fecal stable I increased in almost direct proportion to increased supplemental I (Miller and Swanson, 1973).

Secretion into Milk

Important species differences exist in secretion of I into milk. In the cow, unlike the rat (Grosvenor, 1960), entry of I into the mammary gland is not dependent on active secretion of milk. On the contrary, ^{131}I concentrations were higher in halves of cow's udders distended by 24 hr accumulations of milk and in a non-secretory condition than in opposite udder halves milked out before intravenous radioiodine administration (Miller and Swanson, 1963).

Amounts of radioiodine secreted into milk of the ruminant species compared in a recent review averaged 8% of the dose for cows, 22% for goats, and 39% for sheep (Miller et al, 1975). Reabsorption of radioiodine from the udder, measured as that not recovered in milk 7 to 19 hr after intramammary infusion, averaged 82% (Miller and Swanson, 1963) to 94% (Miller et al, 1965) in cows and 90% in goats (Knutsson, 1961). I enters milk primarily as iodide (Lengemann, 1963) and as naturally secreted is <10% bound. Radioactivity was found only as iodide in goat's milk after administration of ^{131}I either as labeled iodide or iodinated casein (Wright et al, 1955). Milk from thyroprotein-fed cows produced no rise in metabolic rate when fed to humans or to guinea pigs.

Stable I content in milk varies linearly within the normal dietary range if other conditions are equal (Binnerts, 1956; Hemken et al, 1972; Miller and Swanson, 1973). The capacity of the cow's mammary gland to secrete additional I appears to be reduced at I intakes between 162 and 405 mg daily (Iwarsson et al, 1972; Miller and Swanson, 1973). Massive I intakes (1-4 g/day) reduced ^{131}I concentrations in milk by one-third to one-half (Lengemann and Swanson, 1957; Bustad et al, 1963; Miller et al, 1965).

Attempts to relate I concentrations in milk to stage of lactation (Binnerts, 1956; Iwarsson, 1973), amount of milk produced (Garner et al, 1960; Miller and Swanson, 1963) and to seasonal effects (Binnerts, 1956, 1964; Lengemann et al, 1957; Garner et al, 1960; Iwarsson, 1974) have not been consistent. Effects of production or stage of lactation can be obscured by seasonal effects, which in turn are complicated by dietary variations. I concentrations are higher in colostrum than in normal milk (Iwarsson et al, 1973) and may rise in normal milk with declining yield as lactation progresses (Iwarsson, 1973). However, when the diet is deficient in I, depletion of I reserves may mask the normal tendency for I concentration to increase in milk with advancing lactation (Swanson, 1972).

There is evidence for an inverse relationship between the amount of blood thyroxine and secretion of radioiodine into milk. Markedly hyperthyroid cows yielded only about half as much milk that contained almost twice as much of a radioiodine dose as their normal controls. Treating the hypothyroid cows with exogenous thyroxine increased milk and reduced secretion of radioiodine into the milk (Miller et al, 1969). Goitrogenic substances in feed may also influence I concentrations in milk. One class of goitrogens, including perchlorate (Lengemann, 1973), thiocyanate (Piironen and Virtanen, 1963; Iwarsson, 1973) and nitrate (Moss et al, 1972) blocks uptake of inorganic iodide and reduces secretion of I into milk. Methylthiouracil, which is goitrogenic due to its inhibition of organic binding of I by the thyroid gland, increased milk I concentrations (Binnerts, 1963). Although the goitrogens thiocyanate and perchlorate reduced the plasma to milk I concentration gradient similar to thyroxine but to a greater extent. Other important differences suggest that the mechanisms are different (Miller et al, 1969).

Fetal Concentration of Iodine

Measurements in the developing bovine fetus have shown negligible I content prior to 60 days of gestation but from 60 to 138 days fetal thyroid I content was almost directly proportional to thyroid mass and body weight. By day 140, however, fetal thyroids had accumulated more I than could be accounted for by increased thyroid mass. Fetal thyroids contained I concentrations comparable to the adult level by 240 days of development (Wolff et al, 1949). Radioiodine uptakes averaged 19% by near term fetal and 17% by maternal thyroids 7 days after oral administration to the dam (Aschbacher, 1966; Miller et al, 1967, 1968). Apparently, I turnover is more rapid in fetal than in maternal thyroids since the much larger maternal gland contained only about half as much radioiodine 24 hr after dosing (Gorbman et al, 1952) but about the same amount by 7 days (Aschbacher et al, 1966).

I concentrations were 4-8X higher in bovine fetal plasma and amniotic fluid than in corresponding maternal plasma (Aschbacher et al, 1966; Miller et al, 1967, 1968). High total I concentrations in fetal plasma were partially reflected in thyroxine which increased from about one-third at day 90 to more than double the maternal concentration in second and third trimesters (Hernandez et al, 1972). Elevated circulating radioiodine and thyroxine in the neonatal calf cleared rapidly during the first few days after birth, indicating that the fetus may not be able to excrete I efficiently. After parturition, accumulated I is eliminated by normal urinary and fecal excretions.

Tissue Distribution

The primary physiological requirement for I is for synthesis by the thyroid gland of hormones which regulate the rate of energy metabolism. In the thyroid, I is found as thyroglobulin and its constituent iodinated amino acids, principally tri-, di-, and mono-iodotyrosine or di- and tri-iodothyronine (Gross, 1962). The thyroid accumulates more I than the entire remaining body and the amount taken up is partly a function of the I status of the animal. Research with radio-iodine has shown that as I intakes near the minimum requirement, cattle commonly bind 30% of more of their daily consumption in the thyroid (Lengemann and Swanson, 1957; Miller et al, 1975). With very low I intakes it is possible for the thyroid to bind 65% or more of the daily intake but intakes above the requirement greatly reduce I uptake by the thyroid (Lengemann and Swanson, 1957; Swanson et al, 1957).

Thyroid secretion rates of cattle, measured by many investigators using different methods (Premachandra et al, 1958; Post and Mixner, 1961; Mixner et al, 1962, 1966; Vohnout et al, 1968; Anderson, 1971; Swanson, 1972), have been within the range of 0.2 to 0.3 mg/100 kg of body weight. Thyroxine secretion rate is depressed by elevated environmental temperature (Thompson et al, 1963) and is influenced more by seasonal effects than by stage of lactation (Mixner et al, 1962). Thyroid function is inhibited by a number of naturally occurring goitrogens, including those in plants of the genus *Brassica* (Iwarsson, 1973) and when large amounts of soybean meal are fed (Hemken et al, 1971). Certain forages also contain factors which induce adjustments in thyroid activity when the forage fed is changed suddenly (Vandersall et al, 1962).

Both thyroid I uptake and thyroxine secretion rate were lower in lactating than in non-lactating goats (Flamboe and Reineke, 1959). These results and studies with rats have led to the suggestion that under conditions of minimal I intake, lactation could be self-limiting because I in milk would be unavailable for thyroid hormone production (Anonymous, 1962). Dairy cattle apparently can adapt to low I intakes by reducing losses in milk, urine and feces (Swanson, 1972; Miller and Swanson, 1973) and when dietary I is adequate, lactation has little effect on the percentage bound by the thyroid (Swanson et al, 1957; Blinco, 1975).

Uptake of radioiodine by other organs and tissues in the bovine averaged only 0.006 to 0.04% as much per unit weight as in the thyroid gland (Miller et al, 1973, 1975). Non-thyroid tissue and fluid radioiodine concentrations, in descending order, were blood plasma, uterus, cartilage, skin with hair, ovary, mammary gland, lung, kidney, lymph node, salivary gland, pancreas, adrenal, hoof, heart, spleen, liver and skeletal muscle. Inflamed or diseased tissues concentrated 24 to 218% more radioiodine than corresponding normal tissues (Miller et al, 1973), possibly because of infiltrating leucocytes. Pincus and Klebanoff (1971) have suggested a microbicidal involvement of I by phagocytosing leucocytes. This may be another important function of I in the body in addition to its role as a necessary component of thyroxine.

Deficiency in Animals

I deficiency may be a geographical problem where feeds and water are low in I or conditioned by presence of goitrogens. More than a year on low I diets may be required before deficiency symptoms are observed (Hemken et al, 1971; Swanson, 1972). Usually the first obvious sign is enlarged thyroid (goiter) in the newborn even though the dam may appear normal (Hemken et al, 1971). Goiter results from changes in thyroid tissue cells (Fig. 5-14) which enlarge the gland (Fig. 5-15) as a result of the deficiency of I. Deficiency during pregnancy may result in birth of hairless (or wool-less) weak or dead young but only moderate goiter, or hyperplasia of thyroid gland follicles without gross enlargement, may be observed in young animals with normal hair or wool (Aschbacher, 1968; Hemken et al, 1971).

Obvious goiter has been observed in adult sheep (Fig. 5-16) but usually is not seen in adult cattle. Other signs of I insufficiency, including decreased milk yield and reduced reproductive performance, as evidenced by irregular breeding intervals, low conception rate, and retained placentas may result from long term deficiencies (Hemken, 1970). Milk concentrations below 20 μg/l. are typical from cows in I deficient areas (Alderman and Stranks, 1967).

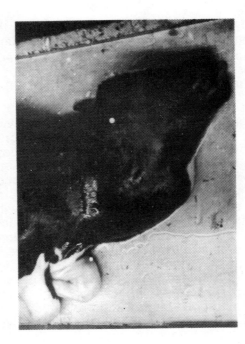

Fig. 5-15. I-deficient calf. Note massive goiter. Calf was born about one month prematurely. Courtesy of J.H. Vandersall, Univ. of Maryland.

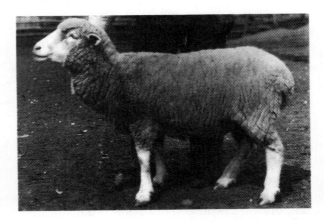

Fig. 5-16. Ewe showing a goiter due to I deficiency. Courtesy of W.W. Hawkins, Vet. Res. Lab., Montana State Univ.

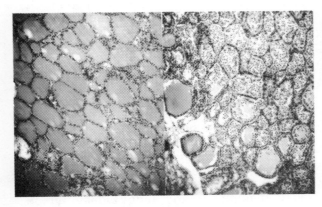

Left   Right

Fig. 5-14. Microphotographs from thyroids of day-old lambs. That on the left is from a lamb whose dam had been supplemented with I. The picture on the right is from a deficient lamb. The section of the normal gland shows typical cells filled with colloid and flat epithelial cells. The deficient gland has few colloid-filled cells and many high columnar-type cells. Courtesy of P.W. Aschbacher, N. Dakota State Univ.

Dietary Requirements

Theoretical dietary requirements for I can be calculated based on feed intake, thyroid uptake efficiency, daily thyroxine secretion rate, and amount of thyroxine recycled. A daily thyroxine secretion rate of 0.2 to 0.3 mg/100 kg body weight (Swanson, 1972) would utilize about 0.7 mg I if the thyroid accumulated 30% of the dietary intake. Recycling of 15% of the thyroxine I (Miller et al, 1975) would reduce the I requirement to 0.6 mg/100 kg body weight at dry matter intakes of 2.5% of body weight. Feed should contain 0.25 ppm I to supply this amount. This calculation indicates currently recommended I contents in ration dry matter of 0.6 ppm (NRC, 1971) to 0.8 ppm (ARC, 1965) should be adequate for dairy cattle. Requirements may be somewhat higher during stress or lactation or when availability of dietary I to the thyroid has been reduced by lactation or by a supply of goitrogenic feeds (Hemken et al, 1971; Iwarsson et al, 1973).

Utilization of Iodine Sources

The need for I supplementation to the diet of farm animals in certain areas has been well established. Various I sources have been compared with iodide to determine their comparative nutritional availability to ruminants (Table 5-4). In this respect, Ca iodate and pentacalcium orthoperiodate (Miller et al, 1968), potassium iodate (Lengemann, 1969), sodium iodate (Bretthauer et al, 1972) and ethylenediaminedihydriodide (EDDI) (Miller and Swanson, 1973) were comparable to NaI or KI. Unfortunately, iodide and iodate were rapidly lost from the surface layer of block salt when exposed to outdoor weather conditions (Shuman and Townsend, 1963). While physically stable, I from 3,5-diiodosalicylic acid (DIS) was found to be only about 20% as available to cattle as I from iodide (Aschbacher et al, 1963; 1966),

Table 5-4. Thyroid uptakes by dairy cows and their neonatal calves of radioiodine following single prepartum doses with different radioiodine labeled compounds.[a]

Compound	Uptake, % of dose	
	Cows	Calves
Diiodosalicylic acid[b]	2.2	1.9
Calcium iodate[c]	17.1	14.5
Calcium periodate[c]	17.6	13.8
EDDI[d]	19.8	--
Sodium Iodide[e]	17.3	13.8

[a] ^{125}I-labeled compounds were compared with ^{131}I-labeled NaI by simultaneous within animal dosing in each experiment. Values from different experiments were expressed on a common basis by multiplying the ^{125}I/^{131}I ratio in each experiment by the ^{131}I average for all experiments.
[b]Aschbacher et al (1966); [c]Miller et al (1968); [d]Miller and Swanson (1973); [e]Average of all experiments.

and when fed to ewes it did not prevent subsequent I deficiency symptoms in their newborn lambs (Aschbacher, 1968). Although rats utilize DIS efficiently, cows have much less ability to remove I atoms from the DIS molecule before it is excreted (Aschbacher and Feil, 1968). Pentacalcium orthoperiodate combines physical stability with nutritional availability to cattle (Miller et al, 1968).

Toxicity

Iodine has been fed to cattle at levels much higher than the nutritional requirement for prevention or the systemic treatment of mycotic infections. Recommended daily I intakes range from prophylactic 40 mg (Miller and Tillapaugh, 1967) to therapeutic doses of over 2000 mg (Long et al, 1956). Care must be taken therefore that prophylactic levels of I are not provided simultaneously in two or more carriers (e.g., mineral mixture and protein supplement), since toxic signs may appear when the diet consistently contains 50 to 100 ppm I (Newton et al, 1974). Young stock are more sensitive to excess I than are lactating cows (Miller and Swanson, 1973). Toxicity signs include excessive salivation, watery nasal discharge, tracheal congestion which causes coughing, excessive lacrimation, and subnormal feed intake and growth rate. However, rapid recovery follows removal of the excess I from the diet.

IRON (Fe)

The frequency of Fe deficiency anemia in many human populations has stimulated a tremendous amount of research on Fe nutrition and metabolism. Much more information is available for humans, laboratory animals and in vitro enzyme systems than for ruminant species. Thus, much of the information in subsequent paragraphs stems from non-ruminant sources. It is included because of the importance of Fe in animal nutrition and it is basically applicable to ruminants. Pertinent reviews include those of Thomas (1970), Forth and Rummel (1973), Forth (1974), Christopher et al (1974), Jacobs (1977), Linder and Munro (1977) and Underwood (1977).

Absorption and Excretion

The amount of Fe absorbed is dictated by body needs, so absorption plays the determining role for the homeostasis of Fe metabolism (Forth, 1974). Only 2-20% of oral radioiron is absorbed by normal individuals and 5-10% of the Fe from food sources. Deficient individuals, however, may absorb 20-60% of an ingested dose. Previously, it was believed Fe was absorbed only in the ferrous (Fe++) form because of the low solubility of Ferric (Fe+++) ions at neutral pH. Neither oxidation state of Fe exists in ionic form to any appreciable extent under physiological conditions. Still the relationship between solubility in the digestive tract and absorption of Fe is important. Natural chelates which can be transported intact across the mucosal cells may be involved in Fe absorption. Several studies with man and experimental animals have shown chelates of ferric Fe were absorbed better than ferrous sulfate (Christopher et al, 1974), the form once considered to be the most readily absorbed. Agents which form stable Fe chelates in the GI tract may prevent uptake of Fe by acceptor sites on mucosal cells, thus inhibiting absorption of Fe. However, weaker agents which form Fe chelates of lower stability may release their Fe to the acceptor sites (Forth, 1974). These weaker agents may keep Fe available for absorption by reducing formation of poorly absorbed hydroxides and phosphates.

As proposed by Linder and Munro (1977) and Forth (1974), Fe in the intestinal lumen absorbs to specific receptors in the brush border of the mucosal cell. From these receptors, Fe is transferred to the cytoplasm of mucosal cells by an active process. Within the cells, Fe exists mainly in two pools, a rapidly exchangeable one (probably identical to the transferrin-like, Fe-binding protein 2), and a slowly exchangeable one (probably the ferritin-like, Fe-binding protein 1). Normally, Fe exchanges with the slowly exchangeable pool, but in Fe deficiency the rapidly exchangeable pool predominates (Wheby, 1966). Exchange of Fe between the two pools and the degradation of Fe chelates may occur in the cytoplasm. At the serosal surface of the cell, Fe becomes attached to transferrin for transport in the plasma. This transfer mechanism probably involves receptors in the cell membrane and may be independent of cell energy. Jacobs (1977) has reviewed evidence for an intracellular pool of low molecular weight Fe compounds which acts as an intermediate between extracellular Fe and a wide variety of intracellular processes.

Current thoughts are that the rate of erythropoiesis and the state of body Fe stores act to control absorption, particularly at the level of serosal transfer. Populations of receptors during mucosal cell formation may be controlled by homeostatic mechanisms within the body. Receptors on the brush border change slowly over several days in response to Fe status. Changes in transport across the serosal surface, which may be more responsive to changes in Fe status, occur with a somewhat shorter time lag. The intermediaries in these regulatory processes have not been identified but serum ferritin could be involved (Linder and Munro, 1977). Fe not transported to plasma is retained in the cell until it is sloughed off, thus returning to the lumen of the GI tract.

Oral ^{59}Fe doses excreted by sheep ranged from 84 to 98% in feces and 0.04 and 0.09 in urine (Fig. 5-17), depending on chemical form of Fe administered (Ammerman et al, 1967). Most of the Fe in feces represents that unabsorbed from food. Fe once absorbed, is tenaciously retained by the body. However, daily fecal excretion of hemoglobin Fe increased from 1 mg in control sheep to over 9 mg by sheep infected with the parasite *Schistosoma mattheei* (Dargie and Preston, 1974). Neither normal nor infected sheep were able to reutilize significant amounts of Fe derived from red cells passed into the gut.

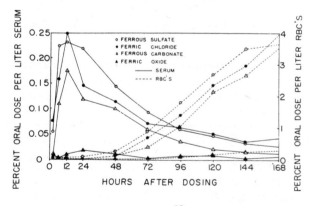

Fig. 5-17. Effect of form of ^{59}Fe on uptake by red cells and serum by sheep following an oral dose. Note the negligible uptake from ferric oxide. From Ammerman et al (1967).

Fe in the Tissues

The body of a 70 kg man contains 4 to 5 g of Fe (Underwood, 1977). Of this, 60-70% is accounted for as a constituent of hemoglobin; 3% in myoglobin; 26% in storage; and less than 1% in Fe transport compounds and Fe-enzyme complexes. Hemoglobin is a complex of globin and four ferroprotoporphyrin moieties with a molecular weight close to 65,000 and an Fe content of about 0.35%. Hemoglobin functions as an oxygen carrier because the bonds between Fe and globin stabilize Fe in the ferrous state and allow it to be reversibly bonded to oxygen. When the Fe atom is oxidized to the ferric state (as in methemoglobin), it loses its capacity to carry oxygen. Blood hemoglobin values vary with age, sex, and species; in the ruminant normal values are about 11-12 g per 100 ml (Hansard and Foote, 1959). Myoglobin, the heme-protein in muscle, has an Fe content of about 0.12%. Its structure is like that of hemoglobin, but it contains only one ferrous porphyrin group per molecule and has a molecular weight of only 16,500. Myoglobin has a greater affinity for oxygen than hemoglobin and thus can accept oxygen released by hemoglobin and serve as an oxygen reservoir (Moore and Dubach, 1962).

Fe is present in blood serum in a non-hemoglobin form called transferrin or siderophilin. Transferrin is a glycoprotein which binds two atoms of ferric Fe per molecule and appears to serve as a carrier for Fe in the same way that hemoglobin acts as a carrier for oxygen. A second important function of transferrin may be its participation in defense mechanisms of the body against infection. Normal plasma contains 240-280 mg transferrin per 100 ml. Transferrins are also found in other extracellular fluids such as cerebrospinal fluid. Plasma transferrin is measured by the amount of Fe plasma will bind before saturation. In normal individuals of most species only 30-40% of the transferrin carries Fe, the remainder representing an unbound reserve. The sum of serum Fe plus the additional Fe required to reach the saturation limit is its total Fe-binding capacity. Plasma Fe concentrations and total Fe-binding capacities in mcg/100 ml average, respectively, 146 and 492 in bovine and 171 and 346 in ovine adults (Underwood and Morgan, 1963).

The reserve or storage Fe of the body occurs predominantly in two non-heme compounds, ferritin and hemosiderin. Ferritin contains up to 20% Fe. Its central Fe nucleus is surrounded by a spherical protein shell of 24 subunits with a combined molecular weight of 445,000 (Jacobs, 1977). Hemosiderin consists mainly of ferric hydroxide in an essentially protein-free aggregate and may contain up to 35% Fe (Underwood, 1977). Ratio of ferritin to hemosiderin is determined by total level as well as by rate of Fe storage. In most mammals, ferritin is the primary Fe storage compound when the total level of stored Fe is low; at higher storage levels, hemosiderin may predominate.

Fe is found in a number of enzymes. Catalases and peroxidases are heme enzymes which liberate oxygen from peroxides. Hemoglobin also has peroxidase action. The cytochromes are heme enzymes occurring in the cell mitochondria which provide a system for electron transfer through the capacity of the Fe atom to undergo reversible oxidation. Other Fe-containing enzymes include non-heme metalo-flavoproteins such as xanthine oxidase, succinic dehydrogenase and NADH-cytochrome reductase (Moore and Dubach, 1962). The muscle proteins, myosin and actomysin, have been shown to contain small amounts of Fe, the function of which remains to be shown .

Fe Research with Ruminants

Hansard et al (1959) and Hansard and Foote (1959) have studied the tissue uptake of ^{59}Fe in calves fed grass hay and a commercial dairy feed. The mean half-time of plasma ^{59}Fe disappearance was 2.7 hr, somewhat slower than the 1.55 hr reported earlier by Baker and Douglas (1957) but in agreement with the 2.5 hr found by Giles et al (1977). Gibbons et al (1976) found plasma ^{59}Fe clearance rates in goats could be analyzed into two exponential components with half times of 2-4 hr and 20-60 hr. ^{59}Fe administered intravenously either as the chloride or specifically bound to transferrin was not distinguishable as separate pools by this technique.

Uptake of intravenously administered ^{59}Fe by red blood cells ranged from 52 (Giles et al, 1977) to 84% (Hansard et al, 1959). Rate of Fe incorporation into the red cells, presumed to represent rate of erythropoiesis since ^{59}Fe does not enter the mature red cells directly, was 0.45 mg/kg body weight/day. Red blood cell lifespan, calculated by dividing total red blood cell Fe by red cell Fe incorporation rate, was 47 days, less than half the 112 days reported by Giles et al (1977) and only about one-third the lifespan of sheep erythrocytes measured using methylene-labeled ^{14}C glycine (Judd and Matrone, 1962).

Fe status has a major influence on its percentage utilization. Fe deficiency in calves shortened half time of plasma Fe clearance, lowered plasma Fe concentration and red cell uptake of injected ^{59}Fe, and raised unsaturated Fe binding capacity (Mollerberg et al, 1975). Matrone et al (1957) calculated 60% utilization of Fe in calves each given 30 mg daily but only 30% utilization with a 60 mg intake.

Table 5-5. Fe concentrations in bovine serum and tissues.[a]

Tissue and unit	Age, years		
	1-3	4-6	7-9
Blood serum, mcg/100 ml	143	146	141
Liver, mcg/g dry weight	128	235	223
Spleen, mcg/g dry weight	3067	20614	30740
Bone marrow, mcg/g dry weight	28	62	100

[a] From Blum and Zuber (1975)

Radioiron concentrations were highest in trabecular bone and in liver tissue 168 hr after intravenous administration (Hansard et al, 1959). Concentrations in liver reached a peak 4-6 hr after dosing and receded gradually to about one-fourth of peak level after 24 hr. Radioactivity in the sternum and vertebral bones of calves reached an initial peak at 10-12 hr after dosing and after 24 hr, bone appeared to serve as the principal metabolic pool for Fe storage. In Fe depleted calves, Ammerman et al (1967) found that relative ^{59}Fe depositions 96 hr after oral administration as ferric chloride were liver > spleen > kidney > heart > rib. Blum and Zuber (1975) measured Fe in blood serum and tissues of clinically healthy cows and heifers. Much higher storage Fe concentrations were found in the spleen than in liver or bone in 104 animals (Table 5-5). Fe concentrations in all three tissues increased markedly after 3 yr of age, and remained constant or increased further between 6 and 9 yr. In contrast, serum Fe from 285 animals remained relatively constant between 1 and 8 yr of age.

Underwood and Morgan (1963) measured total non-heme (storage Fe), water-soluble (presumably ferritin), and water-insoluble (hemosiderin) Fe in ovine and bovine livers and found large variability in both sexes of each species. From two-thirds to three-fourths of total storage Fe was water soluble. Both total storage and ferritin Fe were significantly higher in sheep than in cattle, and somewhat higher in females than in males of each species. Percentage saturation of plasma transferrin was also significantly higher in sheep and was higher in ewes than in rams.

Fe traversed the placenta of sheep (Hoskins and Hansard, 1964) and cattle (Hansard, 1966) at all stages of gestation and was apparently related directly to the amount of Fe actually required for incorporation into growing tissues. Although total fetal ^{59}Fe content 48 hr after intravenous administra-tion to ewes was only 0.09, 0.31 and 0.66% of the retained maternal dose at 47, 94 and 141 days of gestation, the fetus had accumulated 2.3, 28.7 and 123 mg of total Fe by these stages of development. Fetal stable Fe and ^{59}Fe as percentages of that in the whole fetal complex (fetus, fluids, and placental membranes) increased from 4.9 and 14.1 at day 47 to 37.6 and 42.3 at day 94 and 60.8 and 68.3 at day 141.

Radiochemical procedures with lactating ewes (Hansard and Glenn, 1964) indicated only about 0.3% of the absorbed oral ^{59}Fe dose appeared in milk. Milk ^{59}Fe did not peak until 6-8 days after oral dosing. In contrast, following intravenous injection, milk ^{59}Fe concentrations plateaued at 8-12 hr, near the time of highest plasma radioactivity. The peak in milk ^{59}Fe occurred approximately 100 hr before maximum red blood cell uptake suggesting plasma to be the carrier. Concentrations of Fe in milk average about 0.5 mg/ml but colostrum may contain 3-5 times more Fe than true milk (Underwood, 1977).

Plasma Fe concentrations in dairy calves increased considerably between 1 and 3 wk after birth, but declined within the next few days to levels similar to those in adult cattle (Bremner, 1966). Total Fe-binding capacity increased sharply after birth, reaching maximum values between 1 and 5 wk of age. Plasma Fe of female calves decreased with age after 3 mo and was lower than in male calves of the same age by 15 mo. Average hemoglobin levels in lambs were about 14.1-14.3 g/100 ml at birth (Holz et al, 1961) compared to fetal levels of 6.0, 7.4 and 10.4 g/100 ml at 47, 94 and 141 days of gestation (Hoskins and Hansard, 1964). Hemoglobin values declined, reaching minimal values at 14-21 days of age and then gradually increased to about 11 g/100 ml by 56 days of age. Soliman and El Amrousi (1965) reported a similar pattern in sheep, cattle, buffaloes and camels. Generally, values for Fe and hemoglobin were high at birth and then fell, rising significantly when weaned animals had access to green feed. Values were lower in pregnant animals than in open females or those with inactive ovaries.

Deficiency

Underwood (1977) states that an uncomplicated Fe deficiency has not been demonstrated clearly in sheep or cattle grazing under natural conditions. Although these may be exceptions, reports from Florida have shown that supplementation with Fe corrected anemia in grazing cattle in some areas (Becker et al, 1965) and helped to maintain milk yields of newly developed pastures (Wing and Ammerman, 1965). Exhaustion of Fe reserves in calves infected with the parasite *Oesophagostomum radiatum* reduced blood hemoglobin to 6 g/100 ml and plasma Fe to less than 70 µg/100 ml (Bremner, 1969).

Fe reserves of the neonatal calf are variable, but are usually sufficient to prevent serious anemia if dry feeds are provided within the first few weeks of age. It is when young animals are fed exclusively on a milk diet for several weeks that Fe deficiency anemia develops (Blaxter et al, 1957; Matrone et al, 1957; Bremner and Dalgarno, 1973). In fact, the pale color considered characteristic of good veal is caused by Fe deficiency (MacDougall et al, 1973). They found the myoglobin content of veal from calves fed milk powder with 100 ppm of Fe was twice that of veal from calves fed 40 ppm. There was no difference in myoglobin content between calves receiving 10 and 40 ppm of Fe but blood hemoglobin content was reduced at the lower intake.

Calves fed milk diets unsupplemented with Fe develop a microcytic, normochromic anemia (Blaxter et al, 1957; Bremner and Dalgarno, 1973). Blaxter et al (1957) reported the anemia was associated with poikilocytosis (large red cells of irregular shape), lowered resistance to circulatory stresses, anorexia, and atrophy of the papilla of the tongue. There were also reductions in tissue concentrations of Fe and cytochrome C (Bremner and Dalgarno, 1973). Matrone et al (1957) and Bremner and Dalgarno (1973) found that hemoglobin levels of unsupplemented calves declined to 5-6 g/100 ml, and serum Fe to 20-30 mcg/100 ml by 11 to 40 wk of age. A higher than normal pulse rate in anemic calves may partially compensate for the deficiency of hemoglobin (Settlemire et al, 1964). Hematocrit values dropped to about half of normal. No bone marrow abnormalities were reported. Weight gains may (Blaxter et al, 1957; Matrone, 1957) or may not (Getty et al, 1968; Bremner and Dalgarno, 1973) be reduced, depending on duration and severity of Fe deficiency. Symptoms reported in lambs included anorexia, depressed growth (Fig. 5-18), and emaciation (Lawlor et al, 1965). Although no significant hematological changes developed, in contrast to calves, hemoglobin, RBC count, and packed cell volume values tended to be

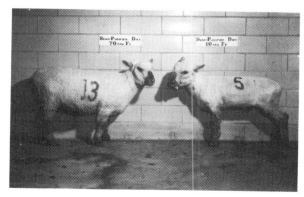

Fig. 5-18. Lamb on right was fed 10 ppm Fe and developed symptoms of Fe deficiency. Normal lamb on left received 70 ppm Fe. From Lawlor et al (1965).

higher in deficient lambs, suggesting hemoconcentration.

Requirements

Fe requirements are defined more precisely for the young calf than for adult sheep or cattle. Daily addition of 20 mg of Fe as the citrate to the diet of milk-fed calves was not sufficient to prevent a deficiency (Blaxter et al, 1957). Normal growth and hemoglobin levels were maintained in calves raised on milk containing 1 ppm Fe by daily drenching with 30 or 60 mg Fe, but serum Fe tended to be lower in those given 30 mg in one of two trials (Matrone et al, 1957). Ellendorff and Smith (1967) fed 0, 20, 40 or 50 mg of Fe to Holstein calves. Results were somewhat inconclusive but indicated that even 60 mg was inadequate for optimum blood levels of hemoglobin or hematocrit values. St. Laurent and Brisson (1968) observed that 50 mg/day in the form of ferrous sulfate was inadequate to maintain liver reserves in Holstein male calves. Using values from a ferrokinetic study, Mollerberg et al (1975) estimated the total daily Fe requirement for a 100 kg calf gaining 1 kg/day to be 160-180 mg. If whole milk is fed at 10% of body weight, 30 mg of supplemental Fe (Matrone et al, 1957) would correspond to dry milk concentrations of approximately 22 and 44 ppm for 50 and 100 kg calves. Bremner and Dalgarno (1973) found that 40 ppm Fe in milk on a dry basis prevented all but a very mild anemia in calves. Khouri and Pickering (1969) found that dried milk supplemented with about 47 ppm Fe and fed at 2% of body weight maintained blood hemoglobin levels.

Getty et al (1968) have compared Fe-dextran injection (500 mg on the 7th and 21st days), daily oral supplementation with 30 mg of ferrous sulfate, and no supplemental Fe in calves fed whole milk for 11 weeks. Dextran treatment resulted in the highest serum Fe but other measures (hematocrit, hemoglobin, rate of gain) indicated little difference in response. Mollerberg et al (1975a) fed veal calves a milk substitute containing 19 mg Fe/kg for 12 weeks. Injection with 800-900 mg Fe dextran at 3 week intervals resulted in 136 g higher daily gains per calf and maintained serum Fe and blood hemoglobin values whereas these measurements decreased significantly in untreated calves. Treatment of calves suckling their dams on the range with Fe-dextran had little effect on their performance (Raleigh and Wallace, 1962; Lesperance et al, 1966). However, there was some indication that suckling lambs may benefit from injections of Fe-dextran compounds (Hardman et al, 1959; Holz et al, 1961), both in terms of blood hemoglobin and improved gain. In older lambs, Lawlor et al (1965) fed partially purified diets with various supplemental levels of Fe as the sulfate. Their data indicate that 25 ppm of Fe did not support maximum growth, but that 40 ppm was adequate as compared to 70 ppm or higher. These values are equivalent to about 20, 48 and 78 mg of Fe/day for lambs with average weights of 22, 26 and 26 kg, respectively.

Fe requirement is greatly influenced by the criteria of adequacy chosen (Miller and Stake, 1974). Although 40 ppm of Fe in the dry diet prevented severe anemia in veal calves (Bremner and Dalgarno, 1973a), it resulted in a much lower transferrin saturation than when 100 ppm Fe was given (Bremner and Dalgarno, 1973). However, it might be noted that calves raised for veal are intentionally kept in an anemic state because of the premium paid for pale meat of such animals. Provided other complications do not affect performance, such anemic calves appear to grow almost as well as do Fe-supplemented animals.

From a practical point of view, Fe deficiency does not appear to be a problem in ruminants consuming food other than milk, with rare exceptions. Fe requirements are probably modified to a considerable extent by other nutrients in the diet. At least this is so with respect to Mn, since research (Hartman et al, 1955) has shown that high levels of Mn will depress serum and liver Fe as well as hemoglobin in lambs. An Fe level in the dry diet of 100 ppm should be adequate for calves to 3 mo of age with 35 ppm sufficient for other cattle (NRC, 1978). Based on the data reviewed, these levels should also be adequate for sheep. If pale veal is of crucial importance, 30-40 ppm may be more desirable.

Sources of Fe

Underwood (1977) points out that leguminous plant species are generally richer in Fe than grass species grown in the same sites. The normal range in legume forage is considered to be 200-400 ppm (dry basis) although values as high as 700-800 ppm have been reported for uncontaminated alfalfa. Grasses grown on sandy soils may contain 40 ppm or less. The level of Fe in pastures and forage can be affected greatly by contamination with soil and dust (Campbell et al, 1974). Cereal grains contain between 30 and 60 ppm and oilseed meals from 100 to 200 ppm. Most feeds of animal origin and some mineral supplements including ground limestone, oyster shell, and many forms of calcium phosphate are excellent sources of Fe. Milk is the one dietary exception, having an average concentration of about 0.5 mg/l. Colostrum, however, may contain 3-5X more Fe than true milk (Underwood, 1977).

There have been a number of experiments in which oral sources of Fe have been compared with Fe-dextran sources. These suggest a much greater utilization of the injected compounds. Different Fe salts given orally have also been compared (Ammerman et al, 1967; Bremner and Dalgarno, 1973). Ammerman et al (1967) administered ^{59}Fe in the form of ferric oxide, ferric chloride, ferrous carbonate or ferrous sulfate as a single oral dose to calves and lambs. Their results generally showed that Fe sulfate, ferrous carbonate and ferric chloride ranked in decreasing order of availability, but were not statistically different when evaluated on the basis of ^{59}Fe deposition. Ammerman (1970) later pointed out that the ferrous carbonate used in these studies was freshly prepared and suggested such preparations may be more available than the naturally occurring ore. Tissue levels of ^{59}Fe were greater in calves partially depleted of Fe before dosing. Ferric oxide was much less available. Excretion of ^{59}Fe, when fed to sheep (Fig. 5-19), shows that only small amounts of Fe are recovered in the urine.

Bremner and Dalgarno (1973) compared the effectiveness of 30 ppm supplemental Fe as ferrous sulfate, ferric citrate, Fe-EDTA or Fe phytate in preventing hematological changes in milk-fed calves. Hemoglobin concentrations were higher in Fe-supplemented than in control calves within 2 weeks, and differences increased as the

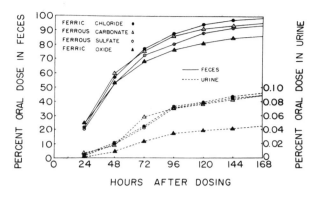

Fig. 5-19. Accumulative fecal and urinary excretion by sheep of ^{59}Fe as influenced by form of Fe. Note the difference in urinary excretion of ferric oxide. From Ammerman et al (1967).

experiment proceeded. Fe availability, as indicated by hemoglobin, was higher from Fe-EDTA and lower from Fe phytate than from other sources. No significant differences in plasma total Fe-binding capacity were noted between treatments, but the 30 ppm level of supplemental Fe increased dietary Fe to only 40 ppm, an amount which resulted in a low transferrin saturation in a subsequent experiment (Bremner and Dalgarno, 1973).

Toxicity

Sufficiently high levels of dietary Fe can reduce weight gains and feed consumption in ruminants. Measurable effects have been produced by as little as 210-400 ppm dietary Fe (Lawlor et al, 1965; Standish et al, 1969), while in other studies calves were able to tolerate 1,000 to 2,000 ppm (Hartley et al, 1959; Koong et al, 1970). Coup and Campbell (1964) found that cattle grazing pastures irrigated with water containing 17 ppm of Fe showed loss of body weight and condition and a reduced milk yield. Similar results were noted the next year with 5 pairs of non-lactating twins. In controlled studies massive doses (40-60 g) of Fe (OH$_3$) resulted in scouring and a rapid decline in milk yield and body weight. Lambs receiving 210 and 280 ppm of Fe developed rather severe diarrhea and some died, but postpartum examination revealed no particular cause other than severe generalized edema (Lawlor et al, 1965). Hartley et al (1959) have reported that cows grazing pastures containing 1,300-1,800 ppm of Fe developed an intense siderosis of the liver and of the hepatic and pancreatic lymph nodes. Feeding 1,000-1,600 ppm Fe as ferrous sulfate to steers increased Fe concentrations in liver, spleen,

heart, kidney, and skeletal muscle and reduced liver Ca, Cu and Zn (Standish et al, 1969, 1971). Plasma P was increased in one study (Standish et al, 1969) and reduced in others (Koong et al, 1970; Standish et al, 1971). Liver Fe content was also increased in sheep by feeding 1,600 ppm Fe but tissue Ca, Cu and Zn or plasma Ca and P were not influenced (Standish and Ammerman, 1971). The feeding of consecutively decreasing 3,200, 2,400 and 0 ppm levels of supplemental Fe for 21, 28 and 35 days indicated that the effects of high Fe levels were transient in nature (Standish et al, 1969).

MANGANESE

Manganese has been a recognized required trace element for some 50 years. Although a considerable amount of research has been reported on Mn, much remains to be learned about Mn-containing compounds in the animal body and its vital functions. Fortunately, since this volume was first published in 1971 there have been a number of reports dealing with Mn in ruminant animals. For detailed reviews on the subject, refer to Cotzias (1962), Thomas (1970) or Underwood (1977).

Functions

Mn is known to activate a variety of enzymes, but many, if not all, of these may be activated by other divalent ions in vitro. Mn is a constituent of arginase and the biotin dependent pyruvate decarboxylase of chicken liver. Mn has been postulated to play a role in protein synthesis, in oxidative phosphorylation and the metabolism of fatty acids and cholesterol synthesis. The mitochondria are the principal sites for Mn uptake. In blood, Mn is transported in the trivalent form by a globulin protein called transmanganin where one metal ion binds more than one protein molecule. In bone Mn appears to be necessary for production and maintenance of the organic matrix.

Tissue Mn

Mn is present in very small amounts in the tissues that have been examined, although like other trace elements, it is found in relatively high concentrations in liver, kidney and pancreas. Bone, gonadal tissues, hair and wool may also contain appreciable amounts. Red hair contains more than black or white hair.

Normal liver Mn in cattle is on the order of 9-12 ppm on a dry basis (Bentley and Phillips, 1951; Rojas et al, 1965; Miller et al,

132

1973). Other tissues showing lesser amounts include kidney, heart and spleen (Miller et al, 1973). Underwood (1977) indicates that a typical Mn level in sheep liver is about 6-8 ppm; apparently young lambs may be similar as Lassiter and Morton (1968) reported values of 1.9 and 2.6 ppm on a fresh basis. German data suggest that body organs of female goats contain more Mn, particularly in the ribs, than those of male goats (Anke et al, 1973).

When using neutron activation analyses, Rojas et al (1965) found cows to have whole blood Mn values on the order of 2.8 mcg/100 ml. Bentley and Phillips (1951) gave values of 4.6-6.6 mcg/100 ml of whole blood in older animals and Miller et al (1973) gave values of 0.2 ppm in whole blood and 0.13 ppm in plasma from calves 6+wk of age. In one study market milk contained 33-210 (av. 91) mcg/l. (Murthy et al, 1973) and colostrum is said to have 130-160 mcg/l. as an organic complex, some of which is in the fat globule membrane (Thomas, 1970).

Absorption and Metabolism

Data on monogastric species indicate that Mn is excreted via the bile and that the feces are the major route of excretion. The pancreatic juice probably also serves as a means of excretion. Other data on monogastric species indicate a very low net absorption of Mn and, furthermore, loading of the tissues results in in a rapid excretion.

In a study with sheep which were fed 0-4,000 ppm of supplementary Mn, Watson et al (1973) found a linear increase in fecal Mn which accounted for essentially all of the increased Mn intake. Urinary Mn ranged from 0.17 mg/day at the basal level (25 ppm) to 3.2 mg at the 4,000 ppm level. Apparent absorption and net retention values for the basal diet were 1.3 and 0.4%, but these values were negative at all of the supplementary levels of Mn. In a second experiment apparent absorption and net retention values were 10.3 and 9.3%, respectively, on an intake of 25 ppm. Plasma Mn (9-15 mcg/100 ml) was not affected by treatment. They also observed that a very high percentage of Mn was excreted via the feces and only negligible amounts via urine. High dosage levels (4,030 ppm) did not greatly alter the excretion curves (Fig. 5-20).

In studies with calves ca. 6 mo. of age, Miller et al (1972) administered [54]Mn via a duodenal catheter. The Mn was absorbed rapidly by small intestinal tissues and the cranial sections of the small intestine

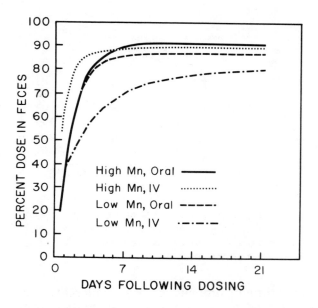

Fig. 5-20. Accumulative excretion (% of dose) of [54]Mn in feces when administered I.V. or orally. From Watson et al (1973).

absorbed considerably more than the other sections. In other work from this laboratory (Miller et al, 1973; Abrams et al, 1977) it has been demonstrated that I.V. dosing with [54]Mn results in the predominant amount of the Mn being excreted via the feces. Giving the dose via the duodenum resulted in very small recoveries in the bile, suggesting that enterohepatic circulation of Mn is not an important factor in Mn metabolism.

Miller et al (1973) suggest that uptake of Mn by the gut limits Mn absorption into the blood stream, particularly since studies with I.V. administration show much higher blood levels of protein-bound Mn than when animals were dosed orally or via the duodenum (Abrams et al, 1977). Although as much as 50% of Mn may be excreted via the bile (Abrams et al, 1977), it must first be absorbed before it can be excreted via the bile (or pancreatic juice). The content of [54]Mn in various segments of the small intestine, cecum or colon are quite similar after I.V. dosing, suggesting that excretion may occur over an extended area in the gut (Miller et al, 1973; Abrams et al, 1977). However, analyses on contents of the GI tract suggested that net secretion of Mn was primarily in the small intestine and cecum (Ivan and Grieve, 1976).

Mn absorption is also greatly affected by dietary levels. In one case feeding supplemental Mn (15 ppm in milk) reduced Mn

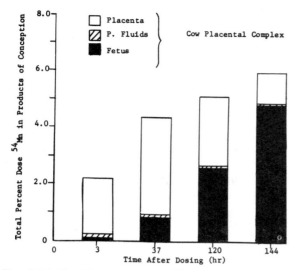

Fig. 5-21. Partition of retained ⁵⁴Mn in the placental complex of gravid heifers after 270 day gestation (Hansard, 1972).

retention from 18 to 2%. Supplemental Mn resulted in a 2 fold increase in liver Mn and a 30 fold increase in bile and increased the rate of turnover of liver ⁵⁴Mn (Carter et al, 1974). In other work with male goats, Anke et al (1972) recovered 33% of a ruminal dose of ⁵⁴Mn ammoniumphosphate in body tissues within 96 hr. The liver took up 44% of the dose and 35% was recovered in the skeleton. Lesser amounts were found in other tissues.

Absorption studies with pregnant sheep have demonstrated that 6% of absorbed ⁵⁴Mn was transferred to placental tissues, fluid and fetal tissues (Hansard et al, 1970). In pregnant cows comparable amounts were deposited in placental and fetal tissues (Fig. 5-21; Hansard, 1972). Reserves in the liver of new-born animals are low. However, supplementation results in a rapid and marked increase in liver Mn (Howes and Dyer, 1971). Odynets et al (1975) concluded that thyroidectomy did not affect Mn retention in sheep.

Interactions with Other Minerals

There are several indications that Ca and P are antagonistic to Mn in ruminants (Gallup et al, 1952; Hawkins et al, 1955; Wilson, 1966; Anke et al, 1973). Suttle and Field (1970) found that increasing dietary Ca from 1 to 2% increased fecal excretion of Mn but changes in dietary P were without effect. Fain et al (1952) suggest an antagonism with Mg. However, Lomba et al (1977) observed that K was the principal element which influenced utilization of Mn by increasing fecal losses. Other minerals were not a factor in this study.

Bremmer (1970) determined that soluble complexes of Zn and Mn occur in the rumen and lower regions of the small intestine. Soluble Mn in the abomasum, duodenum and upper jejunum appeared to exist in ionic form which was affected by pH. Odynets et al (1975) found that giving supplements of $CuSo_4$, $CoCl_2$, or KI resulted in reduced Mn retention. In a trial with cattle, supplemental Zn, Cu and Mn were fed alone or in combination (Ivan and Grieve, 1975). The trace minerals did not affect apparent digestibility but a negative Zn-Mn interaction in digestion of N and energy was observed. Supplementing with Mn increased organ content of Zn while the Cu content of liver was decreased by dietary Mn.

Mn Deficiency

Mn deficiency has been studied in a number of experimental situations with ruminants. Bentley and Phillips (1951) found that Mn-deficient heifers were slower to exhibit estrus and were slightly and consistently slower to conceive upon breeding. They noted that deficient animals had only about half as much Mn in the ovaries as adequately-fed animals. In addition to lower levels of Mn in organs such as liver and kidney, a variety of degenerative changes were seen in the liver of affected cows, including fatty infiltration, abscesses, and reduced bile volume. Anke et al (1973) also observed that Mn deficiency leads to a decreased Mn content in liver, hair, kidneys, spinal cord, ribs, heart, spleen and ovaries and reproductive problems were always seen when Mn content of the ovaries was low. Groppel and Anke (1971) also reported that deficient animals show no signs of estrus despite normal ovulation. Several services were required for conception. Hidiroglou et al (1978) confirmed with sheep that Mn deficiency results in more services per conception. They also observed that the ovarian cortical stroma of dairy cows with cystic ovaries had lower Mn contents than those cows that did not have cystic ovaries. In studies with goats on Mn-deficient diets, more inseminations were required for breeding and 23% of the does on a low Mn diet aborted in the 3rd-5th mo. of pregnancy. Of the kids born alive, a higher percentage were males (Anke and Groppel, 1970).

Severe Mn deficiency has a pronounced effect on the new-born animal. Rojas et al (1965) found that common symptoms in calves were deformities of the bones. Enlarged joints, stiffness, twisted legs and general physical weakness were observed

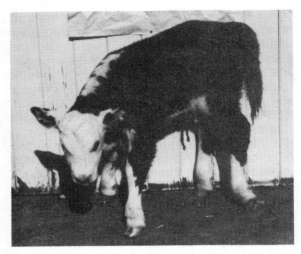

Fig. 5-22. Mn-deficient calf born to a cow receiving 15 ppm of dietary Mn. Typical symptoms noted included enlarged joints, "knuckled-over" pasterns, and twisted fore limbs. Courtesy of I.A. Dyer, Washington State Univ.

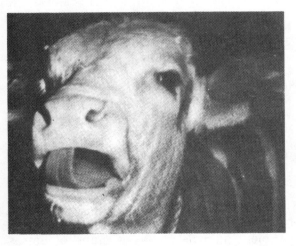

Fig. 5-23. A Mn-deficient calf. This peculiar action of the tongue is said to be one characteristic of deficient animals. Courtesy of Dr. A. Henning, Karl Marx Univ., Leipzig, G.D.R.

(Fig. 5-22). The deficient calves had shorter humeri and the breaking strength was reduced. Mn content of the tissues examined were also reduced to about 60% of controls and the alkaline phosphatase values of serum were reduced. Other similar findings have been reported by Groppel and Anke (1971) and Schellner (1975). Anke and Groppel (1970) produced deficiencies in calves fed milk and grain. The first symptom noted was a nervous tremor of the tongue (Fig. 5-23). Later, they observed a general ataxia and trembling of muscles. After 14

weeks changes in the tarsal joints were noted.

In studies with lambs symptoms seen included evidence of joint pains and poor locomotion (Lassiter and Morton, 1968). Lambs showed a peculiar disturbance of gait and reluctance to move voluntarily. When exercise was forced, movements were described as "rabbit hops." Tibias were shorter and had reduced breaking strength. Hennig et al (1972) reported signs of paralysis in young lambs and reduced rate of gain in both female and male lambs. Birth weights of Mn-deficient goats were lower than those of controls. In kids or lambs born to deficient mothers, Anke and Groppel (1970) observed that ca. 10% showed nervous disturbances as a first symptom, and, later, paralysis of hind limbs and ataxia generally followed. The paralysis was not reversible and led to death after variable time intervals. However, animals which were not paralyzed had no skeletal abnormalities. About 30% of the kids had bony excrescences (abnormal outgrowth) on the front tarsal joint which were visible in some by 6 weeks of age (Fig. 5-24). About 20% of the does showed similar symptoms. Theriez et al (1977) also reported reduced rate of gain in Mn-deficient lambs.

There are also several reports which indicate Mn deficiencies of cattle from field studies. For example, Grashuis et al (1953) described symptoms in cattle from the Netherlands that were believed to be deficient in Mn. Munro (1957) has also indicated that cattle in England may be deficient at times. He reported that cows showed low

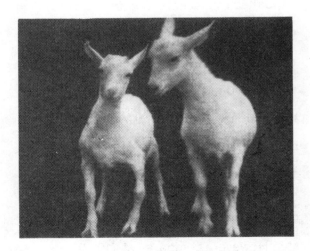

Fig. 5-24. Malformations of fore legs of a Mn deficient goat. Courtesy of Dr. A. Henning, Karl Marx Univ., Leipzig, G.D.R.

conception rates, there were weak joints in new-born calves and depraved appetites which were corrected by Mn supplementation. Wilson (1966) has also reported deficiencies in England; fertility was improved by feeding Mn. Krolak (1969) found that extra Mn significantly reduced the intervals between pregnancies of cows.

Mn Requirements

In studies with cows, Bentley and Phillips (1951) found that deficiency symptoms were produced on an intake of natural feedstuffs that contained <10 ppm of Mn they suggested that 20 ppm would be a satisfactory level. Rojas et al (1965) fed levels of 15.8, 16.9 and 25.1 ppm to beef cows. Deficiencies in calves were produced from cows on the two lower levels, thus indicating that the requirements under these conditions were >17 ppm. Howes and Dyer (1971) did not find any differences in growth of beef heifers fed 13 or 21 ppm of Mn and Hartmans (1974) fed identical twin cattle 16-21 ppm for 2.5-3.5 years without any evidence of a deficiency. However, Lomba et al (1975) suggested that the minimum requirements might be as low as 5 ppm for adult lactating cows to as high as 50 ppm for young fattening cattle.

In studies with goats, Schellner (1975) observed some deficiency symptoms in kids born to females that received 20 ppm of Mn and Anke and Groppel (1970) produced deficiencies in goats on 8 ppm of Mn. Hennig et al (1972) concluded that natural selection will result in animals (cattle and goats) which have lower requirements of Mn when the dietary Mn is low. With respect to lambs, data are not sufficient to quantitate the Mn requirement. Lassiter and Morton (1968) produced deficiency symptoms on a diet with 0.8 ppm and felt that the control diet (30 ppm) was adequate. Thus, it would appear that the requirements of ruminants are on the order of 20 ppm, although other dietary factors may alter this level.

Mn Excess

One of the earliest reports indicated that feeding of high levels of Mn (0-2,000 ppm) resulted in increased fecal excretion of both P and Ca, although plasma values were unaffected. When lower levels were fed (75-200 ppm), Fain et al (1952) found no effect on blood glucose, Ca, K or Fe but did indicate that 100 ppm depressed serum Mg. Hartman et al (1955) fed lambs levels up to 4,000 ppm. They reported that as low a level as 45 ppm resulted in a decrease in

concentration of hemoglobin and serum Fe. Higher levels decrease Fe in the liver, spleen and kidney. On the basis of liver and blood data they suggested that Mn decreased Fe absorption. Cunningham et al (1966) have fed up to 4,900 ppm to calves. Results were variable since gain was depressed in one experiment but not in another; the same comments apply to hemoglobin and other blood components. Robinson et al (1960) found that excess Mn (up to 1,000 ppm) had no effect on Ca or P retention by calves, but it decreased Fe absorption and fiber digestibility. Grace (1973) fed 250 and 500 mg of supplementary Mn/day as the sulfate to sheep consuming pastures with 140-200 ppm of Mn. Increasing the dietary Mn depressed growth rate. Liver Cu and Mn levels and plasma Mn levels were increased. In the case of water with high Mn levels (500 ppm), Weeth (1962) found no evidence of toxicity in cattle although serum alkaline phosphatase was higher and plasma and liver Fe were reduced. Neathery and Miller (1977) conclude that both sheep and cattle can tolerate 1,000 ppm or more.

Availability of Mn

Analytical data on feedstuffs generally indicate that most feeds have sufficient Mn (Adams, 1975), assuming that 20 ppm is accepted as a dietary requrement. In Canada, Miltimore et al (1970) found that only 40% of the samples were <40 ppm of Mn. Based on laboratory analyses in the eastern USA, Adams (1975) concludes that Mn is likely to be the least limiting of the various trace minerals.

With regard to supplemental sources, there is not enough information to evaluate efficiency of utilization. Watson et al (1969) did not detect any appreciable differences in utilization by lambs which were fed reagent grade $MnCO_3$ and $MnSO_4$ or feed grade MnO and $MnCO_3$.

NICKEL (Ni)

The presence of Ni in animal tissues and its in vitro biochemical functions have been known for years (Wacker and Vallee, 1959), but only recently has its essential physiological role in animals been established (Nielsen, 1974; Nielsen and Ollerich, 1974). Earlier work with Ni in ruminants concentrated on its excretion and tissue concentrations (O'Dell et al, 1970; 1971). Recent studies were conducted with lambs to establish whether Ni has an essential role in the ovine (Spears et al, 1977; 1978). For reviews on metabolism and role of Ni, see Miller (1973), Nielsen (1974), and Spears and Hatfield (1977).

Absorption, Excretion and Tissue Concentration

O'Dell et al (1971) measured excretion of Ni by calves fed natural rations supplemented with 62.5, 250 or 1000 ppm Ni as $NiCO_3$. If, as indicated by Ni content of individual ingredients, the basal ration contained about 1 ppm, Ni excretions as percentages of intake averaged 82% in feces and 2.4% in urine and were not affected by dietary Ni content. Spears et al (1978) measured ^{63}Ni excretion by lambs fed a basal semi-purified diet containing 65 ppb Ni with or without 5 ppm supplemental Ni as $NiCl_2$. Percentages of oral $^{63}NiCl_2$ doses excreted by lambs fed basal and Ni supplemented rations, respectively, averaged 74.4 and 64.7 in feces and 0.8 and 2.0 in urine. Whether measured as stable Ni of dietary origin or as ^{63}Ni from single oral doses, feces accounted for >97% of the total Ni excreted by ruminants. Since urine has been shown to be the primary route of excretion after intravenous injection (Smith and Hackley, 1968), these results indicate absorption of Ni is quite low.

O'Dell et al (1971) measured tissue Ni concentrations in 21-week-old Holstein calves which had been fed diets containing 1 to 1001 ppm Ni for 8 weeks. Ni was not detected in blood serum of calves fed 1 or 63.5 ppm and was only 0.25 μg/ml in plasma of those fed 251 ppm Ni. When 1001 ppm was fed, Ni content in serum was 12X greater than in calves fed 251 ppm. Tissue Ni contents were much higher in lung and kidney than in other tissues sampled. Few tissues from the 193 kg calves fed 63.5 ppm or less exceeded 2 μg Ni/g dry weight, a much lower concentration than the 12-38 μg/g fresh tissue found in 33 kg lambs fed 65 ppb or 5 ppm diets (Spears et al, 1978). Compared to stable Ni contents, ^{63}Ni concentrations were much lower in lung than in kidney tissue. High Ni concentrations in kidney may have been due to residual urine. Inhaled feed dust could account for much of the higher stable Ni in calf lung (O'Dell et al, 1971) since ^{63}Ni was given to lambs by gelatin capsule.

Ni content of milk was not measurably increased, even when cows were fed over 1800 mg of supplemental Ni daily (O'Dell et al, 1970). They found that when special precautions were taken to prevent contamination from handling equipment, normal cows milk contained <0.1 ppm Ni, the lower limit for reliable measurement.

Physiological Role

The specific physiological role(s) of Ni in the mammalian system is presently unclear (Spears and Hatfield, 1977). It can activate numerous enzymes but it has not been shown to be specifically required for the in vitro activation of any enzyme (Nielsen, 1974). Spears et al (1977) reported that ruminal urease activity was much lower when lambs were fed only 60 ppb rather than 5 ppm Ni. They concluded that the bacterial enzyme must be specific for Ni since all other known trace elements were supplied in the diet. Martinez and Church (1970) did not find any improvement in cellulose digestion when Ni was added to washed cell preparations. Even very low levels (0.5 ppm) were toxic.

Ni is also thought to contribute to membrane and nucleic acid metabolism or structure for several reasons. Purification of RNA preparations increases their Ni concentration by many times (Wacker and Vallee, 1959). Ni may stabilize the structure of RNA (Fuwa et al, 1960), DNA (Eichhorn, 1962) and ribosomes (Tal, 1968). Involvement of Ni with various hormones includes inhibition of insulin (Clay, 1975; Dormer et al, 1977) and prolactin release (La Bella et al, 1973) and stimulation of glucagon secretion (Horak and Sunderman, 1975). If physiological concentrations of Ni have similar effects in intact animals, these investigations suggest Ni may be involved in carbohydrate metabolism and lactation. Reduced serum alanine transaminase activity in lambs fed only 65 ppb Ni (Spears et al, 1978) also suggests Ni may contribute to gluconeogenesis since alanine is a major gluconeogenic substrate for ruminants (Brockman et al, 1975). Supplementation with Ni has partially alleviated changes associated with deficiencies of Zn (Spears et al, 1978) and Cu (Spears and Hatfield, 1977).

Nickel Deficiency

Ni deficiency has been produced and described in chicks (Nielsen and Ollerich, 1974; Nielsen et al, 1975), rats (Nielsen et al, 1975) and swine (Anke et al, 1974). Gross deficiency symptoms in these species included increased prenatal mortality, unthriftiness, decreased growth rate and several biochemical changes. Although visual symptoms were less obvious in lambs fed a diet containing only 60-65 ppb Ni, supplementation with 5 ppm Ni reduced urinary N and increased N retention, total serum proteins, serum alanine transaminase, and rumen bacterial urease (Spears et al, 1977, 1978). Minimum requirements of Ni have not been established for ruminants. There is presently no information to suggest that a deficiency would be a practical problem.

Nickel Toxicity

O'Dell et al (1970) supplemented the total rations of calves with 0, 62.5, 250 or 1000 ppm Ni as $NiCO_3$ for 8 weeks. Feed intake and growth rate were retarded slightly by 250 ppm and markedly by 1000 ppm (Fig. 5-25). The lower dietary levels of Ni had little effect on Ni levels in several tissues but Ni concentration increased somewhat with 250 ppm and sharply when 1000 ppm was fed (O'Dell et al, 1971). Miller (1973) suggested a homeostatic control mechanism for Ni in ruminants may break down differentially in different tissues with increasing Ni intake. Feeding lactating cows over 1800 mg Ni as $NiCO_3$ per cow daily did not significantly affect milk production, milk composition, animal health or feed consumption (O'Dell et al, 1970). In a cafeteria experiment with heifers (O'Dell et al, 1970) ration palatability was definitely reduced by 100 ppm Ni as the chloride or 500 ppm as the carbonate but not by one-half of these amounts. Nickel is relatively non-toxic to ruminants, probably because of its very low absorption and tissue deposition (Miller, 1973).

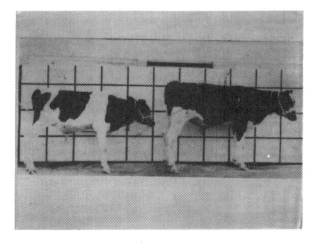

Fig. 5-25. Maintained on normal rations to 12 wks of age. Calf on right served as control and calf on left received 1000 ppm nickel daily for 8 weeks (O'Dell et al, 1970).

SELENIUM (Se)

Until 1957 the only nutritional significance for Se was thought to be related to its toxicity. However, within the last two decades attention has been focused primarily upon its nutritional value as an essential element. There are many publications dealing with Se in the nutrition of ruminant animals, as indicated by the book edited by Muth et al (1967), the NRC report by Oldfield et al (1971), and some review articles by Ammerman and Miller (1975), Andrews et al (1968), and Jenkins and Hidiroglou (1972). For excellent sources of information on many different aspects of Se, the book by Rosenfeld and Beath (1964) or the NAS monograph (1976) are recommended.

Tissue Distribution

The tissue distribution in sheep of physiological doses of ^{75}Se has been reported from a number of laboratories (Cousins and Cairney, 1961; Wright, 1965; Paulson et al, 1966; Ehlig et al, 1967; Ewan et al, 1968; Hidiroglou et al, 1968; Lopez et al, 1969; and Handrick and Godwin, 1970). In general, these reports show the kidney to have the highest concentration of Se followed by the liver and other glandular tissues such as spleen and pancreas. Intestinal and lung tissues can be relatively high. Cardiac muscle contains appreciably more than skeletal muscle. Wool and hair may be relatively high but nervous tissue is low. Some typical values reported by Handrick and Godwin (1970) are shown (ppm wet weight); kidney cortex, 1.38-1.46; liver, 0.48-0.97; cardiac muscle, 0.15-0.20; skeletal muscle, 0.04-0.06; pancreas, 0.34-0.44; ovary, 0.19-0.25; cerebrum, 0.07-0.09; and wool, 0.21-0.49.

Blood levels of Se are quite variable, depending upon dietary intake and possibly other factors as well. Typical values for sheep of an adequate Se status may be in the range of 0.1 to 0.2 ppm. Some data indicate that a large part of blood Se is associated with globulins and a lesser amount with albumins (Handrick and Godwin, 1970). Se is also taken up slowly by the red blood cells (Wright, 1967). The majority of the Se in red cells is associated with the selenoenzyme, glutathione peroxidase (GSH-Px; Oh et al, 1974).

Some of the variation in the reported values for tissue Se concentration could be due to the chemical form of this element in the diet. Ullrey et al (1977) found the tissue

Table 5-6. Effect of natural and inorganic dietary Se on tissue content of Se in lambs and steers.[a]

Item	Michigan Diets		South Dakota diets	
	1	2	1	2
Natural Se	85	85	200	200
Selenite Se	100	200	---	100
Muscle				
Sheep	92	110	167	160
Cattle	86	100	135	136
Liver				
Sheep	380	533	618	656
Cattle	384	435	498	500
Kidney				
Sheep	1261	1223	1300	1351
Cattle	1372	1366	1458	1578

[a] From Ullrey et al (1977); all Se values are given on ppb basis.

Se content to be higher when lambs or steers were fed diets with natural Se (corn grown in S. Dakota) than when the same level of Se was supplied in low Se diets (feed ingredients grown in Michigan) as sodium selenite (Table 5-6). However, the Se concentration even in organs from animals fed the natural Se sources did not reach very high levels. Furthermore, injections of commercial vitamin E and Se preparations in lambs and calves have been shown to moderately increase (up to 5-fold) the liver and kidney levels 1 to 14 days afterwards, but returned to near baseline values 30 days later (Van Vleet, 1975). These injections had no effect upon the muscle Se concentrations at any time after injection.

Metabolic Functions of Se

Even though the first evidence for Se essentiality was presented in 1957, it was 16 years later before its metabolic function was established. Rotruck et al (1973) presented the first evidence that GSH-Px was a seleno-enzyme using rats and sheep. Subsequent work by Oh et al (1974), who purified GSH-Px from ovine erythrocytes, revealed the presence of 4 g atoms of Se per mole enzyme with a molecular weight of about 90,000. The enzyme can be broken down into 4 apparently identical subunits, presumably one Se atom per subunit. Thus, one of the metabolic functions of Se is in GSH-Px, in which it acts to destroy damaging peroxides that accumulate in tissues. Some work by other investigators with lambs indicate that Se is necessary for the formation of a low molecular weight protein, but its metabolic function has not been identified (Black et al, 1978).

Since Se is required for the activity of GSH-Px, various investigators have determined the correlation of tissue GSH-Px activity and Se content. As shown in tables 5-7 and 5-8, there is a correlation between tissue GSH-Px activity and Se content. However, tissues respond differently to various levels of dietary Se, and this response is dependent upon the type of diet fed. For example, GSH-Px activity was almost undetectable in liver of lambs fed the basal artificial milk diet (Table 5-7), but this activity was present in liver of lambs from ewes fed the practical basal diet (0.02 ppm

Table 5-7. Effect of dietary Se on glutathione peroxidase activity and Se content in tissues of lambs fed an artificial milk.[a]

Tissue	Basal Diet		+ 0.05 ppm Se		+ 0.50 ppm Se	
	GSH-Px[b]	Se[c]	GSH-Px[b]	Se[c]	GSH-Px[b]	Se[c]
Heart	130	40	295	90	1240	256
Lung	289	45	815	99	1870	220
Kidney	298	233	1270	436	2380	1015
Liver	4	49	83	104	344	557
Pancreas	37	54	140	88	935	247
Muscle	14	21	38	31	148	80
Testis	658	125	648	176	1070	246

[a] Data of Oh et al (1976). The basal diet was shown by analysis to Contain 10 ppb Se.

[b] Activity is expressed as described by Rotruck et al (1973).

[c] Concentration is expressed as ppb.

Table 5-8. Effect of dietary Se on glutathione peroxidase activity and Se content in tissues of lambs fed a practical type diet.[a]

Dietary Se	Muscle		Heart		Liver	
	GSH-Px[b]	Se[c]	GSH-Px[b]	Se[c]	GSH-Px[b]	Se[c]
Basal (0.02 ppm Se)	28	23	70	37	126	49
0.05 ppm Se	46	34	258	72	139	95
0.07 ppm Se	66	36	410	80	190	96
0.09 ppm Se	64	42	682	126	138	152
0.12 ppm Se	132	55	1100	190	204	181
0.52 ppm Se	225	97	1450	257	427	575

[a] Data of Oh et al (1976).

[b] GSH-Px activity is expressed as indicated by Rotruck et al (1973).

[c] Concentration is expressed as ppb.

Se) at higher concentration (Table 5-8) than in even those given 0.05 Se in the artificial milk. The GSH-Px activity in tissues like the lungs, kidney and testis was almost as high in the deficient lambs as this activity in the liver of lambs given 0.5 ppm Se (Table 5-7). Thus, GSH-Px activity in liver appears to be the most sensitive to the Se status of the animal.

A highly significant correlation between erythrocyte GSH-Px and Se concentration in whole blood has been reported for sheep (r = 0.94, Oh et al, 1976; r = 0.92, Thompson et al, 1976; and r = 0.87, Whanger et al, 1977) and cattle (r = 0.91, 1975; r = 0.60, Thompson et al, 1976; and r = 0.78, Hoffman et al, 1978). Thus, it appears that the Se status of ruminants can be estimated by the erythrocyte GSH-Px activity. A simple test for GSH-Px activity has been described by Board and Peter (1976) for field studies. The activity of GSH-Px has been linked to the oxidation of NADPH via a coupled enzyme procedure, using the fluorescent spot procedure. Defluorescence occurs within 5 min with blood from a Se-treated animal, but fluorescence is still present after 60 min in blood from Se-deficient animals.

Metabolism of Se

Absorption and Excretion. Wright and Bell (1966), using chromic oxide as a marker and ^{75}Se, found very little absorption of Se in the abomasum but considerable absorption occurred in the small intestine. Wright (1965) demonstrated that a substantial amount of absorption occurred between the duodenum and ileum and between the ileum and cecum. Se concentrations in relation to markers or other compartments of the GI tract (Wright, 1965; Wright and Bell, 1966) indicate that some excretion occurs via bile since an increase of Se was observed in digesta between the abomasum and duodenum. Jacobsson and Oksanen (1967) concluded that about 50% of Se excreted via the feces entered the GI tract via the bile.

The route of excretion (urine or feces) of Se given in various forms and when administered via different routes (oral, I.V., sub-Q) has been studied in several laboratories. In general, data indicate that oral administration will result in the bulk of Se being excreted via feces (Butler and Peterson, 1961; Peterson and Spedding, 1963; Paulson et al, 1966; Wright and Bell, 1966; and Lopez et al, 1969), which is in contrast to monogastric animals in which urine is the main excretory route. There is an age effect also, since Ewan et al (1968) observed that ^{75}Se given as the selenate was recovered to the extent of 66-75% in urine and 34-25% in feces in young lambs (8-10 wk of age) fed a synthetic liquid diet. Data on older animals (Cousins and Cairney, 1961; Paulson et al, 1966; Wright and Bell, 1966) show that lesser amounts are excreted in urine than via feces when given single doses of Se. A continual dose provided by dense pellets containing elemental Se (given intraruminally) was shown to result in 0.8% recovered via respiratory gases, 41% in urine and 58% in feces (Handrick and Godwin, 1970).

Doses administered I.V. or sub-Q are generally excreted to a greater extent in urine than is the case for oral doses. For example, Wright (1965) found that 12% of an I.V. was recovered in urine and 10% in feces.

Wright and Bell (1966) recovered 4.5% in feces and 29% in urine from an I.V. dose and 66% in feces and 4.5% in urine after an oral dose. Other workers (Jacobsson and Oksanen, 1967) found that I.V. and sub-Q doses were excreted primarily via urine, whereas intraruminal doses were excreted to a greater extent in feces. When sheep were fed red clover grown with ^{75}Se, 53% of the radioactivity was recovered in the feces but only 2% of this in the urine. (Peterson and Spedding, 1963).

When Se was given orally as Se-methionine or Na-selenite, Ehlig et al (1967) found that fecal excretion was comparable in animals given these compounds but urinary excretion was reduced in those animals given the Se-methionine. Se given as Se-methionine or Se-cysteine resulted in higher levels in the pancreas of sheep than when given as selenite. In other work by these investigators the administration of seleno-amino acids to pregnant ewes resulted in comparable levels of radioactivity in the tissues of the ewes and their lambs; however, when Na-selenite was given, placental transfer was less, resulting in about half as much radioactivity in the tissues of the lambs as in the ewes.

Peak excretion of Se has been reported to occur within 2-3 days after administration of the dose (Wright, 1965; Jacobsson and Oksanen, 1967; Muth et al, 1967; Paulson et al, 1968; Hidiroglou et al, 1968). The size of the dose as well as the Se status of the animal also influence the speed of excretion and the relative amounts that may be excreted via urine (Jacobsson and Oksanen, 1967; Lopez et al, 1969; Kincaid et al, 1977). In both lambs (Lopez et al, 1969) and calves (Kincaid et al, 1977) the retention of Se was found to be inversely related to the dietary intakes of this element.

Se Metabolism by Rumen Microbes. The low net absorption of Se by ruminants observed by several investigators (Cousins and Cairney, 1961; Wright and Bell, 1966; Peterson and Spedding, 1963) is apparently due to the rumen microbes. Up to 40% of the Se is converted to insoluble Se when rumen microbes are incubated with selenite in vitro (Whanger et al, 1968). The chemical form apparently affects this since less of the Se was converted to insoluble Se when the source was selenomethionine. Even though Se is converted to insoluble forms, the Se content of rumen microbes in sheep fed various diets was found to average about

46-fold its dietary level on a dry matter basis, about 11-fold on a N basis, or 26-fold on a S basis (Whanger et al, 1978). If Se-deficient lambs survive to become ruminants, their chances of recovery are improved (Whanger et al, 1970). Thus, one of the reasons for this apparent spontaneous recovery could be the accumulation of Se in the rumen microbes, but there is no information on the availability of Se incorporated into the cells of the rumen microbes.

With respect to Se excretion in the feces, published data indicate that most of it is present in forms which are insoluble in water or organic solvents (Cousins and Cairney, 1961; Butler and Peterson, 1961; Peterson and Spedding, 1963). Most of the Se is apparently present in an inorganic state (Cousins and Cairney, 1961; Peterson and Spedding, 1963). The poor availability of Se in the feces was demonstrated with 3 pasture species of plants by growing them for 75 days in the presence of ^{75}Se in feces; less than 0.3% of the added radioactivity was recovered in the herbage (Peterson and Spedding, 1963). Greater uptake of ^{75}Se in calves fed milk than those given a concentrate supplement was demonstrated by Hidiroglou et al (1969), providing further evidence for the influence of rumen microbes on Se metabolism. The concentrate supplement promotes the propagation of rumen microbes. Thus, ruminant animals could contribute to a loss of this element to the Se cycle, and may explain why Se deficiency is becoming a problem in heavily grazed areas of the USA where no known deficiency problems had been encountered in the past.

Experimental results show that rumen microbes are capable of incorporating Se into seleno-amino acids (Hidiroglou et al, 1968; Paulson et al, 1968), but the latter investigators indicated that incorporation of selenomethionine into microbial protein resulted in a more firmly bound product than when selenite or selenate were the sources of Se. Hidiroglou et al (1968) found the incorporation of ^{75}Se into the rumen microbes to be inversely proportional to the previous dietary intake of Se by the host animal, indicating a dietary factor which affects Se incorporation into these microbes. Se can also affect the metabolism of rumen microbes. With sheep fed purified diets, Se or vitamin E treatments were found to affect the volatile fatty acid content in rumen fluid (Hidiroglou and Lessard, 1976). In addition, some evidence is available to indicate that Se increases the synthesis of rumen bacterial protein, as indicated by increased S incorporation in sheep fed purified diets (Hidiroglou and Zarkadas, 1976).

Effect of Vitamin E on Se Retention. Conflicting data are available on the influence of vitamin E on Se retention. Ewan et al (1968) found lambs to excrete oral ^{75}Se more rapidly when supplemented with vitamin E than when not given this vitamin. In contrast, Wright and Bell (1964) presented data which indicated that vitamin E to improved retention of Se by lambs given a low-Se purified diet. However, Buchanan-Smith et al (1971) reported vitamin E administration had no consistent effect on tissue Se levels in sheep fed purified diets.

In the reverse situation Boyazogu et al (1967) found ewes which were treated with Se to have depressed serum vitamin E levels, and suggested this indicated a sparing effect of Se on tissue vitamin E. This is consistent with data of Hogue and Aydin (1972), who showed that as the dietary Se level increased a decreased level of vitamin E was found in the plasma, with an increased deposition in tissues such as skeletal muscle, pancreas and kidney. They suggested that Se was involved in tocopherol transport from blood to certain tissues. In contrast, Hidiroglou et al (1969) found very little effect of Se on tocopherol metabolism. Perhaps the reasons for some of these differences could be due to the route of administration, the relative amounts of Se and vitamin E given, the diets fed the animals, and the age of experimental animals.

Effect of S on Se Retention. Although S has been implicated in the production of white muscle disease, the literature is not consistent regarding its effect on Se utilization. Paulson et al (1966) found little difference in the Se uptake by tissues when lactating ewes fed rations of either 0.28 or 0.62% were dosed intraruminally with ^{75}Se-selenate. However, there appeared to be a greater uptake of ^{75}Se by the small intestine in sheep fed the high S diet. When dosed intraruminally with ^{75}Se, Pope et al (1968) found that wethers fed a low-S diet (0.05%) maintained higher blood Se and excreted less Se in urine than animals fed higher levels of S (up to 0.20%). This is consistent with work by White and Somers (1977), who showed that sheep fed a low-S diet (0.07% S) had significantly higher plasma and wool levels of Se when given selenomethionine. In the reverse situation the Se status of sheep was found to have no significant effect on

the distribution of ^{35}S in blood and tissues of animals dosed with ^{35}S-methionine (Hidiroglou and Zakardas, 1976). Although no information was given on Se, Boyazoglu et al (1967) reported high level of S to have a depressing effect on blood vitamin E in ewes, which may be the result of the influence of S on Se metabolism.

Selenium Deficiency

Ruminant species, as well as other domestic livestock, are affected with a condition known as nutritional muscular dystrophy (i.e., white muscle disease, stiff lamb disease). This condition, which has been known for more than two decades, is at least partially due to a deficiency of Se in the diet. However, there are other complicating factors that will be mentioned in subsequent sections.

White muscle disease (WMD) occurs in many different areas of the world, occasionally causing very severe losses in young animals. Occurrence has frequently been related to consumption of hay or forage produced in irrigated areas or where rainfall is relatively high. The incidence is sporadic; outbreaks may be very severe in a given year but of little consequence the next. It has occurred on many different soil types, but is probably more prevalent on soils of volcanic origin. Reviews on the symptoms and occurrence of WMD that might be of interest to the reader would include those of Muth (1955, 1963), Oldfield et al (1971), or Underwood (1977).

Clinical Symptoms. WMD is characterized by a degeneration of the striated skeletal and cardiac muscles. In skeletal muscle there is a bilaterally symmetrical distribution of the lesions. Skeletal muscles most affected include those involved with movements of the legs and neck (Muth, 1955). In very severe cases the muscle is bleached to the point where it is almost white (see Fig. 5-26). The right ventricle of the heart is usually the most severely affected part.

The result of degeneration of the muscle is stiffness and difficulty in locomotion. Animals tend to carry their rear feet farther forward than normal and the front feet farther back than normal (see Fig. 5-27, 28). In general, lambs tend to show more severe skeletal damage, whereas calves show more cardiac involvement (Muth, 1963). WMD occurs primarily in the young animal. In field studies WMD is said to often occur in lambs of 3-4 weeks of age and in calves at 4-6 weeks of age. WMD may also occur in older

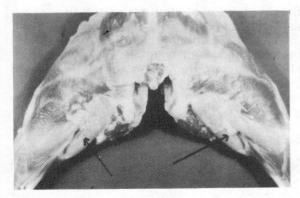

Fig. 5-26. Rear quarters of a lamb carcass showing the marked bleaching of normal myoglobin color of some of the muscles that occurs in WMD. The arrows point to severely affected muscles. Courtesy of O.H. Murth, Oregon State Univ.

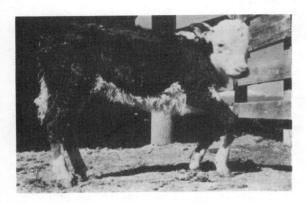

Fig. 5-27. A calf with WMD which occurred on a ranch in central Oregon. Note the marked dystrophy of muscles of the forelegs. Courtesy of O.H. Muth, Oregon State Univ.

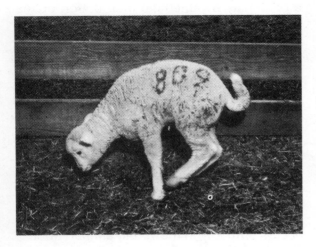

Fig. 5-28. A lamb with WMD which was produced under experimental conditions. Courtesy of O.H. Muth, Oregon State Univ.

sheep, weaned lambs and wethers up to several months of age. WMD may occasionally occur in pregnant and lactating ewes but it is rare in adult cows (Andrews et al, 1968). The muscle lesions that are produced apparently vary in different situations since some reports indicate a high incidence of mineralization yet others do not (Muth, 1963). For example, Schubert et al (1961) found that affected muscles had greatly elevated levels of Ca, P and Na and moderate increases in Mg (see Table 5-9). Others have indicated little or no mineralization (Hartley and Grant, 1961). This may be an indication of the severity of the condition. An example of the high degree of calcification that may occur is shown in Figure 5-29.

Table 5-9. Effect of WMD in lambs on mineral composition of skeletal muscle.[a]

Mineral[b]	Adequate diet	Deficient diet[c]
Ca	25	25-4772
P	574	558-2391
Mg	123	93-332
Na	371	360-1237
K	1800	464-1773

[a] From Schubert et al (1961)
[b] Mg/100 g of fat-free dry matter
[c] Values shown are ranges in concentration

Some biochemical changes reported include marked increases in plasma glutamic-oxaloacetic transaminase (GOT), creatine phosphokinase (CPK), and lactic dehydrogenase (LDH) in WMD lambs (Pauson, 1966; Whanger et al, 1969; 1976). CPK activities, however, appear to be the most reliable as far as assessing muscle damage in WMD lambs (Whanger et al, 1976). Increases of the free activities of the lysosomal enzymes (Buchanan-Smith et al, 1969; Whanger et al, 1970) and collagenase activity (Broderius et al, 1973) have been observed in muscle of WMD lambs. Presumably, this is one of the reasons for degeneration of the muscle. Other biochemical changes include a significant decrease of total and protein sulfhydryl groups and a significant increase of non-protein sulfhydryl groups and reduced glutathione content in muscle of WMD lambs as compared to normals (Broderius et al, 1973). In addition, lower respiratory rates of mitochondria from WMD lambs have been observed by Godwin et al (1974), and

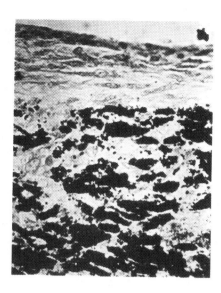

Fig. 5-29. A microsection of cardiac muscle from a lamb with severe WMD. The black areas are stained with silver nitrate to show Ca deposits. Courtesy of O.H. Muth, Oregon State Univ.

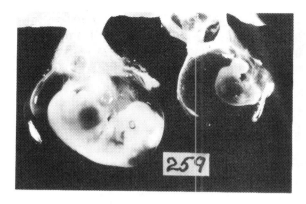

Fig. 5-30. Embryos from sheep. The one on the right is from a ewe which was deficient in Se and was obtained 3 weeks after breeding. Note that resorption is taking place. The embryo on the left is a normal one. Courtesy of W.J. Hartley, Univ. of Sidney.

changes in the free plasma amino acid levels in WMD lambs have been reported (Whanger et al, 1972).

Reports from some laboratories indicate that Se-deficient lambs or calves may have depressed growth and that Se supplementation will improve gain (Oldfield et al, 1960; Hartley and Grant, 1961; and McDonald, 1975). However, Se deficiency does not always result in decreased growth rates (Whanger et al, 1972). Some evidence is available to indicate that persistent diarrhea in older animals may be due to Se deficiency, since Se treatments have been reported to clear up some cases of this disorder (Hartley and Grant, 1961). Also, wool production has been reported to be greater (up to 39%) in Se-supplemented than Se-deficient sheep (Hartley and Grant, 1961; McDonald, 1975).

Se and Reproduction. Most of the work on Se and reproduction has been done with the female. The New Zealand workers have reported that Se deficiency lowers reproductive performances (Hartley and Grant, 1961; Scales, 1974). However, this has not been observed in studies in the USA or Canada (Mitchell et al, 1975). Hartley and Grant (1961) indicated that a high incidence of open ewes occurred on some ranches and Se supplementation returned the incidence of infertile animals to normal. An example of an embryo from a Se-deficient ewe is shown in Figure 5-30. In contrast, Mitchell et al (1975) found no adverse effects on ewe conception rates, embryonic mortality or numbers of lambs born as the result of Se deficiency, results which are consistent with work at Oregon State University (Oldfield, 1971). With use of purified diets, Buchanan-Smith et al (1969) found that vitamin E improved conception and birth rates more than Se alone in ewes fed purified diets, but satisfactory reproductive performance was obtained only in ewes treated with both vitamin E and Se.

Various workers have demonstrated placental transmission of Se in ruminants but the amount is dependent upon the chemical form of Se. Wright and Bell (1964) injected pregnant ewes with ^{75}Se-selenite and showed that the distribution of ^{75}Se in fetal tissues was similar to that in maternal tissues. However, ^{75}Se content in the single fetus was twice that of twins. Jacobsson and Oksanen (1967) injected ewes during late gestation with either ^{75}Se-selenite, ^{75}Se-selenocystine, or ^{75}Se-selenomethionine, and found the two organic forms of Se to be more easily transferred across the placenta than ^{75}Se-selenite. The serum Se levels in calves from cows fed Se in the diet was higher at birth than those from unsupplemented cows (Perry et al, 1978), demonstrating placental transfer in cattle.

Some evidence is available to indicate that retained placenta may be due to Se deficiency. Trinder et al (1973) found that the injection of both vitamin E and Se in cows one month before the estimated calving date reduced the incidence of retained placenta from 39-47% to 2-4%, but injection of Se alone was slightly less effective (reduced to 10-12%). However, Julien et al (1976) found the overall incidence of retained placenta to be reduced by Se administration from 38% to 0% in a controlled study, and this effect was achieved regardless of whether vitamin E was supplemented as well. In a field study with herds with chronic problems of retained placenta, Se and vitamin E administration reduced the incidence from an average of 51% in control cows to an average of 8%. Other workers (Oh, 1972; Swanson, 1978) found very little effect of Se on retained placenta when the incidence of this disorder was low (10 to 18%). Thus, it appears that Se may reduce the incidence of retained placenta when this disorder is abnormally high, but not when it is relatively low.

Se in Milk. Se has been shown to be secreted in the milk of sheep (Jacobsson et al, 1965; Gardner and Hogue, 1967; Godwin et al, 1971) and cows (Bengtsson et al, 1974). The excretion of ^{75}Se in milk was markedly higher when ^{75}Se-selenomethionine was administered to ewes than when ^{75}Se-selenite was given (Jacobsson et al, 1965), demonstrating an influence of the chemical form of Se on secretion. When ^{75}Se-selenite was given to lactating ewes, Godwin et al (1971) presented evidence that it was incorporated into milk proteins as seleno-methionine as well as other selenoamino acid-like fractions which were not identified.

The Se content of casein from milk of cows was shown to drop off from 210 ppb to 30-50 ppb after they were changed to a Se-deficient diet (Bengtsson et al, 1974). When this Se deficient casein was fed as the source of protein in diets for pigs, they died of liver necrosis, a Se deficiency sign. Thus, milk can be a source of Se to the suckling animals in addition to that received during fetal development.

Se-Vitamin E Interrelationships in WMD. Early research with young ruminants showed that WMD could be produced by feeding diets that were low in vitamin E and high in unsaturated fatty acids. This type of WMD is responsive to dietary vitamin E, but not to Se (Kutter and Marble, 1960). Many of the research papers dealing with WMD indicate that it is more apt to occur on diets that are low in both Se and vitamin E, although some of the papers do not give information on both of these nutrients. On the basis of data published on ruminants and on monogastric species (see Oldfield et al, 1971), it can be assumed that Se and vitamin E have a sparing effect on one another. A proposed metabolic interrelationship of vitamin E and

Se has been presented by Hoekstra (1975). He proposes that Se, as GSH-Px, guards against oxidative damage to the cell membranes by converting organic hydroperoxides to the less harmful alcohols, whereas vitamin E functions to protect against oxidant damage to membranes by preventing the formation of these organic hydroperoxides. Thus, since both of these nutrients affect a common intermediate, the physiological effects would appear identical.

Some of the initial work at Oregon State University indicated that Se was highly effective in the prevention of WMD but vitamin E was not (Muth et al, 1958). However, these results appear to be due to the use of a vitamin E preparation which was not available to the animal since preparations of readily available vitamin E are highly effective in the prevention of WMD in lambs from ewes injected with this vitamin during pregnancy (Whanger et al, 1976). Other work had shown vitamin E to be effective in the prevention of WMD when administered directly to the lamb (Oldfield et al, 1960; Hogue et al, 1962; and Hopkins et al, 1964).

Information from the Wisconsin (Hopkins et al, 1964; Ewan et al, 1968; Paulson et al, 1966), Oklahoma (Buchanan-Smith et al, 1969), and Oregon experiment stations (Whanger et al, 1977) with sheep or lambs fed purified diets indicates that a combination of vitamin E and Se is more effective in prevention of WMD than either nutrient given alone. For example, Hopkins et al (1964) found that Se supplementation prevented clinical signs of WMD but serum GOT values became elevated and red blood cells became susceptible to hemolysis when lambs were fed a synthetic milk. The muscles showed microscopic lesions of WMD upon autopsy, suggesting that Se moderated the course of this disorder. Vitamin E alone or with Se was found to restore LDH, GOT or CPK activities to normal levels, whereas Se alone only had a transient effect on their activities (Paulson et al, 1966; Buchanan-Smith, 1969; Whanger et al, 1977). Very few data are available on cattle, but there is no reason to suspect that this is not also true for these animals. In support of this the supplementation of cattle with both Se and vitamin E was found to be more effective than with either one alone (Jenkins and Hidiroglou, 1972). Thus, this may be one of the reasons researchers do not always agree on the response of Se because they have not also taken into consideration the vitamin E status of animals. In support of this, the Se requirement of chicks and rats have been shown to be dependent upon the vitamin E content of the diet.

Se-S Interrelationships in WMD. Although there are a number of fairly well known interrelationships between Se and S in monogastric species, information on ruminant species is less well defined. Some work reported from Oregon by Schubert et al (1961) hinted that fertilization of forages with gypsum might result in more WMD in sheep. Hintz and Hogue (1964) found that S added at a level of 0.33% of the diet resulted in an increased incidence of clinical WMD. Boyazoglu et al (1967) found some suggestions that supplementary S resulted in pathological tissue changes similar to those seen in WMD. Whanger et al (1969) reported data to indicate that S supplementation (K sulfate or methionine) resulted in a delay of the development of WMD as indicated by plasma activities of LDH, GOT or malic dehydrogenase. They concluded that the S and Se interaction was at the plant-soil level and not at the plant-animal level. This is consistent with the report of Allaway and Hodgson (1964), who were unable to demonstrate a consistent effect of increased S content of forages in contributing to WMD in livestock. Sulfate supplementation, but not methionine, did increase cardiac calcification significantly in WMD lambs (Whanger et al, 1969) which was shown in later work to be prevented by Se (Whanger et al, 1970).

Effect of Other Nutritional Factors. Hogue et al (1962) found that cooking a basal dystrogenic diet (kidney beans) decreased the incidence of WMD, implicating a heat-labile factor in the diet. Similar observations have been made by Tripp et al (1979) with alfalfa hay. The incidence of WMD was reduced when low-Se autoclaved hay was fed in comparison to untreated hay. The incidence of WMD has been found to be consistently higher when legume hay was fed than when non-legumeous hay was fed, even though the Se content was the same (Whanger et al, 1972). Interestingly, the vitamin E content of the legume hay was found to be higher than grass hay. This effect of forage types has also been observed with beef calves (Hidiroglou et al, 1968). Even though the Se content was deficient in all diets, no cases of WMD were observed in calves from cows fed either alfalfa-timothy hay or grass-legume silage. Furthermore, Cartan and Swingle (1959) found a succinoxidase inhibitor in dystrogenic feeds; its action could be reversed by vitamin E. In addition, exercise will appar-

ently influence the development of WMD (Godwin, 1972). Thus, a number of factors must be taken into consideration in addition to the dietary levels of vitamin E and Se.

There are some reports that other trace minerals may be associated with Se as related to WMD. Blaxter (1963) concluded that there was no indication of a synergism between Se and Co in Scotland which is in contrast to Andrews et al (1964) in New Zealand. The latter investigators reported a greater accumulation of Se in the kidneys of Co-deficient sheep. In the reverse situation, Wise et al (1968) reported no difference in the Co levels in sheep tissues due to Se intake, but did observe a lower Co level in kidney of WMD lambs. In other work Cu administration was found to increase live weight, fleece weight, and incidence of twinning only in Se-treated sheep (Hill et al, 1969), suggesting an interaction of Cu and Se, but these investigators found no clinical signs of either Se or Cu deficiency in their untreated sheep. In contrast, Canadian workers (Hidiroglou and Jenkins, 1975) found no evidence for an interaction of Se and Cu with beef cattle, suggesting that other dietary factors must be considered.

Selenium Requirement

The NRC recommended dietary Se requirement for ruminants is 0.1 ppm, but sufficient data are available to indicate that this level does not meet requirements under all dietary regimes. Early experimental data (Kuttler and Marble, 1960; Schubert et al, 1961) and field observations in the Western USA or in Canada (Jenkins and Hidiroglou, 1972) have indicated that WMD occurs on natural rations which have <0.1 ppm Se. A level of 0.1 ppm Se in the diet for ewes and cows was indicated in these early reports to prevent the development of WMD in the young. However, results from other areas of the USA were not consistent with these findings. For example, Shirley et al (1966) found the Se content of various forages in Florida to range between 0.02 to 0.06 ppm, yet supplementation with Se of either lambs or cattle resulted in no improvement and no evidence of WMD was found. In contrast, the work from New York (Hogue et al, 1962) in which the rations were based on mixed hay and raw cull kidney beans, 1 ppm Se in the ewe's diet was not completely adequate for protection. Subsequently, it was reported from this station that 0.17 ppm Se in the diet of ewes during lactation reduced the high GOT values in lambs but there were a significant number of lambs affected with WMD (Hintz and Hogue, 1964). However, recent data from Wisconsin indicated the Se requirement of reproducing ewes and their lambs fed a practical type diet (legume-grass silage plus hay and corn pellets) to be approximately 0.12 ppm (Oh et al, 1976).

The incidence of WMD has been observed to be greater when legumes are fed as compared to non-leguminous forages (Muth 1963; Whanger et al, 1972). A level of 0.1 ppm Se appears to be sufficient to protect against WMD when grass hay is fed (Whanger et al, 1972). However, recent results from Oregon indicate that the requirement of Se is greater than 0.1 ppm when legume hay is fed (Whanger et al, 1978). In fact, 0.2 ppm Se in this diet did not completely prevent the elevation of some of the indicator enzymes of WMD, and the Se requirement for sheep was suggested to be raised to at least 0.2 ppm Se when legume forages are fed. Furthermore, hay grown on a certain ranch in Oregon appeared to contain some antagonistic factors against Se, thus raising the amount of Se required to prevent WMD (Tripp et al, 1979). These studies are consistent with the Washington studies where evidence was obtained indicating that the Se requirements for pregnant cows are above the NRC recommended level of 0.1 ppm (Moramarco et al, 1977). In contrast, Perry et al (1976) presented evidence that the addition of 0.1 ppm Se to a basal diet containing 0.08 ppm Se met the requirements of beef cattle. Thus, from this discussion it is evident that the Se requirements are influenced markedly by the diet. It seems unlikely that the dietary level of vitamin E is the primary difference (see section on interrelationships). Further research will be required to determine what other modifying factors (S, trace minerals, organic compounds, inhibitors, etc.) change the Se requirements.

Methods of Se Administration

Since ruminants are not usually raised under confined conditions like monogastric animals, the supplementation of Se for these animals is more difficult. To evaluate Se in a fertilizer, this element was applied with a liquid fertilizer and the harvested alfalfa hay fed to pregnant ewes (Allaway et al, 1966). Protection of lambs against WMD from feeding this hay to their dams was evident. However, it was estimated that less than 2% of the Se applied to the soil was taken up by the alfalfa over a 2-year period of time. Therefore, it was concluded that application of Se to soil is an inefficient method in terms of the amount of Se required to meet the Se requirement of animals.

Various means have been studied for giving Se to ruminants. These include inclusion in salt, injections, implantation, with the drench, or as ruminal pellets. Injections of 5 mg Se in gravid ewes at 90, 60 and 30 days before estimated parturition have been shown to prevent WMD in lambs (Whanger et al, 1972, 1978), but this is not a practical method because of the extra labor involved. The inclusion of Se with the drench is a convenient and practical way of giving this element. Optimally, sheep should be drenched four times per year to control gastrointestinal parasitism. If 10 mg of Se were included with the anthelmintic, this would likely prevent Se deficiency within the scope of usual management practices (Whanger et al, 1978). New Zealand workers (Andrews et al, 1968) have also shown the beneficial effects of including Se in the drench for sheep. Se drenches have also been shown to improve the growth of beef calves (Davis, 1974). Implantations at the base of the ear of slow-release Se pellets have been shown to reduce WMD in both sheep and cattle (Jenkins and Hidiroglou, 1972). The Australian workers (Kuchel and Buckley, 1969 and Godwin, 1975) indicated that the placement of one Se pellet (composed of 0.5 g elemental Se and 9.5 g Fe) plus a binder in the rumen of sheep would prevent all signs of WMD for 3+ years. Although other workers found these pellets to be effective in the prevention of WMD, problems were encountered in keeping these in the rumen of sheep (Whanger et al, 1978). If this can be overcome, it would appear to be a practical way of giving Se to ruminants.

Probably one of the most practical means for giving Se to ruminants is in salt. Wisconsin workers (Paulson et al, 1968) reported the feeding of selenized salt (26 to 264 ppm Se in salt) to sheep prevented WMD as indicated by reduced serum LDH activity. The prevention of WMD by giving Se in the salt for sheep is in agreement with Oregon (Whanger et al, 1978) and Michigan workers (Ullrey et al, 1977, 1978). The results indicate that 30 to 65 ppm Se in the salt proved safe and effective in preventing subclinical Se deficiency.

Se for Wild Ruminants

While domestic livestock fed diets composed of ingredients from Se deficient areas of the USA develop WMD, very little is known about the manner in which native wild ruminants survive in the same areas. As far as is known the Michigan group are the only ones who have investigated this problem by studying the effects of vitamin E and Se on various biochemical parameters and survival of young among the captive white-tailed deer (Brady et al, 1978). Thirty-two female deer were assigned to 4 complete pelleted diets with (45 ppm) or without vitamin E or with (0.2 ppm) or without Se. The Se and vitamin E contents in the unsupplemented diet were respectively 0.04 and 5.5 ppm, respectively. Plasma Se and vitamin E were significantly lower among unsupplemented adults within 5 mo. of treatment and remained essentially constant at low levels from 10 mo. until the end of the experiment at 2 years. In vitro hemolysis of erythrocytes and mortality of young deer were affected by dietary vitamin E but not by Se. Tissue GSH-Px was correlated with tissue Se in the tissues measured (erythrocytes, liver and muscle) and tissue Se was in turn related to dietary Se. Thus, they concluded that dietary Se deficiency (at 0.04 ppm) resulted in a biochemical deficiency but not in gross lesions among these experimental animals. The Se requirements, therefore, appear to be <0.04 ppm for deer.

ZINC (Zn)

Zn was established as an essential nutrient for mammals over 40 years ago but the value of supplemental Zn in practical rations for farm animals was not recognized until much later. Positive proof that Zn was a required nutrient for ruminants was not published until 1960. Reviews concerning Zn metabolism in ruminants include those of Herrick (1974), Miller (1969, 1970, 1973), Mills et al (1969) and Underwood (1977).

Absorption and Excretion

Early [65]Zn tracer studies showed feces to be the primary route of Zn excretion (Feaster et al, 1954). Gravid cows consuming 100 mg Zn daily excreted 78 mg in feces and 4 mg in urine (Hansard et al, 1968). During 144 hr after dosing with [65]Zn, 70% was recovered in feces and 0.2% in urine. Similar values were found in sheep (Hansard and Mohammed, 1968) except the rate of Zn movement was more rapid. Urinary excretion of Zn is very low, usually not exceeding 0.3% of a [65]Zn dose (Miller et al, 1966) but the relative percentage of Zn in urine can be greatly increased by feeding a chelating agent such as EDTA (Powell et al, 1967).

Since absorption of Zn in ruminants is a dynamic process influenced by many dietary and physiological factors (Miller, 1970; 1973) selection of a figure representative of fecal excretion is difficult. The percentage absorbed increases with decreasing dietary Zn and is reduced with high Zn intakes (Table 5-10). Clinically Zn-deficient animals will also absorb a higher percentage of their Zn intake than normal animals. Although younger calves absorbed a higher percentage of dietary Zn than older ones (Miller and Cragle, 1965), this may have reflected deposition of larger amounts of Zn in body tissue relative to intake rather than a reduced ability to absorb Zn with increasing age (Miller, 1970). Stake et al (1973) noted that lower weight gains and nitrogen balances in calves during restricted energy and protein intake were accompanied by reduced Zn absorption and retention and suggested that Zn homeostasis is controlled at the tissue level and is closely related to protein deposition changes. Endogenous fecal Zn is also

Table 5-10. Effect of zinc deficiency and dietary zinc concentration on fecal excretion of [65]Zn by ruminants.[a]

Species, age, Zn status and dietary Zn level	Method of dosing	
	Oral	Intravenous
	% of dose in 7 days	
Goats up to 6 months		
4-6 ppm, Zn deficient	24	4
4-6 ppm, normal	34	4
Calves up to 6 months		
3-6 ppm, Zn deficient	25	7
3-6 ppm, normal	37	--
8.5 ppm, normal	41	--
33-46 ppm, normal	52	10
240 ppm, normal	64	12
640 ppm, normal	77	13
Cows	% of intake	
6 ppm, Zn deficient[b]	25	--
17 ppm, normal	45	--
40 ppm, normal	65	--

[a] Data summarized from Miller et al (1966, 1967, 1968, 1970, 1971), Neathery et al (1972, 1973), Powell et al (1967), Roberts et al (1973), and Stake et al (1975).

[b] Stable Zn measurements (Kirchgessner et al, 1978)

reduced by both low dietary Zn and Zn deficiency (Miller et al, 1966; Miller, 1970). These changes in Zn absorption are important for the homeostatic control of body Zn in accordance with needs (Miller, 1969).

Sites of Zn absorption and excretion in the GI tract of ruminants have been investigated by several methods. Studies with re-entrant cannulae in sheep (Grace, 1975) and cows (Bertoni et al, 1976) indicated net secretion of Zn into the forestomachs and net absorption from the small and large intestines. In relation to non-absorbed reference materials, the small intestine was the primary site of [65]Zn absorption (Hiers et al, 1968) although as much as one-third of the daily intake may be absorbed from the abomasum (Miller and Cragle, 1965). Arora et al (1969) reported over 70% in vitro uptake by rumen mucosal tissue of [65]Zn from buffered nutrient solutions but did not establish whether this was absorbed or adsorbed. Net secretion of [65]Zn occurred in the rumen-reticulum and small intestine. The appreciable Zn content of bovine saliva (0.5-1.0 mg/l.) would contribute to the apparent net secretion into the rumen (Bertoni et al, 1976). Apparently, Zn is secreted across the small intestinal mucosa since the cannulated pancreas accounted for one-fourth or less of the total endogenous loss in calves (Stake et al, 1974).

Absorption, defined as [65]Zn unrecovered in intestinal contents and feces after injection directly into the calf duodenum, was very rapid during the first hour (Pate et al, 1970). Thereafter, it diminished progressively with little absorption after 8 hr.

Relating these results to intestinal movement suggested that little Zn absorption occurred in the cecum or beyond. Hampton et al (1976) determined GI sites of Zn absorption by injecting [65]Zn into various sections and comparing tissue [65]Zn content. They found that Zn absorption, per unit of intestinal length, was similar throughout the small intestine of calves fed either low (9 ppm) or generous (55 ppm) amounts of Zn. Absorption was negligible when [65]Zn was injected directly into the large intestine. Available data indicate the small intestine is the primary site of both absorption and excretion of Zn in ruminants.

Tissue Distribution of Zn

Studies with cattle using [65]Zn (Feaster et al, 1954; Hansard et al, 1968; Miller et al, 1967; Neathery et al, 1974; Stake et al, 1975) indicated concentrations in soft tissues ranked liver, pancreas, pituitary, kidney, adrenal, lung, heart and skeletal muscle. Bones and teeth had relatively high levels of Zn. Other reports have shown that the testicles and accessory sex glands of the male contain high concentrations of Zn; the digestive tract secretions also were relatively high (Miller et al, 1968).

Total Zn content of bovine tissues and organs appears to be under close homeostatic control and is reduced only slightly when a Zn-deficient ration is fed (Table 5-11). In some tissues, including the liver, pancreas and bone, Zn content may be reduced 30-60% when clinical deficiency symptoms are apparent (Miller, 1969). In calf and sheep

Table 5-11. Effect of dietary Zn content on bovine tissue Zn concentrations.[a]

Tissue	Dietary Zn, ppm				
	2	17	33-40	233	633
	------------ mg/kg dry wt ----------				
Liver	84	109	114	213	870
Pancreas	--	80	108	228	1887
Spleen	--	93	90	--	--
Lung	72	88	80	--	--
Kidney	76	78	82	105	615
Heart	--	75	80	81	88
Skeletal muscle	78	109	95	75	84
Rib	62	71	76	97	125
Tibia	63	63	69	80	88

[a] Data summarized from Miller et al (1968, 1970) and Neathery et al (1973).

livers, Zn was found with Cu in three main protein fractions with approximate molecular weights of >75,000, 35,000 and 12,000 (Bremner and Marshall, 1974). Zn was usually absent from the low molecular weight fraction in Zn-deficient or high Cu livers. Much higher tissue Zn contents when 633 ppm dietary Zn was fed indicated a failure of the homeostatic control mechanism at this high level (Miller et al, 1970).

Whole blood of the ruminant contains approximately 2 mg Zn/l. of which about half is in serum or plasma. Supplemental Zn had little effect on bovine blood serum Zn levels unless the dietary level was extremely high (300 mg/kg or above; Miller et al, 1970; Beeson et al, 1977). Serum Zn of dairy cows was decreased by hyperthermal stress or ketosis and higher in older cows and those with evidence of mastitis (Wegner et al, 1973). Dufty et al (1977) found that cow plasma Zn levels remained relatively constant from conception until late pregnancy when a decline occurred followed by a more marked decline during the periparturient period. Zn levels were even lower in cows with dystocia. Unlike cattle, sheep with dystocia did not exhibit a fall in plasma Zn (McSparran and Lorentz, 1977). Serum Zn concentrations in sheep increased with advancing pregnancy and decreased with increasing age in both sexes (Singh and Mehta, 1975). Of the total Zn in lamb plasma, 66% was bound to albumin, 22% was bound to α_2 macroglobulin and 12% was unbound and presumably immediately available for physiological activity (Parry, 1977). During Zn deficiency, bound Zn decreased by half in albumin and by 83% in α_2 macroglobulin.

Gestation effects on fetal Zn accumulation were similar in cows (Hansard et al, 1968) and ewes (Hansard and Mohammed, 1968). Bovine fetal Zn increased by 13 times between the first and second thirds of pregnancy and by another 7 times during the final third. At 270 days, total accumulated Zn averaged 135 mg in placenta, 3 mg in placental fluids and 551 mg in the fetus. Of the [65]Zn absorbed by the cows, 14% was transferred to the fetus, placenta and fluids. Similarly, gravid ewes transferred 16% of the absorbed [65]Zn dose to the products of conception (Fig. 5-3), over half of which was deposited in the fetus (Hansard and Mohammed, 1968). Bremner (1976) reported that approximately 80% of the Zn in the 80-day ovine fetus was in the liver; thereafter the liver Zn contribution declined rapidly. At 140 days, the total fetal burden of the ewe contained approximately 180 mg of Zn.

Although the Zn concentration of fetal bovine plasma was equal to or lower than maternal plasma Zn at 270 days (Hansard et al, 1968) samples from calves 24 hr after delivery contained Zn at concentrations more than double that of their dams (Dufty et al, 1977). Between the 85th and 140th days of gestation, average fetal plasma Zn was 65% higher than maternal in sheep and 41% higher in goats (Lichti et al, 1970).

Lactation represents a major homeostatic demand for Zn in cattle (Miller, 1969) despite the relatively low Zn content (4 mg/l.) of milk (Neathery et al, 1973, Schwarz and Kirchgessner, 1978). Colostrum contains 3-4 times more Zn than milk (Underwood, 1977). Milk Zn concentrations can be increased with high dietary Zn and reduced when Zn intake is low but the percentage of the Zn intake appearing in milk declines rapidly as dietary Zn is increased (Neathery et al, 1973). Most of the Zn in cow's milk is associated with high molecular weight protein fractions (Eckbert et al, 1977).

Functions of Zn

A primary role of Zn in the animal body is related to its presence as a component and activator of enzymes. Vallee (1962) has listed a variety of Zn-containing enzymes which have been isolated from different animal tissues. Such enzymes include: carbonic anhydrase, alcohol dehydrogenase, glutamic dehydrogenase, lactic dehydrogenase and

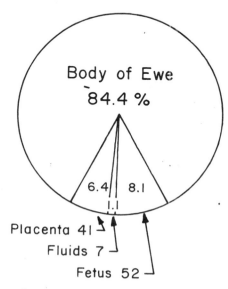

Products of Conception (15.6%)

Fig. 5-31. Calculated partition of retained [65]Zn in the 140-day gravid ewe; 7 days after dosing. From Hansard and Mohammed (1968).

alkaline phosphatase. Zn is also capable of activating a wide variety of enzymes in vitro, although many of these can be activated by other divalent cations.

In addition to its critical role in enzymes, Zn has also been associated with DNA and RNA functions (Chesters, 1974) and related to the actions of insulin, glucagon, corticotropin and other hormones (Halsted et al, 1974). Actions of follicle stimulating and luteinizing hormones appear to be enhanced by Zn and there is some evidence Zn plays a role in both keratinization and calcification. Zn content in protein fractions of bovine occular tissue is light dependent and is stoichiometrically related to rhodopsin (Tam et al, 1976). Furthermore, Zn has been associated with somatic and sexual development (Underwood, 1977), taste acuity (Cohen et al, 1973), wound healing (Miller et al, 1965), vitamin A transport and utilization (Arora et al, 1969), sulfate metabolism (Nielsen et al, 1970; Quarterman et al, 1976) and brain development (Lokken et al, 1973). The cell mediated immune system may also be adversely affected when Zn is lacking (Andresen et al, 1973) because of its critical role in the metabolism of nucleic acids and protein.

Zn deficiency

The first report of a naturally occurring deficiency of Zn in ruminants was that of Legg and Sears (1960) from British Guinea. The deficiency was seen in cattle grazing forage on sandy soils, particularly where the predominant grass was Pangola grass (*Trachypagan polymorphus* or *Digitaria decumbens*). Other reports of naturally

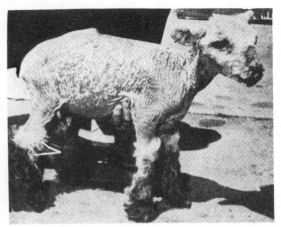

Fig. 5-32. A naturally occurring Zn deficiency in a young lamb. This 6-wk old lamb is showing loss of wool over the body, thick, wrinkled skin, and lesions around the mouth and eyes. From Pierson (1966).

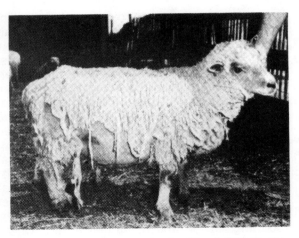

Fig. 5-33. A naturally occurring Zn deficiency in a Southdown ewe. Note the loss of wool on the belly, flank and quarter. From Pierson (1966).

occurring deficiencies in cattle include those of Haaranen (1963) in Finland, Grashuis (1964) in the Netherlands, Spais and Papasteriadis (1974) in Greece, and Rickard (1975) in New Zealand. Pierson (1966) also reported naturally occurring Zn deficiency in sheep in the USA (Fig. 5-32, 33).

A hereditary Zn deficiency in Dutch Friesian cattle apparently caused by a simple recessive gene has been reported in Denmark (Andresen et al, 1973) and in the Netherlands (Kroneman et al, 1975). Calves appear normal at birth but characteristic skin lesions appear at 4 to 6 weeks of age. The disorder is lethal if left untreated. Homozygous calves appear to have an unusually high requirement for Zn which can be met by oral supplementation if the dose is large enough. Flagstad (1976, 1977) presented evidence that the defect may be due to absence of a transepithelial transport mechanism for Zn. When Zn intake is high enough, diffusion may allow sufficient Zn to pass without the transport mechanism.

Research reports dealing with production of Zn deficiencies in sheep on purified diets include those of Ott et al (1964, 1965), Mills et al (1967), Arora et al (1969), Underwood and Somers (1969), Somers and Underwood (1969), Mann et al (1974) and Parry (1977). Papers reporting work on goats include those of Miller et al (1964, 1966, 1968) and Neathery et al (1973); and those on cattle include Miller and Miller (1960, 1962), Miller et al (1965, 1966, 1967, 1968), Mills et al (1967), Pitts et al (1966) and Kirchgessner et al (1978).

Deficiency Symptoms. Itching eczema is said to be a clinical symptom of naturally occurring Zn deficiency in cattle (Haaranen, 1963; Rickard, 1975) and it has responded to Zn treatment. Hyppola (1966) reported that itching cows had a greater incidence of difficult conceptions and abnormal estrus and that there was a tendency for cystic degeneration of the ovary; retention of the placenta after calving was more prevalent than in non-itching cows. Other clinical symptoms in mature animals included unthrifty appearance, rough coat, hair loss and eczematous lesions with thickening and folding in various parts of the skin in severe cases (Spais and Papasteriadis, 1974). Legg and Sears (1960) observed a parakeratosis which rapidly spread over about 40% of the body surface of cattle—muzzle, vulva, anus, top of tail, ears, back of hind legs, knee fold, flanks and neck. Animals gained very little. Symptoms in sheep included loss of body

wool and development of thick, wrinkled pink skin (see Fig. 5-32, 33). Miller (1970) has suggested that responses in feed intake and growth after feeding supplemental Zn are perhaps the best indicators for diagnosing a deficiency.

Experimantelly induced Zn deficiency has been well characterized in ruminants. Early deficiency symptoms in calves include decreased feed consumption and body weight gain and excessive salivation (Fig. 5-34). The calves developed a rough hair coat followed by the development of swelling of the feet and legs, loss of hair on the rear legs, and breaks in the skin around the hooves. Symptoms seen later included a stiff gait, swelling of the hocks and knees; creased, wrinkled appearance of the skin; red, scabby and shrunken skin (Fig. 5-35), and in some calves, impairment of vision. Inflammation of the skin around the nose and mouth with submucosal hemmorrhages has also been observed. Similar symptoms have been reported for sheep (Fig. 5-36) and goats. Parakeratotic changes have been observed in the skin, papillae of the rumen and of the esophageal mucosa. Clinical Zn deficiency symptoms occurred in

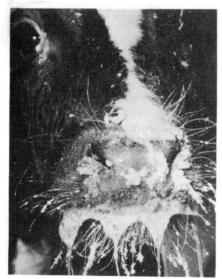
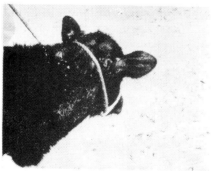

Fig. 5-34. Zn deficient calves. The young calf (top) shows excessive salivation, an early symptom; from Mills et al (1967). The calf on the bottom shows the typical dermatitis seen about the head and neck in a deficiency of longer duration. Courtesy of W.J. Miller, Georgia Agr. Expt. Sta.

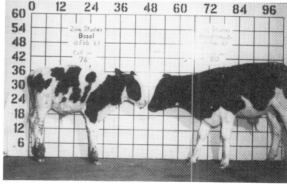
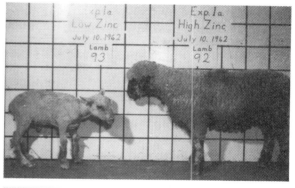

Fig. 5-35. Zn-deficient lamb and calf. The deficient animals (on the left) received diets with 3 ppm of Zn and the normals received 103 ppm. Courtesy of W.M. Beeson, Purdue Univ.

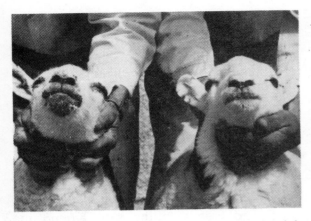

Fig. 5-36. Zn-deficient Cheviot lamb on the left showing loss of hair and development of skin lesions around the eyes and mouth. The lamb on the right had the same ration plus a drench providing 0.7 mg of Zn per kg of weight/day. From Mills et al (1967).

lactating cows after 3 weeks of dietary Zn depletion (Kirchgessner et al, 1978). Parakeratotic skin lesions, initially around the fetlock and pastern, spread over the hocks and inner surfaces of the shanks and finally the udder.

Digestibility of the diet is impaired very little, if any (Miller et al, 1966), but N and S retention may be reduced in deficient lambs due to increased urinary excretion of these elements (Somers and Underwood, 1969). These latter data indicate a marked reduction in the ability of the deficient animal to utilize protein (see Table 5-12). Feed conversion is reduced considerably—providing futher evidence—and the concentration of rumen VFA is reduced (Ott et al, 1964, 1965).

Serum or plasma Zn may drop from normal levels of 0.8-1.2 mg/l. to very low levels of 0.15-0.2 mg/l. Serum albumin and blood glucose may decrease and globulin may increase (Ott et al, 1964, 1965). Zn depletion of animals has been shown to reduce blood hemoglobin levels and activities of serum and bone alkaline phosphatase, liver alcohol dehydrogenase, muscle malate dehydrogenase, pancreatic carboxypeptidase A and B, and erythrocyte carbonic anhydrase (Miller and Miller, 1962; Miller et al, 1965; Arora et al, 1969; and Roth and Kirchgessner, 1974; Kirchgessner et al, 1978). Zn deficiency apparently reduced the mobilization of liver vitamin A in lambs (Arora et al, 1969). Liver alcohol dehydrogenase activity remained higher in control lambs or those which did not develop impaired vision when subjected to deficient diets. Liver Zn dropped rapidly, more so than in many other organs.

A number of reports showed that testicular size was reduced in calves and goats during Zn deficiency (Miller and Miller, 1960, 1962; Pitts et al, 1966; Neathery et al, 1973) but after 43 weeks on a normal ration, testicle size and activity and reproductive performance of initially Zn deficient Holstein bulls had returned to normal (Pitts et al, 1966). Underwood and Somers (1969) reported complete cessation of spermatogenesis when lambs were fed a diet with 2.4 ppm of Zn. Complete remission of testicular changes was observed when the lambs were given a diet with adequate Zn.

Zinc Requirements

Some of the early reports of Miller and co-workers from the Georgia Experiment Station with calves and kids indicated that addition of 40 ppm Zn to semipurified diets containing around 4 ppm Zn prevented Zn deficiency signs. In studies with older calves fed semi-practical diets, 25 ppm (Miller et al, 1962) and even 9 ppm (Miller et al, 1963) were adequate as indicated by weight gain, feed consumption, testicle size and Zn content, blood Zn content and clinical examination. Mills et al (1967) suggested that 10-14 ppm was sufficient to maintain blood plasma Zn levels in calves fed a synthetic diet containing no plant protein sources. However, Zn requirements may be somewhat higher with growth rates more rapid than obtained in calves fed semipurified diets (Stake et al, 1973).

Although Zn requirements of cattle under experimental conditions have usually been met by rations near 20 ppm (Neathery et al, 1973; Kirchgessner et al, 1978), deficiencies have occurred in the field with higher Zn levels (Legg and Sears, 1960; Spais and Papasteriadis, 1974). Addition of 73-346 ppm

Table 5-12. Effect of Zn deficiency in lambs on digestibility and retention of some nutrients.[a]

Item	Zn-deficient	Restricted-fed controls
Gain in 2 wk, kg	0.26	0.47
Dry matter intake, g	489	489
Dry matter digestibility, %	64.5	66.8
Nitrogen		
intake, g	12.4	12.4
fecal excretion, g	4.6	4.5
urinary excretion, g	5.8	3.7
balance, g	2.0	4.2
Sulfur balance, g	0.25	0.49
Zn intake, mg	1.17	15.8
Zn balance, mcg	70.6	1357

[a] From Somers and Underwood (1969)

supplemental Zn to natural rations containing 18-29 ppm Zn increased daily gain of beef steers in 2 of 4 experiments (Perry et al, 1968). In later work from the same station (Beeson et al, 1977), gain of growing beef cattle fed basal diets containing approximately 20 ppm Zn was increased by supplemental Zn (75 ppm) in only 1 out of 7 experiments.

Zn levels considered adequate for lambs depend on the measurement of adequacy chosen. Mills et al (1967) suggested that only 7 ppm maintained growth and 15 ppm maintained blood Zn levels. In contrast, Holod et al (1969) found that growth was stimulated in sheep when dietary Zn was increased from 9 to 34 ppm for 61 days and then to about 74 ppm for 46 days. Arora et al (1969) found that 23 ppm of Zn did not maintain blood enzyme activity and reduced liver vitamin A mobilization when compared to a Zn level of 50 ppm. Requirements for reproduction in sheep appeared to be greater than the 17 ppm adequate for growth of lambs (Underwood and Somers, 1969). Normal testicular development and function were significantly improved by a dietary intake of 32 ppm Zn.

Interfering Factors. Dynna and Harve (1963) reported a disorder similar to parakeratosis in young cattle fed herbage containing 4.6 ppm Cu and 37 ppm Zn. Treatment of the animals with both Zn and Cu was more efficient than Zn alone. In 30 field cases, treatment with Cu sulfate and Zn sulfate cured the disorder. A relationship between Zn and Mo was suggested by Holod et al (1969) who found that a large increase in the Mo content of sheep rations was accompanied by decreased Zn content in liver, intestines and heart and increases in kidney and blood.

The antagonistic effect of Ca on Zn utilization in swine is well known. A similar relationship in dairy cattle has been suggested by Haarenen (1963). He calculated that 45 ppm Zn was required to prevent itching and hair slicking in cows if the dietary Ca level was 0.3% of the dry matter and that, for each increase of 0.1% Ca above this level, Zn should be increased by 16 ppm. Grashuis (1964) believed that Zn deficiency occurred in cattle when hay, grass and silage contained 20-80 ppm Zn and about 0.6% Ca. However, Anke et al (1976) found that Zn content of sheep blood serum, rib, liver, brain and wool was not influenced by dietary Ca levels ranging from 1 to 3.8% of dry matter.

The lower availability to non-ruminants of Zn from soybean protein than from casein diets has been demonstrated in numerous reports. O'Dell et al (1964) have postulated that a 3-way interaction among Ca, Zn and phytate forms a complex less available than is formed by any of the two ions alone. After an extensive literature review, however, Hartmans (1965) concluded that such an interaction is unlikely in ruminants. In fact, data published by Ott et al (1964) indicated that inclusion of 0.6% phytic acid to a diet containing no plant protein appeared to reduce the severity of Zn deficiency symptoms in lambs, although blood components or tissue Zn concentrations were little different from deficient lambs. Further evidence against a Zn-phytate interaction in ruminants was presented by Miller (1967) who found apparent absorption of ^{65}Zn by calves fed rations containing isolated soybean protein, a source of phytate, was comparable to that of calves fed casein supplemented diets. However, when isolated soybean protein was deposited directly into the abomasum, ^{65}Zn absorption was reduced 35%. Soy protein thus reduced ^{65}Zn absorption only when the rumen was by passed. These results are not surprising since phytin phosphorus is essentially as available to ruminants as that supplied by monocalcium phosphate. Hydrolysis of phytin in the rumen would most likely destroy its Zn binding capacity.

Cadmium is highly toxic to ruminants and its effects can be partially offset by feeding supplemental Zn (Powell et al, 1964). In other work, Cd increased fecal excretions of Zn in calves but not in goats which were more mature (Miller et al, 1968). Livers of Cd-fed, Zn-deficient calves had an increased concentration of Zn but this was not observed in goat livers.

The chelating agent, EDTA, improves utilization of Zn by non-ruminants fed rations containing soybean meal. However, EDTA did not appear to have this Zn sparing effect in calves or goats fed semi-purified diets containing no plant proteins. Addition of 300 ppm EDTA to the ration had no clear cut effects on absorption and tissue retention of ^{65}Zn (Powell et al, 1967), ^{65}Zn secretion and reabsorption in the GI tract (Hiers et al, 1968) or fecal Zn excretion (Miller et al, 1968) although urinary ^{65}Zn excretion was markedly increased. It is questionable that EDTA would improve utilization of Zn by ruminants even if the ration contained soybean protein since dietary protein source did not affect Zn availability to calves unless the rumen was bypassed (Miller, 1967). Clearly, caution should be used in extrapolating results of Zn metabolism studies with non-ruminants to ruminants.

Zn Toxicity

Early research by Feaster et al (1954) showed that steers fed rations containing 1000 ppm of supplemental Zn for as long as 18 mo. continued to grow. Although feed intake and body weight were lower than when 50 ppm was fed, no other symptoms were reported. Gains and feed efficiency were subnormal in cattle fed 900 ppm Zn and depraved appetite resulted when rations contained 1,700 ppm and above (Ott et al, 1966). In dairy cows, the only apparent effect of dietary Zn levels up to 1,279 ppm was increased blood Zn concentration (Miller et al, 1965). Ott et al (1966) also studied Zn toxicity in lambs. No ill effects were found in lambs fed rations containing 500 ppm Zn but Zn consumption above 1000 ppm caused reduced gains, decreased feed efficiency and increased mineral consumption. Force feeding 4 to 6 g of Zn daily depressed water intake and resulted in eventual death. Suckling lambs fed a milk substitute containing 840 ppm Zn (dry basis) for 4 weeks developed symptoms of Zn toxicity including poor growth, low appetite and extensive renal damage (Davies et al, 1977).

High levels of Zn increased serum and tissue Zn, particularly in the liver, pancreas and kidney (Ott et al, 1966; Kincaid et al, 1976). Liver Cu was depressed and liver Fe increased. Elevated liver and duodenal Zn in calves fed 600 ppm Zn was confined largely in the soluble cell fraction (Kincaid et al, 1976) and was associated with a 10,000 molecular weight protein (Kincaid et al, 1976). A comparable increase of dietary Zn did not affect organ Zn content or alter its intracellular distribution in mature cows. It was suggested that homeostatic control mechanisms regulating Zn content of tissues are much more effective in mature cows than in calves.

Incorporation of Zn in the diet is more applicable to more intensive farming rather than to pastoral conditions such as in New Zealand where trace elements are often administered as drenches. Wethers drenched with 180 mg Zn/kg body weight/day suffered severe diarrhea, rapid weight loss and death in 7 to 8 days (Smith, 1977). Diarrhea and weight loss were less severe in those given 60 mg Zn/kg/day but they died in 4 weeks.

Zn in the drench solution, similarly to Cu salts, stimulated closure of the reticular groove mechanism and channeled the dose directly to the abomasum where considerable damage to the mucosa could result (Smith et al, 1977).

Exposure of cattle to fumes when galvanized metal was cut and welded inside the barn resulted in acute pulmonary emphysema although Zn levels in tissues were not increased (Hilderman and Taylor, 1974).

Sources of Zn

Plant species vary widely in Zn content. Legumes are generally higher than grasses and cereals, and Zn levels decrease with age of the plant (Gladstones and Loneragan, 1967). It was observed that application of other trace elements in fertilizer increased forage Zn content but yield responses did not affect concentration. Species adapted to sandy soils also usually had higher concentrations than those not adapted to such soils. However, in Georgia, Coastal Bermuda grass contained twice as much Zn when grown on sandy clay loam in the Piedmont than when grown on sandy loam soil in the Coastal plain (Miller and Miller, 1963). Forage analyses from Western Canada (Miltimore et al, 1970) indicated that over 90% of hays, silages and grains are below 48 ppm of Zn; mean values for forage and silage were on the order of 21-23 ppm and grain averaged about 33 ppm. Reported Zn contents of several feedstuffs include 7-11 ppm in beet or citrus pulp, 20-26 in corn, 62 in soybean meal and 104 in sesame meal (Miller and Miller, 1963).

When fed at relatively high levels (384-633 ppm), Zn oxide or Zn sulfate did not differ appreciably in their effects on rate of wound healing in heifers (Miller et al, 1967) or on tissue Zn content in calves (Miller et al, 1970). Unfortunately, data of this type are not adequate to evaluate the utilization of these sources of Zn. Neathery et al (1972) compared metabolism of [65]Zn chloride with [65]Zn in the natural form in forage fed to calves. Chemical form did not affect [65]Zn excretion or total retention but [65]Zn in the metabolically more active tissues was higher when given as forage than as chloride. It was theorized that the two sources of [65]Zn were metabolized differently after absorption due to different [65]Zn-ligand combinations being transported from the intestine to the tissues.

OTHER MINOR ELEMENTS

Although evidence for the essentiality of

arsenic, vanadium, tin, silicon, and cadmium has been presented for rats, arsenic (As) is the only one in which evidence for essentiality has been obtained for ruminants (Anke et al, 1976, 1977). Growing, pregnant and lactating goats were fed semisynthetic rations with <50 ppb or this diet with additions of 350 ppb As. Only 58% of the deficient goats gave birth and the average body weight was 13% less than controls. Rations with <50 ppb As had no direct influence on growth of the first generation, but the second generation grew significantly slower (Anke et al, 1976). As deficiency lowered the ash content of the skeleton and the Mn content in the organs, but increased the Cu content of the organs. However, the tissue Zn and Fe levels were not affected. These investigators suggested 50 ppb As and less as deficient, 350 to 500 ppb As as meeting requirements and therapeutic doses as 3.5 to 5.0 ppm (Anke et al, 1977). Although, at present the likelihood of any of these other minor elements becoming of nutritional significance in ruminants under field conditions appears very remote, the same sentiment for Se was prevalent when its essentiality was first presented. Thus, all possible mineral deficiency must be kept in mind regardless of how impractical they may seem.

SUMMARIZATION

The information on the trace elements is too detailed to summarize in a paragraph or so. However, it might be in order to briefly summarize some of the data in tabular form as shown in Table 5-13. In this table are shown typical tissue (blood serum, liver) concentrations of normal, adequately-fed animals. Information is also shown, where available, on the site of absorption from and excretion into the GI tract, route of excretion when given as oral or I.V. doses, the authors' estimate of dietary requirements, and probable toxic levels.

The reader must keep in mind that the values shown may vary widely. The dietary intake of nearly every given element will greatly influence the blood and liver concentrations as will many of the various interfering factors that have been discussed. Likewise, the relative amount that may be excreted via urine or feces can be influenced to a considerable degree by the dietary intake. At any rate, a summary of this type will give an approximation of these various items and the values shown in the table are within the ranges that may be found in published literature.

Table 5-13. Summary of data on trace minerals—normal tissue levels, site of absorption, route of excretion, probable dietary requirements and toxic concentration.

| Mineral | Tissue concentration | | Site of absorption and excretion in the GI tract | | Route of excretion, % | | Probable dietary require-ment, ppm | Toxic level, ppm |
	Blood serum, mcg/100 ml	Liver, ppm	Absorption	Excretion	Oral doses via feces	I.V. doses via urine		
Co	0.1-0.3 [a]	0.1-0.2	S.I., ?	bile, gut	85	65-80	0.1	<75**
Cu	100	200+	S.I., L.I.	bile, abomasum	90	50	10+	20-40**
Fe	150	200+	S.I., ?	?	?	?	35-100	< 400*
I	5-10	negligible	rumen, S.I., L.I.	abomasum, bile	85-95	60	0.6-0.8	> 50
Mn	2-3	9-12	S.I.	bile, S.I.	?	70-90	20+	>100**
Mo	1-5	2-4	abomasum, S.I.	?	40-95	60-70	<0.01 ?	< 20**
Ni	?	?	?	?	65-90	?	?	> 100
Se	10-20	0.5+	S.I.	bile	50-60	60-90	0.1-0.3	5**
Zn	80-120	50+	S.I.	abomasum, bile, S.I.	95+	1-5	30-40+	> 100**

[a] As Vitamin B

*Cattle

**Sheep

General References

Comar, C.L. and F. Bronner. 1964. Mineral Metabolism. Vol. II-A,B. Academic Press, NY.

Csaky, T.Z. 1975. Intestinal Absorption and Malabsorption. Ravin Press, NY.

Harper, H.H. 1971. Review of Physiological Chemistry - 14th ed. Lange Med. Pub., Los Altos, California.

Hoekstra, W.G., J.W. Suttle, H.E. Ganther and W. Mertz. 1974. Trace Element Metabolism - 2. In: Proc. 2nd Int. Trace Element Symp. University Park Press, Madison, Wisconsin.

Mills, D.F. 1970. Trace Element Metabolism in Animals. Proc. WAAP/IBP Int. Symp. Trace Element Metabolism-2, Aberdeen, Scotland.

Mitchell, H.H. 1962. Comparative Nutrition of Man and Domestic Animals. Vols. 1,2, Academic Press, NY.

Mortvedt, J.J., P.M. Giordano and W.L. Lindsay. 1972. Micronutrients in Agriculture. Soil Science Soc. of America, Inc., Madison, WI.

Nicholas, D.J.D. and A.R. Egan. 1975. Trace Elements in Soil-Plant-Animal Systems, Academic Press, NY.

Nutrition Reviews. 1976. Present Knowledge in Nutrition. 4th ed. Nutrition Foundation, NY.

Prasad, A.S. and D. Oberleas. 1976. Trace Elements in Human Health and Disease. Vol. I-II, Academic Press, NY.

Underwood, E.J. 1977. Trace Elements in Human and Animal Nutrition. 4th ed. Academic Press, NY.

Wacker, W.E.C. and B.L. Vallee. 1959. J. Biol. Chem. 234:3257.

Wohl, N.S. and R.S. Goodhart. 1968. Modern Nutrition in Health and Disease. Lea & Febiger, Philadelphia, PA.

Wynick, M. 1972. Nutrition and Development. John Wiley and Sons, NY.

References Cited

Cobalt

Ammerman, C.B. 1970. J. Dairy Sci. 53:1097.

Andrews, E.D. 1956. N.Z. J. Agr. 92:239.

Andrews, E.D., L.I. Hart and B.J. Stephenson. 1959. N.Z. J. Agr. Res. 2:274.

Andrews, E.D. and B.J. Stephenson. 1966. N.Z. Agr. Res. 9:491.

Andrews, E.D. et al. 1958. N.Z. J. Agr. Res. 1:125; N. Z. Vet. J. 6:140.

Becker, D.E. and S.E. Smith. 1951. J. Animal Sci. 10:266.

Comar, C.L. and G.K. Davis. 1947. Arch. Biochem. 12:257; J. Biol. Chem. 170:379.

Comar, C.L. et al. 1946. Arch. Biochem. 9:149; J. Nutr. 32:61.

Dewey, D.W., H.J. Lee and H.R. Marston. 1958. Nature 181:1367.

Dickson, J. and M.P. Bond. 1974. Aust. Vet. J. 50:236.

Dunn. K.M., R.E. Ely and C.F. Huffman. 1952. J. Animal Sci. 11:326.

Ely, R.E., K.M. Dunn and C.F. Huffman. 1948. J. Animal Sci. 7:239.

Ely, R.E. et al. 1952. J. Animal Sci. 12:394.

Gardiner, M.R. and M.E. Nairn. 1969. Aust. Vet. J. 45:215.

Gawthorne, J.M. 1968. Aust. J. Biol. Sci. 21:789.

Gille, G., E.R. Graham and W.H. Pfander. 1971. Proc. Fed. Amer. Soc. Expt. Biol. 30:295 (abstr).

Griffiths, J.R., R.J. Bennett and R.M.R. Bush. 1970. Animal Prod. 12:89.

Hine, D.C. and M.C. Dawbarn. 1954. Aust. J. Expt. Biol. Med. Sci. 32:641.

Holmes, E.G. 1965. Quart. J. Expt. Physiol. 50:203.

Hopper, J.H. and B.C. Johnson. 1955. J. Animal Sci. 14:273.

Ibbotson, R.N., S.H. Allen and C.W. Gurney. 1970. Aust. J. Expt. Biol. Med. Sci. 48:161.

Irving, E.A. 1959. Aust. Vet. J. 35:88.

Jones, O.H. and W.B. Anthony. 1970. J. Animal Sci. 31:440.

Keener, H.A., R.R. Baldwin, G.P. Percival. 1951. J. Animal Sci. 10:428.

Keener, H.A., G.P. Percival and K. S. Morrow. 1954. N. Hampshire Agric. Expt. Sta. Bul. 411.

Kercher, C.J. and S.E. Smith. 1955. J. Animal Sci. 14:458.

Kercher, C.J. and S.E. Smith. 1956. J. Animal Sci. 15:550.

Lanigan, G.W. and J.H. Whittem. 1970. Aust. Vet. J. 46:17.

Lee, H.J. 1950. Aust. Vet. J. 26:152.
Lee, H.J. and R.E. Kuchel. 1953. J. Agr. Res. 4:88.
Lee, H.J. and H.R. Marston. 1969. Aust. J. Agr. Res. 20:905.
Li, V.V. and A.A. Abdrakhmanov. 1975. Nutr. Abstr. Rev. 46:825.
MacPherson, A. and F.E. Moon. 1974. In: Trace Element Metabolism in Animals-2. University Park
    Press, Baltimore.
MacPherson, A., F.E. Moon and R.C. Voss. 1973. Brit. Vet. J. 129:414.
Marston, H.R. 1970. Brit. J. Nutr. 24:615.
Marston, H.R., S.H. Allen and R.M. Smith. 1961. Nature. 190:1085.
Marston, H.R., S.H. Allen and R.M. Smith. 1972. Brit. J. Nutr. 27:131.
Monroe, R.A., H.E. Sauberlich, C.L. Comar and S.L. Hood. 1952. Proc. Soc. Expt. Biol. Med.
    80:250.
Neathery, M.W. and W.J. Miller. 1977. Feedstuffs 49(38):22.
Odynets, R.N., E.M. Tokobaev and G.S. Lysenko. 1972. Nutr. Abstr. Rev. 42:1028.
Owen, E.C., S.E. Ellis, R.C. Voss, A.L. Wilson and J. Robertson. 1960. Proc. Nutr. Soc. 19:xxi.
Pearson, P.B., L. Struglia and I.L. Lindhal. 1953. J. Animal Sci. 12:213.
Phillipson, A.T. and R.L. Mitchell. 1952. Brit. J. Nutr. 6:176.
Ray, S.N., W.C. Weir, A.L. Pope, G. Bohstedt and P.H. Phillips. 1948. J. Animal Sci. 7:3.
Rothery, P., J.M. Bell and J.W.T. Spinks. 1953. J. Nutr. 49:173.
Rozybakiev, M.A. 1967. Nutr. Abstr. Rev. 37:757.
Russel, A.J.F., A. Whitelaw, P. Moberly and A.R. Fawcett. 1975. Vet. Rec. 96:194.
Sahaski, K. et al. 1953. J. Biochem. (Tokyo) 40:227.
Smith, E.L. 1962. In: Mineral Metabolism, Vol. 2, part B. Academic Press.
Smith, R.M. and H.R. Marston. 1970. Brit. J. Nutr. 24:879.
Smith, S.E., D.E. Becker, J.K. Loosli and K.C. Beeson. 1950. J. Animal Sci. 9:221.
Somer, M. and J.M. Gawthorne. 1969. Aust. J. Expt. Med. Sci. 47:227.
Tribe, D.E., J.M. Bond and A.D. Osborne. 1954. Nature 173:728.

Cu and Mo

Adamson, A.H., D.A. Volks, M.A. Appleton and W.B. Shaw. 1969. Vet. Rec. 85:368.
Amer, M.A., G.T. St-Laurent and G.J. Brisson. 1973. Can. J. Physiol. Pharmacol. 51:649.
Anke, M. et al. 1971. Arch. Tierernahrung 21:505.
Arneson, R.M. 1970. Arch. Biochem. Biophys. 136:352.
Askew, H.O. 1958. N.Z.J. Agr. Res. 1:447.
Awad, Y.L., A.A. Ahmed, A.Y. Lofti and F. Fahny. 1973. Zentrabl. Veterinaermed. (A)20:742.
Barden, P.J. and A. Robertson. 1962. Vet. Rec. 74:252.
Barlow, R.M. et al. 1976. Vet. Rec. 98:86.
Beck, A.B. 1962. Aust. J. Expt. Agr. Animal Hus. 2:40.
Bell, M.C., B.G. Diggs, R.S. Lowrey and P.L. Wright. 1964. J. Nutr. 84:367.
Bell, M.C., N.N. Sneed and R.F. Hall. 1966. Proc. 7th Int. Cong. Nutr. 1-5:765. Hamburg,
    West Germany.
Bertoni, G., M.J. Watson, G.P. Savage and D.G. Armstrong. 1976. Zoot. Nutr. Animal 2:185.
Bingley, J.B. and J.H. Dufty. 1973. Res. Vet. Sci. 15:379.
Bremner, I. 1975. Proc. Nutr. Soc. 34:10A.
Bremner, I. 1976. Proc. Nutr. Soc. 35:21A.
Bremner, I., B.W. Young and C.F. Mills. 1976. Brit. J. Nutr. 36:551.
Bull. L.B. et al. 1956. Aust. Vet. J. 32:229: Aust. J. Agr. Res. 7:281.
Butler, E.J., R.M. Barlow and B.S.W. Smith. 1964. J. Comp. Path. 74:419.
Camargo, W.V., H.J. Lee and D.W. Dewey. 1962. Proc. Aust. Soc. Animal Prod. 4:12.
Chapman, H.L. et al. 1962. J. Animal Sci. 21:960.
Claypool, D.W. et al. 1975. J. Animal Sci. 41:911.
Clegg, F.G. 1956. Vet. Rec. 68:332.
Comar, C.L., G.K. Davis and L. Singer. 1948. J. Biol. Chem. 174:905.
Cook, G.A., A.L. Lesperance, V.R. Bohman and E.H. Jensen. 1966. J. Animal Sci. 25:96.
Corrigall, W., A.C. Dalgarno, L.A. Ewen and R.B. Williams. 1976. Vet. Rec. 99:396.
Cragle, R.G., M.C. Bell and J.K. Miller. 1965. J. Dairy Sci. 48:793 (abstr).
Cunningham, I.J. 1946. N.Z.J. Sci. Tech. 27A:372, 381.
Cunningham, I.J., and K.G. Hogan. 1959. N.Z.J. Agr. Res. 2:134.

Cunningham, I.J., K.G. Hogan and B.M. Lawson. 1959. N.Z.J. Agr. Res. 2:145.

Dick, A.T. 1953. Aust. Vet. J. 29:18, 233.

Dick, A.T. 1954. Aust. J. Agr. Res. 5:511; Aust. Vet. J. 30:196.

Dick, A.T. 1956. Soil Sci. 81:229.

Doherty, P.C., R.M. Barlow and K.W. Argus. 1969. Res. Vet. Sci. 10:303.

Dowdy, R.P. and G. Matrone. 1968. J. Nutr. 95:191,197.

Ellis, W.C., W.H. Pfander, M.E. Muhrer and E.E. Pickett. 1958. J. Animal Sci. 17:180.

Evans, G.W. 1973. Physiol. Revs. 53:535.

Fell, B.F., D. Dinsdale and C.F. Mills. 1975. Res. Vet. Sci. 18:274.

Fell, B.F., C.F. Mills and R. Boyne. 1965. Res. Vet. Sci. 6:170.

Fisher, G.L., C.A. Hjerpe and C.W. Qualls. 1976. Bioinorg. Chem. 6:11.

Flynn, A., A.W. Franzmann, P.D. Arneson and J.L. Oldemeyer. 1977. J. Nutr. 107:1182.

Gallagher, C.H. and V.E. Reeve. 1976. Aust. J. Exp. Biol. Med. Sci. 54:593.

Goodrich, R.D. and A.D. Tillman. 1966. J. Nutr. 90:76; J. Animal Sci. 25:484.

Goold, G.J. and B. Smith. 1975. N.Z. Vet. J. 23:233.

Gopinath, C., G.A. Hall and J. McC. Howell. 1974. Res. Vet. Sci. 16:57.

Grace, N.D. 1975. Brit. J. Nutr. 34:73.

Gracey, J.F. and J.R. Todd. 1960. Brit. Vet. J. 116:405.

Gubler, C.J., M.E. Lahey, G.E. Cartwright, and M.M. Wintrobe. 1953. J. Clin. Invest. 32:405.

Hankinson, D.J. 1975. J. Dairy Sci. 58:326.

Harker, D.B. 1976. Vet. Rec. 99:78.

Harvey, J.M. 1953. Aust. Vet. J. 29:261.

Hemingway, R.G. and A. MacPherson. 1967. Vet. Rec. 81:695.

Hill, C.H., B. Starcher and C. Kim. 1967. Fed. Proc. 26:129.

Hill, M.K., S.D. Walker and A.G. Taylor. 1969. N.Z. J. Agr. Res. 12:261.

Ho, S.K. et al. 1977. Can. J. Animal Sci. 57:727.

Hodge, R.W. and N.C. Palmer. 1973. Aust. Vet. J. 49:369.

Hogan, K.G., D.F. L. Money and A. Blayney. 1968. N.Z. J. Agr. Res. 11:435.

Howell, J.M. 1968. Vet. Rec. 83:226.

Huber, J.T., N.O. Price and R.W. Engel. 1971. J. Animal Sci. 32:364.

Huisingh, J., G.G. Gomez and G. Matrone. 1973. Fed. Proc. 32:1921.

Huisingh, J., D.C. Milholland and G. Matrone. 1975. J. Nutr. 105:1199.

Idris, O.F. and G. Tartour. 1975. Trop. Anim. Health Prod. 7:12.

Irwin, M.R., P.W. Poulos, B.P. Smith and G.L. Fisher. 1975. J. Comp. Path. 84:611.

Ishizaki, H. and K.T. Yasunobu. 1976. Adv. Exp. Med. Biol. 74:575.

Ivan, M. and C.M. Grieve. 1976. J. Dairy Sci. 59:1764.

Lassiter, J.W. and M.C. Bell. 1960. J. Animal Sci. 19:754.

Leigh, L.C. 1975. Res. Vet. Sci. 18:282.

Lesperance, A.L. and V.R. Bohman. 1963. J. Animal Sci. 22:686.

Lorentz, P.P. and F.M. Gibb. 1975. N.Z. Vet. J. 23:1.

MacPherson, A. and R.G. Hemingway. 1965. J. Sci. Food Agr. 16:220.

MacPherson, A. and R.G. Hemingway. 1968. J. Sci. Food Agr. 19:53.

Maddox, I.S. 1973. Biochem. Biophys. Acta 306:74.

Marcilese, N.A. et al. 1969. J. Nutr. 99:177.

Marcilese, N.A. et al. 1970. J. Nutr. 100:1399.

Mason, J. and C.J. Cardin. 1977. Res. Vet. Sci. 22:313.

McCleod, N.S.M. and J.A. Watt. 1970. Vet. Rec. 86:375.

McCord, J.M. and I. Fridovich. 1969. J. Biol. Chem. 244:6049.

McCosker, P.J. 1968. Res. Vet. Sci. 9:91,103.

Miller, J.K., B.R. Moss, M.C. Bell and N.N. Sneed. 1972. J. Animal Sci. 34:846.

Miller, L.R. et al. 1970. J. Animal Sci. 30:1032 (abstr).

Mills, C.F. 1954. Biochem. J. 57:603.

Mills, C.F. 1958. Soil Sci. 85:100.

Mills, C.F., A.C. Dalgarno and G. Wenham. 1976. Brit. J. Nutr. 35:309.

Morgan, K.T. 1973. Res. Vet. Sci. 15:83.

Moss, B.R., F. Madsen, S.L. Hansard and C.T. Gambel. 1974. J. Animal Sci. 38:475.

Mylrea, P.J. and D.T. Byrne. 1974. Aust. Vet. J. 50:169.

Neethling, L.P., J.M.M. Brown and P.J. DeWet. 1968. J.S. African Vet. Med. Assoc. 39:13.

O'Dell, B.L., R.M. Smith and R.A. King. 1976. J. Neurochem. 26:451.

Osaki, S., J.A. McDermott and E. Frieden. 1964. J. Biol. Chem. 239:3570.

Osaki, S., D.A. Johnson and E. Frieden. 1966. J. Biol. Chem. 241:2746.

Patterson, D.S.P. et al. 1974. J. Neurochem. 23:1245.

Patterson, D.S.P. and D. Sweasey. 1975. Biochem. Soc. Trans. 3:118.

Pearson, J.K.L. 1956. Vet. Rec. 68:766.

Pierson, R.E. and W.A. Aanes. 1958. J. Amer. Vet. Med. Assoc. 133:307.

Pitt, M.A. 1976. Agents Actions 6:758.

Pointevint, A.L. and J.D. Nelson. 1978. Proc. Georgia Nutr. Conf. Feed Industry. Feb. 15-17. p 36.

Pryor, W.J. 1959. Aust. Vet. J. 35:366.

Roberts, H.E. 1976. Vet. Rec. 99:496.

Roberts, H.E., B.M. Williams and A. Harvard. 1966. J. Comp. Path. 76:279.

Robinson, G.A. et al. 1964. Amer. J. Vet. Res. 25:1040.

Rogers, P.A.M. and D.B.R. Poole. 1978. Proc. 3rd Int. Symp. Trace Element Metab. Man Animals. p. 481. M. Kirchgessner, ed. Friesing Weihenstephan, West Germany.

Ross, D.B. 1964. Vet. Rec. 76:875.

Ross, D.B. 1966. Brit. Vet. J. 122:279.

Scaife, J.F. 1956. N.Z. J. Sci. Tech. 38A:285.

Sharoyan, S.G. et al. 1977. Biochim. Biophys. Acta 493:478.

Sheriha, G.M., R.J. Sirny and A.D. Tillman. 1962. J. Animal Sci. 21:53.

Smith, B. 1975. N.Z. Vet. J. 23:73.

Smith, B. and M.R. Coup. 1973. N.Z. Vet. J. 21:252.

Smith, B., D.A. Woodhouse and A.J. Fraser. 1975a. N.Z. Vet. J. 23:109.

Smith, B.P., G.L. Fisher, P.W. Poulos and M.R. Irwin. 1975b. J. Amer. Vet. Med. Assoc. 166:682.

Smith, B.S.W., A.C. Field and N.F. Suttle. 1968. J. Comp. Path. 78:449.

Smith, B.S.W. and H. Wright. 1975. J. Comp. Path. 85:299.

Soli, N.E. and I. Nafstad. 1976. Acta. Vet. Scand. 17:316.

Spencer, V.E., R.E. Reading and L.W. Thran. 1958. Nevada Agr. Expt. Sta. Bul. 202.

Sutter, M.D., D.C. Rawson, J.A. McKeown and A.R. Haskell. 1958. Amer. J. Vet. Res. 19:890.

Suttle, N.F. 1973. Proc. Nutr. Soc. 32:24A,69A.

Suttle, N.F. 1974a. In: Trace Element Metabolism in Animals-2. University Park Press, Baltimore, MD.

Suttle, N.F. 1974b. Brit. J. Nutr. 32:395.

Suttle, N.F. 1974c. Brit. J. Nutr. 32:559.

Suttle, N.F. 1974d. Proc. Nutr. Soc. 33:299.

Suttle, N.F. 1975a. In: Trace Elements in Soil-Plant-Animal Systems. Academic Press, NY.

Suttle, N.F. 1975b. Brit. J. Nutr. 34:411.

Suttle, N.F. 1975c. Proc. Nutr. Soc. 34:76A.

Suttle, N.F. 1978. In: Proc. 3rd Int. Symp. Trace Element Metab. Man Animals-3. Freising-Weihenstephan, West Germany.

Suttle, N.F. and K.W. Angus. 1976. J. Comp. Path. 86:595.

Suttle, N.F., K.W. Angus, D.I. Nisbet and A.C. Field. 1972. J. Comp. Path. 82:93.

Suttle, N.F. and A.C. Field. 1968. J. Comp. Path. 78:351,363.

Suttle, N.F. and A.C. Field. 1974. Vet. Rec. 95:166.

Suttle, N.F., A.C. Field and R.M. Barrow. 1970. J. Comp. Path. 80:151.

Suttle, N.F. and M. McLauchlan. 1976. Proc. Nutr. Soc. 35:22A.

Tabor, C.W., H. Tabor and S.M. Rosenthal. 1954. J. Biol. Chem. 208:645.

Tait, R.M. et al. 1971. Can. Vet. J. 12:73.

Thomas, J.W. and S. Moss. 1951. J. Dairy Sci. 34:929.

Thompson, R.H. and J.R. Todd. 1974. Res. Vet. Sci. 16:97.

Thompson, R.H. and J.R. Todd. 1967a. Brit. J. Nutr. 36:299; Res. Vet. Sci. 20:257.

Todd, J.R. 1969. Proc. Nutr. Soc. 28:189.

Todd, J.R. 1978. In: Proc. 3rd Int. Symp. Trace Element Metab. Man Animals-3. Freising-Weihenstephan, West Germany.

Todd, J.R. and J.F. Gracey. 1959. Vet. Rec. 71:145.

Todd, J.R., J.F. Gracey and R.H. Thompson. 1962. Brit. Vet. J. 118:482.

Todd, J.R. and H.J. Griblen. 1965. Vet. Rec. 77:498.

Todd, J.R. and R.H. Thompson. 1963. Brit. Vet. J. 119:161.

Togyesi, G. and I.A. Elmotz. 1967. Acta Vet. Acad. Sci. Hung. 17:39.

Tulloch, J.D. 1973. N.Z. Vet. J. 21:177.

160

Underwood, E.J. 1977. Trace Elements in Human and Animal Nutrition. 4th ed. Academic Press, NY.

Vanderveen, J.E. and H.A. Keener. 1964. J. Dairy Sci. 47:1224.

Ward, G.M. 1978. J. Animal Sci. 46:1078.

Wasfi, I.A. and S.E.I. Adam. 1976. J. Comp. Pathol. 86:387.

Weiss, E. and P. Baur. 1968. Nutr. Abstr. Rev. 38:1412.

Wiener, G., A.C. Field and J. Wood. 1969. J. Agr. Sci. 72:93.

Wiener, G., D.I. Sales and A.C. Field. 1976. Vet. Rec. 98:115.

Williams, R.B., I. McDonald and I. Bremner. 1978. Brit. J. Nutr. 40:377.

Whitelaw, A., R.H. Armstrong, C.C. Evans and A.R. Fawcett. 1977. Vet. Rec. 101:229.

Wynne, K.N. and G.L. McClymont. 1956. Aust. J. Agr. Res. 7:45.

Iodine

Alderman, G. and M.H. Stanks. 1967. J. Sci. Food Agr. 18:151.

Anderson, R.R. 1971. J. Dairy Sci. 54:1195.

Anonymous. 1962. Nutr. Rev. 20:20.

ARC. 1965. The Nutrient Requirements of Farm Livestock. No. 2. Ruminants. Agricultural Research Council, London.

Aschbacher, P.W. 1968. J. Animal Sci. 27:127.

Aschbacher, P.W., R.G. Cragle, E.W. Swanson and J.K. Miller. 1966. J. Dairy Sci. 49:1042.

Aschbacher, P.W. and V.J. Feil. 1968. J. Dairy Sci. 51:762.

Aschbacher, P.W., J.K. Miller and R.G. Cragle. 1963. J. Dairy Sci. 46:1114.

Barua, J., R.G. Cragle and J.K. Miller. 1964. J. Dairy Sci. 47:539.

Bauman, T.R. and C.W. Turner. 1965. J. Dairy Sci. 48:1353.

Binnerts, W.T. 1956. Med. Lanbouwhogesch. 56(4). Wageningen, The Netherlands.

Binnerts, W.T. 1963. Neth. Milk Dairy J. 17:87.

Binnerts, W.T. 1964. Neth. Milk Dairy J. 18:227.

Binnerts, W.T., F.W. Lengemann and C.L. Comar. 1962. J. Dairy Sci. 45:327.

Blincoe, C. 1975. J. Animal Sci. 40:342.

Bretthauer, E.W., A.L. Mullen and A.A. Moghissi. 1972. Health Phys. 22:257.

Bustad, L.K. et al. 1963. Health Phys. 9:1231.

Cline, T.R., M.P. Plumlee, J.E. Christain and W.V. Kessler. 1969. J. Dairy Sci. 52:1124.

Daburon, R., A. Cappelle, Y. Tricaud and P. Nizza. 1968. Revue Med. Vet. 119:323.

Flamboe, E.E. and E.P. Reineke. 1959. J. Animal Sci. 18:1135.

Garner, R.J., B.F. Sansom and H.G. Jones. 1960. J. Agr. Sci. 55:283.

Gross, J. 1962. Mineral Metabolism. Vol. 2 Part B:221. Academic Press, NY.

Grosvenor, C.E. 1960. Amer. J. Physiol. 199:419.

Hemken, R.W. 1970. J. Dairy Sci. 53:1183.

Hemken, R.W., J.H. Vandersall, M.A. Oskarsson and L.R. Fryman. 1972. J. Dairy Sci. 55:931.

Hemken, R.W., J.H. Vanderall, B.A. Sass and J.W. Hibbs. 1971. J. Dairy Sci. 54:85.

Hernandez, M.V. et al. 1972. J. Animal Sci. 34:780.

Iwarsson, K. 1973. Acta Vet. Scand. 14:570.

Iwarsson, K. 1974. Nord. Veterinaermed. 26:39.

Iwarsson, K. et al. 1973. Acta Vet. Scand. 14:254,610.

Iwarsson, K., J.A. Nyberg and L. Elman. 1972. Nord. Vet. Med. 24:559.

Knutsson, P.G. 1961. Nature 192:977.

Lengemann, F.W. 1963. J. Agr. Sci. 61:375.

Lengemann, F.W. 1969. Health Phys. 17:565.

Lengemann, F.W. 1973. J. Dairy Sci. 56:753.

Lengemann, F.W. and E.W. Swanson. 1957. J. Dairy Sci. 40:216.

Lengemann, F.M., E.W. Swanson and R.A. Monroe. 1957. J. Dairy Sci. 40:37.

Long, J.F., L.O. Gilmore and J.W. Hibbs. 1956. J. Dairy Sci. 39:1323.

Meier-Ruge, W. and R. Fridrich. 1969. Histochemie. 19:147.

Miller, J.I. and K. Tillapaugh. 1967. Cornell Feed Service No. 62:11.

Miller, J.K. 1966. Proc. Exp. Biol. Med. 121:291.

Miller, J.K. et al. 1965. J. Dairy Sci. 48:888,1118.

Miller, J.K. et al. 1968. J. Dairy Sci. 51:1831.

Miller, J.K. et al. 1970. J. Animal Sci. 41:369.

Miller, J.K. et al. 1971. J. Dairy Sci. 54:397.

Miller, J.K., B.R. Moss and E.W. Swanson. 1969. J. Dairy Sci. 52:677.

Miller, J.K. and E.W. Swanson. 1963. J. Dairy Sci. 46:927.

Miller, J.K. and E.W. Swanson. 1973. J. Dairy Sci. 56:378.

Miller, J.K., E.W. Swanson, P.W. Aschbacher and R.G. Cragle. 1967. J. Dairy Sci. 50:1301.

Miller, J.K., E.W. Swanson and W.A. Lyke. 1973. J. Dairy Sci. 56:1344.

Miller, J.K., E.W. Swanson and G.E. Spalding. 1975. J. Dairy Sci. 58:1578.

Mixner, J.P., D.H. Kramer and K.T. Szabo. 1962. J. Dairy Sci. 45:999.

Mixner, J.P. and H.D. Lennon, Jr. 1960. J. Dairy Sci. 43:1480.

Mixner, J.P., K.T. Szabo and R.E. Mather. 1966. J. Dairy Sci. 49:199.

Moss, B.R., R.F. Hall, J.K. Miller and E.W. Swanson. 1968. Proc. Soc. Exp. Biol. Med. 129:153.

Moss, B.R. et al. 1972. J. Dairy Sci. 55:1487.

NRC. 1971. Nutrient Requirements of Dairy Cattle. Nat. Acad. Sci., Washington, D.C.

Newton, G.L., E.R. Barrick, R.W. Harvey and M.B. Wise. 1974. J. Animal Sci. 38:449.

Piironen, E. and A.I. Virtanen, 1963. Z. Ernaehrungswiss. 3:140.

Pincus, S.H. and S.J. Klebanoff. 1971. New Eng. J. Med. 284:744.

Fe

Ammerman, C.B. 1970. Personal communication to D.C. Church. Florida Agr. Exp. Sta.

Ammerman, C.B. et al. 1967. J. Animal Sci. 26:404.

Baker, N.F. and J.R. Douglas. 1957. Amer. J. Vet. Res. 18:295.

Becker, R.B. et al. 1965. Florida Agr. Expt. Sta. Tech. Bul. 699.

Blaxter, K.L., G.A.M. Sharman and A.H. MacDonald. 1957. Brit. J. Nutr. 11:234.

Blum, J.W. and U. Zuber. 1975. Res. Vet. Sci. 18:294.

Bremner, K.C. 1966. Aust. J. Expt. Biol. Med. Sci. 44:259.

Bremner, K.C. 1969. Exptl. Parasitol. 24:184.

Bremner, I. and A.C. Dalgarno. 1973. Brit. J. Nutr. 29:229; 30:61.

Campbell, A.G. et al. 1974. N.Z. J. Agr. Res. 17:393.

Christopher, J.P., J.C. Hegenauer and P.D. Saltman. 1974. In: Trace Element Metabolism in Animals-2. University Park Press, Baltimore.

Coup, M.R. and A.G. Campbell. 1964. N.Z. J. Agr. Res. 7:624.

Dargie, J.D. and J.M. Preston. 1974. J. Comp. Pathol. 84:83.

Ellendorff, F.W. and A.M. Smith. 1967. J. Dairy Sci. 50:995 (abstr).

Forth, W. 1974. In: Trace Element Metabolism in Animals-2. University Park Press, Baltimore.

Forth, W. and W. Rummel. 1973. Physiol. Rev. 53:724.

Getty, S.M. et al. 1968. J. Animal Sci. 27:712.

Gibbons, R.A. et al. 1976. Biochim. Biophys. Acta. 437:301.

Giles, R.C. et al. 1977. Amer. J. Vet. Res. 38:535.

Hansard, S.L. 1966. Proc. 7th Int. Nutr. Cong. Hamburg, Germany.

Hansard, S.L. and L.E. Foote. 1959. Amer. J. Physiol. 197:711.

Hansard, S.L., L.E. Foote and G.T. Dimopoullos. 1959. J. Dairy Sci. 42:1970.

Hansard, S.L. and J.C. Glenn. 1964. J. Animal Sci. 23:905 (abstr).

Hardman, G.V. et al. 1959. J. Animal Sci. 18:1558 (abstr).

Hartman, R.H., G. Matrone and G.H. Wise. 1955. J. Nutr. 57:429.

Hartley, W.J., J. Mullins and B.M. Lawson. 1959. N.Z. Vet. J. 7:99.

Holz, R.C., T.W. Perry and W.M. Beeson. 1961. J. Animal Sci. 20:445.

Hoskins, F.H. and S.L. Hansard. 1964. J. Nutr. 83:10.

Jacobs, A. 1977. Fed. Proc. 36:2904; Blood 50:433.

Judd, J.T. and G. Matrone. 1962. J. Nutr. 77:264.

Khouri, R.H. and F.S. Pickering. 1969. N.Z. J. Agr. Res. 12:509.

Koong, L.J., M.B. Wise and E.R. Barrick. 1970. J. Animal Sci. 31:422.

Lawlor, M.J., W.H. Smith and W.M. Beeson. 1965. J. Animal Sci. 24:742.

Lesperance, A.L., C.M. Bailey and V.R. Bohman. 1966. J. Animal Sci. 25:595 (abstr).

Linder, M.C. and H.N. Munro. 1977. Fed. Proc. 36:2017.

MacDougall, D.B., I. Bremner and A.C. Dalgarno. 1973. J. Sci. Fd. Agr. 24:1255.

Matrone, G. et al. 1957. J. Dairy Sci. 40:1437.

Mollerberg, L. et al. 1975. Acta Vet. Scand. 16:197,205.

Miller, W.J. and P.E. Stake. 1974. Proc. Georgia Nutr. Conf. Feed Industry, p. 25.

Moore, C.V. and R. Dubach. 1962. In: Mineral Metabolism, Vol. 2, Part B. Academic Press.

NRC. 1978. Nutrient Requirements of Dairy Cattle. Nat. Acad. Sci., Washington, DC.

Raleigh, R.J. and J.D. Wallace. 1962. Amer. J. Vet. Res. 23:296.

Settlemire, C.T., J.W. Hibbs and H.R. Conrad. 1964. J. Dairy Sci. 47:875.

Soliman, M.D. and S. El Amrousi. 1965. Indian Vet. J. 42:831.

Standish, J.F. and C.B. Ammerman. 1971. J. Animal Sci. 33:481.

Standish, J.F. et al. 1969. J. Animal Sci. 29:496.

Standish, J.F. et al. 1971. J. Animal Sci. 33:171.

St. Laurent, G.J. and G.J. Brisson. 1968. J. Animal Sci. 27:1426.

Thomas, J.W. 1970. J. Dairy Sci. 53:1107.

Underwood, E.J. 1977. Trace Elements in Human and Animal Nutrition. 4th ed. Academic Press, New York.

Underwood, E.J. and E.H. Morgan. 1963. Aust. J. Exp. Biol. Med. Sci. 41:247.

Wheby, M.S. 1966. Blood 22:416.

Wing, J.M. and C.B. Ammerman. 1965. J. Animal Sci. 24:911 (abstr).

Manganese

Abrams, E. et al. 1977. J. Animal Sci. 45:1108.

Adams, R.S. 1975. J. Dairy Sci. 58:1538.

Anke, M. 1967. Nutr. Abstr. Rev. 37:243.

Anke, M. et al. 1972. Arch. Tierernahrung. 22:347.

Anke, M. and B. Groppel. 1970. In: Trace Element Metabolism in Animals. E. & S. Livingstone, Edinburgh.

Anke, M., B. Groppel and M. Grun. 1973. Arch. fur. Tierernahrung. 23:483.

Bentley, O.G. and P.H. Phillips. 1951. J. Dairy Sci. 34:396.

Bremner, I. 1970. Brit. J. Nutr. 24:769.

Carter, J.C. et al. 1974. J. Animal Sci. 38:1284.

Cotzias, G.C. 1962. In: Mineral Metabolism. Vol. 2, part B. Academic Press.

Cunningham, G.N., M.B. Wise and E.R. Barrick. 1966. J. Animal Sci. 25:532.

Fain, P., J. Dennis and F.C. Harbough. 1952. Amer. J. Vet. Res. 13:348.

Gallup, W.D., A.B. Nelson and A.E. Darlow. 1952. J. Animal Sci. 11:783 (abstr).

Grace, N.D. 1973. N.Z. J. Agr. Res. 16:177.

Grashuis, J., J.J. Lehr, L.L.E. Beuvery and A. Beuvery-Asman. 1953. Nutr. Abstr. Rev. 24:480 (abstr).

Groppel, B. and M. Anke. 1971. Arch. fur. Experiment. Vet. 25:52.

Hansard, S.L. 1972. IAEA-SM 156/19:351.

Hansard, S.L., C.T. Gamble, B.M. Moss and D.J. Davis. 1970. Fed. Proc. 29:2936; J. Animal Sci. 19:655.

Hartmans, J. 1974. In: Trace Element Metabolism in Animals. Univ. Park Press, Baltimore.

Hartman, R.H., G. Matrone and G.H. Wise. 1955. J. Nutr. 57:429.

Hawkins, G.E., G.H. Wise, G. Martone and R.K. Waugh. 1955. J. Dairy Sci. 38:536.

Hennig, A. et al. 1972. Arch. fur. Tierernahrung. 22:601.

Hidiroglou, M. et al. 1978. Can. J. Animal Sci. 58:35; Can. J. Compar. Med. 42:100.

Howes, A.D. and I.A. Dyer. 1971. J. Animal Sci. 32:141.

Ivan, M. and C.M. Grieve. 1975. J. Dairy Sci. 58:410.

Ivan, M. and C.M. Grieve. 1976. J. Dairy Sci. 59:1764.

Krolak, M. 1969. Nutr. Abstr. Rev. 39:970 (abstr).

Lassiter, J.W. and J.D. Morton. 1968. J. Animal Sci. 27:776.

Lomba, F., G. Chauvaux and A. Bienfet. 1977. Nutr. Abstr. Rev. 47:393 (abstr).

Miller, W.J. 1975. J. Dairy Sci. 58:1549.

Miller, W.J. et al. 1972. J. Animal Sci. 34:460.

Miller, W.J. et al. 1973. J. Animal Sci. 37:827.

Miltimore, J.E., J.L. Mason and D.L. Ashby. 1970. Can. J. Animal Sci. 50:293.

Munro, I.B. 1957. Vet. Rec. 69:125.

Murthy, G.K., U.S. Rhea and J.T. Peeler. 1973. J. Dairy Sci. 55:1666.

Neathery, M.W. and W.J. Miller. 1977. Feedstuffs 49(36):18.

Odynets, R.N. et al. 1975. Nutr. Abstr. Rev. 45:624 (abstr).

Robinson, N.W., S.L. Hansard, D.M. Johns and G.L. Robertson. 1960. J. Animal Sci. 19:1290 (abstr).
Rojas, M.A., I.A. Dyer and W.A. Cassatt. 1965. J. Animal Sci. 24:664.
Schellner, G. 1975. Nutr. Abstr. Rev. 45:367 (abstr).
Suttle, N.F. and A.C. Field. 1970. Proc. Nutr. Soc. 29:33A (abstr).
Theriez, M., M. Lamand and J.P. Brun. 1977. Nutr. Abstr. Rev. 47:928 (abstr).
Thomas, J.W. 1970. J. Dairy Sci. 53:1107.
Watson, L.T., C.B. Ammerman, J.P. Feaster and C.E. Roessler. 1973. J. Animal Sci. 36:131.
Watson, L.T., C.B. Ammerman, W.G. Hills and C.B. Aulsbrook. 1969. J. Animal Sci. 29:174 (abstr).
Weeth, H.J. 1962. Proc. West. Sec. Amer. Soc. Animal Sci. 13:1.
Wilson, J.G. 1966. Vet. Rec. 79:562.

Nickel

Anke, M. et al. 1974. Trace Element Metabolism in Animals-2. University Park Press, Baltimore.
Brockman, R.P., E.N. Bergman, P.K. Joo and J.G. Manns. 1975. Amer. J. Physiol. 229:1344.
Clay, J.J. 1975. Toxicol. Appl. Pharmacol. 31:55.
Dormer, R.L. et al. 1973. Biochem. J. 140:135.
Eichhorn, G.L. 1962. Nature 194:474.
Fishbein, W.N., M.J. Smith, K. Nagarajan and W. Scurzi. 1976. Fed. Proc. 35:1680 (abstr).
Fuwa, K. et al. 1960. Proc. Nat. Acad. Sci. 46:1928.
Horak, F. and F.W. Sunderman. 1975. Toxicol. Appl. Pharmacol. 33:383.
LaBella, F.S. et al. 1973. Nature 245:330.
Martinez, A. and D.C. Church. 1970. J. Animal Sci. 31:982.
Miller, W.J. 1973. Fed. Proc. 32:1915.
Nielsen, F.H. 1974. Trace Element Metabolism in Animals-2. University Park Press, Baltimore.
Nielsen, F.H. and D.A. Ollerich. 1974. Fed. Proc. 33:1767.
Nielsen, F.H. et al. 1975. J. Nutr. 105:1607,1620.
O'Dell, G.D. et al. 1970. J. Nutr. 100:1447; J. Dairy Sci. 53:1266,1545.
O'Dell, G.D. et al. 1971. J. Animal Sci. 32:769.
Smith, J.C. and B. Hackley. 1968. J. Nutr. 95:541.
Spears, J.W. and E.E. Hatfield. 1977. Feedstuffs 49(24):13.
Spears, J.W., C.J. Smith and E.E. Hatfield. 1977. J. Dairy Sci. 60:1073.
Spears, J.W. et al. 1978. J. Nutr. 108:307,313.
Tal, M. 1968. Biochim. Biophys. Acta 169:564.
Wacker, W.E.C. and B.L. Vallee. 1959. J. Biol. Chem. 243:3257.

Selenium

Allaway, W.H., D.P. Moore, J.E. Oldfield and O.H. Muth. 1966. J. Nutr. 88:411.
Allaway, W.H. and J.F. Hodgson. 1964. J. Animal Sci. 23:271.
Allen, W.M. et al. 1975. Vet. Rec. 96:360.
Ammerman, C.E. and S.M. Miller. 1975. J. Dairy Sci. 58:1561.
Andrews, E.D., A.B. Grant and B.J. Stephenson. 1964. N.Z. J. Agr. Res. 7:17.
Andrews, E.D., W.J. Hartley and A.B. Grant. 1968. N.Z. Vet. J. 16:3.
Bengtsson, G. et al. 1974. Acta Vet. Scand. 15:135.
Black, R.S. et al. 1978. Bioinorganic Chem. 8:161.
Blaxter, K.L. 1963. Brit. J. Nutr. 17:105.
Board, P.G. and D.W. Peter. 1976. Vet. Rec. 99:144.
Brady, P.S. et al. 1978. J. Nutr. 108:1439.
Boyazoglu, P.A., R.M. Jordan and R.J. Meade. 1967. J. Animal Sci. 26:1390.
Broderius, M.A., P.D. Whanger and P.H. Weswig. 1973. Proc. Soc. Exptl. Biol. Med. 143:297; J. Nutr. 103:336.
Buchanan-Smith, J.G., B.A. Sharp and A.D. Tillman. 1971. Can. J. Physiol. Pharm. 49:619.
Butler, G.W. and P.J. Peterson. 1961. N.Z. J. Agr. Res. 4:484.
Cartan, G.H. and K.F. Swingle. 1969. Amer. J. Vet. Res. 20:235.
Cousins, F.B. and I.M. Cairney. 1961. Aust. J. Agr. Res. 12:927.
Davis, G.H. 1974. N.Z. J. Expt. Agr. 2:393.
Ehlig, C.F., D.E. Hogue, W.H. Allaway and D.J. Hamm. 1967. J. Nutr. 92:121.
Ewan, R.C., C.A. Baumann and A.L. Pope. 1968. J. Agr. Food Chem. 16:216.

Gardner, R.W. and D.E. Hogue. 1967. J. Nutr. 93:418.

Godwin, K.O. 1972. Aust. J. Expt. Agr. Animal Hus. 12:473.

Godwin, K.O., R.E. Kuchel and C.N. Fuss. 1974. Aust. J. Biol. Sci. 27:633.

Godwin, K.O., K.A. Handrick and C.N. Fuss. 1971. Aust. J. Biol. Sci. 24:1251.

Godwin, K.O. 1975. In: Trace Elements in Soil-Plant-Animal Systems. Academic Press, NY.

Handrick, K.A. and K.D. Godwin. 1970. Aust. J. Agr. Res. 21:71.

Hartley, W.J. and A.B. Grant. 1961. Fed. Proc. 20:679.

Hidiroglou, M. et al. 1968. Can. J. Physiol. Pharm. 46:229,853; Can. J. Animal Sci. 48:335.

Hidiroglou, M. et al. 1969. Ann. Biol. Anim. Bioch. Biophys. 9:161: Can. J. Physiol. Pharm. 47:953.

Hidiroglou, M. and K.J. Jenkins. 1975. Can. J. Animal Sci. 55:307.

Hidiroglou, M. and J.R. Lessard. 1976. Intern. J. Vit. Nutr. Res. 46:458.

Hidiroglou, M. and C.G. Zakardas. 1976. Can. J. Physiol. Pharm. 54:336.

Hill, M.K., S.D. Walker and A.G. Taylor. 1969. N.Z. J. Agr. Res. 12:261.

Hintz, H.F. and D.E. Hogue. 1964. J. Nutr. 82:495.

Hoekstra, W.G. 1975. Fed. Proc. 34:2083.

Hoffman, C., B. Rivinus and L. Swanson. 1978. J. Animal Sci. 47:192.

Hogue, D.E., J.F. Proctor, R.G. Warner and J.K. Loosli. 1962. J. Animal Sci. 21:25.

Hogue, D.E. and A. Aydin. 1972. Proc. Cornell Nutr. Conf., p. 64.

Hopkins, L.L., A.L. Pope and C.A. Baumann. 1964. J. Animal Sci. 23:674.

Jacobsson, S.O., H.E. Oksanen and E. Hansson. 1965. Acta. Vet. Scand. 6:299.

Jacobsson, S.O. and H.E. Oksanen. 1967. Nutr. Abst. Rev. 37:136.

Jenkins, K.J. and M. Hidiroglou. 1972. Can. J. Animal Sci. 52:591.

Julien, W.E., H.R. Conrad, J.E. Jones and A.L. Moxon. 1976. J. Dairy Sci. 59:1954.

Kincaid, R.L. et al. 1977. J. Animal Sci. 44:147.

Kuchel, R.E. and R.A. Buckley. 1969. Aust. J. Agr. Res. 20:1099.

Kuttler, K.L. and D.W. Marble. 1960. Amer. J. Vet. Res. 21:437.

Lopez, P.L., R.L. Preston and W.H. Pfander. 1969. J. Nutr. 97:123.

McDonald, J.W. 1975. Aust. Vet. J. 51:433.

Mitchell, D., M. Hidiroglou and K.J. Jenkins. 1975. Can. J. Animal Sci. 55:513.

Moramarco, M.A.. J.A. Froseth and T.A. Bray. 1977. 69th Amer. Sco. Anim. Sci, Meeting. p. 248.

Muth, O.H. 1955. J. Amer. Vet. Med. Assoc. 126:355.

Muth, O.H. 1963. J. Amer. Vet. Med. Assoc. 142:272.

Muth, O.H., J.E. Oldfield, L.F. Remmert and J.R. Schubert. 1958. Science 128:1090.

Muth, O.H., J.E. Oldfield and P.H. Weswig (ed.). 1967. Selenium in Biomedicine AVI Pub. Co.

Muth, O.H. et al. 1967. Amer. J. Vet. Res. 28:1397.

Oh, S.H. 1972. M.S. Thesis, Univ. of Wisconsin. Madison, WI.

Oh, S.H., H.E. Ganther and W.G. Hoekstra. 1974. Biochemistry 13:1825.

Oh, S.H. et al. 1976. J. Animal Sci. 42:977,984.

Oldfield, J.E. et al. 1971. Selenium in Nutrition. Nat. Acad. Sci. Washington, D.C.

Oldfield, J.E., O.H. Muth and J.R. Schubert. 1960. Proc. Soc. Exptl. Biol. Med. 103:799.

Paulson, G.D. et al. 1968. J. Animal Sci. 27:195,497.

Paulson, G.D., A.L. Pope and C.A. Baumann. 1966. Proc. Soc. Exptl. Biol. Med. 122:321.

Perry, T.W., W.M. Beeson, W.H. Smith and M.T. Mohler. 1976. J. Animal Sci. 42:192.

Perry, T.W., R.C. Peterson, D.D. Griffith and W.H. Beeson. 1978. J. Animal Sci. 45:562.

Peterson, P.J. and D.J. Spedding. 1963. N.Z. J. Agr. Res. 6:13.

Pope, A.L., R.J. Moir, M. Somers and E.J. Underwood, 1968. J. Animal Sci. 27:1771.

Rosenfeld, I. and O.A. Beath. 1964. Selenium. Geobotany, Biochemistry, Toxicity and Nutrition. Academic Press.

Rotruck, J.T. et al. 1974. Science 179:588.

Scales, G.H. 1974. Proc. N.Z. Soc. Animal Prod. 34:103.

Schubert, J.R., O.H. Muth, J.E. Oldfield and L.F. Remmert. 1961. Fed. Proc. 20:689.

Shirley, R.L. et al. 1966. J. Animal Sci. 25:648.

Thompson, R.H., C.H. McMurray and W.J. Blanchflower. 1976. Res. Vet. Sci. 20:229.

Tripp, M.J., P.D. Whanger, J.A. Schmitz and J.E. Oldfield. 1979. J. Agr. Food Chem. (Submitted).

Trinder, N., R.J. Hall and C.P. Renton. 1973. Vet. Rec. 93:641.

Ullrey, D.E. et al. 1977. J. Animal Sci. 45:559.

Ullrey, D.E. et al. 1978. J. Animal Sci. 46:1515.

Underwood, E.J. 1977. Trace Elements in Human and Animal Nutrition. Academic Press.

Van Vleet, J.F. 1975. Amer. J. Vet. Res. 36:1335.

Whanger, P.D., P.H. Weswig and O.H. Muth. 1968. Fed. Proc. 27:418.

Whanger, P.D., P.H. Weswig, O.H. Muth and J.E. Oldfield. 1969. J. Nutr. 97:353; 99:331

Whanger, P.D., P.H. Weswig, O.H. Muth and J.E. Oldfield. 1970. Amer. J. Vet. Res. 31:965; J. Nutr. 100:73.

Whanger, P.D., P.H. Weswig, J.A. Schmitz and J.E. Oldfield. 1977. J. Nutr. 107:1288,1298.

Whanger, P.D. et al. 1972. J. Nutr. 102:435; Nutr. Rep. Intern. 6:21.

Whanger, P.D. et al. 1976. Nutr. Rep. Intern. 13:159.

Whanger, P.D. et al. 1978. J. Animal Sci. 46:515; 47:1157.

White, C.L. and M. Somers. 1977. Aust. J. Biol. Sci. 30:47.

Wise, W.R., P.H. Weswig, O.H. Muth and J.E. Oldfield. 1968. J. Animal Sci. 27:1462.

Wright, E. 1965. N.Z. J. Agr. Res. 8:284,297.

Wright, P.L. 1967. In: Selenium in Biomedicine. AVI Pub. Co.

Wright, P.L. and M.C. Bell. 1964. J. Nutr. 84:49.

Wright, P.L. and M.C. Bell. 1966. Amer. J. Physiol. 211:6.

Zinc

Andresen, E., A. Basse, E. Brummerstedt and T. Flagstad. 1973. Lancet 1(808):839.

Anke, M., M. Grun, M. Hoffman and A. Dittrich. 1978. Naturwiss. 25:271.

Arora, S.P. et al. 1969. J. Nutr. 97:25.

Beeson, W.M., T.W. Perry and T.D. Zurcher. 1977. J. Animal Sci. 45:160.

Bertoni, G. et al. 1976. Zoot. Nutr. Animal 2:185.

Bremner, I. 1976. Proc. Nutr. Soc. 35:86A.

Bremner, I. and R.B. Marshall. 1974. Brit. J. Nutr. 32:283.

Chesters, J.K. 1974. In: Trace Element Metabolism in Animals-2. University Park Press, Baltimore.

Cohen, I.K., P.J. Scheclter and R.I. Henkin. 1973. J. Amer. Med. Assoc. 112:914.,

Davies, N.T. et al. 1977. Brit. J. Nutr. 38:153.

Dufty, J.H., J.B. Bingley and L.Y. Cove. 1977. Aust. Vet. J. 53:519.

Dynna, O. and G.N. Harve. 1963. Acta Vet. Scand. 4:197.

Eckbert, C.D. et al. 1977. Science 195:789.

Feaster, J.P. et al. 1954. J. Animal Sci. 13:781.

Flagstad, T. 1976. Nord. Vet. Med. 28:160.

Flagstad, T. 1977. Nord. Vet. Med. 29:96.

Gladstones, J.S. and J.F. Lonergan. 1967. Aust. J. Agr. Res. 18:427.

Grace, N.D. 1975. Brit. J. Nutr. 34:73.

Grashuis, J. 1964. Nutr. Abstr. Rev. 34:900.

Haaranen, S. 1963. Nord. Vet. Med. 15:536.

Halsted, J.A., J.C. Smith and M.I. Irwin. 1974. J. Nutr. 104:345.

Hampton, D.L. et al. 1976. J. Dairy Sci. 59:712,1963.

Hansard, S.L. and A.S. Mohammed. 1968. J. Animal Sci. 27:807.

Hansard, S.L., A.S. Mohammed and J.W. Turner. 1968. J. Animal Sci. 27:1097.

Hartmens, J. 1965. Versl. Landbouwk. Onderz. 664.

Herrick, J.B. 1974. Vet. Med. Small Animal Clin. 69:85.

Hilderman, E. and P.A. Taylor. 1974. Can. Vet. J. 15:173.

Hires, V.M., G.E. Spak and J.L. Butkovic. 1969. Nutr. Abstr. Rev. 39:976.

Hyppola, K. 1966. J. Sci. Agr. Soc. Finland 38:180.

Kincaid, R.L. et al. 1976. J. Dairy Sci. 59:552,1580.

Kirchgessner, M., W.A. Schwarz and H.P. Roth. 1978. In: Trace Element Metabolism in Man and Animals-3. University Park Press, Baltimore.

Kroneman, J. et al. 1975. Zbl. Vet. Med. A. 22:201.

Legg, S.P. and L. Sears. 1960. Nature 186:1061.

Lichti, E.L. et al. 1970. Amer. J. Obstet. Gynecol. 106:1242.

Lokken, P.M., E.S. Halas and H.H. Sandstead. 1973. Proc. Soc. Exp. Biol. Med. 144:680.

Mann, S.O., B.F. Fell and A.C. Dalgarno. 1974. Res. Vet. Sci. 17:91.

McSparran, K.D. and P.P. Lorentz. 1977. Res. Vet. Sci. 22:393.

Mills, C.F., A.C. Dalgarno, R.B. Williams and J. Quarterman. 1967. Brit. J. Nutr. 21:751.

Mills, C.F. et al. 1969. Amer. J. Clin. Nutr. 72:1240.

Miller, J.K. 1967. J. Nutr. 93:386.

Miller, J.K. and R.G. Cragle. 1965. J. Dairy Sci. 48:370.

Miller, J.K. and W.J. Miller. 1960. J. Dairy Sci. 43:1854.

Miller, J.K. and W.J. Miller. 1962 J. Nutr. 76:467.

Miller, J.K., W.J. Miller and C.M. Clifton. 1962. J. Dairy Sci. 45:1536.

Miller, W.J. 1969. Amer. J. Clin. Nutr. 22:1323.

Miller, W.J. 1970. J. Dairy Sci. 53:1123.

Miller, W.J. 1973. Fed. Proc. 32:1915.

Miller, W.J., D.M. Blackmon, R.P. Gentry and F.M. Pate. 1970. J. Nutr. 100:893.

Miller, W.J., C.M. Clifton and N.W. Cameron. 1963. J. Dairy Sci. 46:715.

Miller, W.J. and J.K. Miller. 1963. J. Dairy Sci. 46:581.

Miller, W.J., W.J. Pitts, C.M. Clifton and S.C. Schmittle. 1964. J. Dairy Sci. 47:556.

Miller, W.J. et al. 1965. J. Dairy Sci. 48:450, 1091, 1329; Proc. Soc. Expt. Biol. Med. 118:427.

Miller, W.J. et al. 1966. J. Dairy Sci. 49:1012,1446; J. Nutr. 90:335.

Miller, W.J. et al. 1967. J. Nutr. 92:71; J. Dairy Sci. 50:715.

Miller, W.J. et al. 1968. J. Nutr. 94:391; J. Dairy Sci. 51:82.

Miltimore, J.E., J.L. Mason and D.L. Ashby. 1970. Can. J. Animal Sci. 50:293.

Neathery, M.W., W.J. Miller, D.M. Blackmon and R.P. Gentry. 1974. J. Animal Sci. 38:854.

Neathery, M.W. et al. 1972. Proc. Soc. Exp. Biol. Med. 139:953.

Neathery, M.W. et al. 1973. J. Dairy Sci. 56:98,212,1526; J. Animal Sci. 37:848.

Nielsen, F.H., R.P. Dowdy and Z.Z. Ziporin. 1970. J. Nutr. 100:903.

O'Dell, B.L., J.M. Yohe and J.E. Savage. 1964. Poultry Sci. 43:415.

Ott, E.A., W.H. Smith, M. Stob and W.M. Beeson. 1964. J. Nutr. 82:41.

Ott, E.A. et al. 1965. J. Animal Sci. 24:735.

Ott, E.A. et al. 1966. J. Animal Sci. 25:414,419,424,432.

Parry, W.H. 1977. Nutr. Metab. 21 (suppl. 1):48.

Pate, F.M. et al. 1970. J. Nutr. 100:1259.

Perry, T.W. et al. 1968. J. Animal Sci. 27:1674.

Powell, G.W., W.J. Miller and D.M. Blackmon. 1967. J. Nutr. 93:203.

Powell, G.W., W.J. Miller, J.D. Morton and C.M. Clifton. 1964. J. Nutr. 84:205.

Pierson, R.E. 1966. J. Amer. Vet. Med. Assoc. 149:1279.

Pitts, W.J. et al. 1966. J. Dairy Sci. 49:995.

Quarterman, J., F.A. Jackson and J.N. Morrison. 1976. Life Sci. 19:979.

Roth, P. and M. Kirchgessner. 1974. In: Trace Element Metabolism in Animals-2. University Park Press, Baltimore.

Rickard, B.F. 1975. N.Z. Vet. J. 23:41.

Roberts, K.R. et al. 1973. Proc. Soc. Exp. Biol. Med. 144:906.

Schwarz, F.J. and M. Kirchgessner. 1978. Z. Lebensm. Unters. Forsch. 166:6.

Singh, K. and R.K. Mehta. 1975. Indian J. Exp. Biol. 13:496.

Smith, B.L. 1977. N.Z. Vet. J. 25:310.

Smith, B.L., G.W. Reynolds and P.P. Embling. 1977. N.Z. J. Expt. Agr. 5:261.

Somers, M. and E.J. Underwood. 1969. Aust. J. Agr. Res. 20:899.

Spais, A.G. and A.A. Papasteriadis. 1974. In: Trace Element Metabolism in Animals-2. University Park Press, Baltimore.

Stake, P.E., W.J. Miller and R.P. Gentry. 1973. Proc. Soc. Expt. Biol. Med. 142:494.

Stake, P.E. et al. 1974. J. Nutr. 104:1279.

Stake, P.E. et al. 1975. J. Animal Sci. 40:132; J. Dairy Sci. 58:78.

Tam, S.W., K.E. Wilber and F.W. Wagner. 1976. Biochem. Biophys. Res. Comm. 72:302.

Tucker, H.E. and W.D. Salmon. 1955. Proc. Soc. Expt. Biol. Med. 88:613.

Underwood, E.J. 1977. Trace Elements in Human and Animal Nutrition. 4th ed. Academic Press, NY.

Underwood, E.J. and M. Somers. 1969. Aust. J. Agr. Res. 20:889.

Vallee, B.L. 1962. In: Mineral Metabolism, Vol. 2, part B. Academic Press, NY.

Wegner, T.N., D.E. Ray, C.D. Lox and G.H. Stott. 1973. J. Dairy Sci. 56:748.

Chapter 6 - Lipid Utilization and Requirements

Over the years a considerable amount of information has been accumulated on utilization of lipids by ruminants. Rumen metabolism, digestion and absorption, transport from the GI tract to other tissues, tissue components and tissue metabolism and secretion by the mammary gland have been studied. Recent reviews on some of these topics include several in the books edited by Phillipson (1970) and by McDonald and Warner (1975) and a review by Garton (1977). Other reviews on specific topics will be mentioned from time to time.

This chapter must be quite selective in the material to be covered because of the large amount of literature. Only slight reference is made to topics dealing with cellular metabolism and lipid synthesis and the enzymes involved, since this information seems more appropriate in biochemistry texts.

DIETARY LIPIDS

Since grass and other plants (forbs, browse, harvested crops) make up a high percentage of the diet of most ruminant animals, the lipid content is of interest. The lipid content of forage leaf tissues ranges from 3-10% of dry weight and most of it is located in the chloroplasts. The important lipid classes are mono- and diglyactosyldiglycerides, sulpholipids, and phosphatidylglycerols. In alfalfa and perennial ryegrass these three lipid classes are partitioned as shown: alfalfa, 40, 51 and 7% (Kuiper, 1970); ryegrass, 23, 70 and 7% (Roughan and Batt, 1968).

Lipid content may vary with stage of growth, plant species, and other factors. Fatty acid composition also varies considerably between species. Linolenic acid (C18:3) usually is the major component followed by C16:0 and C18:2. These three acids make up 70-80% of the fatty acids in some grasses, but C18:3 by itself may account for 60-75% of total fatty acids (Hawke, 1973). Leaf lipids may provide as much as 225-360 g/day of fatty acids for an animal consuming 9 kg of grass (dry basis) with a lipid content of 5-8% (Hawke, 1973).

The surface of the leaf of forage plants is covered with waxes and other compounds usually comprised of hydrocarbons, esters of long chain alcohols and minor amounts of other components. The leaf waxes make up <1% of dry matter in most plants. Although the waxes are important to the plant, they are presumed to be of no use to animals.

Volatile oils are present in high concentrations in some plant species (sage, peppermint, etc.). Their value to the animal remains in question. Other lipids make up very minor amounts of herbage or browse. Silages retain most of the original plant lipid and appreciable amounts of volatile fatty acids may be added by fermentation.

With regard to other dietary sources, the amount of lipids in grains and other concentrates varies considerably depending on the nature of processing to which the feeds have been exposed. The seed oils are primarily triglycerides with high concentrations of unsaturated C18 acids. Volatile fatty acids are found in low amounts in a number of feed ingredients, particularly in instances where propionic acid or mixtures of acids have been used as preservatives for high-moisture feeds. Feeding fats are used in many animal rations and are often added to fattening rations for cattle, occasionally to rations for lactating dairy cows, and they are used in all milk replacers.

RUMEN METABOLISM

Details of rumen metabolism of dietary lipids have been reviewed in Ch. 14 of Vol. 1, thus only a brief recapitulation will be given here. Most dietary lipids, whether galactosyl esters, triglycerides, phospholipids, etc., are hydrolyzed by rumen microorganisms at a relatively rapid rate to produce free fatty acids and glycerol or other moieties, depending on the particular lipid. An exception to this statement occurs if added dietary fat is in sufficient supply to "saturate" the system; then more of the lipids may pass into the lower GI tract without being hydrolyzed.

Rumen microorganisms may bring about a number of alterations to long-chain unsaturated fatty acids following hydrolysis to free fatty acids. A relatively rapid saturation occurs with the result that a high percentage of the double bonds are saturated (biohydrogenated). However, complete biohydrogenation does not normally occur. In the process a variety of isomers are produced. Nearly all plant unsaturated fatty acids have the *cis* configuration between unsaturated carbon atoms. Rumen microorganisms produce a variety of *trans* isomers of which some may be hydrogenated eventually, but also many are absorbed and either deposited in the tissues or given off in milk fat. Positional isomers (where migration of the double bond occurs) are also produced.

Rumen microorganisms synthesize a moderate amount of long-chain fatty acids with odd lengths (13, 15, 17 carbon atoms) which originate from volatile fatty acids such as propionic or valeric acids. Branched-chain acids are also produced which originate from isobutyric or isovaleric acids. Small amounts of keto-acids, cyclopropane acids, or aldehydes are also produced.

The amount of fat contained in and produced by rumen microorganisms is not well documented. In one study lipid (primarily free fatty acids) content of bacteria ranged from 5.4-8.8% and that in protozoa (primarily phospholipids) was 9.6% of dry matter (Kurilov et al, 1976). In a recent paper Czerkawski (1976) gives lipid composition of protozoa, large bacterial species and small bacterial species on a carbohydrate-free basis and when animals were fed three different rations and sampled before and after feeding. The lipid content of protozoa did not vary greatly with conditions of feeding and diet. In large and small bacteria the amounts of lipid increased with the amount of concentrate in the rations. If a certain amount of liberty is taken with Czerkawski's data and assuming a distribution of microbial protoplasm of 1:3:5 for large bacteria, small bacteria and protozoa as suggested by the author, the mean lipid composition was 15.6% of dry weight. Composition of the total lipids in rumen microorganisms after feeding was (weighted mean): phospholipids and other complex lipids, 36.3%; diglycerides, 1.5 %; free fatty acids, 58.4%; and sterol esters, 3.6%.

A number of reports (Ch. 14, Vol. 1) show that there is a net synthesis of long-chain fatty acids in the rumen and/or secretion into the stomach. Other papers giving data on this topic include those of Hogan (1973) and Outen et al (1974). With sheep fed subterranean clover Hogan calculated that the amount of long-chain acids passing into the small intestine was 127% of consump-

tion. With sheep fed dried grass, Outen et al found that total fatty acids leaving the stomach were almost twice the amount in the diet. Thus, it is evident that either an appreciable amount of synthesis occurs in the rumen or that some synthesis occurs along with secretion into the stomach.

ABSORPTION FROM THE GUT

There is some secretion into the small intestine via bile (Heath and Hill, 1969); most of which comes from phospholipids containing a high proportion of C18:2 (Lennox et al, 1968). The majority of fatty acids absorbed from the small intestine is accounted for by C18:0. In sheep fed clover hay, Hogan (1973) calculated that ca. 5-6 g of C18:1 and 5-6 g of 18:2 + 18:3 were absorbed from the small intestine when the total disappearance was 38 g of fatty acids. Outen et al (1974) calculated that the C18 unsaturated acids accounted for ca. 21% of long-chain acids absorbed in sheep fed ground or chopped dried grass.

Studies with sheep having re-entrant cannulas between the abomasum and duodenum show that >70% of the fatty acids entering the duodenum were unesterified (Table 6-1; Lennox et al, 1968); they are unionized and are not bound to proteins but are adsorbed on particulate matter in the gut. The remaining lipid was esterified and about 50% was phospholipid; about 3 g of phospholipid enter the duodenum of the sheep daily. Nearly all of the esterified lipid is found in rumen microorganisms (Garton, 1977). Bile salts and phospholipids solubilize the adsorbed fatty acids resulting in micell formation from which the fatty acids are then absorbed. Further along the small

Table 6-1. Source of fatty acids by lipid class (% of total weight) in the GI tract of sheep.[a]

Lipid class	Source of digesta		
	Rumen	Aboma-sum	Upper jejenum
Free fatty acids	71.5	77.1	53.4
Neutral lipids	23.6	19.7	22.1
Phospholipids	4.9	3.2	24.5

[a] From Lennox et al (1968)

intestine a lower percentage may be free acids (Table 6-1), presumably because of the influx of bile lipids (Garton, 1977).

In pre-ruminants some hydrolysis of triglycerides occurs in the abomasum (Felinski and Toullec, 1973; Flatlandsmo, 1973), probably because of hydrolysis by pregastric esterase secreted in saliva. However a much higher percentage of the fatty acids in the abomasum are esterified compared to ruminant animals (Table 6-2). Digestion in pre-ruminants is similar to monogastric animals in that lipid digestion occurs in a biphasic medium, namely an oil phase and a micellar phase. Digestion occurs as a result of transfer of fatty acids from the esterified oily phase to the soluble phase which results from action of pancreatic lipase, bile salts and bile phospholipids. In ruminant animals there is a two phase system—the insoluble particulate phase and the micellar phase. Pancreatic lipase produces lysolecithin (a detergent) from bile phospholipid. Lysolecithin solubilizes the fatty acids on particulate matter (Leat and Harrison, 1975).

Table 6-2. Lipids in abomasal and duodenal contents of the suckling lamb.[a]

| Lipid class | Amount, mM | |
	Abomasum, pH 3.8	Duodenum, pH 5.8
Triglycerides	28.0	3.0
1:2 diglycerides	5.1	1.8
1:3 diglycerides	22.8	1.0
Monoglycerides	11.2	3.2
Free fatty acids	72.8	95.2

[a] From Leat and Harrison (1975)

Studies with ^{14}C-labeled fatty acids or triglycerides show that they are absorbed to the extent of 85-90%. Other studies with animals with cannulas in the gut show that most of the absorption occurs in the upper half of the small intestine (Lennox and Garton, 1968; Sutton et al, 1970). However, absorption apparently occurs in the lower gut. For example, Hogan's (1973) data show the disappearance of 59% (of acids entering the duodenum) occurred between the duodenum and end of the ileum and 11% in the large gut. Aliev and Kafarov (1974) calculated that in cattle 42% of dietary phospholipids were absorbed in the small intestine and 15% in the large intestine. Comparable values for buffalo were 29% in both sections of the gut. In another example when corn oil was infused into the abomasum, 56% was digested and from 34-49% when infused into the cecum (Warner et al, 1972). Leat and Harrison (1975) point out that most of the fatty acids are absorbed from an area of the gut where the pH is still distinctly acid (pH 3-6), as contrasted to monogastric species where absorption usually occurs in a neutral or slightly acid medium.

Fatty acids in micellar solution are incorporated into segments of sheep intestine (in vitro) at a rate of up to 300 nmol/100 mg of intestinal tissue. Speed of uptake decreases with increasing chain length and increasing saturation. Unsaturated acids with trans bonds and branched-chain acids are effectively absorbed (Garton, 1977). After uptake by the intestinal cells, the lipids are resynthesized into normal blood lipids. The major pathway of resynthesis of triglycerides is the α-glycerophosphate pathway. Synthesis from the monoglyceride pathway appears to be of minor importance, although it can occur (Leat and Harrison, 1975).

LYMPH LIPIDS

The lymphatic system is important in absorption and transport of lipids. In one example where ^{14}C-labeled palmitic, stearic and oleic acids were injected into the duodenum, 71, 60 and 80%, respectively, were recovered in lymph (Harrison and Leat, 1972), values which were believed to be minimal. Absorption of free fatty acids is rapid and maximum activity from labeled acids occurred 1-1.5 hr after injections into the duodenum. Absorption also favors acids with shorter chain length and unsaturated structures as with intestinal absorption. Most of the palmitic, stearic and monoenoic acids are resynthesized into triglycerides, while phospholipids contain most of the C18:2 and C18:3 acids. The composition of lymph lipids is illustrated in Table 6-3.

Chylomicron particle size (750 Å) is smaller than intestinal particles of non-ruminants (1000-5000 Å). Triglyceride content is lower, and phospholipid (which comprises surface coating material) is higher. The small particle size reflects both the low fat content of ruminant diets and the continuous nature of absorption. Thus, the absence of typical intestinal chylomicrons

Table 6-3 Composition of thoracic duct lymph lipids.

Lipid Class	Sheep[a]		Cow[b]	
	mg/dl	%	mg/dl	%
Triglyceride	659	67.3	772	67.9
Diglyceride	12.9	1.3	--	--
Cholesteryl ester	55.7	5.7	89.8	7.9
Free cholesterol	22.3	2.2	21.6	1.9
Phospholipid	219	22.4	225	19.8
Non-esterified fatty acid	8.5	.9	17.1	1.5

[a] Leat and Harrison (1974)
[b] Hartmann and Lascelles (1966)

(1000-5000 Å diameter) from ruminant lymph and plasma is explained. Typical chylomicrons are readily demonstrated in lymph and blood of suckling preruminants, where fat may constitute 50% of the calories.

Triglyceride fatty acids in lymph are much more saturated than diet fatty acids (Table 6-4), a reflection of the biohydrogenating activity of the rumen microorganisms. The distribution of linoleic acid among the lipid classes is of particular significance. Although phospholipid is only 20% of the total lipid, it contains half of the essential fatty acid, reflecting the specificity of acyl-CoA transferase in the gut mucosa.

Generally, feeding of fat increases lipid concentration and rate of lymph flow (Shannon and Lascelles, 1967; Beitz et al, 1971). In calves concentration of neutral lipid (predominantly triglyceride) is 1-3% and makes up 80% of the total lipid; phospholipid is 10-12% of total lipid (Shannon and Lascelles, 1967). Lymph flow shows a diurnal pattern with once-a-day feeding of calves, but not with twice-a-day (Shannon and Lascelles, 1967). This may reflect trapping of lipid by the firm casein curd formed in the abomasum, since Gooden et al (1971) showed much more rapid lipid output in lymph of calves fed a casein-free diet than in those fed milk. Hartmann et al (1966) reported greater increases in total output of lymph lipid than in lymph flow of cows fed up to 480 g safflower oil. Thus, concentration of lipid in the lymph increased.

LIPID TRANSPORT

Lipids are transported in lymph as chylomicrons (25%) and as lipoprotein (75%) designated as very low density lipoprotein (VLDL). The chylomicrons are also high in triglycerides and have a central core of triglycerides, cholesterol ester and some free cholesterol, and the whole is covered with a thin coating of hydrophilic lipoprotein (Allen, 1976).

In blood, lipids are transported as chylomicrons, lipoproteins designated as VLDL, low density (LDL) or high density (HDL) and as non-esterified fatty acids which are a complex of fatty acids and albumin. Proportions vary according to lipid intake and metabolic activity of the animal. In the blood of adult sheep HDL accounts for ca. 70% of the lipids, LDL account for ca. 17% and VLDL for <5% although the VLDL makes up more of the total lipid (9-23% in suckling lambs; Leat and Harrison, 1975). Triglycerides of VLDL and chylomicrons are transported to extrahepatic tissues where they are hydrolyzed by lipoprotein lipase and the liberated fatty acids are taken up by the tissues and are either incorporated into the tissues or oxidized as an energy source. Glycerol released by lipolytic activity is utilized by the liver for lipid synthesis or gluconeogenesis. The LDL appear to be metabolic products of VLDL and chylomicrons degradation in the

Table 6-4. Fatty acid composition of diet and lymph lipid classes[a].

Lipid class	Fatty acid, % of total weight					
	16:0	18:0	18:1	18:2	18:3	20:4
Total diet lipid	25.9	3.1	16.1	29.2	9.2	0
Lymph						
Triglyceride	30.7	38.6	15.1	1.9	0.5	trace
Cholesteryl ester	14.1	26.5	31.4	16.3	2.2	1.0
Phospholipid	21.5	22.4	16.4	23.9	4.6	5.3
Nonesterified fatty acid	17.3	20.7	36.6	9.0	3.9	0.4

[a] Leat and Harrison (1974)

plasma and they contain high levels of cholesterol esters and phospholipids. The HDL are synthesized by the liver and in plasma and contain even more cholesterol esters and phospholipid than LDL (Raphael et al, 1973). The half life of chylomicrons and VLDL is short, ranging from 1.5-2.5 and 7-11 min., respectively, as contrasted to a much longer half life for LDL of 60-360 min. (Glascock and Welch, 1974; Palmquist and Mattos, 1977). Although few data are available on protein content of ruminant lipoproteins, it is ca. 3% of chylomicrons, 10% of VLDL, 20% of LDL and 45% of HDL (Hartmann et al, 1966; Leat et al, 1976).

The phospholipid content of ruminant intestinal lipoprotein is more than double that of human chylomicrons (Leat and Harrison, 1974). It is interesting to note that the ratio of free/esterified cholesterol in ruminants is ca. 4, compared to ca. 1 in humans. This probably reflects the smaller particle size and relatively greater surface area of ruminant lipoproteins, as free cholesterol is found at the surface of the particle.

Hepatic synthesis of VLDL (endogenous triglyceride carrier) is very similar to intestinal synthesis, except that the particles are smaller, due to lower triglyceride content. The source of fatty acids for triglyceride synthesis is either synthesis by the liver or from the blood free fatty acid pool. Synthesis of fatty acids in ruminant liver is not great (Ballard et al, 1969), so that its contribution to VLDL triglyceride fatty acid is probably small. Thus VLDL synthesis is mainly dependent upon plasma fatty acid concentration and availability of glycerol (from glucose) for esterification. Contribution of liver VLDL synthesis in ruminants to total circulating triglyceride has not been quantitated.

METABOLISM OF LIPOPROTEINS

The triglycerides of lipoproteins may be taken up by all tissues of the body, depending upon the nutritional and physiological state. Liver does not take up chylomicrons or VLDL until they have been metabolized extensively by other tissues.

The majority of interest in metabolism of lipoproteins in ruminants has centered in their utilization for milk fat synthesis. The combination of low fat diet, continuous absorption and rapid removal rate explains the

nearly undetectable levels of chylomicron triglyceride in ruminants (Palmquist, 1976). Furthermore, the ratio of LDL removal/VLDL removal explains the much higher concentration of LDL than VLDL in ruminants.

Although plasma concentrations of chylomicrons and VLDL are extremely low in lactating cows (Wendlandt and Davis, 1973), they are the predominant precursors of long-chain fatty acids in milk fat. Glascock and Welch (1974) concluded on the basis of radioisotope data that all lipoproteins of density <1.039 g/ml contributed equally to milk fat.

The relative contribution of dietary chylomicron (exogenous) and liver VLDL (endogenous) lipoproteins to milk fatty acids has not been established with certainty. Palmquist and Mattos (1977) estimated that 88% of milk long-chain fatty acids were of exogenous origin in 5 mid-lactation cows. This value would likely be reduced in early lactation when cows were mobilizing tissue fat to meet energy demands and in late lactation when increased proportions of exogenous fat would be stored in adipose tissues.

Serum NEFA arise predominantly from mobilization of adipose triglyceride fatty acids; however, up to one third of serum NEFA may be obtained from chylomicrons and VLDL triglyceride during active lipolysis by lipoprotein lipase (Scow et al, 1975). NEFA may be taken up and oxidized by all tissues of the body except brain and testes (Lindsay, 1975). Liver is very active in metabolism of serum NEFA, esterifying them into VLDL triglyceride in the fed state and oxidizing them to ketone bodies in the fasting condition. NEFA have the highest turnover (shortest half life) of all the plasma lipids.

Factors Affecting Plasma Lipids

The largest single factor affecting total lipoprotein concentration in preruminant and ruminant animals appears to be the quantity of dietary fat. Plasma lipid content of ruminants at maintenance feed intake is relatively low (<100 mg/dl, Nelson, 1973). Leat et al (1976) showed the highest lipoprotein concentration occurred in 21-28 day-old lambs, corresponding to maximum milk intake. They reported that HDL transported 52% of cholesterol, 73% of cholesteryl esters, 66% of phospholipid and 4% of the triglyceride in sheep plasma. Similar relationships can be computed from the data of Raphael et al (1973) for lactating cows. As dietary fat increases, the LDL cholesterol and phospholipid concentration increases dramatically (Bitman et al, 1973; Scott and Cook, 1975).

Plasma total lipid increases at onset of lactation in dairy cows with concentration trends following total feed intake (Raphael et al, 1973). Of particular significance, VLDL (the primary transporter of triglyceride) increased during the dry period. Although dietary intake of fat would be low during this time (confirmed by lower plasma total lipid), an increase in VLDL would be explained by absence of mammary uptake. In kinetic terms input decreased moderately and output decreased extensively, causing an increase in VLDL pool size.

All plasma lipid classes (triglyceride, cholesterol, phospholipid) except NEFA are decreased in ketosis. This is probably due to decreased feed intake and impaired mobilization of lipoproteins from the liver (Ch. 12).

Diets high in forage (high production of 18:3) increase 18:3 content of plasma cholesteryl esters and phospholipids (Moore et al, 1968). A diet of grass silage fed to steers for three months increased plasma phytanic acid (3,7,11,15-tetramethylhexadecanoic acid) from normal values of 1% to 8% of the total fatty acids. In lactating cows it increased to 13%. In both cows and steers phytanic acid was a substantial proportion of triglyceride and phospholipid fatty acids; but only traces (<1%) were found in cholesteryl esters, milk fat or tissue lipids (Lough, 1977). Phytanic acid is a metabolite of the isoprenoid alcohol, phytol, which represents about 30% of the chlorophyll content of forage (Body, 1977).

The fatty acid composition of maternal and neonatal plasma are compared in Table 6-5. The most striking differences are seen in the small quantities of polyunsaturated (18:2 and 18:3) fatty acids in plasma of the newborn. This is due apparently to low proportions of these fatty acids in the maternal NEFA fraction (see section on Essential Fatty Acids). Neonatal plasma has increased quantities of 16:0, 16:1, and 18:1, which can be synthesized in the fetal tissues.

TISSUE METABOLISM

This is a very complex topic and not one particularly suited to this book. Thus, only a very brief review will be given with some emphasis on how ruminant animals differ from non-ruminant species. An overall review has been presented by Allen (1976) and more specific reviews have been published by Bauman and Davis (1975), Bauman (1976) and Volpe and Vagelos (1976).

Ruminant animals are capable of synthesizing large quantities of long chain fatty acids. Fatty acid synthesis is minimal in liver but may be very active in adipose and mammary tissues. In non-ruminants the pre-

Table 6-5. Percentage composition of the total fatty acids of maternal and newborn blood plasma [a].

Fatty Acid	Fatty acid composition, weight %							
	Sow	Pig	Cow	Calf	Doe	Kid	Ewe	Lamb
14:0	1.3	2.1	1.5	1.5	1.5	2.2	1.2	1.8
16:0	19.4	23.1	11.5	32.3	17.5	24.1	16.7	22.5
16:1	4.2	10.5	3.1	11.0	2.9	13.0	3.3	8.4
18:0	14.0	11.8	9.5	10.2	12.7	6.8	12.2	9.3
18:1	18.7	36.9	15.4	39.5	27.6	49.5	28.3	50.0
18:2	34.2	5.5	24.9	2.0	29.5	0.5	26.1	0.9
18:3	1.3	--	30.3	0.5	3.4	--	4.6	0.5
20:3	--	--	--	--	--	1.4	--	2.0
20:4	1.8	6.3	1.0	1.2	3.0	0.5	2.1	1.2
Triene/ Tetraene	--	--	--	--	--	2.8	--	1.7

[a] Leat (1966)

dominant dietary source of acetyl-CoA (the immediate precursor for fatty acid synthesis) is glucose. In ruminants most of the glucose in the diet is fermented to volatile fatty acids in the rumen and acetate and β-hydroxyl-butyrate (β-HBA) are the precursors for fat synthesis. The first step in synthesis of fatty acids is the carboxylation of acetyl-CoA to form malonyl-CoA. Studies with mammary gland tissue show that butyrate is the preferred primer for fatty acid synthesis. This is particularly significant to ruminants as rather large quantities of βHBA are available which originate from metabolism of butyrate by the ruminal wall. In the absence of butyrate or βHBA, butyrate is synthesized by the reversal of the β-oxidation pathway, a pathway which does not utilize malonyl-CoA but proceeds by way of crotonyl-CoA.

Synthesis of fatty acid requires large amounts of NADPH. In non-ruminants NADPH is generated from the pentose cycle and the malate transhydrogenation cycle. The latter cycle has negligible activity in ruminants. Instead, in ruminants NADPH is generated from the pentose cycle and by cystolic NADP-isocitrate dehydrogenase. The latter enzyme has the advantage of generating NADPH from oxidation of acetate and provides a minimum of one-fourth of the NADPH necessary to support lipogenesis (Bauman, 1976); the remaining three-fourths is derived from the pentose cycle. Thus, the fatty acid synthesis in ruminants differs from non-ruminants in that the acetyl units and some of the NADPH are derived from different sources, allowing the animal to conserve glucose for other uses.

Microorganisms in the rumen and gut are relatively efficient in saturating long chain unsaturated acids. However, enzymes are present in the intestinal mucosa which can desaturate C18:0 to C18:1, and it is likely that similar enzymes are present in adipose and mammary tissues (Kinsella, 1972; Seifreid and Gaylor, 1976).

Liver Metabolism

As indicated previously, lipogenic activity in ruminant liver is relatively low. The principal activity appears to be incorporation of free cholesterol, cholesteryl esters, triglycerides and phospholipids into VLDL for export and to fatty acid oxidation. Some synthesis of cholesterol occurs, but activity is less than that in intestinal or adipose tissue (Liepa et al, 1978). VLDL synthesis is dependent upon the rate of triglyceride synthesis which is, in turn, dependent on availability of long chain fatty acids. It is probable that liver VLDL synthesis contributes relatively more to total triglyceride turnover in high producing cows during early than during late lactation. During this time high producing cows are incapable of consuming sufficient energy to maintain body weight and large amounts of adipose tissue are mobilized and utilized, at least in part, for milk fat synthesis. Such conditions do not usually occur in non-lactating animals so that liver VLDL synthesis is probably always low in them.

When energy expenditure exceeds intake, long chain fatty acids are mobilized from adipose tissues as long as there are reserves. Under these conditions plasma concentrations may increase from normal levels of ca. 100-400 to levels exceeding 1000-1500 μmol/liter. Liver takes up and oxidizes these acids in direct proportion to plasma concentration (Lindsay, 1975). In some cases fatty acid oxidation may exceed the capacity of the liver to oxidize the NADH and acetyl-CoA resulting from fatty acid oxidation. When this occurs, the acetyl-CoA is shunted into acetoacetate and βHBA. Free acetate may also be released from the liver (Lindsay, 1975). These ketones are not utilized by liver tissues because the required mechanisms are not present. Rather, utilization occurs in extrahepatic tissues (Bush and Milligan, 1971; Williamson et al, 1971) and this may result in production of significant amounts of acetate in fed animals (Bergman and Wolff, 1971).

Studies with radioisotopes show that appreciable amounts of acetate may be produced by non-hepatic tissues and that quantities produced increased in fasted animals (Annison and White, 1962). More recent data on labeled palmitic acid demonstrated that up to 65% of plasma acetate was derived from fatty acid oxidation in fasted animals but <10% in fed animals, and the amounts decreased with increasing plane of nutrition (Palmquist, 1972).

Adipose Tissue Metabolism

Adipose tissue activity takes up fatty acids from plasma lipoprotein triglycerides, and it is the most active site of fatty acid synthesis in non-lactating ruminant animals (Ingle et al, 1972). Precursors for synthesis are acetate, lactate, and possibly βHBA (Bauman, 1976). Adipose tissue also is an active site of cholesterol synthesis. Synthesis of fat in adipose tissues is affected by increased glucose and insulin levels (Bauman, 1976); thus high starch diets, which increase rumen propionate and lead to increased blood glucose, tend to result in increased fat deposition in the tissues and reduced milk fat production (see later sections).

Mobilization of fatty acids from adipose tissues is stimulated by action of a number of hormones acting on hormone sensitive lipase. Studies with dairy cows have shown that lipolytic activity of adipose tissue was higher in lactating than in non-lactating cows (Yang and Baldwin, 1973). However, the small response of ruminants to lipolytic hormones as well as the negligible increase in rate of fatty acids synthesis after feeding have lead Bauman (1976) to conclude that these small changes are related to the nature of the ruminant diet and to digestion, which result in a relatively constant supply of nutrients being supplied to the tissues.

Milk Fat

Milk fat is characterized by a high concentration of short-chain fatty acids (Table 6-5) which serves to maintain the fat in a fluid state at body temperature. Synthesis of milk fatty acids of 4-16 carbon atoms occurs in the mammary gland; 16-carbon fatty acids may be synthesized there or be of blood origin, but all 18-carbon and longer acids are taken from the blood and may be derived from the diet or from adipose tissues. There is little evidence for significant chain lengthening in the mammary gland. Various investigators have suggested that the relative concentrations of malonyl-CoA and acetyl-CoA may affect the characteristics of milk fat (Smith and Dils, 1966; Bartley et al, 1967); i.e., that higher ratios of malonyl-CoA would promote longer chains. Much additional information is available on milk fat synthesis, but it is not unique to ruminants and will not be discussed here.

FACTORS AFFECTING ADIPOSE TISSUES

Although triglycerides, phospholipids and other lipids occur in most tissues, adipose tissue is concentrated in certain areas such as subcutaneous, inter- and intramuscular spaces, around the viscera, as a major part of bone marrow and on the walls of the thoracic and abdominal cavities. Preferential sites of deposition generally are in the order of the

Table 6-6. Fatty acid content (% of weight of methyl esters) of butter samples [a].

Acid	%	Acid [b]	%
4	4.0-4.2	17br	0.6
6	2.5-2.7	18br	0.0-0.1
8	1.4-1.6	18	9.7-10.0
10	3.0-3.3	t18:1	1.8
12	3.2-3.4	c18:1	22.0-22.5
14br	0.1-0.2	ct18:2	0.0-0.2
14	10.3-10.6	cc18:2	3.7-4.1
t14:1	0.0-0.1	18:3	tr-0.1
c14:1	1.2-1.5	18:3	1.0-1.1
15br	0.6-0.7	20	0.1-0.2
15	1.2-1.3	c20:1	0.0-0.1
16br	0.3-0.4	20:3	0.1-0.2
16	27.2-28.1	20:4	0.1-0.2
c16:1	2.4-2.6		

[a] From Smith et al (1978)
[b] t = trans; c = cis

viscera and around the kidney, intermuscular fat, subcutaneous fat and last in intramuscular deposits (marbling). In starved animals the last visible fat is found around the kidney and on the heart. Bone marrow fat is usually the last to be depleted. Many different factors affect the amount or fatty acid composition of adipose tissues (Oltjen and Dinius, 1975). These will be reviewed briefly.

Non-Dietary Factors

It has been known for many years that fat from different species varies in composition. Comparative values for the pig and several ruminant species are given in Table 6-7. In ruminants >80% of the fatty acids in triglycerides of subcutaneous fat is made up of 14:0, 16:0, 18:0 and 18:1 acids. Other acids are found in lesser amounts as shown in Table 6-8. Cis and trans unsaturated acids are both present as well as very small amounts of other isomers (Duncan et al, 1974). Note (Table 6-7) that ruminants differ from the pig in that the pig has less 18:0, more 18:1 and much more 18:2. As a general rule, the fat of ruminants is much less subject to variation in composition than that of monogastric species because of the stabilizing effect of rumen fermentation which results in a rather stable supply (quantity and quality) being provided to the tissues.

Table 6-7. Fatty acid composition of fats from different species, molar % [a].

Fatty acid	Butter	Beef	Sheep	Deer	Camel	Pig
Myristic (14:0)	11	4	5	3	5	1
Palmitic (16:0)	29	30	27	24	31	28
Palmitoleic (16:1)	5	5	3	3	4	3
Stearic (18:0)	9	25	27	31	31	15
Oleic (18:1)	27	35	35	36	28	42
Linoleic (18:2)	4	1	2	2	1	9
Linolenic (18:3)	tr	--	1	1	tr	2

[a] Mattson et al (1964)

There are also breed differences in deposition of fat. For example, Holsteins tend to have more internal fat, Herefords more subcutaneous fat and Angus more muscle fat (Hecker, 1973). Holsteins tend to have more unsaturated depot fats than Angus (Leat, 1977). However, there is little, if any, difference in fatty acid composition that can be attributed to genetic factors within breeds (Berry et al, 1966; Link et al, 1970; Rumsey et al, 1972).

Sex may have some slight effect on fatty acid composition. One example is illustrated in Table 6-8. Some reports suggest no differences related to sex (Clemens et al, 1973; Vesely, 1973) and others show minor differences (Cramer and Marchello, 1964, Roberts, 1966; Terrell et al, 1969). Heifers tend to produce fat that is more unsaturated than steers (Terrell et al, 1969). Castration of lambs results in some minor changes (Tichenor et al, 1970; Course et al, 1972). Hormones such as diethylstilbestrol may (Edwards et al, 1961) or may not (Church et al, 1967) result in any changes in fat composition.

The fatty acid composition of subcutaneous samples varies somewhat from site to site (Marchello and Cramer, 1963), and the percentage of unsaturated fatty acids in subcutaneous fat increases as the animals' weight, age and fatness increase (Waldeman et al, 1968; Link et al, 1970; Dryden et al, 1973; Clemens et al, 1974; Leat, 1977). In addition, the saturated fatty acids increase from external to internal sampling sites (Waldeman et al, 1968) and fatty acids tend to be more saturated in winter than in summer (Cramer and Marchello, 1964; Link et al, 1970).

Age and growth have a major effect on amount, distribution and quality of fat. For example, there is a complete absence of linoleic acid in the depot fat of the lamb at

Table 6-8. Effect of sex on fatty acid composition of subcutaneous adipose tissue [a].

Fatty acid [b]	Source	
	Steers	Heifers
8:0	.05	.06
9:0	.06	.08
10:0	.10	.12
11:0	.02	.02
12:0	.28	.34
13:0	.07	.08
14:0	8.48	9.24
14:1	3.92	4.80***
15:0	1.37	1.51
16:0	29.49	29.34
16:1	7.04	7.28
17:0	1.46	1.44
18:0	8.23	7.70
18:1	36.44	35.32
18:2	1.90	1.64**
18:3	.94	.88

[a] From Link et al (1970)

[b] Expressed as % of weight of total methyl esters

** Statistically different

176

birth although some unsaturated fatty acids are found in phospholipids (Noble et al, 1971). Fatty acid composition of the tissues in the pre-ruminant lamb as in monogastric species tends to be similar to dietary fat (Stokes and Walker, 1970; Noble et al, 1971). As the young ruminant develops, there is an increased deposition of 14:0, 18:2, 17:0 and 17:1 in depot triglycerides in addition to branched chain acids and trans 18:1 (Garton and Duncan, 1969). The effect of age on amount and distribution of fat in different depots is illustrated in Tables 6-9 and 6-10.

Leat et al (1977) have demonstrated the effect of the rumen on tissue fatty acids with the use of gnotobiotic lambs. No hydrogenation of dietary lipids occurred in the rumen and this was reflected in the virtual absence of trans acids in depot lipids. Also, the 18:0 content of perirenal fat was similar to that in newborn lambs.

Effect of Diet

Of the several dietary factors which affect fatty acid composition or fat deposition, the energy level fed to the animal has one of the more pronounced effects. This is illustrated in Fig. 6-1 using data from animals slaughtered at the same weights. Those animals fed a higher energy level had appreciably larger amounts of body fat, presumably because they were fed more energy over and above maintenance requirements. In sheep a reduced plane of nutrition results in increased 18:1 and reduced 18:0 (Bensadoun and Reid, 1965).

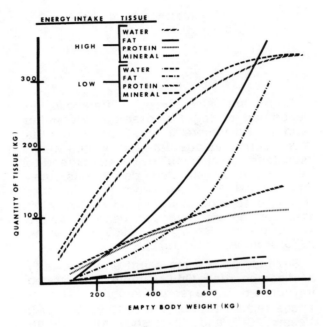

Figure 6-1. Quantity of tissue gain as function of energy intake and body size. Data adapted by Byers et al (1977) from Moulton and Trowbridge (1922).

Table 6-9. Distribution of carcass fat in ewe lambs at different ages, % of total [a].

Fat Depot	Age, days		
	120	197	225
Subcutaneous	48	42	42
Intermuscular	29	38	36
Intramuscular	11	7	8
Perirenal (kidney)	12	13	14
Total carcass fat, %	28	37	39

[a] Allen et al (1976)

Table 6-10 Composition of gain in cattle.[a]

Slaughter weight [b]	Carcass components, %		
	Water	Fat	Protein
273	59.1	17.2	19.2
458	49.9	29.4	16.8
642	45.9	34.8	15.9
685	41.3	40.2	15.4

[a] Adapted from Haecker (1920) by Marchello and Hale (1976)
[b] Initial weight 47-52 kg.

Some dietary components (other than added fats) have a minor effect on fatty acid composition of adipose tissues. In studies with young lambs, which received a lipid-free diet other than colostrum for a few days, Duncan and Garton (1971) observed that perinephric fat contained about 10% less stearic acid than that of those lambs receiving a more normal diet. In other studies it was shown that continued consumption of milk by calves increased the amount of 14:0, 18:2, 17:0 and 17:1 as compared to calves which were raised on solid feed from 60 to 100 kg; the latter animals had increased amounts of 18:0 and large amounts of trans 18:1 (Garton and Duncan, 1969).

A number of experiments have shown that addition of corn grain to a forage diet or increasing the amount of corn results in some changes in composition of the long-chain fatty acids (Bensadoun and Reid, 1965; Cabezas et al, 1965; Clemens et al, 1974; Ray et al, 1975). Wheat results in somewhat different composition than barley, and beet pulp also causes some modifications as compared to alfalfa hay or corn silage (Church et al, 1967). Corn silage apparently does not alter fatty acid composition (Skelley et al, 1973) but differences have been noted in lambs fed white clover as compared to perennial ryegrass (Cramer et al, 1967). Feeding an all-concentrate diet increased unsaturated acids as compared to an all-forage diet (Rumsey et al, 1972), and high grain diets have been shown to increase the amount of odd-numbered (15:0, 17:0, 17:1) and branched-chain acids in adipose tissue of lambs (Garton et al, 1972). Fattening cattle on barley vs hay results in minor differences in composition (Leat, 1977). Pelleted forages, steamed corn, or gelatinized corn (Shaw et al, 1960; Cramer et al, 1967; Clemens et al, 1974) also caused some minor changes and the antibiotic bacitracin resulted in increased deposition of unsaturated fatty acids (Cramer and Marchello, 1962). Added dietary fat also has a demonstrable effect on fat composition.

FACTORS AFFECTING MILK FAT

It has been recognized for years that the quantity of milk fat is affected by breed, species, age, stage of lactation, season of the year, fasting, and heat stress (Schultz, 1974). High grain diets usually increase 18:1 and decrease 16:0 and 18:0 (Davis and Brown, 1970; Qureshi et al, 1972) and short-chain acids may also be decreased (Storry et al, 1974). A change from a dry feed to pasture may result in decreased 18:2 and increased 18:3 (Boatman et al, 1965).

The most pronounced changes in quantity of milk fat related to diet result from feeding rations in which roughages make up less than one-third of the total dry matter, roughages and grain with low fiber content, finely ground and pelleted roughages, or heat-treated grains (Chalupa et al, 1970; Askew et al, 1971; Schultz, 1974). An example of the effect of feeding a diet with 75% pelleted concentrate is illustrated in Table 6-11. The cause in each case seems to

Table 6-11. Effect of a high concentrate diet on milk fat % [a].

Item	Prelim., 3 wk	Experimental, 8 wk	Post, 4 wk
Milk fat, %	3.3	1.7	3.3
Milk yield, kg	25.6	20.7	19.7
Rumen acids, molar %			
Acetic	55.9	37.2	59.6
Propionic	26.2	38.9	22.5
C2/C3 ratio	2.13	0.96	2.65

[a] From Bringe and Schultz (1969)
[b] Experimental diet was 75% pelleted concentrate, 25% alfalfa hay; before and after cows were fed corn silage, hay and grain.

be a reduction in acetic acid and an increase in the proportion of propionic acid in the rumen, although this change is mediated by different mechanisms. Pelleted or finely ground roughages appear to cause this change because of more rapid passage out of the rumen resulting in less fiber digestion and relatively less acetic acid production. Heat treated grain or high levels of grain result in the same change in rumen acids (see Ch. 16, Vol. 1). Added dietary fat also results in significant changes (see later section).

ESSENTIAL FATTY ACIDS

Linoleic (18:2) and linolenic (18:3) acids are considered to be essential in the diet since arachidonic is synthesized in the liver from 18:2 by chain elongation and desaturation. The essentiality of 18:3 is suggested since it has some growth promoting effects and causes some alteration in tissue levels of 20:3 as does 18:2. Payne (1978) suggests that 18:3 derivatives should also be considered essential.

For rats the requirement of essential fatty acids is estimated to be 0.5-2% of dietary GE. In sheep fed a diet of hay and concentrates (Leat and Harrison, 1972) the quantity of 18:2 and 18:3 acids entering the duodenum amounted to 0.3 and 0.1%, respectively. Deficiencies have been produced in pre-ruminant calves, lambs and kids by feeding purified diets devoid of or low in fat (Fig.

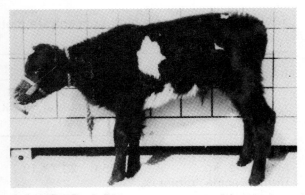

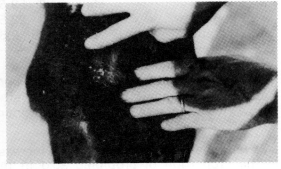

Figure 6-2. Male calf exhibiting fat deficiency symptoms at 56 days of age. Note the scaly dandruff. Other symptoms included loss of part of the hair over the back, shoulders and tail. From Lambert (1953). Courtesy of N.L. Jacobson, Iowa State University, Ames, Iowa.

6-2). In one case calves developed weakness and muscular twitches within 1 to 5 weeks and died unless a source of fat was supplied. Lambs or kids on a similar diet did not show symptoms other than loss of weight and death (Cunningham and Loosli, 1954). In another instance calves showed symptoms such as a marked reduction in growth, scaly dandruff, long dry hair, excessive loss of hair on the back, shoulders and tail, and diarrhea (Lambert et al, 1954). Symptoms were partially prevented by feeding butter oil or hydrogenated soybean oil plus lecithin. More recent information suggests that healthy calves could be raised on diets which provided as little as 0.01% of the caloric intake as 18:2. The low fat content of this diet (0.2%) resulted in reduced feed utilization but otherwise the calves were normal (Sklan et al, 1972).

Ruminants are born with very low reserves of 18:2 and 18:3, presumably a reflection of low placental transfer. However, significant amounts of C22 polyunsaturated acids (derived from 18:3) have been found in fetal tissues (Noble et al, 1971, 1972), particularly in brain tissues where fetal levels are comparable to adults (Payne, 1978). The young lamb (Noble et al, 1972) or calf (Payne, 1978) are very effective in retaining 18:2 in their tissues during the first few days of life; thus tissues attain levels comparable to adults at a fairly early age. In the adult animal intake of 18:3 is low compared to 18:2, but preferential uptake by the brain allows the maintenance of high levels of 22:6 (Payne, 1978). Gnotobiotic lambs (those reared without rumen microorganisms) appear to have a substantially higher requirement for 18:2 than normal lambs (Bruckner et al, 1977).

Older animals appear to be resistant to loss of 18:2 from their tissues (Palmquist et al, 1977). Adult (ruminating) animals are also efficient at absorbing 18:2. With the use of ^{14}C-labeled acid, Mattos and Palmquist (1977) found that one-third of dietary 18:2 escaped hydrogenation. Of that which was absorbed, half was secreted into milk fat, leaving 16% of dietary 18:2 available for uptake by the tissues. When uptake by the tissues was expressed in proportion to metabolic weight, lactating cows had available 225 mg of 18:2/kg BW $^{0.75}$. This compares to a requirement of 88 mg/kg BW $^{0.75}$ for rats. Lindsay and Leat (1977) have shown that C18:2 is incorporated into plasma phospholipids and cholesteryl esters to a much greater degree than C18:0. Furthermore, they have shown that C18:2 is less likely to be oxidized than C18:0 and, when animals were starved, other acids (C16:1, C18:0, C18:1) were preferentially mobilized compared to C18:2.

Long-term studies (70-90 weeks) with sheep and cattle on purified diets said to be almost lipid free indicated very little effect on performance. There were negligible effects on rumen microbes and rumen and blood lipids were lower than supplemented animals (Øltjen and Williams, 1974). Thus, it would appear that the ruminant animal has an adequate supply of essential fatty acids in most situations.

FAT AS A FEED INGREDIENT

Fats are now commonly used in several situations in ruminant rations. Relatively large amounts (% of diet) are used in most milk replacers and smaller amounts are often used in finishing rations for fattening cattle; occasionally, some fat is used in rations for lactating cows and sometimes in other situations.

A variety of fat sources are usually available. Most of the animal fats are classed as inedible (for human use). Beef tallow or animal fat (mixtures of animal sources) may be available from slaughterhouse waste, trimmings or boning operations. Feeding fats are also produced from rendering plants which process waste and dead animals. Mixtures of animal-vegetable fats are often used as well as hydrolyzed fats which are by-products of the soap industry, and used cooking fats are available in increasing quantities. Other fats such as lard, high grade tallows, and high quality seed oils (corn, safflower, soy, etc.) are usually too expensive to use in feed even though a considerable amount of research has been done with them. Based on a survey of 40 rendering plants in the USA, the raw material used for producing feeding fats was composed of (%): restaurant grease, 40; shop fat and bone, 21; packing house offal, 19; fallen animals (dead or sick), 9; poultry offal, 6; other materials (garbage grease, pigskin oil, etc.), 4. However, the ingredients from any particular rendering plant may be appreciably different (Boehme, 1978).

Although the type of fat may vary considerably depending on the source, usual specifications state that feeding fats shall contain not less than 90% total fatty acids, not more than 2.5% unsaponifiable matter and not more than 1% insoluble matter. Data on the 40 fat sources mentioned in the previous paragraph are shown in Table 6-12 to give the reader an idea of values characteristic of feeding fats. Quality is reflected by color, odor, rancidity, and water content as well as by the amount of non-fat materials such as foreign matter, hair, dirt, etc. Free fatty acids may make up a substantial percentage of total in some poor quality feeding fats although they may also make up 50% or more of high quality hydrolyzed animal-vegetable fats. Fats which are rancid, off flavor and unpalatable are not, of course, desirable feed ingredients. Most feeding fats have antioxidants added to prevent deterioration during storage or after addition to mixed rations.

Scott and co-workers (1970, 1971) developed procedures for protecting polyunsaturated fatty acids from hydrogenation in the rumen. Originally, oils such as linseed, soy or safflower were homogenated with casein, spray-dried and treated with formaldehyde. More recent modifications use a mixture of finely-ground whole soybeans or other

Table 6-12 Analyses of feed grade fat from 40 rendering plants.[a]

Component	Mean	Range
Moisture and volatiles, %	0.44	0.01-1.99
Insolubles, %	0.21	0.01-2.97
Unsaponifiables, %	0.68	0.24-3.48
Total, M, I, U, %	1.33	0.48-7.33
Free fatty acids, %	6.50	0.70-36.81
Capillary melting point, °C	39.8	27.8-45.3
F.A.C. color	25	11-45
A.O.M. stability		
<20 hr	23	
>20 hr	77	
Peroxide value at 20 hr	105.2	1.5-340

[a] Data provided by Boehme (1978).

high-oil seeds treated with alkali and formaldehyde. These processes create an oil core surrounded by protein. Formaldehyde treatment causes methylene (-CH-) bridges to be formed between amino acids. This cross-linked protein structure is not degraded to any degree in the rumen at pH 6-7. In the acid conditions of the abomasum (pH 2-3), the methylene bridges are broken and the oil is released to be digested and absorbed in the small intestine. However, excessive use of formaldehyde will result in very poor digestion in the gut. These protected fats can be used to increase the content of polyunsaturated fatty acids in milk or adipose tissues. At this time the application remains largely experimental and has not yet found much use in practical situations.

Another source of fat is the high-oil seeds such as soybean and cottonseed. These have found favor by dairymen for use with lactating cows. Prices paid for the seeds compared to normal feedstuffs determine whether or not it is feasible to use these seeds for feed. They are often called full-fat feeds in the trade.

Fats serve a number of useful purposes in ruminant rations. They are high in energy and can be used to increase ration energy density and they generally improve absorption of fat-soluble vitamins and other fat-soluble compounds. Fats are also useful to reduce dustiness and usually increase palatability when used in limited amounts.

Lubricating properties result in less wear and tear on milling equipment. In addition, fats result in some reduction in methane production in the rumen (see Ch. 14, Vol. 1). More specific effects will be discussed in later sections.

Digestibility of Added Fat

A considerable number of digestibility trials have been reported in the literature, but most of the recent information has been obtained with sheep or calves fed milk replacers. Examples are given in Table 6-13. Note that pre-ruminants digest fat more completely when given in a milk replacer than do ruminating animals given dry diets.

This appears to be a reflection of the physical form of the diet rather than age of the animal. Chiou and Jordan (1973) did not notice any affect of age (1-31 days) with lambs nor did Bjornstad and Hansen (1974) with calves. In preruminants the data suggest that digestibility of fats decreases with increasing chain length of the acids and that unsaturated fats are utilized more completely than saturated analogues (Flatlandsmo, 1972; Bjornstad and Hansen, 1974), although Bedo et al (1974) found that utilization of saturated fatty acids declined with age while that of unsaturated acids increased. This is difficult to verify since bacterial synthesis occurs and a high percentage of unsaturated

Table 6-13. Digestibility of different fat sources by ruminants.

Fat source	Milk replacers Lambs[a]	Milk replacers Calves[b]	Sheep with 40-50% roughage rations	Cattle with 20-25% roughage rations	Lactating dairy cows*
Butterfat		96.5			
Coconut oil	99.5				
Corn oil	97.2		78.3[c]		
Cottonseed oil	97.5		93.6[d]		
Herring oil			83.8[c]		
HEF**			74.2[c]		81[g]
Lard	89.1				
Olive oil	99.0				
Peanut oil	97.7				
Rapeseed oil	61.9			80.2[e]	
Saflower oil	98.5			41.3[f]	
Soybean oil	98.2		83.1[c]		
Sunflower oil				65.8[e]	
Tallow, beef			85.1[c]		
Tallow, animal	77.8	88.7		78.6[e]	
Tallow, Int.***		93.1			
Tallow, Int. + trimyristin and triolein		89.9			

* Corrected for fat excretion on low-fat basal diet.

**HEF = hydrolyzed animal/vegetable fat.

*** Interesterified fat prepared by hydrolyzing the fat and re-esterifying.

[a] Walker and Stokes (1970); [b] Hamilton and Raven (1972); [c] Andrews and Lewis (1970); [d] Shell et al (1978); [e] Roberts and McKirdy (1964); values were derived using crude fat extracts which include fecal soaps; [f] Cuitin et al (1975); [g] Palmquist and Conrad (1978); rations contained 42% concentrate and 2.5% added fat. When fat content was increased to 8.4%, the increased fat was only 56% digestible.

fatty acids are hydrogenated in the gut, even in pre-ruminants, so that balance data on individual acids are rather meaningless.

In older animals (ruminating) digestibility of saturated fats tends to be higher than in non-ruminants but digestibility of unsaturated fats tends to be lower (Andrews and Lewis, 1970). Hydrogenation or poor physical dispersion of fat in a dry diet reduces digestibility (Macleod and Buchanan-Smith, 1972). Lactation tends to increase absorption of lipids in cows (Klinskaya, 1976). Protection of oils with protein-formaldehyde improves fat digestion substantially (Cuitin et al, 1975).

All animals excrete some metabolic fecal fat (fat derived from the tissues). Metabolic fecal fat is determined by feeding a fat-free diet for a few days and measuring excretion. In pre-ruminant animals Cunningham and Loosli (1954) estimated that it amounted to 19-29 mg/kg of BW/day in calves 7-8 weeks of age and Veen (1974) found it to be an average of 35 mg/kg of BW. With lambs Walker and Stokes (1970) reported 4.1 g/100 g of fecal DM. In older animals there is little information. Digestibility of ether soluble materials tends to be low (50-70%) in typical ruminant diets that contain 2-5% lipids. When added fats were given, digestibility is generally higher for the test fats (Table 6-13). This statement applies to most but not all studies where added fat has been used in moderation.

The possible occurrence of significant quantities of insoluble fatty acid soaps (Ca, Mg salts of fatty acids) in fecal matter of ruminants must be taken into consideration in determining digestibility of fat. In one example fat digestibility was 91% for a diet with ca. 4% tallow when ether was used to determine fat content of feed and feces; when crude fat (including soaps) was determined, fat digestibility dropped to 79% (Roberts and McKirdy, 1964). Insoluble soaps are not extracted by ether; this problem can be overcome by including 10% acetic acid in the extracting ether to lower the pH and free the bound fatty acids. To determine digestibility of "true fat", the saponifiable material (fatty acids) of both feed and feces must be determined. This is particularly important for forages.

Energy Values of Fats

Surprising as it may seem, there is relatively little recent information which gives some basis for establishing energy values for feeding fats. As a result there is confusion as to the values which are appropriate for use. The NRC publications, in particular, give a wide range in energy values for feeding fats.

Some values on GE are given in Table 6-14. There is not information at hand to know how well these values correspond to feed grade fat values. It should be pointed out that the energy value (GE or heat of combustion) of a fatty acid increases as the chain length increases. For example, palmitic acid (16:0) has a defined value of 9.353 and stearic has a value of 9.533 Kcal/g. A double bond decreases the value (18:1 has 9:406 Kcal/g). Thus, a fat such as butterfat, which has appreciable amounts of short-chain acids, will have a lower GE value than tallow. On the other hand, it is usually more digestible, so the ME value would normally be higher than tallow.

There is also relatively little information in the nutrition literature on composition of feeding fats. Important variables which affect energy value are moisture, insoluble material, non-saponifiable ether-soluble lipids (cholesterol, waxes, hydrocarbons, etc.) and variations in proportions of animal/vegetable fats.

Tabulated NRC values are given in Table 16-15. The NE_m and NE_g values were based

Table 6-14. Gross energy values of fats and fatty acids.[a]

Source	Kcal/g
Corn oil	9.43
Soybean oil, crude	9.43
Rapeseed oil, crude	9.43
Acidulated soapstock	9.25
Animal/vegetable blend,	
feed grade	9.38
edible	9.45
Butterfat	9.1
Lard	9.43
Tallow	9.42
Oleic acid, distilled	9.32
Palm oil fatty acids, distilled	9.33
Stearic acid	9.42
Acetic acid	3.49
Propionic acid	4.96
Butyric acid	5.95

[a] Data from Sibbald and Kramer (1977) or Merck Index.

on one report by Lofgreen (1965) which gave averages for three fat sources fed at three levels. It is assumed by the writer that the other values were calculated by use of some formula(s). It seems obvious that some of these must be incorrect. Some suggested DE, ME and TDN values are given based on certain assumptions as to digestibility and fat content of the fat source. These may not be highly accurate, but at least they give a starting point which seems to be more realistic than some of the NRC values. ME is calculated by multiplying DE X .82; TDN is calculated by dividing DE by 4.4 and multiplying by 100, both standard methods of converting energy values. The equations that have been presented by various authors to calculate NE_m, NE_g or NE_{milk} of different feedstuffs seemingly give very high values for fat and, thus, were not used in this illustration. It seems likely, however, that the ME values are probably low in relation to DE, since there would be little energy loss in urine or gases as a result of feeding fat (Czerkawski et al, 1966). Use of fat might increase ME of the remaining part of the ration since it does, at times, reduce methane production in the rumen. Likewise, the heat increment of feeding for fat is lower than for any other energy source (see Ch. 8), so the loss between ME and NE should be less than for proteins or carbohydrates. In poultry, fats or blends of fats often result in higher ME values than anticipated, presumably because of a positive associative effect which has not been explained (Sibbald and Kramer, 1977). Whether this occurs with ruminants remains to be seen.

Effect of Added Fat on Other Nutrients

Fats serve a number of useful functions in ruminant diets but there are also some detrimental aspects which should be mentioned. One of these is that free fatty acids (Steele and Moore, 1968) or fats (Devendra and Lewis, 1974; Phillips and Church, 1975) generally, although not always, result in some reduction in fiber digestibility. The mechanism for this action has not been clearly explained. It may be a result of microbial inhibition or a physical coating of fibrous material in the rumen. At any rate the effect appears to be a consequence of rumen function since feeding a liquid supplement to bypass the rumen did not result in a depression in digestibility or feed consumption as fat did when fed in dry form (Kowalczyk et al, 1977). Reduced digestibility

Table 6-15. Energy values of feeding fats.

Source of Value	Energy Term					
	DE	ME	NEm	NEg	NEmilk	TDN
	— — — — — — — — Mcal/kg — — — — — —					
NRC Sheep	5.68	4.66	--	--	--	129
Beef	--	4.66	4.57	2.62	--	--
Dairy	8.00	7.50	--	--	5.25	--
Preston[a]	8.73	--	4.56	2.87	--	198
Devendra and Lewis[b]	7.00	--	--	--	--	--
Palmquist and Conrad[c]	7.52	6.00	--	--	--	--
Suggested Values						
Pre-ruminants[d]	8.75	7.18	--	--	--	199
Ruminants[e]	7.65	6.30	4.53[f]	2.59[f]	--	174

[a] As tabulated in Feedstuffs 49(41):A2 (1977).

[b] (1974). Value for beef tallow fed at 8% level to sheep where digestibility was 74.5%.

[c] (1978); cows fed rations containing 42% roughage and 2.5% added fat.

[d] Assumes digestibility of 95%, GE value of 9.4 Kcal/g of fat content and that fat source is 98% fat or hydrolyzed fat.

[e] Assumes digestibility of 83% and same parameters as [d].

[f] Values reported by Lofgreen (1965) for three fat sources fed at three levels.

of fiber caused by addition of corn or soybean oil can usually be alleviated by addition of moderate amounts of Ca but may not be by larger amounts (Davison and Woods, 1963; Phillips and Roberts, 1966; Devendra and Lewis, 1974). Protection of oils with protein-formaldehyde relieves some of the depressing effects on digestibility (Cuitin et al, 1975).

Ca and P utilization may be decreased by tallow or corn oil. Mg utilization has been reduced by feeding animal fat (Kemp et al, 1966), hydrogenated marine fat (Sundstol, 1974) or corn oil (Devendra and Lewis, 1974) and liver Mn was higher in cattle fed corn oil as compared to tallow (Lassiter, 1968). This effect on minerals appears to be the result of formation of insoluble soaps of fatty acids (Roberts and McKirdy, 1964). Tallow appears to be less responsive than oils to additions of Ca or Ca and P (Hubbert et al, 1961), as measured by growth or digestibility, but it does not usually have as severe effects on fiber or minerals when moderate levels have been added.

Another problem related to fat utilization is that fat-urea interactions have been observed which result in reduced digestibility or performance of animals (Bradley et al, 1966; Hatch et al, 1972; Buchanan-Smith et al, 1974; Phillips and Church, 1975). This negative effect can be overcome to some extent by adding higher levels of urea (Phillips and Church, 1975; Kezar and Church, 1976) or by feeding protected tallow (Aseltine and Church, 1976). The exact nature of the interaction remains to be explained but a given level of fat results in higher rumen ammonia and lower production of volatile fatty acids than a comparable ration without the fat. This shows that the N is not utilized as well and that fermentation of substrate is inhibited by the fat under some conditions. In a recent report Kowalcyk et al (1977) found that a tallow-dried milk-lecithin supplement fed with dried grass resulted in reduced rumen ammonia and increased free fatty acids. The data suggest, then, that rumen urease activity is not inhibited but that other enzymes, perhaps deaminases, are inhibited in the rumen by high fat levels.

EFFECT OF ADDED FAT ON PERFORMANCE

This topic is more suited to Vol. 3, but a very brief summary will be given here. When fats are added to feedlot rations at low levels (1-4%), there is generally some improvement in efficiency as measured by gain per unit of dry matter consumption. Even moderate levels may result in some reduction in consumption, and levels approaching 10% will cause a marked decrease in consumption and, in most instances, in digestibility. In studies with lactating dairy cows, the results of feeding fats are variable. Generally, the data suggest that feeding of unsaturated oils (soy, fish, etc.) results in some reduction in milk fat percentage. More saturated fats such as tallow are not likely to have much effect, and feeding of protected fats or full-fat seeds tends to increase fat percentage. However, a long-term study with protected fat demonstrated that fat and milk yield increased early in the lactation but this was more than offset by a subsequent depression in milk yields and shortening of lactation in several cows (Yang et al, 1978). With both feedlot and dairy animals the use of added fats results in some modifications of fatty acid composition in the tissues, but particularly so for milk fat.

References

Aliev, A.A. and M. Sh. Kafarov. 1974. Nutr. Abstr. Rev. 44:168.

Allen, C.E. 1976. Fed. Proc. 35:2323.

Allen, C.E. et al. 1976. Biology of Fat in Meat Animals. N.Central Regional Res. Pub. 234. U. of Wisconsin, Madison.

Andrews, R.J. and D. Lewis. 1970. J. Agr. Sci. 75:47;55.

Annison, E.F. and R.R. White. 1962. Biochem. J. 84:546.

Aseltine, M.S. and D.C. Church. 1976. Proc. West. Sec. Amer. Soc. Anim. Sci. 27:345.

Askew, E.W., J.D. Benson, J.W. Thomas and R.S. Emery. 1971. J. Dairy Sci. 54:854.

Ballard, F.J., R.W. Hanson and D.S. Kronfeld. 1969. Fed. Proc. 28:218.

Bartley, J.C., S. Abraham and I.L. Chaikoff. 1967. Biochem. Biophys. Acta 144:51.

Bauman, D.E. 1976. Fed. Proc. 35:2308.

Bauman, D.E. and C.L. Davis. 1975. In: Digestion and Metabolism in the Ruminant. Univ. of New England Pub. Unit, Armidale, N.S.W., Australia.

Bedo, S., D. Lukacs, J. Harczi and A. Vutskic. 1974. Arch. fur Tierernahrung. 24:159.

Beitz, D.C., M. J. Magat, R.S. Allen and A.D. McGilliard. 1971, J. Dairy Sci. 54:1681.

Bensadoun, A. and J.T. Reid. 1965. J. Nutr. 87:239.

Bergman, E.N. and J.E. Wolff. 1971. Amer. J. Physiol. 221:586.

Berry, B.W. et al. 1966. Proc. West. Sec. Amer. Soc. Anim. Sci. 17:133.

Bitman, J. et al. 1973. J. Amer. Oil Chem. Soc. 50:93.

Bjornstad, J. and P.J. Hansen. 1974. Tierernahrung. Futtermitte. 33:126.

Boatman, C., D.K. Hotchkiss and E.G. Hammond. 1965. J. Dairy Sci. 48:34.

Boehme, W.R. 1978. Personal Communication. Fats and Proteins Research Foundation, Inc., Des Plaines, Ill.

Body, D.R. 1977. Lipids 12:204.

Bradley, N.W. et al. 1966. J. Animal Sci. 25:480.

Bringe, A.N. and L.H. Schultz. 1969. J. Dairy Sci. 52:465.

Bruckner, G.G., G.E. Mitchell and K.K. Grunewald. 1977. Proc. 69th Ann. Meet. Amer. Soc. Anim. Sci., p. 225 (abstr).

Buchanan-Smith, J.G., G.K. Macleod and D.N. Mowat. 1974. J. Animal Sci. 38:133.

Bush, R.S. and L.P. Milligan. 1971. Can. J. Animal Sci. 51:129

Cabezas, M.T. et al. 1963. J. Animal Sci. 24:57.

Chalupa, W., G.D. O'Dell, A.J. Kutches and R.Lavker. 1970. J. Dairy Sci. 53:208.

Chiou, P.W.S. and R.M. Jordan. 1973. J.Animal Sci. 36:597

Church, D.C., A.T. Ralston and W.H. Kennick. 1967. J. Animal Sci. 26:1296.

Clemens, E., W.Woods and V. Arthand. 1974. J. Animal Sci. 38:640.

Course, J.D. et al. 1973. J. Animal Sci. 34:384.

Cramer, D.A. and J.A. Marchello. 1962. Proc. West. Sec. Am. Soc. Anim. Sci. 13:38

Cramer, D.A. and J.A. Marchello. 1964. J. Animal Sci. 23:1002.

Cramer, D.A., R.A. Barton, F.B. Shorland and Z. Czochanska. 1967. J. Agr. Sci. 29:367.

Cuitin, L.L. et al. 1975. J. Animal Sci. 40:691.

Cunningham, H.M. and J.K. Loosli. 1954. J. Animal Sci. 13:265; J Dairy Sci. 37:453.

Czerkawski, J.W. 1976. J.Sci Fd. Agr. 27:261.

Czerkawski, J.W.. K.L. Blaxter and F.D. Wainman. 1966. Brit. J. Nutr. 20:485.

Davis, C.L. and R.E. Brown. 1970. In: Physiology of Digestion and Metabolism in the Ruminant. Oriel Press, Newcastle upon Tyne, England.

Davison, K.L. and W.Woods. 1963. J. Animal Sci. 22:919.

Devendra, C. and D. Lewis. 1974. Animal Prod. 19:67.

Dryden, F.D., J.A. Marchello, W.C. Figroid and W.H. Hale. 1973. J. Animal Sci. 36:19.

Duncan, W.R.H. and G.A. Garton. 1971. Proc. Nutr. Soc. 30:48A (abstr).

Duncan, W.R.H., A.K. Lough and G.A. Garton. 1974. Lipids 9:669.

Edwards, R.L., S.B. Tove, T.N. Blumer and E.R. Barrick. 1961. J. Animal Sci. 20:712.

Felinski, L. and R. Tollec. 1972. Nutr. Abstr. Rev. 42:515.

Flatlandsmo, K. 1972. Acta. Vet. Scand. 13:260.

Flatlandsmo, K. 1973. Acta. Vet. Scand. 14:673.

Garton, G.A. 1969. Proc. Nutr. Soc. 28:131.

Garton, G.A. and W.R.H. Duncan. 1969. Brit. J. Nutr. 23:421; J.Sci. Fd. Agr. 20:39.

Garton, G.A., F.D. Deb. Hovell and W.R.H. Duncan. 1972. Brit. J. Nutr. 28:409.

Glascock, R.F. and V.A. Welch. 1974. J. Dairy Sci. 57:1364.

Gooden, J.M., M.R. Brandon, P.E. Hartmann and A.K. Lascelles. 1971. Aust. J. Biol. Sci. 24:1309.

Hartmann, P.E. and A.K. Lascelles. 1966. J. Physiol. 184:193.

Hatch, C.F., T.W. Perry, M.T. Mohler and W.M. Beeson. 1972. J. Animal Sci. 34:483.

Hawke, J.C. 1973. In: Chemistry and Biochemistry of Herbage, Vol. 1. Academic Press, New York.

Heath, T.J. and L.N. Hill. 1969. Aust. J. Biol. Sci. 22:1015.

Hecker, A.L. 1973. Dissert. Abstr. Int. B. 33:558.

Hogan, J.P. 1973. Aust. J. Agr. Res. 24:587.

Hubbert, F. et al. 1961. J. Animal Sci. 20:669.

Ingle, D.L., D.E. Bauman and U.S. Garrigus. 1972. J. Nutr. 102:609;617.

Kemp, A. W.B. Deijs and E. Kluvers. 1966. Neth. J. Agr. Sci. 14:290.

Kezar, W.W. and D.C. Church. 1976. Proc. West. Sec. Amer. Soc. Anim. Sci. 27:342.

Kinsella, J.E. 1972. Lipids 7:349.

Klinskaya, M.M. 1976. Nutr. Abstr. Rev. 47:311.

Kowalczyk, J., E.R. Orskov, J.J. Robinson and C.S. Stewart. 1977. Brit. J. Nutr. 37:251.

Kuiper, P.J.C. 1970. Pl. Physiol., Lancaster. 45:684.

Kurilov, N.V. et al. 1976. Livestock Prod. Sci. 3:57.

Lambert, M.R. 1953. Ph.D. Thesis, Iowa State University.

Lambert. M.R., N.L. Jacobson, R.S. Allen and J.H. Zaletel. 1954. J. Nutr. 52:259.

Lassiter, J.W. 1968. J. Animal Sci. 27:1466.

Leat, W.M.F. 1966. Biochem. J. 98:598.

Leat, W.M.F. 1977. J. Agr. Sci. 89:575.

Leat, W.M.F. and F.A. Harrison. 1972. Proc. Nutr. Soc. 31:70A (abstr).

Leat, W.M.F. and F.A. Harrison. 1974. Quart. J. Expt. Physiol. 59:131.

Leat, W.M.F. and F.A. Harrison. 1975. In: Digestion and Metabolism in the Ruminant. Univ. of New England Pub. Unit., Armidale, N.S.W., Australia.

Leat, W.M.F., P. Kemp, R.J. Lysons and T.J.L. Alexander. 1977. J. Agr. Sci. 88:175.

Leat, W.M.F., F.O.T. Kubasek and N. Buttress. 1976. Quart. J. Expt. Physiol. 61:193.

Lennox, A.M. and G.A. Garton. 1968. Brit. J. Nutr. 22:247.

Lennox, A.M., A.K. Lough and G.A. Garton. 1968. Brit. J. Nutr. 22:237.

Liepa, G.U., D.C. Beitz and J.R. Lindner. 1978. J. Nutr. 108:535.

Lindsay, D.B. 1975. Proc. Nutr. Soc. 34:241.

Lindsay, D.B. and W.M.F. Leat. 1977. J. Agr. Sci. 89:215.

Link, B.A., R.W. Bray, R.G. Cassens and R.G. Kauffman. 1970. J. Animal Sci. 30:722.

Lofgreen, G. P. 1965. J. Animal Sci. 24:480.

Lough, A.K. 1977. Lipids 12:115.

MacLeod, G.K. and J.G.Buchanan-Smith. 1972. J. Animal Sci. 35:890.

Marchello, J.A. and D.A. Cramer. 1963. J. Animal Sci. 22:380.

Marchello, J.A. and W.H. Hale. 1976. In: Fat Content and Composition of Animal Products. Nat. Acad. Sci., Washington, D.C.

Mattos, W. and D.L. Palmquist. 1977. J. Nutr. 107:1755.

Mattson, F.H.. R.A. Volpenhein and E.S. Sutton. 1964. J. Lipid Res. 5:363.

McDonald, I.W. and A.C.I. Warner. (eds.) 1975. Digestion and Metabolism in the Ruminant. The Univ. of New England Pub. Unit, Armidale, N.S.W., Australia.

Moore, J.H., R.C. Noble and W. Steele. 1968. Brit. J. Nutr. 22:681.

Nelson, G.J. 1973. Comp. Biochem. Physiol. 46B:81.

Noble, R.C., W. Steele and J.H. Moore. 1971. Lipids 6:26.

Noble, R.C., W. Steele and J.H. Moore. 1972. Brit. J. Nutr. 27:503.

Oltjen, R.R. and D.A. Dinius. 1975. J. Animal Sci. 41:703.

Oltjen, R.R. and P.P. Williams. 1974. J. Animal Sci. 38:915.

Outen, G.E., D.E. Beever and D.F. Osbourn. 1974. J. Sci. Fd. Agr. 25:981.

Palmquist, D.L. 1972. J. Nutr. 102:1401.

Palmquist, D.L. 1976. Fed. Proc. 35:2300; J. Dairy Sci. 59:355.

Palmquist, D.L. and H.R. Conrad. 1978. J. Dairy Sci. 61: (in press)

Palmquist, D.L. and W. Mattos. 1977. Fed. Proc. 36:1140.

Palmquist, D.L., W. Mattos and R.L. Stone. 1977. Lipids 12:235.

Payne, E. 1978. Brit. J. Nutr. 39:45;53.

Phillips, G.D. and W.K. Roberts. 1966. Can. J. Animal Sci. 46:59.

Phillips, R.L. and D.C. Church. 1975. J. Animal Sci. 41:588.

Phillipson, A.T. (ed.). 1970. Physiology of Digestion and Metabolism in the Ruminant. Oriel Press. Newcastle upon Tyne, England.

Qureshi, S.R. et al. 1972. J. Dairy Sci. 55:93.

Raphael, B.D., P.S. Dimick and D.L. Puppione. 1973. J. Dairy Sci. 56:1025.

Ray, E.E., R.P. Kromann, and E.J. Cosma. 1975. J. Animal Sci. 41:1767.

Roberts, W.K. 1966. Can. J. Animal Sci. 46:181.

Roberts, W.K. and J.A. McKirdy. 1964. J. Animal Sci. 23:682.

Roughan, P.G. and R.D. Batt. 1969. Anal. Biochem. 22:74.

Rumsey, T.S., R.R. Oltjen, K.P. Bovard and B.M. Priode. 1972. J. Animal Sci. 35:1069.

Schultz, L.H. 1974. J. Dairy Sci. 57:729.

Scott, A.M. and A.K. Lough. 1971. Brit. J. Nutr. 25:307.

Scott, T.W. et al. 1970. Aust. J. Sci. 32:291.

Scott, T.W. and L.J. Cook. 1975. In: Digestion and Metabolism in the Ruminant. Univ. of New England Pub. Unit. Armidale, N.S.W., Australia.

Scott, T.W., L.J. Cook and S.C. Mills. 1971. J. Amer. Oil Chem. Soc. 48:358.

Scow, R.O. et al. 1975. Mod. Prob. Paediat. 15:31.

Seifried, H.E. and J.L. Gaylor. 1976. J. Biol. Chem. 251:7468.

Shannon, A.D. and A.K. Lascelles. 1967. Aust. J. Biol. Sci. 20:669.

Shaw, J.C., W.L. Ensor, H.F. Tellechea and S.D. Lee. 1960. J. Nutr. 27:365.

Shell, L.A. et al 1978. J. Animal Sci. 46:1332.

Sibbald, I.R. and J.K.G. Kramer. 1977. Poultry Sci. 56:2079.

Skelley, G.C., W.C. Stanford and R.L. Edwards. 1973. J. Animal Sci. 36:576.

Sklan, D., R. Volcani and P. Budowski. 1972. Brit. J. Nutr. 27:365.

Smith, L.M., W.L. Dunkley, A. Franke and T. Dairiki. 1978. J. Amer. Oil Chem. Soc. 55:257.

Smith, S. and R. Dils. 1966. Biochem. Biophys. Acta 116:23.

Steele, W. and J.H. Moore. 1968. J. Dairy Res. 35:371.

Stokes, G.B. and D.M. Walker. 1970. Brit. J. Nutr. 24:435.

Storry, J.E. et al. 1974. J. Dairy Sci. 57:61,1046; J. Dairy Res. 41:165.

Sunastol, F. 1974. Meldinger Norges Landskogskole. 53:50.

Sutton, J.D., J.E. Storry and J.W.G. Nicholson. 1970. J. Dairy Res. 37:97.

Terrell, R.N., G.G. Suess and R.W. Bray. 1969. J. Animal Sci. 28:449.

Tichenor, D.A. et al. 1970. J. Animal Sci. 31:671.

Ulyatt, M.J. and J.C. Macrae. 1974. J. Agr. Sci. 82:295.

Veen, W.A.G. 1974. Nutr. Abstr. Rev. 44:977.

Vesely, J.A. 1973. Can. J. Animal Sci. 53:187,673.

Volpe, J.J. and P.R. Vagelos. 1976. Physiol. Rev. 56:339.

Waldeman, R.G., G.G. Suess and V.H. Brungardt. 1968. J. Animal Sci. 31:296.

Walker, D.M. and G.B. Stokes. 1970. Brit. J. Nutr. 24:425.

Warner, R.L., G.E. Mitchell and C.O. Little. 1972. J. Animal Sci. 34:161.

Wendlandt, R.M. and C.L. Davis. 1973. J. Dairy Sci. 56:337.

Williamson, D.H., M.W. Bates, M.A. Page and H.A. Krebs. 1971. Biochem. J. 121:41.

Yang, Y.T. and R.L. Baldwin. 1973. J. Dairy Sci. 56:366.

Yang, Y.T., R.L. Baldwin and J. Russell. 1978. J. Dairy Sci. 61:180.

Chapter 7 - Carbohydrate Metabolism

by T.E. C. Weekes

The adult ruminant derives considerable benefit from the anaerobic fermentation of dietary components which occurs in the reticulo-rumen. In particular, the breakdown of cellulose and other polysaccharides to volatile fatty acids (VFA) allows the ruminant to meet a large proportion of its energy needs from these sources. However, glucose and starch are also rapidly fermented in the reticulo-rumen, so that only small amounts of glucose are absorbed from the gut under most dietary conditions. This means that ruminants are liable to suffer from a shortage of glucose, particularly during periods of high metabolic activity, since glucose is an essential metabolite for some tissues and biochemical pathways. The process of gluconeogenesis (glucose synthesis) is therefore of great importance in ruminants. For example, Young (1977) has calculated that a high producing dairy cow may have to synthesize 6.6 kg of glucose daily. The need to meet this formidable requirement results in some differences in ruminant intermediary metabolism from the well-defined monogastric pattern. This chapter outlines some of these differences. For reviews on the subject the reader is referred to Ballard et al (1969), Leng (1970), Lindsay (1970, 1971), Sutton (1971), Bergman (1973), Bassett (1975) and Young (1977).

A thorough treatment of carbohydrate metabolism in monogastric species is not attempted; for this the reader should consult a biochemistry textbook such as Newsholme and Start (1973). Likewise, data specifically relating to metabolic disorders (ketosis) are presented in Ch. 12 of this volume and the digestion and absorption of carbohydrates in the ruminant GI tract is covered in Ch. 9 and 12 of Vol. 1.

Glucose Turnover in Ruminants

It is well known that blood glucose levels are considerably lower in ruminants than in monogastric species. Prefeeding whole blood glucose levels in adult non-pregnant ruminants are generally between 35-45 mg/100 ml (1.9-2.8 mM), compared to levels of 80 mg/100 ml for man, 90-100 mg/100 ml for rats and 250-300 mg/100 ml for birds. Ruminants are also unusual in that their red cells contain virtually no glucose. Prefeeding

plasma glucose levels are therefore 55-65 mg/100 ml (3.0-3.6 mM; Reid, 1968). This does not mean that glucose is a relatively unimportant metabolite in ruminants, since plasma glucose levels merely reflect the point of balance between glucose input into the plasma (derived from gluconeogenesis, glycogenolysis and any glucose absorbed from the gut) and glucose uptake by the tissues. An apparently static plasma glucose concentration represents a precisely balanced 'dynamic steady state.' This important concept applies equally to other blood metabolites. Changes in plasma metabolite levels may represent changes in input or uptake or in both processes at different rates. Quantitative information is therefore required about the *turnover* of glucose in the whole animal and the production and utilization of glucose by the different organs of the body.

Methodology

Two general approaches have been used. The turnover of glucose in the whole body is estimated using isotope dilution methods, while the metabolism of specific organs is measured from the rate of blood flow through the organ and the blood glucose concentration difference across the organ.

The principle of the isotope dilution method is remarkably simple. A small quantity of radioactively labeled glucose (^{14}C or ^{3}H-labeled) is injected or infused into the blood stream, generally into the jugular vein, and the specific radioactivity (radioactivity/g glucose) of plasma glucose is followed over several hours. The rate of dilution of labeled glucose (tracer) by non-labeled (i.e. endogenous) glucose is measured. The quantity of tracer used is too small to affect the metabolism of endogenous glucose and it is assumed that the labeled glucose is metabolized at the same rate as endogenous plasma glucose. These measurements represent the flow or *entry* of glucose into the blood from all sources, or glucose production. If the animal is in a dynamic steady state with a constant blood glucose concentration, the glucose entry rate will equal the rate of glucose utilization; the term *glucose turnover rate* is therefore used (Bergman, 1963). A large number of these measurements have now been made with adult ruminants.

Despite the apparent simplicity of this approach, accurate interpretation of the results can be exceedingly complex, requiring the use of computer-assisted multi-exponential or multicompartmental analyses (Kronfeld et al, 1971; Horsfield et al, 1974). Young (1977) has outlined the possible pitfalls in this work. We include a brief discussion of these problems, since without an understanding of what is being measured it is impossible to grasp the biological significance of the values quoted by different authors.

Most early experiments used uniformly labeled [^{14}C]-glucose. However, [^{14}C]-glucose can give rise to ^{14}C-labeled glycogen, lactate, pyruvate and amino acids, which may be reincorporated into glucose in the course of the experiment, following glycogenolysis or gluconeogenesis. This recycling of label will lead to an underestimate of the rate of glucose synthesis, giving instead the apparent replacement rate, or *irreversible loss rate.* This is the most commonly measured parameter of glucose metabolism, but does not indicate the rate of glucose production by the liver and kidney, nor utilization of glucose by body tissues. This is given by the *total glucose entry rate* or glucose outflow rate, which represents the rate of glucose-6-phosphate formation from glucose.

The total glucose entry rate can be obtained by analysis of [U - ^{14}C]-glucose kinetics following a single injection of labeled glucose (White et al, 1969; Kronfeld et al, 1971). These calculations indicate that about 20% of the total glucose production is recycled in sheep and dairy cows. More simply and probably more accurately, [^{3}H]-glucose can be used as the tracer. Complete recycling of glucose through lactate via the Cori cycle will remove almost all ^{3}H from all positions in glucose. This complete recycling is measured using [6 - ^{3}H]-glucose and [U - ^{14}C]-glucose, the tritium being lost at the level of pyruvate and phosphoenolpyruvate. The tritium from [2 - ^{3}H]-glucose is lost at an earlier stage of metabolism, in the reversible phosphohexose isomerase reaction, allowing correction for all forms of recycling, including that via glycogen. However, tritium will also be lost from [2 - ^{3}H]-glucose by 'futile cycling' taking place within the liver. Futile cycling reactions, such as glucose $\rightarrow$ glucose-6-phosphate $\rightarrow$ glucose result in ^{3}H loss without any net metabolism of glucose, so would overestimate the requirement for net glucose synthesis.

Total glucose entry rates have now been measured in sheep using [6 - ^{3}H]-glucose (Brockman et al, 1975) and [2 - ^{3}H]-glucose (Evans and Buchanan-Smith, 1975; Judson et al, 1976). In fact, chemical recycling appears to be less important in ruminants than in monogastric species. Recycling accounted for only 11% of total glucose entry rate in sheep when [2 - ^{3}H]-glucose and [U - ^{14}C]-glucose were compared and only 4% when [6-^{3}H]-glucose was used (Judson and Leng, 1972). This contrasts with 29% recycling of glucose carbon in rabbits fasted overnight and 36% in rats, estimated with [2 - ^{3}H]-glucose (Katz et al, 1974). Interconversion with liver glycogen is relatively unimportant in ruminants (Judson and Leng, 1972), since ruminant liver lacks the enzyme glucokinase and never displays a net glucose uptake from the blood. The extent of futile cycling in ruminants is unknown; in rats this accounts for 10% of the glucose entry rate measured with [2 - ^{3}H]-glucose (Clark et al, 1975).

This chemical recycling should be distinguished from recirculation of labeled glucose between different body glucose pools, termed *reflux*. Reflux is sometimes included in estimates of total glucose entry rates obtained by multicompartmental analysis (Horsfield et al, 1974), accounting for the very high values obtained. Although reflux is physiologically important (Kronfeld et al, 1971), it does not impose any extra demands on the liver's capacity to produce glucose.

Finally, the assumption of steady-state conditions prevents conventional entry-rate measurements when that rate is changing. Alternative procedures for non-steady-state conditions have been used with sheep (Brockman et al, 1975; Judson et al, 1976).

Thus, it is possible to determine glucose turnover in the whole animal with good precision. Most of the values quoted in this chapter are irreversible loss rates, since this has been most frequently measured, but total glucose entry rates are unlikely to be more than 10-20% higher.

In order to determine the sites of glucose production and utilization within the body, blood vessels supplying and draining a particular organ are catheterized. The blood glucose concentration difference across the organ multiplied by the blood flow through the organ gives the net glucose uptake or output. In the case of the liver, glucose inputs via both the hepatic portal vein and the hepatic artery must be considered. The technical problems of surgical implantation of catheters means that this valuable approach is used in relatively few laboratories. The liver and kidney both utilize and produce glucose, so that only net glucose production is measured directly. Therefore, a combination of this technique and isotope infusion has been used in the elegant studies of Bergman and his colleagues (Bergman, 1975) to measure total glucose production and utilization.

Effect of Feeding and Fasting

In non-ruminants glucose is absorbed from the small intestine after a meal, when the liver has a net uptake of glucose. The process of gluconeogenesis only becomes important during fasting, exercise or in disease. The situation is radically different in the ruminant, with gluconeogenesis taking place at all times. Glucose irreversible loss rates, which represent gluconeogenesis, are decreased rather than increased on starvation, as shown by the data in Table 7-1. These values are comparable to the rates of glucose synthesis found in man after a prolonged fast, when expressed on a metabolic body weight basis. Total glucose entry rates after an overnight fast (post absorptive) are considerably higher than this, reaching 300 mg/hr/kg $^{0.75}$ in the rabbit and 450 mg/hr/ kg $^{0.75}$ in the rat, estimated using [2 - ^{3}H]- glucose (Katz et al, 1974) and 330 mg/hr/ kg $^{0.75}$ in the dog, estimated using [3 - ^{3}H]-glucose (Altszuler et al, 1975). However, much of the glucose synthesis is derived from glycogenolysis rather than gluconeogenesis. Ballard et al (1969) concluded that the rate of glucose turnover in ruminants was only slightly less than that in other mammals, on a metabolic body weight basis, and more recent evidence generally supports this conclusion.

In monogastric species the Cori (lactate) and glucose-alanine cycles (Felig, 1973) are particularly important in starvation. These cycles do not provide any extra glucose, but enable the animal to conserve glucose precursors to meet the needs of glucose-dependent tissues (Krebs, 1973). It might be expected that these cycles would be well developed in the fasting ruminant, but this does not appear to be the case. Indeed, early studies using monoexponential analysis suggested that recycling became progressively more important as sheep were starved for 6 days (Steel and Leng, 1973). However, when [6 - ^{3}H]-glucose was used, the proportion of glucose recycled remained at the same low level in sheep starved for 3 days as in fed animals (Brockman et al, 1975). It appears that these cycles via tricarbon intermediates are of less use to the ruminant than to animals subject to intermittent reliance upon gluconeogenesis.

Effect of diet

The quantity of glucose synthesized by ruminants is affected by the quantity and quality of the diet. As expected, glucose entry rates increase with increasing DE (digestible energy) intake (Fig. 7-1), reflecting an increased supply of glucose precursors. Judson and Leng (1968) found that on roughage diets an extra 14 g of glucose were synthesized daily for every MJ increase in DE intake. The relation between glucose entry rate and protein intake is less good

Table 7-1. Glucose irreversible loss rates in fed and fasted ruminants.

Species	Period of fasting, days	Prefasting diet	Live-weight, kg	Glucose irreversible loss		References
				g/hr	mg/hr/kg $^{0.75}$	
1. Sheep	0	800 g alfalfa pellets	55	4.7	235	Brockman et al (1975)[a]
	3		59	2.4	114	
2. Sheep	0	800 g chopped alfalfa hay	37	3.5	232	Steel and Leng (1973)
	2		31	1.9	141	
	4		31	1.4	110	
	6		30	1.4	112	
3. Sheep	0	alfalfa hay ad lib	53	4.6	240	Bergman et al (1974)
	3-4		53	3.0	150	
4. Cattle	0	Restricted grain	584	39.4	332	Head et al (1965)
	4		500	19.8	187	

[a] Total entry rate, estimated using [6 - ^{3}H] - glucose

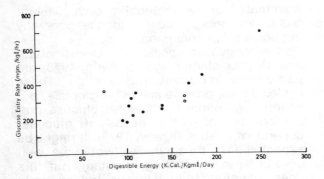

Fig. 7-1. Relationship between glucose entry rate and digestible energy intake in sheep. From Lindsay (1970) with permission of the author and Oriel Press Ltd.

(Lindsay, 1970), probably because amino acids are a less important glucose precursor than propionate (see below). The relationship between glucose precursor supply and glucose entry rate has also been demonstrated by abomasal infusion of casein or amino acids in sheep (Judson and Leng, 1973b; Lindsay and Dyke, 1974) and cattle (Spires et al, 1973) and by intraruminal infusion of propionate (Judson and Leng, 1973b).

These considerations would lead one to expect that isoenergetic replacement of roughage by concentrate in a ruminant's diet would increase the glucose entry rate, since the supply of propionate would be increased and some glucose may also be absorbed from the small intestine on the concentrate diet. This prediction has been fulfilled in studies with both sheep (Evans and

Buchanan-Smith, 1975) and lactating dairy cows (Evans et al, 1975; Table 7-2). Substitution of roughage with concentrate has increased plasma glucose concentration in several studies with sheep (Trenkle, 1970) and dairy cows (Jenny and Polan, 1975). The well known depression in milk fat yield when cows are fed high-grain, low-fiber diets (low milk fat syndrome) has also been ascribed to an increased supply of glucose and the glucose precursor propionate when large amounts of readily available carbohydrate are fed (McClymont and Vallance, 1962).

However, in other studies glucose entry rate in sheep was unaffected by varying the relative proportions of roughage and cereal in the diet (Judson et al, 1968; Ulyatt et al, 1970). These conflicting results may in part reflect methodological differences: Evans' animals were fed 2X daily while Judson and Ulyatt employed more frequent feeding. This may have minimized any response to diet.

Increasing supplies of glucose and glucose precursors do not have a simple additive effect on the glucose entry rate. Thus, although propionate infusions increase gluconeogenesis in well-fed animals, glucose synthesis from sources other than propionate is depressed (Judson and Leng, 1973b). Glucose infusions also depress gluconeogenesis in ruminants (Bartley and Black, 1966; Judson and Leng, 1973a; Thompson et al, 1975), although the total glucose entry rate (sum of exogenous infusion and endogenous gluconeogenesis) was elevated during glucose infusions. Thus, the effects of ration composition on

Table 7-2. Effects of low-(LR) and high-roughage (HR) diets at two intake levels on glucose metabolism in sheep. [a]

Item	Diet [b]				Statistical effect	
	LR-1X	LR-2X	HR-1X	HR-2X	Diet	Intake
Plasma glucose, mM/l.	3.40	4.27	2.86	3.07	*	*
Body pool size of glucose, mg/kg BW	119	152	98	108	*	*
Body glucose space, % of BW	19.0	19.8	19.0	19.5	NS	NS
Glucose turnover rate, mg/hr/kg$^{0.75}$	295	460	232	295	*	*

[a] From Evans and Buchanan-Smith (1975)

[b] IX = fed at a level equivalent to maintenance; 2X = fed at twice this level (DE basis). Diets were based on ground, shelled corn and hay, either ground (LR) or chopped (HR).

* P<.05, NS, not significant

glucose entry rate are not clearcut, although in general a low-fiber ration increases the glucose entry rate.

Dietary N source may also affect glucose synthesis. Somewhat tentative evidence suggests that gluconeogenesis may be slower in urea-fed lambs than in lambs fed plant proteins, at least when animals are fed 2X daily (Prior et al, 1972; Leonard et al, 1977). More research is required on this topic in view of the importance of NPN sources in practical rations (see Ch. 3).

Effect of Exercise

Most studies of glucose metabolism are conducted using housed animals. The requirement for gluconeogenesis may be considerably higher under field conditions, since glucose turnover rate in sheep was doubled during a 2-hr exercise period (Judson et al, 1976). Much of the extra glucose produced was oxidized by musculature (see below). Further research is clearly required in this area.

Effect of Cold Stress

Exposure to cold causes an increase in whole body oxygen consumption and heat production in ruminants, as in other mammals (see Ch. 8, 16). This is accompanied by increases in plasma glucose concentration and in the rates of glucose production and oxidation in sheep (McKay et al, 1974) and steers (Bell et al, 1975). Glucose output by the liver was doubled when sheep were exposed to a moderately cold environment (0-54°C) for 3 hr (Thompson et al, 1978). Some of this extra glucose probably originates from liver glycogen stores, at least in the early stages of cold stress, but gluconeogenesis in the liver also increases (Thompson et al, 1978). Prolonged cold stress is therefore likely to considerably increase the animal's requirement for glucose precursors.

Effect of Pregnancy

Glucose entry rates in pregnant ruminants have been well documented, particularly for sheep. These studies have been stimulated by the occurrence of hypoglycemia and ketosis during late pregnancy in sheep (pregnancy toxemia, see Ch. 12).

Glucose appears to be the major energy source for the fetus. Uptake by the pregnant uterus and its contents accounts for between 43% (Prior and Christenson, 1978) and 70% (Setchell et al, 1972) of the total glucose entry rate in pregnant sheep. Uterine glucose uptake also increases with stage of gestation and the number of fetuses. Prior and Christenson (1978) calculate a uterine glucose uptake of about 1 g/kg of fetus/hr.

Table 7-3. Glucose entry rates in pregnant sheep, $mg/hr/kg^{0.75}$.[a]

Diet	Days from lambing		
	63-71	42-52	5-11
Alfalfa chaff, ad lib	323	332	401
Alfalfa chaff, 800 g/day	262	280	315
Alfalfa chaff 250 g + wheaten chaff, 250 g/day	208	220	265
Starved 4 days	160	174	152

[a] From Steel and Leng (1973)

Despite this large increase in glucose demand during pregnancy, glucose entry rate is still determined more by the food intake than by stage of gestation (Table 7-3). Glucose production on a fixed ration does increase slightly as gestation advances, but the effect is small compared with the response to an increased level of feeding. Glucose oxidation by other tissues of the body is depressed during pregnancy (Setchell et al, 1972), but starved pregnant ewes are unable to synthesize glucose at any greater rate than starved non-pregnant sheep (compare Tables 7-3 and 7-1). The glucose demands of the fetus take precedence over that of the ewe unless starvation is severe, when abortion may occur. Thus, the pregnant ewe is highly susceptible to fluctuations in her food supply.

When the supply of glucose precursors is reduced, the ewe is unable to meet the fetal glucose demands from her own resources and maternal hypoglycemia and ketosis results (Ch. 12). The fetal calf also has a high glucose demand, but pregnacy ketosis is not a problem in the dairy cow. This is, presumably, because only one fetus is carried and the normal practice of concentrate feeding before calving (steaming up) ensures an adequate supply of glucose precursors for dairy cows.

Effect of Lactation

Glucose entry rates increase dramatically in early lactation in ewes, goats and dairy cows (Table 7-4). The glucose economy of the entire animal is dominated by the udder's

Table 7-4. Glucose irreversible loss rates in lactating ruminants, mg/hr/kg $^{0.75}$.[a]

Species	Stage of lactation or milk yield, kg/day	Glucose entry rate	Reference
Sheep	Early lactation	550	Bergman & Hogue (1967)
	Peak lactation	680	
	Late lactation	500	
	Non-lactating	230	
Goat	Early lactation	740	Annison & Linzell (1964)
	Late lactation	550	
Cow	14-18 weeks, 20	780	Bickerstaffe et al (1974)
Cow	4	690	Kronfeld et al (1971)
	20	708	
Ccw	12-15	310	Horsfield et al (1974)
	28-30	825	

[a] Glucose irreversible loss rates calculated from multicompartmental analyses; figures for glucose outflow rate were 15-45% higher.

requirement for glucose. Lactose production alone may account for 60% of the glucose entry rate (Bergman et al, 1974).

Glucose is also required for other processes in the udder, so that the udder may account for 60-85% of the total glucose entry rate. The relationship between glucose entry rate and plasma glucose concentration is clearly altered during lactation (Fig. 7-2). The steep slope of this regression line is a further indication of the powerful influence glucose supply has on milk lactose synthesis (Bergman, 1973).

An adequate supply of glucose is vital for continued milk synthesis. In some situations milk yield may be limited by glucose supply (Linzell, 1967). This is not always true, particularly when the dietary supply of glucose precursors is elevated (Ørskov et al, 1977). The major determinant of the increased glucose production in lactation is probably the increased food intake. Changes in the hepatic extraction of lactate (Baird et al, 1978) and in the activities of key gluconeogenic enzymes (Mackie and Campbell, 1972) may also increase the efficiency of conversion of glucose precursors into glucose. Starvation reduces the glucose entry rate in lactating cows (Kronfeld et al, 1971), with no indication of an improved capacity to maintain gluconeogenesis (Lindsay, 1970). The relationship between glucose demand and the development of bovine ketosis in early lactation is considered in Ch. 12.

In conclusion, glucose entry rates in adult ruminants can be seen to be quite variable, ranging from around 60 g/day in fasted sheep to 350 g/day at peak lactation and in cattle from 500 g/day to over 7 kg/day.

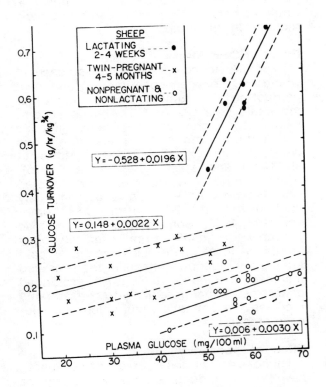

Fig. 7-2. Relationship between glucose turnover per unit of metabolic body weight and plasma glucose concentration in sheep. Dashed lines indicate one standard deviation. All three lines differ from each other in their intercept (P<.001). The slope of the line for lactating sheep also differs from the slopes for pregnant and non-pregnant sheep (P< .001). About half of the pregnant ewes were hypoglycemic. From Bergman (1973) with permission of The Cornell Veterinarian.

GLUCOSE SUPPLY

Sites of Glucose Production

Glucose originates in the body by gluconeogenesis in the liver and kidney cortex and by absorption from the small intestine. Renal gluconeogenesis is relatively unimportant, accounting for only 8-10% of the whole body glucose turnover in fed sheep and 15% during fasting (Bergman, 1973). Figure 7-3 illustrates the relative contributions of the liver and kidney to glucose production in fed sheep.

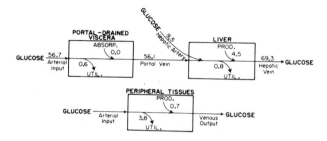

Fig. 7-3. Flow of glucose (g/hr) in portal drained viscera and liver of non-pregnant sheep fed alfalfa hay or hay and grain (800 g/day) at a constant rate. Each number is the mean value for 10 sheep. From Bergman (1975) with permission of The University of New England Publishing Unit.

Post Abomasal Digestion of Carbohydrate in the Adult

It is well recognized that the reticulo-rumen is the major site of carbohydrate digestion in the adult ruminant resulting in the production of VFA, varying amounts of lactic acid and gases (CO_2 and CH_4). The potentially fermentable quantities of structural carbohydrates such as cellulose and hemicellulose which escape fermentation in the rumen undergo further degradation in the cecum and colon (Armstrong and Beevers, 1969). Studies by Heald (1951), Weller and Gray (1954), and Porter and Singleton (1971) among others indicate that on roughage diets, i.e. those virtually free of starch—little α-linked glucose polymer enters the small intestine.

When diets containing grains are fed, depending on the value of the grain, the extent of its processing prior to feeding, and the species of animal fed, appreciable amounts of starch or starch-like material (protozoal glycogen) escape fermentation in the rumen and enter the small intestine. The subject has been reviewed by Ørskov (1969), Armstrong and Beever (1969) and Waldo

(1973). Some overall mean results calculated by Armstrong and Beever are given in Table 7-5.

It can be seen from Table 7-5 that overall digestibility of the ingested starch in these diets is virtually complete and that, for sheep, digestibility prior to the small intestine accounts for some 90% of the digestion. With reference to this last-mentioned value, when the starch was fed as whole or rolled barley, the amount (6%) was significantly lower than that of 10.5% found for a diet of 1 part hay and 2 parts flaked corn.

Table 7-5. Some average values calculated by Armstrong and Beever (1969) from data in the literature relative to the extent and sites of digestion of starch in cereal-containing diets fed to cattle and sheep.

Item	Sheep	Cattle
Diets [a]	Rolled barley or ground corn	Ground corn
Digestibility of starch, %	99.9 ± 0.25	98.5 ± 0.40
Disappearance of digested starch, %		
Before S. Intestine	91.8 ± 0.8	68.0 ± 1.8
In S. Intestine	8.0 ± 0.8	26.7 ± 2.2
In cecum or colon	0.2 ± 0.09	5.3 ± 2.1

[a] Grain components of the rations.

However, when ground corn is fed to cattle, appreciable quantities of α-linked glucose polymer escape fermentation within the rumen and enter the small intestine (Table 7-5). In studies with cows Voight et al (1976) observed that when starch was supplied as corn meal, some 26% of that ingested entered the small intestine compared with 14% of the starch fed as barley meal. In cattle fed diets containing varying proportions of hay and rolled barley or ground corn, Thivend and Journet (1968, 1970) observed mean values for starch digested within the rumen of 95% and 67%, respectively, when expressed as a percentage of that ingested. With reference to overall starch digestibility by cattle, it must be emphasized that it is not always complete. Thus, Morrison (1959) refers to studies in which 18-35% of the whole shelled corn fed to cattle passed through the tract undigested.

Appreciable amounts of the α-linked glucose polymer entering the small intestine are likely to comprise microbial storage polysaccharide. Thus, McAllan and Smith (1974) reported concentrations of an α-dextran glucose up to 140 g/kg of dry matter in rumen bacteria harvested 4-6 hr after feeding calves a diet containing equal parts of concentrate to roughage. The polymer is readily available by an α-amylglucosidase enzyme and exclusively digested in the small intestine.

The Fate of α-linked Glucose Polymer in the Small Intestine

With early weaned lambs Ørskov et al (1969) observed a limited capacity for digestion of starch in the small intestine; the major site of disappearance of that leaving the reticulo-rumen occurred in the cecum and colon. This was also observed in 4 mo. old ewes fed rations containing rolled barley or kibbled corn (Ørskov et al, 1971). From Table 7-5 it would appear that virtually all the α-linked glucose polymer entering the small intestine of mature sheep was digested there and from the mean values for cattle it can be calculated that some 83% of that entering the small intestine was apparently digested therein. However, when cattle are fed high levels of ground corn, the quantity of starch reaching the cecum is appreciable and increases as the level of corn in the ration rises. It would certainly appear that the extent of digestion of starch within the small intestine is not unlimited.

It has to be stated that the fate of such starch which disappears within the small intestine is far from certain at the present time. There is evidence (see Ch. 9, Vol. 1) that in mature cattle pancreatic juices have a high amylase but low maltase activity and that, with reference to pancreatic anylase activity, this increases as the proportion of corn in the diet increases. No data are available on oligo-1, 6-glucosidase activity in ruminant intestinal mucosa but amylase and maltase are present and reach their peak activity in the jejunum; the activity of maltase exceeds that of amylase. From a consideration of the pH of the digesta for maximal activity of these carbohydrates, it would appear that hydrolysis of starch to glucose is likely to occur most effectively in the proximal half of the jejunum.

That the ruminant small intestine can absorb glucose has been shown by White et al (1971), although the importance of active transport relative to passive transport of glucose is not known. While absorptive capacity decreased from pylorus to terminal ileum in young lambs, there was little change in adult sheep. These workers also obtained evidence of increased absorptive capacity for glucose in the proximal half of the small intestine of adult sheep when the diet contained high levels of grain (wheat) than when it contained all forage.

Some indirect evidence for the hydrolysis of starch to glucose and absorption of it from the small intestine is available. Thus, in sheep fed ground corn, Thivend (1974) reported increased concentrations of glucose in portal blood (venous). Symonds and Baird (1975) observed an increase in total reducing substances in the blood from the mesenteric vein of cows when fed corn meal.

Although the importance of the cecum as the site of secondary fermentation is well established, it is relevant to note that in sheep fed diets high in ground corn (Badaway et al, 1958), there was a pronounced rise in concentration of the VFA towards the distal end of the small intestine, suggesting that at least some of the starch entering the small intestine and disappearing therein was being fermented to VFA.

Contribution of Digested Starch to Absorbed Glucose

It will be appreciated from the foregoing discussion that the extent to which starch digestion in the small intestine contributed to overall glucose supply in the ruminant cannot be stated with any certainty. Nevertheless, estimates of such a contribution can be derived if the assumption is made that α-linked glucose polymer which does disappear survive passage of the digesta through the small intestine is absorbed as glucose.

Thus, on the basis of data reviewed by Armstrong and Beever (1969), these workers concluded that the glucose requirement of non-pregnant sheep would be more than provided for by glucose absorbed from the small intestine on diets containing 40-60% ground corn; if barley or flaked corn were used, such glucose would make a substantial contribution (41-59%) of glucose requirement.

Sutton (1976) has made a comparable calculation for a lactating cow receiving a ration of 6 kg hay and of dairy concentrate containing 70% rolled barley (air-dry). In this instance it was assumed that 20% of the starch ingested reached the small intestine and of this some 75% was absorbed as glucose. On the basis of a daily requirement for glucose of 1.5 kg daily for a cow producing 20 kg milk (Armstrong and Beever, 1971), propionic acid absorbed from the rumen and cecum, and glucose from the small intestine would contribute 55 and 50%, respectively, of the daily glucose requirement leaving the balance to be derived from other sources.

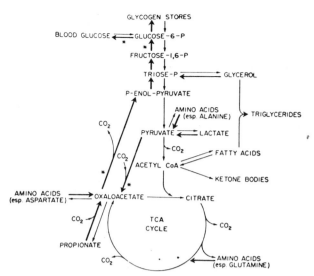

Fig. 7-4. Major metabolic pathways in ruminant liver (and kidney cortex). Heavy arrows indicate pathways for gluconeogenesis and asterisks denote the 4 key irreversible reactions of gluconeogenesis. From Bergman (1973) with permission of The Cornell Veterinarian.

Gluconeogenesis

That portion of the glucose entry rate not supplied by glucose absorption must be provided by gluconeogenesis. The metabolic pathways involved in this process are outlined in Fig. 7-4 . The major precursors used are propionate, the only major VFA which can give rise to net glucose synthesis, amino acids, glycogen, lactate and glycerol. The total supply of these precursors considerably exceeds the rate of glucose synthesis in the fed ruminant, but none of these compounds is quantitatively converted to glucose. Oxidation and conversion into other products, for example, protein synthesis from amino acids, will remove a variable proportion of these potentially glucogenic substrates. Thus, the contributions of these precursors to glucose synthesis are difficult to quantify with any precision since the relative mix of substrates available to the liver varies with diet and physiological state. Some of these precursors will not make any net contribution to glucose supply, since all of the glycogen and a large part of the body lactate and glycerol are themselves derived from glucose. Thus, these compounds contribute to the recycling of glucose, which is relatively rapid in the case of lactate, while recycling through glycerol is slow enough for this compound to be considered a source of 'new' glucose during fasting. Recycling of glucose may also occur through non-essential amino acids, particularly alanine.

Glucose Precursors

Propionate. Propionate is the most important source of glucose in fed ruminants not absorbing glucose from the small intestine. Isotope infusion studies (for references, see Herbein et al, 1978) indicate that between 27 and 59% (mean 42%) of glucose metabolized by fed ruminants originates from propionate. This value may be an underestimate since some of the ^{14}C label will be lost as CO_2 rather than appearing as glucose due to the crossover of label in the tricarboxylic acid cycle (Fig. 7-4). Wiltrout and Satter (1972) attempted to correct for this error and concluded that a maximum of 60% of glucose could be derived from propionate in lactating dairy cows. In fact the correction for crossover may be relatively small, as measurements of hepatic glucose formation and propionate uptake also suggest around 40% of glucose may be derived from propionate (Bergman and Wolff, 1971; Thompson et al, 1978). As already mentioned, the contribution of propionate is by no means constant. The precentage of glucose originating from propionate increases as propionate absorption increases (Bergman et al, 1966; Judson and Leng, 1973) and may also increase in lactation (Wiltrout and Satter, 1972).

The amount of propionate absorbed from the rumen of well-fed ruminants is frequently sufficient to meet the animal's requirement for glucose synthesis (Bergman, 1973). However, the proportion of absorbed propionate actually converted to glucose is generally around 50%, with a range from 19-60% in published values (Herbein et al, 1978). The proportion of propionate converted to glucose does increase slightly in pregnancy (Steel and Leng, 1973), but there is no evidence for an appreciable redirection of propionate metabolism towards glucose synthesis when the supply of glucose precursors is limited. Considerable amounts of propionate are used by the gut wall (Bergman and Wolff, 1971; Weekes and Webster, 1975). The remainder is normally metabolized by the liver, involving both oxidation and conversion to other compounds (Bergman et al, 1966).

Amino Acids. The contribution of amino acids (AA) to gluconeogenesis is particularly difficult to assess. Bergman and Heitmann (1978) have compared the results obtained by two techniques (Table 7-6). The transfer of ^{14}C from AA to glucose gives a minimal estimate of gluconeogenesis, largely because of the problem of crossover of ^{14}C in

Table 7-6. Contribution of amino acids to glucose synthesis in sheep.[a]

Amino Acid	% of glucose derived from amino acid on basis of:	
	[14]C transfer	Net hepatic removal
Alanine	5.5	7.4
Glutamine	4.7	5.9
Glutamate	3.4	-2.9
Serine	0.7	3.1
Glycine	0.9	5.2
Aspartate	0.5	0.0
Other amino acids		13.5
Total	16	32

[a] Bergman and Heitmann (1978). Mean glucose entry rate 4 g/hr. Sheep fed 800 g/day of alfalfa pellets at hourly intervals.

the tricarboxylic acid cycle (Fig. 7-4). The net hepatic uptake of AA gives a maximal value, since the liver also uses AA for protein synthesis and other reactions. These specialized reactions, rather than gluconeogenesis, account for most of the hepatic uptake of serine and glycine (Table 7-6). The results óf Bergman's group, together with other work, suggests that 15-25% of glucose is derived from AA in well-fed sheep, with alanine and glutamine the most important substrates. The essential AA make very little contribution to glucose synthesis, except insofar as their oxidation may spare glucose or glucose precursors from oxidation (Egan and MacRae, 1978).

The contribution of AA to glucose synthesis will be greater in starvation, when propionate and absorbed glucose are unavailable and the AA are provided by tissue breakdown rather than by absorption. Lindsay (1979) concludes that AA may contribute 37% of the glucose irreversible loss in starved sheep. AA make an even higher contribution (53%) to what Lindsay terms the 'irrevocable' loss of glucose, which is the rate of glucose loss by oxidation, rather than recycling through other compounds. Lindsay further concludes that the rate of glucose synthesis from AA is relatively constant, regardless of diet and physiological status, averaging 20-50 mg/hr/kg $^{0.75}$ (compare with glucose entry rates in Tables 7-1 to 7-4). Thus, when the glucose entry rate is elevated, the contribution of AA to glucose synthesis will be low. Indeed, Bruckental et al (1978) calculate that in high-yielding dairy cows only 2% of glucose was derived from AA.

Even though non-essential AA provide an important source of glucose precursors, direct conversion to glucose represents a relatively minor route by which these AA are utilized in the body. Gluconeogenesis only accounts for 25% of the total turnover of alanine in fed sheep (Wolff and Bergman, 1972).

Lactate. L-lactate, together with small amounts of pyruvate, is formed during the anaerobic metabolism of glucose in all types of cells. This process is greatly accelerated during periods of oxygen shortage, as in exercising muscle. Lactate is then transported in the blood to more aerobic tissues to undergo complete oxidation or reconversion to glucose in the liver and kidney. The glucose formed may return to the muscle, for incorporation into glycogen, to be used later as a fuel for anaerobic metabolism (the Cori cycle). Lactate is also absorbed from the rumen (see Vol. 1, Ch. 12) and small amounts are produced by metabolism of propionate in the rumen epithelium (Weekes, 1972; Weigand et al, 1972). Only lactate from the latter two sources can contribute to a net synthesis of glucose. Glucose entry rate measurements will correct for recycling that occurs during the course of the experiment, but longer term recycling will not be allowed for. Recent studies (Reilly and Chandrasena, 1978) suggest that about 15% of glucose is derived from lactate in sheep fasted overnight. Lindsay (1979) calculates that lactate may contribute 40% of total glucose synthesis in sheep fasted for longer periods (3-6 days), but since all of this lactate will itself be derived from glucose, no contribution will be made to the irrevocable loss of glucose. Lactate may make an increased contribution during lactation, since the extraction of lactate by the liver is elevated in lactating cows (Baird et al, 1978).

Glycerol. The contribution of glycerol to glucose synthesis is determined by the rate of fat mobilization. In fed sheep only about 5% of glucose is derived from glycerol, while in starvation 23% of glucose comes from this source, with an even higher contribution in ketotic sheep (Bergman et al, 1968). Since glycerol, like lactate, is largely derived from glucose, a 'glycerol cycle' will operate in the fed animal. In starvation glycerol, like glycogen, can make a net contribution to supplying the animal's immediate glucose needs.

Other Sources. Liver and muscle glycogen provide an important reserve of glucose units in all animals, particularly useful in short term starvation, stress and exercise. Ruminant liver also contains glycogen, which can be mobilized in starvation or by sympathetic nervous stimulation (Baird, 1977). Liver glycogen turnover is much less important in fed ruminants than in other species, since the ruminant liver lacks the enzyme glucokinase and has a net glucose uptake at all times (Bergman et al, 1974). Glucose derived from muscle glycogen can only be used within the muscle, by complete oxidation or anaerobic glycolysis. Further research is required to establish the contribution of muscle glycogen to the immediate demands of the tissue, for example, during exercise (Jarrett et al, 1976).

Small amounts of glucose may be synthesized in fed ruminants from isobutyric and valeric acids produced in the rumen. The maximum theoretical contribution of these acids is surprisingly large; their actual contribution is unknown.

The process of ω-oxidation of long-chain fatty acids may make a small contribution to glucose supply in starvation. The necessary enzymes for this pathway are available in sheep tissue (Wahle et al, 1977) but their quantitative significance is unknown.

Table 7-7. Possible substrates for glucose synthesis in fed and starved sheep.

	Fed	Fasted 3-6 days
Glucose entry rate, mg/hr/kg$^{0.75}$	230[b]	130
% of glucose entry rate derived from:		
Propionate	40-60	-
Valerate & iso-butyrate	?	-
Amino acids	15-30	35
Lactate	15	40
Glycerol	5	23
ω-oxidation	-	2.5

[a]See text for references; data for fasted animals computed by Lindsay (1979) Glucose absorption from the small intestine has been ignored.

[b]From Table 7-1.

The relative contributions of different substrates to glucose supply in sheep are summarized in Table 7-7. These contributions depend primarily on the relative mixture of substrates available to the liver and the extent to which their metabolism is directed towards glucose synthesis rather than other pathways. This will, in turn, depend on the levels of key enzymes in the liver and the hormonal environment.

GLUCOSE METABOLISM BY RUMINANT TISSUES

We have established that the ruminant is able to synthesize large amounts of glucose and that the amount produced varies with physiological state and substrate supply. We now turn to consider the fate of that glucose in different tissues. One might assume that ruminants would have adapted to conserve glucose for essential processes which cannot use any other substrate—the validity of this assumption will be explored. Unless otherwise stated, the metabolic pathways of glucose metabolism are assumed to be the same as those in monogastric species, with which the reader is assumed to be familiar.

Glucose serves 3 major functions in cell metabolism. It may act as a carbon source for the synthesis of other carbohydrates, mucopolysaccharides, amino acids, lipids and other compounds. Secondly, metabolism via the pentose phosphate pathway (hexose monophosphate shunt) provides a source of NADPH required for biosynthetic reactions, in particular, lipogenesis. Finally, glucose may simply act as an energy source. Some of these functions are believed to occur to the same extent in ruminants and monogastrics, for example, nucleic acid and mucopolysaccharide synthesis, while other routes of glucose utilization are modified considerably in the ruminant.

Glucose makes a relatively small contribution to respiratory CO_2 (4-11%) in fed or fasted adult ruminants (Lindsay, 1970). Only about a third of the glucose produced is oxidized, since the major energy sources are fatty acids whereas in the monogastric glucose provides the major energy source. Instead, large amounts of glucose appear to be involved in recycling reactions of various kinds. Recycling occurs through lactate, glycerol, glycogen and amino acids.

Brain, Central Nervous System and Testes
These tissues have an absolute requirement for glucose as an energy source. In

man the nervous system may utilize 80% of the total glucose supply in the postabsorptive period. Very much less glucose is used by the smaller sheep brain, only 5-6% of the glucose entry rate (Lindsay, 1971), with a similar utilization by the testes in rams (Setchell and Waites, 1964). The rat and human brain are able to use ketone bodies as an alternative energy source during starvation, but this opportunity does not exist in the sheep (Lindsay and Setchell, 1976).

Erythrocytes

In humans the blood cells may utilize 15% of the postabsorptive glucose supply. Adult ruminant erythrocytes contain little or no glucose and have much lower rates of glucose utilization, consuming about 3% of the glucose supply (Leng and Annison, 1962).

Gastro-Intestinal Tract

The viscera utilize a surprisingly large amount of glucose, about a fifth of the total glucose turnover (Fig. 7-3; and Weekes and Webster, 1975). Much of this glucose may be recycled as lactate rather than oxidized (Baird, 1977). The high rate of glucose utilization may be related to the rapid cell turnover which occurs in the GI tract (Fell and Weekes, 1975). Utilization by the portal-drained viscera is unimpaired in starved sheep (Bergman, 1975), suggesting a specific glucose requirement.

Liver

Ruminant liver both produces and utilizes glucose. In fed sheep 10% of total glucose entry is removed by the liver (Fig. 7-3), due to exchange of blood glucose with liver glycogen. Glucose utlization is limited by the absence of glucokinase in adult ruminant liver (Ballard et al, 1969). Activities of some enzymes of glucose utilization can be increased by a high concentrate diet (Pearce and Unsworth, 1976) or by duodenal infusions of glucose (Unsworth and Pearce, 1977), but glucokinase activity cannot be increased (Ballard et al, 1972).

The same key enzymes are involved in gluconeogenesis in ruminant and monogastric liver (Fig. 7-4), with the exception that propionyl-CoA carboxylase may also be a rate-limiting enzyme in the ruminant. Pyruvate carboxylase is not required for gluconeogenesis from propionate.

These key enzymes are highly adaptive to gluconeogenic needs in the rat, but they are much less adaptive in the ruminant, where the continuous requirement for gluconeo-genesis may have limited the need for adaptation (Baird and Heitzman, 1971). Changes in activity of glucogenic enzymes have been reported in ruminant liver in response to starvation, feeding a high concentrate diet, glucocorticoid administration and pregnancy (Young et al, 1969; Baird and Heitzman, 1971; Mackie and Campbell, 1972; Baird and Young, 1975; Pearce and Unsworth, 1976), but different studies are frequently contradictory and responses modest. One of the few consistent findings is a decrease in bovine liver phosphoenol-pyruvate carboxykinase activity in response to glucocorticoid injection (Baird and Young, 1975), a finding of practical importance in the treatment of bovine ketosis (see Ch. 12).

Liver enzyme levels per unit of tissue may be of less significance than the supplies of different glucogenic precursors, the rate of blood flow through the liver and liver size. Portal blood flow increases after feeding, during cold exposure (Thompson et al, 1978) and in lactation (Baird et al, 1975), all situations where glucose synthesis is stimulated. The liver also increases in size during lactation (Fell et al, 1972), when glucose synthesis is most rapid.

Synthesis of fatty acids from any source is limited in ruminant liver (Ballard et al, 1969). This eliminates competition in the liver for carbon, reducing equivalents and energy between gluconeogenesis and lipogenesis. For example, propionate is virtually completely removed by the liver, while acetate, the primary lipogenic substrate, undergoes very little hepatic metabolism (Bergman, 1975).

Adipose Tissue and Lipogenesis

Very little glucose is used as a direct precursor for fatty acid synthesis in the ruminant liver, adipose tissue or mammary gland. All three tissues have very low activities of the enzymes ATP-citrate lyase and NADP-malate dehydrogenase (Ballard et al, 1969). Acetate is the major carbon source for fatty acid synthesis in the ruminant, unlike the rat (see Ch. 6). Glucose incorporation into fatty acid and the activities of ATP-citrate lyase and NADP-malate dehydrogenase can be increased in sheep liver and adipose tissue by feeding a high carbohydrate diet or by infusing glucose (Ballard et al, 1972). Even in these circumstances acetate still remains the preferred substrate for fatty acid synthesis. Somewhat surprisingly ruminant adipose tissue is able to use lactate at an appreciable rate for fatty acid synthesis (Prior, 1978), suggesting an indirect route for glucose incorporation into fatty acids. The pathway of incorporation is uncertain.

Lipogenesis in ruminant adipose tissue does, however, still have an essential glucose requirement. Glucose is firstly necessary to supply α-glycerophosphate for triglyceride formation. Glycerol liberated by lipolysis is not reutilized, since glycerokinase activity is very low in adipose tissue. Secondly, glucose is required to supply NADPH by operation of the hexose monophosphate shunt. In the rat NADPH is supplied in part by NADP-malate dehydrogenase, but this enzyme is absent in ruminant adipose tissue. The ruminant has an alternative system, involving NADP-isocitrate dehydrogenase in the cytoplasm. The enzymes of this glucose-independent pathway display considerably higher activities than those of the pentose phosphate pathway in ruminant adipose tissue and mammary gland (Bauman and Davis, 1975). Approximately equal amounts of NADPH are generated by each pathway in the bovine mammary gland, with at least a quarter of the NADPH arising from the glucose-independent pathway in bovine adipose tissue (Baldwin et al, 1973). Tricarbon compounds generated in the pentose phosphate pathway are extensively recycled within both tissues, with very little oxidation of glucose through the tricarboxylic acid cycle.

Thus, the process of lipogenesis shows considerable adaptation in the ruminant to limit glucose utilization. The actual amount of glucose used has not been quantified. Assuming that all glycerol is derived from glucose, glycerol synthesis accounts for 10% of the glucose entry rate in fed sheep (Bergman et al, 1968), only half of which is directly recycled back to glucose.

Muscle

Glucose uptake by the whole musculature cannot readily be calculated from the published data, which only relates to the hind limb. Calculation by difference (Table 7-8) suggests that muscle must use large amounts of glucose, although the value of 42% suggested is a maximal one, including the contribution of other tissues.

Glucose is taken up by the hind limb of fed sheep (Jarrett et al, 1976) and steers (Bell et al, 1975), with a reduced uptake on fasting. Only a small proportion of this glucose is oxidized. Muscle lactate output will account for between 28% (Domanski et al, 1974) and

Table 7-8. Sites of glucose metabolism in fed sheep.[a]

Tissue or pathway	% of glucose entry rate
Brain and central nervous system	5
Testes, rams	5
Erythrocytes	3
Gastro-intestinal tract	25
Adipose tissue-glycerol turnover	10
Liver	10
Total	58
'Muscle,' by difference	42
Oxidation, whole body	33

[a] See text for references. Muscle figure will include contributions of other tissues, e.g. lungs, kidney, skin and connective tissue.

60% (Jarrett et al, 1976) of hind limb glucose uptake in fed sheep and virtually all the glucose uptake in fasting. Glucose may also be recycled through amino acids, particularly alanine and glutamine.

This process, the alanine cycle, operates in a similar manner to the Cori cycle in monogastric species. Alanine and glutamine function as amino group carriers from muscle to liver, where the amino groups are incorporated into urea. The carbon skeletons of the amino acids are derived from glucose breakdown in muscle. Glucose is resynthesized in the liver from the amino acids, completing the cycle. Muscle alanine output increases during fasting and exercise in man.

Release of alanine and glutamine in excess of that expected from simple proteolysis has also been demonstrated in ruminant muscle, with an increased release on fasting (Ballard et al, 1976; Lindsay et al, 1977). If all of the carbon was derived from glucose, it would represent 15% of glucose uptake by muscle of fed sheep (Ballard et al, 1976; Jarrett et al, 1976). Recycling through lactate, alanine and glutamine could, therefore, account for 75% of glucose uptake by hind limb of fed sheep and is more than adequate to account for glucose uptake in fasting. Glucose oxidation would only contribute 5% of the fuel of muscle respiration in the fed animal and nil in fasting (Jarrett et al, 1976). Recycling also occurs in steers, perhaps to a lesser extent than in sheep (Bell et al, 1975).

In exercise, when the whole body glucose entry rate is increased (see above), Jarrett et al (1976) report a 6X increase in hind limb glucose uptake, but lactate output was surprisingly reduced. Alanine release was not measured. Glucose supplied a maximum of 27% of the fuel of muscle respiration during exercise. Glucose uptake by the hind legs of steers is also increased by cold exposure, with a decreased proportion being recycled as lactate or amino acids (Bell et al, 1975). Glucose oxidation could contribute 52% to hind leg oxidative metabolism in cold-exposed steers fasted 20 hr rising to 75% shortly after a meal. Muscle glycogen deposition and utilization has been ignored in these calculations, probably leading to an overestimate of glucose oxidation by muscle of fed anmals and an underestimation in fasting or stressed animals.

The alanine released by muscle may be derived from lactate as well as glucose (Chandrasena, 1976). Glucose, lactate and non-essential amino acids may, therefore, form a common pool, with long-term recycling of glucose carbon through muscle amino acids and protein (Lindsay, 1979). This would explain the limited oxidation of glucose observed in short-term isotope infusion studies (Table 7-8). Thus, although ruminant muscle may utilize large amounts of glucose, little of this is directly oxidized in fed or fasted animals. Once again adaptation is apparent to prevent loss of glucose or its precursors. Only in exercise or exposure to cold is glucose used solely as an energy source.

Pregnancy

Glucose metabolism in the adult ruminant is adapted to limit 'wasteful' loss of glucose. These adaptations are absent in the fetal ruminant, accounting for the high glucose requirement of the pregnant uterus and its contents (see above) and producing a pattern of metabolism reminiscent of a non-ruminant in these tissues. Whereas the non-breeding ewe only derives 10% of its CO_2 from glucose, the pregnant sheep uterus and contents derive about 40% of its CO_2 from glucose and directly oxidize about 45% of the glucose utilized (Setchell et al, 1972). Glucose is also required for synthesis of fructose in the placenta and glycogen and fatty acids in the fetus.

The fetal plasma glucose level is below the maternal concentration in all species and is particularly low (10-25 mg/100 ml) in fetal lambs, less than half of maternal levels (Leat, 1971). Fetal tissues—including the brain—are adapted to operate at these low glucose levels without signs of hypoglycemia. The placenta is freely permeable to glucose by a process of facilitated transfer, delivery of glucose to the fetus being largely dependent on the glucose concentration gradient across the placenta. Fetal blood glucose levels are closely correlated with maternal levels, but can also be regulated, at least in the last third of gestation, by fetal insulin secretion (Bassett, 1977). Although fetal wellbeing is preserved at the expense of maternal hypoglycemia in maternal undernutrition, fetal blood glucose will decline during maternal starvation (Shelley et al, 1975).

Levels of fructose in fetal lamb plasma considerably exceed those of glucose, declining from about 150 mg/100 ml in mid gestation to 90 mg/100 ml near term. However, fructose is a relatively inert metabolite in the fetus, making no significant contribution to fetal energy supply (Warnes et al, 1977). Fructose formation in the placenta, via the sorbitol pathway, equally consumes very little of the total glucose uptake by the uterus. The true function of fetal fructose is uncertain.

The uterus takes up large amounts of glucose, up to 70% of the total glucose entry rate in pregnancy (see above). Christenson and Prior (1978) calculate that the uterus of a twin-bearing ewe will consume 77 g glucose/day at 105 days of gestation and 92 g/day at 121 days. Much of this glucose is metabolized by the uterine tissues, particularly the placenta. In the cow about a third of the glucose taken up by the uterus is transferred to the fetus unchanged, while 50% is metabolized anaerobically to lactate, the majority of which is also utilized by the fetus (Comline and Silver, 1976). Only 13% of the uterine glucose uptake was oxidized by the uteroplacental tissues, which thus resemble other maternal tissues in relying on acetate as the major energy source.

In the fetus almost all the glucose consumption is oxidized, accounting for around 50% of the fetal oxygen consumption. This contribution may be slightly higher in the calf than in the lamb (Comline and Silver, 1976), consistent with the slightly higher maternal blood glucose level in the cow. Most of the remaining fetal oxygen consumption in the calf can be attributed to the oxidation of lactate (43%) and acetate (16%); (Comline and Silver, 1976), while in the lamb lactate and amino acid oxidation could each contribute 25% (Burd et al, 1975) and acetate 10% (Char and Creasy, 1976) to oxygen consumption. This pattern of substrate oxidation is clearly different from that in adult ruminant tissues.

Some of the substrates listed are also used for tissue deposition. Glucose will be used for glycogen synthesis. Glycogen levels in the fetal liver rise throughout the last half of gestation, reaching 80 mg/g wet weight at term, double adult values. Glycogen also accumulates in late gestation in fetal cardiac and skeletal muscle (5X adult values) and lungs. The glycogen is mainly utilized immediately after birth, but can also be mobilized in utero in times of stress (see Leat, 1971).

Glucose carbon may also be incorporated into fetal lipid, both as glycerol and as fatty acid, since the enzymes ATP-citrate lyase and NADP-malate dehydrogenase are present in fetal ruminant liver (Ballard et al, 1969), but the amount of fatty acid synthesis is probably limited.

The enzymes of gluconeogenesis are present in the fetal lamb liver in late gestation (Warnes et al, 1977) and active fetal gluconeogenesis has been claimed (Hodgson and Mellor, 1977; Prior and Christenson, 1977). Other workers strongly dispute this suggestion (Warnes et al, 1977; Anand and Sperling, 1978). Further work is required to resolve this conflict.

There is no doubt that uterine glucose removal places a considerable strain on maternal glucose homeostasis in late pregnancy. Glucose oxidation by extra-uterine tissues is greatly reduced (Lindsay, 1971). Such an adaptation would appear feasible, since the essential body requirements for glucose oxidation are not large (Table 7-8). In monogastric species the elevated levels of progesterone and placental lactogen in late gestation produce a diabetogenic effect to limit maternal glucose utilization, increase reliance on free fatty acids and accelerate the metabolic responses to starvation. Similar adaptations probably occur in the pregnant ewe. It is well known that such adaptations are frequently insufficient to prevent maternal hypoglycemia and pregnancy toxemia in late gestation (see Ch. 12). Even if maternal glucose utilization was limited to essential demands only, the large fixed demand of the uterus and its contents would be difficult to meet when harsh climatic conditions or a decline in voluntary feed intake (see Ch. 11) reduces the supply of glucose precursors.

Lactation

The massive glucose requirements of lactating ruminants have already been de-scribed (Table 7-4). Thus, in dairy cows yielding 12-26 kg/day, 66% of whole body glucose entry was utilized by the udder (Bickerstaffe et al, 1974). Glucose is the major precursor of milk lactose, which accounted for 51% of the total glucose entry rate and 80% of the glucose taken up by the udder in this study. Smaller amounts of glucose are also used for the synthesis of milk citrate, non-essential amino acids and glycerol. Glucose does not contribute carbon for milk fatty acid synthesis (see above).

Around 11% of the glucose taken up by the udder appears as CO_2, accounting for 25% of the total udder CO_2 production, whereas only 7% of whole body CO_2 output was derived from glucose (Bickerstaffe et al, 1974). These figures are misleading, since most of the CO_2 produced from glucose in the udder is derived from the pentose phosphate pathway (Davis and Bauman, 1974). Glucose oxidation via the tricarboxylic acid cycle may be virtually absent in the mammary gland (Smith, 1971), an adaptation of obvious benefit in conserving glucose supplies. This is achieved by extensive recycling of triose phosphates derived from the pentose phosphate cycle, using the enzyme, fructose-1, 6-diphosphatase, which is present in much higher activity in ruminant than in monogastric mammary gland (Davis and Bauman, 1974).

Glucose uptake per unit weight of tissue is twice as great in the ewe mammary gland as in the cow, with a smaller proportion of this glucose being used for lactose synthesis (Davis and Bickerstaffe, 1978). The high fat content of ewe's milk will require additional glucose for synthesis of glycerol and NADPH generation via the pentose phosphate pathway. Whereas in the bovine mammary gland, approximately equal amounts of the NADPH required for fatty acid synthesis are derived from the pentose phosphate pathway and the NADP-isocitrate dehydrogenase pathway, the relative contribution of the pentose phosphate pathway may be higher in the goat and the ewe (Davis and Bickerstaffe, 1978). Glucose utilization by extra-mammary tissues does not appear to be reduced in lactation (Lindsay, 1971), in contrast with the situation in pregnancy.

In some situations milk yield may be limited by glucose supply to the udder (Linzell, 1967), whereas shortages of other precursors are more specific in their effect on mammary gland metabolism. Shortage of glucose precursors is a major factor in the development of bovine ketosis (see Ch. 12). Low blood glucose levels are also associated with reduced fertility in lactating cattle (McClure et al, 1978).

Milk yield in lactating dairy cows can sometimes be increased by post-ruminal infusion of glucose (Vik-Mo et al, 1974; Frobish and Davis, 1977), but in other studies there was no response to glucose but a large response to post-ruminal casein supplementation (Ørskov et al, 1977). Responsiveness to glucose will clearly depend on the relative availability of glucose precursors to supplies of energy and protein. Ørskov (1975) has expressed this concept in terms of the non-glucogenic ratio of VFA's (NGR), defined as (acetic + 2 butyric + valeric)/(propionic + valeric). He calculates that an optimum ratio of 2-4 is required for maximal energetic efficiency. Higher ratios can be tolerated if glucose is absorbed from the small intestine. Responses to glucose would not be expected when NGR is low.

Despite the large requirement for glucose precursors in lactation, NGR ratios below 3 are not recommended, since such diets are associated with a reduction in milk fat percentage and increased body fat deposition (low milk fat syndrome, see Ch. 6). An early theory proposed that high levels of propionate caused an increase in blood glucose levels and an increased secretion of insulin, which in turn would suppress adipose tissue fat mobilization (McClymont and Vallance, 1962). A stimulation of adipose tissue lipoprotein lipase and/or L-α-glycerophosphate dehydrogenase, with no effect on these enzymes in the mammary gland (Rao et al, 1973) would produce this response and may explain the reduced extraction of triglycerides by the udder (Annison et al, 1974). A reduced availability of acetate to the udder has also been implicated, limiting de novo lipogenesis. Annison et al reported a decrease in blood acetate levels and acetate entry rate, but this was mainly due to a fall in endogenous acetate production by the body tissues, rather than a decrease in ruminal acetate production on the high-concentrate diet. The most recent theory to explain the low milk fat syndrome proposes that supplies of vitamin B_{12} may be inadequate to metabolize the increased load of propionate absorbed on low fiber diets (Frobish and Davis, 1977). A build up of methylmalonic acid may result, inhibiting milk fat synthesis. Thus, it is uncertain whether changes in carbohydrate metabolism are directly implicated in the syndrome.

CONTROL OF CARBOHYDRATE METABOLISM

The endocrinological and enzymatic control of carbohydrate metabolism has been well established in monogastric species. Preservation of glucose homeostasis is achieved by the combined action of several hormones, integrated by neural reflex mechanisms and expressed at the tissue level in a delicate control of the amounts and activities of key enzymes of glucose formation and utilization. The continued requirement for glucose synthesis in the ruminant and normal lack of absorbed dietary glucose means that the balance of control mechanisms is different in the ruminant. This topic has been reviewed by Bassett (1975, 1978) and Trenkle (1978). Fig. 7-5 gives an example of the pattern of metabolite changes after feeding in sheep, with a slow increase in plasma glucose levels after feeding, associated with absorption of VFA's from the reticulo-rumen and a decreased reliance on free fatty acids as an energy source.

The major short-term control of glucose homeostasis is exercised by the pancreatic enzymes, insulin and glucagon. The largely opposing actions of these two hormones has led to the suggestion that the molar concentration ratio of the hormones (I/G ratio) may

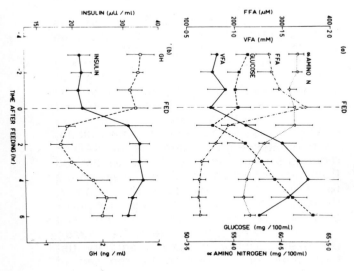

Fig. 7-5. Effect of feeding on plasma metabolites, insulin and growth hormone concentrations in sheep fed 800 g of a 1:1 mixture of alfalfa chaff and oat grain 1X daily. Vertical bars show standard errors of group means. Note the rapid changes in insulin and growth hormone concentrations and the initial decline in plasma glucose after feeding. From Bassett (1974) with permission of The Aust. J. Biol. Sci.

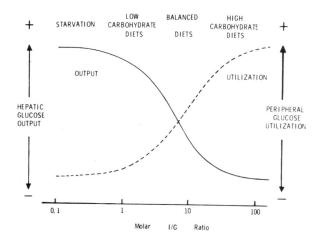

Fig. 7-6. Influence of the molar insulin:glucagon ratio (I/G ratio) in peripheral plasma on glucose metabolism in monogastric species. From Bassett (1975) with permission of The University of New England Pub. Unit.

be more important than the absolute level of either hormone (see Bassett, 1975). Thus, in monogastric species the I/G ratio will be low during starvation or when low-carbohydrate diets are fed (Fig. 7-6), favoring hepatic gluconeogenesis and glycogenolysis and limiting glucose utilization. As carbohydrate supply is increased, elevated levels of glucose result in a raised I/G ratio (Fig. 7-6) with the balance of metabolism shifted towards increased tissue anabolism and glucose utilization. Hepatic gluconeogenesis is inhibited and hepatic glycogen levels increase, stimulated by insulin and glucose itself.

This pattern is considerably modified in the ruminant, although the key role of the endocrine pancreas remains. Insulin levels remain fairly constant in sheep fed at frequent intervals, but at concentrations related to the digestible organic matter intake (Bassett, 1975). A biphasic increase in insulin secretion occurs in sheep (Fig. 7-5) and cattle (Trenkle, 1978) fed 1X or 2X daily. An initial rapid rise in insulin level within 1 hr of feeding is probably mediated by reflex vagal nervous mechanisms (Bassett, 1974) and may result in a moderate fall in plasma glucose concentration at this time (Fig. 7-5). A second, more prolonged insulin peak occurs 4-6 hr after feeding, coincident with increasing absorption of the products of digestion. The magnitude of the response depends on the amount of food consumed and the diet (Bassett, 1975). The hyperinsulinemic response is smaller after feeding hay

rather than concentrates (Ross and Kitts, 1973), probably reflecting a slower rate of digestion and a lower intake of digestible nutrients.

The stimulus for insulin secretion in ruminants is unclear. Plasma glucose concentrations are unlikely to be a normal regulator of insulin secretion in ruminants, unlike in monogastric species (Trenkle, 1978), although intravenous injection of glucose will stimulate insulin secretion. Likewise, although several amino acids can stimulate insulin secretion when injected intravenously, the postprandial changes in peripheral plasma amino acid levels do not correlate with insulin secretion (Fig. 7-5; Bassett, 1974). Insulin secretion is often coincident with the rise in plasma VFA after feeding (Fig. 7-5) and propionate, butyrate and valerate, but not acetate, can stimulate insulin release from ruminant pancreas (see Bassett, 1975). However, it is doubtful whether VFA have a physiological role in regulating insulin secretion (Stern et al, 1970). Bassett (1975, 1978) has suggested that a major stimulus for insulin secretion may be provided by the gastro-intestinal hormones, in particular gastric inhibitory peptide, released by the presence of the products of digestion in the gut. These hormones are known to be important regulators of insulin release in monogastric species, but their involvement in the ruminant is still speculative.

Plasma glucagon levels in ruminants are less well defined, due to difficulties in the assay of this hormone. In sheep fed once daily, plasma glucagon increased after the meal at the same time as insulin, with a decrease on fasting (Bassett, 1972). The stimulus for the rise in glucagon is uncertain. Hyperglycemia reduces plasma glucagon, while acute insulin-induced hypoglycemia increases glucagon levels in sheep (Brockman, 1977) as in other species. However, the latter response, like the stimulation of glucagon secretion by catecholamines and the sympathetic nervous system, may reflect the additional role of glucagon as an 'emergency' hormone, rather than its function in normal metabolic regulation (Brockman et al, 1975).

As a result of the parallel changes in insulin and glucagon secretion after feeding, the I/G ratio remains much more constant in ruminants than in monogastric species (Fig. 7-7), ranging from 1.0 in prolonged fasting to a peak of 3.3 at 2 hr after feeding in one study (Bassett, 1975). Ratios in this region are characteristic of monogastric species fed low carbohydrate diets (Fig. 7-6). Ruminant diets can be considered as low carbohydrate in terms of the absorbed products of digestion.

The metabolic consequences of these changes in hormone levels depends on the responsiveness of ruminant tissues to insulin and glucagon. The hypoglycemic response to insulin injection (insulin sensitivity) is less in ruminants than other species, as is the rate of insulin secretion (Brockman and Bergman, 1975). However, the hormone is no less important in the overall regulation of anabolic metabolism in general. Insulin is the major regulator of glucose disposal, even though plasma glucose concentration may not control insulin secretion in ruminants. Insulin greatly stimulates utilization of glucose and acetate by adipose tissue, as well as inhibiting lipolysis (Bassett, 1978) and stimulating amino acid uptake by muscle . The hepatic actions of insulin are less clear in the ruminant (Brockman et al, 1975). Stimulation of hepatic glycogen synthesis by insulin and glucose is unlikely to be physiologically important, since ruminant liver has a net glucose output at all times. Hepatic gluconeogenesis may be inhibited by insulin in sheep (Bassett, 1978). However, Lomax et al (1978) recently reported that intravenous infusions of glucose into non-lactating cows

produced a 4X increase in insulin production, with no significant effect on hepatic glucose output.

Glucagon stimulates hepatic gluconeogenesis and glycogenolysis in ruminants (Brockman et al, 1975). Glucagon directly stimulates the hepatic uptake of lactate, amino acids and propionate and increases the proportion of alanine converted to glucose (Brockman and Bergman, 1975). Brockman and Manns (1974) reported that the stimulation of gluconeogenesis involved an acute increase in pyruvate carboxylase activity. This contrasts with the action of glucagon in monogastric liver, where inactivation of pyruvate kinase occurs. Glucagon stimulates adipose tissue lipolysis and also increases hepatic ketogenesis in sheep (Brockman and Johnson, 1977). The hormone does not affect muscle protein metabolism directly in the ruminant, but the glucagon-induced fall in plasma amino acid levels will indirectly retard muscle protein synthesis (Brockman and Bergman, 1975).

Thus, the interrelated secretion of insulin and glucagon in the ruminant can be correlated with known changes in glucose turnover and maintenance of glucose homeostasis. The availability of substrates and the secretion of both hormones in fed ruminants will stimulate hepatic gluconeogenesis and the peripheral utilization of glucose, amino acids and acetate for tissue anabolism. During prolonged fasting the fall in I/G ratio will allow gluconeogenesis to be maintained from endogenous substrates and glucagon-stimulated lipolysis will provide free fatty acids and ketone bodies as the major energy source.

This basic system of regulation will be modified by the actions of other hormones. Some of these interactions are shown in Fig. 7-8. Growth hormone (STH in Fig. 7-8) is secreted in an episodic manner (Bassett, 1974), with a clear decrease in levels after feeding in sheep (Fig. 7-5). Prolonged treatment with exogenous growth hormone increases N retention, but the major effects of this hormone in the ruminant are to diminish glucose utilization and stimulate lipolysis, i.e. insulin antagonism (Bassett, 1978). Thus, growth hormone tends to increase when availability of nutrients becomes limiting, mobilizing energy from adipose tissue to satisfy the needs for metabolism. Thus, in fasting growth hormone will augment the effect of the low I/G ratio.

In the short term hepatic glycogenolysis and adipose tissue lipolysis will be stimulated in respone to stress by increased

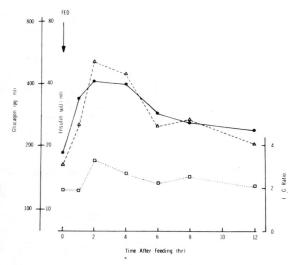

Fig. 7-7. Plasma insulin (Δ) and glucagon (•) concentrations and the molar insulin:glucagon ratio (□) in sheep fed 800 g of a 1:1 ratio of alfalfa chaff and oat grain 1X daily. Note the relatively constant I/G ratio in the ruminant (compare with Fig. 7-6). From Bassett (1975) with permission of The University of New England Pub. Unit.

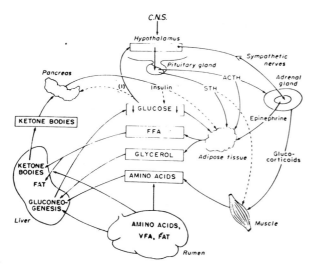

Fig. 7-8. Outline of the major hormonal controls regulating the supply of precursors for hepatic gluconeogenesis and ketogenesis. Dashed lines indicate inhibitory effects. Hypoglycemia triggers a series of hormonal adjustments involving the hypothalmus, pituitary, adrenal and endocrine pancreas. Direct hormonal effects on the liver have been omitted for clarity. These involve stimulation of glycogenolysis and gluconeogenesis by epinephrine and glucagon. Glucagon may stimulate amino acid release from muscle; this action is opposed by insulin. Lactate release from muscle and use in gluconeogenesis has also been omitted. From Bergman (1977); reprinted from Dukes' Physiology of Domestic Animals (9th ed) by permission of The Cornell University Press.

activity of the sympathetic nervous system and output of epinephrine from the adrenal gland. Glucagon secretion will be stimulated and insulin inhibited. These effects on the I/G ratio probably account for the increased hepatic glucose output in sheep during acute cold exposure (Thompson et al, 1978).

Cold exposure and other prolonged stresses, such as fasting, will increase cortisol output (Trenkle, 1978). Cortisol inhibits extra-hepatic glucose utilization and antagonizes insulin action. Exogenous corticosteroids stimulate muscle proteolysis (Fig. 7-8), providing substrate for hepatic gluconeogenesis, and increase the glucose entry rate in sheep (Brockman et al, 1975; Ranawere and Ford, 1976). In cattle the antiketogenic action of exogenous glucocorticoid is associated with decreased phosphoenolpyruvate carboxykinase activity in liver cytoplasm and increased hepatic levels of tricarboxylic acid cycle intermediates (Baird, 1977).

Changes in the hormonal environment will also control glucose metabolism during reproduction. The effects of placental hor-

mones on maternal glucose utilization have already been mentioned. In lactation the balance between insulin and growth hormone may control the division of nutrients between milk and body tissues. Thus, plasma levels of growth hormone are higher and insulin lower in high-yielding dairy cows in negative energy balance than in lactating beef cows (Bines and Hart, 1978). Whether these responses are cause or effect is not established. One could argue that the apparent energy deficit in high-yielding cows would result in lower insulin and higher growth hormone levels.

Plasma levels of hormones only provide a first indication of the manner in which glucose homeostasis is maintained. The actions of hormones at the different tissues involve interaction with specific receptors. Regulation at this level may be as important as changes in circulating hormone concentrations. This area of regulation has not been investigated in ruminants and is likely to be an active field for future research.

CARBOHYDRATE METABOLISM IN THE PRERUMINANT ANIMAL

This topic has been reviewed by Leat (1971) and Shelley et al (1975). Nutritional aspects of carbohydrate metabolism in the young ruminant are covered in Ch. 10. Three phases of carbohydrate metabolism can be distinguished in the preruminant.

Neonatal Period

Rapid changes in carbohydrate metabolism occur to ensure survival following the cessation of maternal glucose supplies at birth. The fetal stores of glycogen are rapidly mobilized, falling to about 10% of fetal values within 2-3 hr (Ballard et al, 1969). Glycogenolysis is accelerated in lambs exposed to cold, when stores of brown adipose tissue are also mobilized. Hepatic gluconeogenesis is initiated within minutes of birth, possibly triggered by increased oxygenation of the blood (Warnes et al, 1977). Neonatal hypoglycemia is thereby avoided and blood glucose levels increase rapidly after birth, reaching 100 mg/100 ml within 48 hr.

Postnatal Period

Fasting blood glucose levels remain elevated, around 80-100 mg/100 ml, with a slow decline towards adult levels by 8-12 weeks in lambs (Bassett, 1974). The decline is due to both replacement of fetal, glucose-containing, red blood cells by adult cells containing very little glucose and to a declining milk consumption. Hepatic glycogen stores are replenished over the first 3 weeks of life, reaching higher levels than in the adult (Ballard et al, 1969).

Carbohydrate metabolism in the postnatal period is similar to that of young monogastric animals and will not be considered in detail. Glucose is derived from absorption of milk lactose and by gluconeogenesis. Thus, blood glucose levels increase rapidly after feeding (Bassett, 1974), in contrast with the immediate hypoglycemic response in adult sheep (Fig. 7-5).

The neonatal calf and lamb can readily utilize glucose, lactose and galactose, but are unable to use fructose, sucrose or starch and have only a limited capacity to digest maltose. Digestion is limited by levels of intestinal and pancreatic digestive enzymes. Pancreatic amylase activity is low at birth but increases with age in calves and intestinal maltase and isomaltase also develop over the first 4 weeks of life, while lactase levels decline with age (see Vol. 1). Sucrose cannot be digested by the preruminant calf, since intestinal activity never develops.

Digestion of starch, maltose and lactose and absorption of glucose and galactose in the preruminant calf have been studied by Coombe and Smith (1973, 1974). Sugars left the abomasum at the same rate as a water-soluble marker but starch was considerably delayed due to its association with the casein clot. With starch, maltose and lactose, some 60, 43 and 97% of the amounts ingested were removed in passage of digesta through the small intestine. The presence of glucose which was rapidly absorbed from the proximal part of the intestine, depressed absorption of galactose in that part of the intestine; however in the more distal intestine, where glucose concentration was lower, galactose was absorbed more rapidly.

Rumen Development

Forestomach development occurs gradually, over a period of 3-9 weeks of age in lambs reared at pasture. During this period additional changes occur in carbohydrate metabolism as the adult pattern of increasing reliance upon gluconeogenesis develops. Blood glucose levels decline to adult values, as does glucose entry rate, glucose tolerance and the hypoglycemic response to exogenous insulin. In the liver glycogen levels decrease, as do the activities of glycogen synthetase and phosphorylase

and the rate of glucose oxidation, while gluconeogenesis increases. The level of ATP-citrate lyase activity declines to the negligible adult value, preventing diversion of glucose carbon into fatty acids (see Leat, 1971). The active transport of glucose in the small intestine also decreases (Scharrer, 1975).

Some of these changes are related to age rather than rumen development per se. Thus, Ponto and Bergen (1974) observed that the decline in plasma glucose levels, glucose tolerance and hepatic pyruvate kinase activity followed the same pattern in conventional and gnotobiotic goats. However, the development of gluconeogenesis from propionate requires increasing supplies of substrate from rumen fermentation (Ballard et al, 1969), while the decrease in intestinal glucose absorption is related to the reduced amount of carbohydrate entering the small intestine (Scharrer, 1975).

GLUCOSE REQUIREMENTS

With regard to the diet, the majority of any ruminant's diet is carbohydrate of one kind or another. The RAC (readily available carbohydrates) content may range from 10% in some poor-quality forages or grass silage to 70-80% in high-grain feedlot rations. Likewise, the fibrous components may vary from 50 to 10% acid detergent fiber. While different proportions of RAC and ADF are more suitable in one situation than another, it is difficult at this time to suggest specific requirements for RAC or ADF. This is so because optimal concentrations appear to depend on various factors such as the amount, kind and solubility of dietary nitrogen sources, density of feedstuffs, feed processing methods, the species of animal and the type of production involved. The rumen microorganisms are quite flexible in their ability to metabolize a wide variety of carbohydrates (see Ch. 12, Vol. 1). On the other hand, over a long-term period ruminants need a bulky diet which is provided by the fibrous carbohydrates. However, it can be said with a high degree of certainty that there is no dietary need for any specific carbohydrate molecule.

Definitive statements cannot yet be made concerning glucose requirements in all physiological states. Glucose entry rates are known fairly precisely, but it is not clear how much of this glucose is essential and how much can be replaced by other metabolites in particular situations. The supply of glucose precursors is most likely to be the limiting factor for performance, or even survival, in late pregnancy and lactation. In these circumstances glucose entry rates (Tables 7-3 and 7-4) probably represent true requirements which must be met by adequate supplies of precursors, bearing in mind that no precursor is quantitatively converted to glucose and that excessive amounts of propionate will reduce the milk fat percentage.

Requirements are less readily determined in non-breeding animals, since so little glucose is directly oxidized or used for defined purposes and glucose entry rates are largely controlled by food intake. The rate of glucose oxidation in fasted animals provides a minimal estimate of requirement for de novo glucose synthesis of 50 mg/hr/kg$^{0.75}$ in sheep. The different hormonal environment of fed and fasted ruminants may result in a higher irrevocable loss in fed animals. Lindsay (1979) has calculated that the minimal requirement in fasting sheep could just be supplied by the known rates of fat and protein breakdown during starvation.

Glucose supplies are unlikely to be a limiting factor when animals are fed at the maintenance level. Provided rumen fermentation patterns are not grossly abnormal, diets supplying adequate energy will also meet the animal's requirement for glucose precursors.

Glucose requirements cannot be considered in isolation. This is particularly obvious in growing ruminants. The efficiency of utilization of metabolizable energy for growth and fattening is determined by the relative proportions of VFA's produced (see Ch. 8). An adequate proportion of glucogenic VFA's must be available to meet the glucose requirement for growth-related processes, such as NADPH, glycerol and nucleic acid synthesis. Ørskov (1975) calculates that the optimum non-glucogenic ratio of VFA's (see above) is 2.25-3.0 for growing sheep. Provided that this ratio is achieved, the relation between energy intake and glucose entry rate means that an adequate supply of glucose precursors will always be provided to support the rate of growth determined by energy and protein supplies.

References Cited

Altszuler, N. et al. 1975. Amer. J. Physiol. 229:1662.

Anand, R.S. and M.A. Sperling. 1978. Amer. J. Physiol. 235:3449.

Annison, E.F., R. Bickerstaffe and J.L. Linzell. 1974. J. Agr. Sci. 82:87.

Annison, E.F. and J.L. Linzell. 1964. J. Physiol. 175:372.

Armstrong, D.G. and D.E. Beever. 1969. Proc. Nutr. Soc. 28:121.

Armstrong, D.G. and J.H.D. Prescott. 1971. In: Lactation. Butterworths, London.

Badawy, A.M., R.M. Campbell, D.P. Cuthbertson and W.S. Mackie. 1958. Brit. J. Nutr. 12:384.

Baird, G.C. 1977. Biochem. Soc. Trans. 5:819.

Baird, G.D. and R.J. Heitzman. 1971. Biochem. Biophys. Acta 252:184.

Baird, G.D., M.A. Lomax, H.W. Symonds and S.R. Shaw. 1978. Proc. Nutr. Soc. 37:94A.

Baird, G.D., H.W. Symonds and R. Ash. 1975. J. Agr. Sci. 85:281.

Baird, G.C. and J.L. Young. 1975. J. Agr. Sci. 84:227.

Baldwin, R.L. et al. 1973. J. Dairy Sci. 56:340.

Ballard, F.J., O.H. Filsell and I.G. Jarrett. 1972. Biochem. J. 126:193.

Ballard, F.J., R.W. Hanson and D.S. Kronfeld. 1969. Fed. Proc. 28:218.

Bassett, J.M. 1972. Aust. J. Biol. Sci. 25:1277.

Bassett, J.M. 1974. Aust. J. Biol. Sci. 27:157,167.

Bassett, J.M. 1975. In: Digestion and Metabolism in the Ruminant. The Univ. of New England Pub. Unit, Armidale, Australia.

Bassett, J.M. 1977. Ann. Rech. Vet. 8:362.

Bassett, J.M. 1978. Proc. Nutr. Soc. 37:273.

Bauman, D.E. and C.L. Davis. 1975. In: Digestion and Metabolism in the Ruminant. The Univ. of New England Pub. Unit, Armidale.

Bell, A.W., J.W. Gardner, W.Manson and G.E. Thompson. 1975. Brit. J. Nutr. 33:207.

Bergman, E.N. 1963. Amer. J. Physiol. 204:147.

Bergman, E.N. 1973. Cornell Vet. 63:341.

Bergman, E.N. 1975. In: Digestion and Metabolism in the Ruminant. The Univ. of New England Pub. Unit, Armidale.

Bergman, E.N. 1977. In: Dukes' Physiology of Farm Animals. 9th ed. Cornell University Press, Ithaca.

Bergman, E.N., R.P. Brockman and C.F. Kaufman. 1974. Fed. Proc. 33:1849.

Bergman, E.N. and R.N. Heitmann. 1978. Fed. Proc. 37:1228.

Bergman, E.N. and D.E. Hogue. 1967. Amer. J. Physiol. 213:1378.

Bergman, E.N., W.E. Roe and K.Kon. 1966. Amer. J. Physiol. 211:793.

Bergman, E.N., D.J. Starr and S.S. Reulin. 1968. Amer. J. Physiol. 215:874.

Bergman, E.N. and J.E. Wolff. 1971. Amer. J. Physiol. 221:586.

Bickerstaffe, R., E.F. Annison and J.L. Linzell. 1974. J. Agr. Sci. 82:71.

Bines, J.A. and I.C. Hart. 1978. Proc. Nutr. Soc. 37:281.

Brockman, R.P. 1977. Can. J. Comp. Med. 41:95.

Brockman, R.P. and E.N. Bergman. 1975. Amer. J. Physiol. 228:1627;229:1338.

Brockman, R.P., E.N. Bergman, P.K. Joo and J.G. Manns. 1975a. Amer. J. Physiol. 229:1344.

Brockman, R.P., E.N. Bergman, W.L. Pollak and J. Brondum. 1975b. Can. J. Physiol. Pharmacol. 53:1186.

Brockman, R.P. and M.R. Johnson. 1977. Can. J. Animal Sci. 77:177.

Brockman, R.P. and J.G. Manns. 1974. Cornell Vet. 64:217.

Bruckenthal, I., J.D. Oldham and J.D. Sutton. 1973. Proc. Nutr. Soc. 37:107A.

Burd, L.I. et al. 1975. Nature 254:710.

Chandrasena, L. 1976. Ph.D. Thesis, Univ. of Liverpool, England.

Char, V.C. and R.K. Creasy. 1976. Amer. J. Physiol. 230:357.

Christenson, R.K. and R.L. Prior. 1978. J. Animal Sci. 46:189.

Clark, D., D. Lee, R. Rognstad and J. Katz. 1975. Biochem. Biophys. Res. Commun. 67:212.

Comline, R.S. and M. Silver. 1976. J. Physiol. 260:571.

Coombe, N.B. and R.H. Smith. 1973. Brit. J. Nutr. 30:331.

Coombe, N.B. and R.H. Smith. 1974. Brit. J. Nutr. 31:227.

Davis, C.L. and D.E. Bauman. 1974. In: Lactation, Vol. 2. Academic Press, New York.

Davis, S.R. and R. Bickerstaffe. 1978. Aust. J. Biol. Sci. 31:133.

Domanski, A., D.B. Lindsay and B.P. Setchell. 1974. J. Physiol. 242:28P.

Egan, A.R. and J.C. MacRae. 1978. Proc. Nutr. Soc. 37:15A.

Evans, E. and J.G. Buchanan-Smith. 1975. Brit. J. Nutr. 33:33.

Evans, E., J.G. Buchanan-Smith, G.K. MacLeod and J.B. Stone. 1975. J. Dairy Sci. 58:672.

Fell, B.F., R.M. Campbell, W.S. Mackie and T.E.C. Weekes. 1975. J. Agr. Sci. 79:397.

Fell, B.F. and T.E.C. Weekes. 1975. In: Digestion and Metabolism in the Ruminant. The Univ. of New England Pub. Unit, Armidale.

Frobish, R.A. and C.L. Davis. 1977. J. Dairy Sci. 60:204,268.

Head, H.H., J.D. Connolly and W.F. Williams. 1964. J. Dairy Sci. 47:1371.

Heald, P.J. 1951. Brit. J. Nutr. 5:84.

Herbein, J.H. et al. 1978. J. Nutr. 108:994.

Hodgson, J.C. and D.J. Mellor. 1977. Proc. Nutr. Soc. 36:33.

Horsfield, S. et al. 1974. Proc. Nutr. Soc. 33:9.

Jarrett, I.G., O.H. Filsell and F.J. Ballard. 1976. Metabolism 25:523.

Jenny, B.F. and C.E. Polan. 1975. J. Dairy Sci. 58:512.

Judson, G.J., O.H. Filsell and I.G. Jarrett. 1976. Aust. J. Biol. Sci. 29:215.

Judson, G.J. and R.A. Leng. 1968. Proc. Aust. Soc. Animal Prod. 7:354.

Judson, G.J. and R.A. Leng. 1972. Aust. J. Biol. Sci. 25:1313.

Judson, G.J. and R.A. Leng. 1973. Brit. J. Nutr. 29:159,175.

Katz, J., A. Dunn, M. Chenoweth and S. Golden. 1974. Biochem. J. 142:171.

Krebs, H.A. 1973. Adv. Enzyme Regul. 10:397.

Kronfeld, D.S., C.F. Ramberg and D.M. Shames. 1971. Amer. J. Physiol. 220:886.

Leat, W.M.F. 1971. Proc. Nutr. Soc. 30:236.

Leng, R.A. 1970. Adv. Vet. Sci. 14:209.

Leng, R.A. and E.F. Annison. 1962. Aust. J. Agr. Res. 13:31.

Leonard, M.C., P.J. Buttery and D. Lewis. 1977. Brit. J. Nutr. 38:455.

Lindsay, D.B. 1970. In: Physiology of Digestion and Metabolism in the Ruminant. Oriel Press, Newcastle upon Tyne.

Lindsay, D.B. 1971. Proc. Nutr. Soc. 30:272.

Lindsay, D.B. 1979. In: Protein Metabolism in the Ruminant. ARC, London.

Lindsay, D.B. and C. Dyke. 1974. Proc. Nutr. Soc. 33:39A.

Lindsay, D.B. and B.P. Setchell. 1976. J. Physiol. 259:801.

Lindsay, D.B., J.W. Steel and P.J. Buttery. 1977. Proc. Nutr. Soc. 39:7A.

Linzell, J.L. 1967. Proc. Nutr. Soc. 27:44.

Lomax, M.A. et al. 1978. Proc. Nutr. Soc. 37:95A.

Mackie, W.S. and R.M. Campbell. 1972. J. Agr. Sci. 79:423.

McAllan, A.B. and R.H. Smith. 1974. Brit. J. Nutr. 31:77.

McClure, T.J., C.D. Nancarrow and H.M. Radford. 1978. Aust. J. Biol. Sci. 31:183.

McClymont, G.L. and S. Vallance. 1962. Proc. Nutr. Soc. 21:xli.

McKay, D.G., B.A. Young and L.P. Milligan. 1974. In: Energy Metabolism of Farm Animals. Univ. Hohenheim Dokumentationstelle, Hohenheim.

Morrison, F.B. 1959. Feeds and Feeding. Morrison Pub. Co., Clinton, Iowa.

Ørskov, E.R. 1969. Rev. Cubana Cienca Agr. 3:1.

Ørskov, E.R. 1975. Wld. Rev. Nutr. Diet. 22:152.

Ørskov, E.R., C. Fraser and R.N.B. Kay. 1969. Brit. J. Nutr. 23:217.

Ørskov, E.R., C. Fraser and I. McDonald. 1971. Brit. J. Nutr. 26:477.

Ørskov, E.R., D.A. Grubb and R.N.B. Kay. 1977. Brit. J. Nutr. 38:397.

Pearce, J. and E.F. Unsworth. 1976. Brit. J. Nutr. 35:407.

Ponto, K.H. and W.G. Bergen. 1974. J. Animal Sci. 38:893.

Porter, P. and A.G. Singleton. 1971. Brit. J. Nutr. 26:75.

Prior, R.L. 1978. J. Nutr. 108:962.

Prior, R.L. and R.K. Christenson. 1977. Amer. J. Physiol. 233:E462.

Prior, R.L. and R.K. Christenson. 1978. J. Animal Sci. 46:201.

Prior, R.L., J.A. Milner and W.J. Visek. 1972. J. Nutr. 102:1223.

Ranawere, A. and E.J.H. Ford. 1976. J. Agr. Sci. 87:417.

Rao, D.R., G.E. Hawkins and R.C. Smith. 1973. J. Dairy Sci. 56:1415.

Reid, R.L. 1968. Adv. Vet. Sci. 12:163.

Reilly, P.E.B. and L. Chandrasena. 1978. Amer. J. Physiol. 235:E487.

Ross, J.P. and W.D. Kitts. 1973. J. Nutr. 103:488.

Scharrer, E. 1975. In: Digestion and Metabolism in the Ruminant. The Univ. of New England Pub. Unit, Armidale.

Setchell, B.P. and G.M.H. Waites. 1964. J. Physiol. 171:411.

Setchell, B.P. et al. 1972. Q.J. Exp. Physiol. 57:257.

Shelly, H.J., J.M. Bassett and R.D.G. Milner. 1975. Brit. Med. Bul. 31:37.

Smith, G.H. 1971. Proc. Nutr. Soc. 30:265.

Spires, H.R. et al. 1973. J. Animal Sci. 37:357 (abstr).

Steel, J.W. and R.A. Leng. 1973. Brit. J. Nutr. 30:451,475.

Stern, J.S., C.A. Baile and J. Mayer. 1970. Amer. J. Physiol. 219:84.

Sutton, J.D. 1971. Proc. Nutr. Soc. 30:243.

Sutton, J.D. 1976. In: Principles of Cattle Production. Butterworths, London.

Symonds, H.W. and G.D. Baird. 1975. Brit. Vet. J. 131:17.

Thivend, P. 1974. Proc. Nutr. Soc. 33:7A.

Thivend, P. and M. Journet. 1968. Ann. Biol. Anim. Bioch. Biophys. 8:449.

Thivend, P. and M. Journet. 1970. Ann. Biol. Anim. Bioch. Biophys. 10:323.

Thompson, G.E., J.M. Bassett and A.W. Bell. 1979. Brit. J. Nutr. 39:219.

Thompson, G.E., W. Manson, P.L. Clarke and A.W. Bell. 1978. Q.J. Exp. Physiol. 63:189.

Trenkle, A. 1970. J. Nutr. 100:1323.

Trenkle, A. 1978. J. Dairy Sci. 61:281.

Ulyatt, M.J., F.G. Whitelaw and F.G. Watson. 1970. J. Agr. Sci. 75:565.

Unsworth, E.F. and J. Pearce. 1977. Proc. Nutr. Soc. 36:127A.

Van Maanen, R.W. et al. 1978. J. Nutr. 108:1002.

Vik-Mo, L., R.S. Emery and J.T. Huber. 1974. J. Dairy Sci. 57:869.

Voigt, J. et al. 1976. Archiv. fur Tierernahrung 26:345.

Wahle, K.W.J. et al. 1977. Proc. Nutr. Soc. 36:30P.

Waldo, D.R. 1973. J. Animal Sci. 37:1062.

Warnes, D.M., R.F. Seamark and F.J. Ballard. 1977. Biochem. J. 162:617,627.

Weekes, T.E.C. 1972. J. Agr. Sci. 79:409.

Weekes, T.E.C. and A.J.F. Webster. 1975. Brit. J. Nutr. 33:425.

Weigand, E., J.W. Young and A.D. McGilliard. 1972. Biochem. J. 126:201.

Weller, R.A. and F.V. Gray. 1954. J. Exp. Biol. 31:40.

White, R.G., T.W. Steel, R.A. Leng and J.R. Luick. 1969. Biochem. J. 114:203.

White, R.G., V.J. Williams and R.H.J. Morris. 1971. Brit. J. Nutr. 25:57.

Wiltrout, D.W. and L.D. Satter. 1972. J. Dairy Sci. 55:307.

Wolff, J.E. and E.N. Bergman. 1972. Amer. J. Physiol. 223:455.

Young, J.W. 1977. J. Dairy Sci. 60:1.

Young, J.S., S.L. Thorp and H.Z. DeLumen. 1969. Biochem. J. 114:83.

Chapter 8 - Energy Metabolism and Requirements

By A.J.F. Webster

Living is hard work. To maintain the same body mass and composition for 1 year, an adult human weighing 70 kg requires about 10^6 Kcal of available (or metabolizable) food energy, an amount equivalent to about 6X the energy content of his own body mass, and all this energy is dissipated as heat. Domestic animals require food energy not only for maintenance but also to support the work of production: growth and fattening, pregnancy and lactation. The greater the level of production the more work is required and the more energy lost as heat.

The conversion by a ruminant of the energy contained in the food it eats to the energy contained in marketable animal produce is a highly complex process. As a first step in its analysis one may identify three stages: (a) The fermentation and digestion of food energy to yield fuel for the processes of metabolism. The digestibility of energy is largely a function of the physical and chemical nature of the food. (b) The metabolism of the nutrients made available by digestion for the maintenance of body structure and function and the synthesis of new tissue. This depends both on the nature of the nutrients and the physiological use to which they are put. (c) The relationship between energy retention and the mass of new material synthesized (as meat, milk or wool). This depends on the proportions of the three major constituents of body tissues and secretions, namely protein, fat and water.

Some examples of what happens to feed energy eaten by cattle are given in Fig. 8-1. A dairy cow producing 20 kg milk a day and getting a typical dairy ration will only yield about 21% of the gross energy of her feed in the form of milk; 27% is lost in the feces and 39% as heat. A yearling steer eating a low quality feed and gaining 0.25 kg/day only retains about 3% of feed energy; 46% is lost in the feces and 41% as heat. Even a veal calf growing rapidly on a highly digestible liquid diet may only retain 37% of feed energy; in this case about 55% is dissipated as heat.

These examples are given at the outset to emphasize three important points. Firstly, energy utilization by even the most productive ruminant is a very inefficient process. Secondly, energy is the most important single nutrient, both in absolute and economic terms. Finally, the two main factors that determine the efficiency of utilization of feed energy are the amounts lost as feces and as heat.

There are three classic textbooks which relate specifically to the energy metabolism of farm animals (Brody, 1945; Kleiber, 1961; Blaxter, 1967). All three provide an excellent foundation but all three have, inevitably, been overtaken by events. Recent developments in this subject appear in the triennial symposia, Energy Metabolism of Farm Animals, published by the European Association of Animal Production. Most of the references given in this chapter are to review

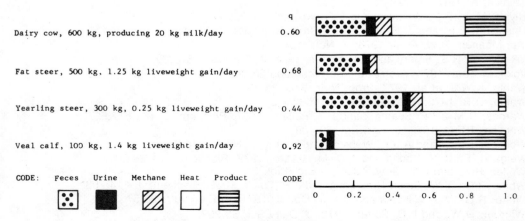

Fig. 8-1. Destinations of feed energy in cattle, expressed as proportions of gross energy intake. Energy in product refers to milk or liveweight gain; q is the ratio of metabolizable energy to gross energy in the feed.

articles or papers summarizing a lengthy series of experiments. Original communications are normally only cited if their conclusions have not yet been incorporated into reviews.

DEFINITIONS AND ABBREVIATIONS

The standard unit of energy is the joule (J). In Europe, the energy content of feeds is now expressed in KJ or MJ (J x 10^6) per kg. In the USA the calorie (cal) is still used (1 cal = 4.184 J) and feed energy is expressed in Kcal or Mcal. The calorie will be used as the standard unit of energy throughout this chapter, and energy intake and expenditure will be expressed in Kcal or Mcal/day. The expressions and conventions used to describe the utilization of energy by ruminants are illustrated in Fig. 8-2.

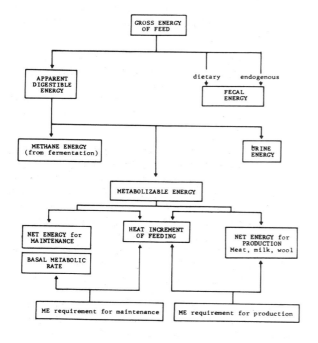

Fig. 8-2. Definitions and conventions used to describe the utilization of energy by ruminants.

Gross Energy (GE) is the heat of combustion of food ingested per unit time (Mcal/day). This is measured in a bomb calorimeter. A sample of the food is placed in a strong metal chamber (the bomb) resting in an insulated tank of water. Oxygen is admitted under pressure, the sample is ignited and the heat of combustion calculated from the rise in temperature that results.

Digestible Energy. Apparently digestible energy (DE) is defined as GE minus fecal energy. The latter (again measured in a bomb calorimeter) is made up of undigested food, bacterial cell residues and material from the cells lining the gut.

Total Digestible Nutrients. (TDN) is a measure of DE, but it is expressed in units of weight or percent rather than as energy *per se*. TDN is based on the traditional methods of proximate analysis of food and feces to obtain digestible protein (DP), digestible crude fiber (DCF), digestible ether extract (DEE) and digestible nitrogen-free extract (DNFE). The formula for this is:

$$TDN = DP + DCF + DNFE + 2.25 \ DEE \quad (1)$$

The 2.25 correction factor is an expression of the greater calorific value of fat relative to carbohydrate and protein. DP and DNFE appear to have been ascribed the same energy content. In fact, the energy content of DP exceeds that of DNFE, but protein is incompletely oxidized in the body so that DP and DNFE have rather similar metabolizable energy values (see below). As a first approximation, the energy equivalent of TDN is 4.4 Kcal/g, or, (conveniently) 2000 Kcal/lb (Swift, 1957).

Metabolizable Energy. (ME) is GE minus the sum of fecal energy, urinary energy and energy lost as combustible gases (principally methane) from the gastro-intestinal tract. Thus, it represents the amount of chemical energy available for metabolism, or the physiological fuel on which the body runs. ME is lost as heat (h) or retained in the body (RE).

Thus, $ME = H \pm RE$ (2).

When ME = H, ME Intake equals *ME requirement for maintenance*. When ME = 0, RE is the sum of H, *fasting metabolism*, or *basal metabolic rate* and the small loss of chemical energy in the urine.

The more an animal eats, the more heat it produces. Reasons for this will be discussed later. At this stage it is necessary only to define the *Heat Increment of Feeding* (HIF) which is the increment in metabolic heat production (Kcal/day) resulting from the ingestion of food and is most conveniently expressed as a proportion of ME intake (Kcal H/Mcal ME).

Net Energy (NE) is defined as ME-HIF. It follows from equation 2 that NE is an expression of the increment in RE produced by a stated increment of food (Kcal/g). Below maintenance, NE for maintenance (NE_m) substitutes for the energy reserves of the body as a source of energy for metabolism but all is finally dissipated as heat. The requirement of NE_m for maintenance is obviously synonymous with basal metabolic rate (Fig. 8-2). Above maintenance, NE is a measure of the amount of chemical energy stored in body tissues.

Thus, *NE for gain* (NE_g, Mcal/kg) defines the energy value of a feed in terms of its capacity to promote energy retention in a growing animal *when fed above maintenance.*

NE for lactation (NE_{milk}, Mcal/kg) defines the energy value of a feed in terms of its capacity to promote the secretion of energy in milk *when fed above maintenance.*

NE is the basis of the newer feeding systems used in the USA (NRC, 1971, 1975, 1976). Scientists in the United Kingdom have adopted a feeding system based on ME (MAFF, 1975) which was proposed by Blaxter (1967) and elaborated by the Agricultural Research Council (ARC, 1965). According to the ME system, the net efficiency of utilization of increments of ME for maintenance, fattening and lactation are described by the constants k_m, k_f, and k_l, respectively. There is no basic theoretical difference between the energy systems used in the USA and the UK since $NE_m = k_m \times ME$; $NE_g = k_f \times ME$; and $NE_{milk} = k_l \times ME$.

The concept of net energy is not easy to grasp when first defined. It is helpful to remember always that it depends on the relationship between ME intake and H, a subject which will be discussed in detail later.

EVALUATING THE ENERGY CONTENT OF FEEDS

The energy value of feeds can be measured quite precisely in terms of DE, TDN or ME since these values are primarily dependent on the physical and chemical nature of the feed itself. NE, on the other hand, is determined to a great extent by the metabolic use to which the feed is put and cannot therefore be regarded as a fixed and absolute property of the feed. A detailed description of the measurement of DE or ME, and the properties of feeds that determine these

things, is outside the scope of this chapter. This topic has been covered very thoroughly in a recent book by Schneider and Flatt (1975).

The direct measurement of DE is a laborious process. Three or four animals are given the same weighed amounts of the same feed or feed mixture for four weeks. During the last 7-10 days of the trial, collections are made of feces, which are weighed, sampled and analyzed, like the feed, for their energy content in a bomb calorimeter. Alternative methods for estimating DE include the use of indicators such as chromic oxide (Faichney, 1972), in vitro fermentation and acid digestion of feed samples (Tilley and Terry, 1963), or laboratory analysis of the structural components of the feed (Van Soest, 1967). None of these alternative methods can yet equal the precision of the direct approach, although they are of real value in circumstances where complete digestibility trials are impossible or impracticable.

To measure ME, it is necessary also to collect and analyze urine and methane produced by fermentation. This is usually measured at the same time as H is estimated from respiratory exchange in a respiration calorimeter.

Table 8-1 presents energy values for some typical feeds for ruminants. Obviously, these are only average values but a recent report from the UK Feedingstuffs Evaluation Unit (1975) suggests that there are only very small differences in ME between different samples of barley, oats or wheat when fed to sheep in combination with forage diets. Table 8-1 also illustrates the extent to which the ME value of grasses decreases if they are allowed to mature and demonstrates the high ME content of good quality silage. Comprehensive tables of the DE and ME contents of feedstuffs are published by NRC (1971, 1975, 1976) and MAFF (1975). Unfortunately, many of the MAFF and most of the NRC values are not based on direct measurements of energy balance. In most normal mixed diets, the ME values of the individual components are additive so that the ME value of the mixture can be estimated directly. For most forages and mixtures of forages and cereals the ratio ME:DE is about 0.82. For fattening diets containing 15% or less of forage, the ratio ME:DE is about 0.9.

The DE and ME contents of feeds are affected by the amount of feed consumed. In the UK, therefore, measurements of ME are

Table 8-1. Energy values of some typical feeds for ruminants, measured at about the maintenance level of nutrition. All values are expressed as Mcal/kg dry matter.

Feed	Gross energy	Loss of energy in			DE	ME
		Feces	Urine	Methane		
Barley †	4.40	0.67	0.16	0.51	3.73	3.06
Oats †	4.68	1.34	0.12	0.37	3.34	2.85
Wheat †	4.38	0.56	0.14	0.49	3.82	3.19
Corn	4.51	0.67	0.16	0.30	3.84	3.38
Dried ryegrass, young	4.65	0.81	0.36	0.39	3.84	3.09
Dried ryegrass, mature	4.53	1.69	0.15	0.33	2.84	2.36
Alfalfa hay	4.38	1.95	0.23	0.31	2.43	1.89
Ryegrass silage	4.64	1.40	0.25	0.35	3.24	2.64
Corn silage	4.50	1.42	0.20	0.30	3.08	2.58

† fed in combination with dried grass or silage

systematically made at about the maintenance level. This is satisfactory for non-lactating, mature animals, moderately satisfactory for growing animals consuming about twice maintenance, but unsatisfactory for a dairy cow consuming perhaps 3-4X her maintenance requirement for ME.

For most ruminant feeds, digestibility decreases as intake, relative to maintenance requirement, increases, probably because the more an animal eats, the faster is the rate of passage of food through the gut. Generally speaking, the less digestible the feed the greater the dependence of digestibility on level of intake. However, the proportion of DE lost as methane declines with increasing intake, which tends to compensate for the decline in digestibility by increasing the ratio ME:DE. Blaxter (1974) has plotted differences in metabolizability of the same feeds given to sheep at maintenance and twice maintenance as a function of metabolizability as conventionally determined at the maintenance level of nutrition. Fig. 8-3 shows that for most feeds the difference was less than 3 percentage units, but for some poorly digestible feeds the further decline in metabolizability with increasing intake above maintenance was very marked. Of course, ruminants are seldom given very poorly digestible feeds in amounts considerably above maintenance. If they were, they would be unwilling or unable to eat them.

Practical rations for growing cattle and sheep may vary widely in their ME content. However, since growing animals seldom eat more than twice their maintenance require-

ment unless given feeds of the highest quality and, since the effect of level of feeding on metabolizability is so variable (Fig. 8-3), there is, in practice, little point in

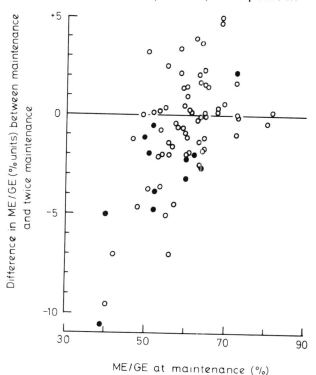

Fig. 8-3. The difference in ME/GE (% units) between measurements made at the maintenace level of feeding and at twice maintenance, expressed as a function of ME/GE as conventionally determined at the maintenance level. Chopped forages and mixed feeds are indicated by open circles, pelleted feeds by closed circles (from Blaxter, 1974).

applying a level of feeding correction to values for ME determined at the maintenance level in formulating rations for lambs or beef cattle.

The dairy cow may consume an amount of ME as great as 4X her maintenance requirement. In this case a level of feeding correction is necessary. However, the range of diets suitable for the high yielding dairy cow is rather small. If ME content is too low, she cannot eat enough to sustain lactation. If it is too high, metabolic disorders may ensue and milk fat content falls (see Ch. 7). When calculating the amount of ME (or NE_{milk}) required to support lactation in a dairy cow, it is recommended that values for ME/GE expressed in percentage units at the maintenance level of nutrition be reduced by 1.8% for each multiple of ME requirement for maintenance consumed by the animal. For example, a feed having a metabolizability of 58% at maintenance would be given a value of 54.4% [58 - (2 x 1.8)] for a cow given an amount of ME equal to 2X her maintenance requirement.

There is general agreement that sheep and cattle digest and metabolize most normal diets with similar efficiency, i.e. ME and DE values are the same for both species. Schneider and Flatt (1975) discuss some differences in digestibility between *Bos taurus* and *Bos indicus*, and there have been suggestions, although little convincing evidence, that deer can utilize forages of very low digestibility better than sheep or cattle. However, for the most part tables of DE and ME for ruminants can be applied with reasonable assurance to all ruminants of economic importance.

TECHNIQUES OF CALORIMETRY

Direct Calorimetry

An animal loses heat to the environment in two ways, usually called sensible and evaporative heat loss. Sensible heat loss is that lost from the body to the environment by the pathways of convection, conduction and radiation. Evaporative heat is lost from the surfaces of the skin and respiratory tract. Heat loss from animals can be measured directly using heat sink or thermal gradient calorimeters. In the heat sink calorimeter, sensible heat loss from an animal is measured as a rise in temperature in an absorbing medium which may be the air stream ventilating the chamber or water cir-

culating outside its walls. Evaporative heat loss can be measured by the increase in relative humidity of the ventilating air stream (Mount, 1968).

The thermal gradient layer calorimeter measures sensible heat loss from the instantaneous temperature across a conducting layer interposed between an animal and a constant temperature source. Evaporative heat loss can be measured with equal rapidity and precision by measuring heat balance across the air conditioning system for the chamber (Pullar, 1969).

Indirect Calorimetry

Metabolic heat production is the result of the oxidation in the body of organic compounds. In the special case of a simple-stomached animal completely oxidizing carbohydrate and fat to CO_2 and H_2O, the rate of oxidizing these substrates, and thus the rate of heat production, could be estimated precisely from a knowledge of the rates of O_2 consumption and CO_2 production. A ruminant getting a complete diet of carbohydrates, fats and proteins does not, however, completely oxidize all substrates; incomplete oxidation of protein yields combustible nitrogenous compounds, principally urea, which are excreted in the urine. Anaerobic fermentation of carbohydrates in ruminants yields combustible gases, principally methane. For ruminants therefore, the equation to predict metabolic heat production from chemical exchange is:

$$H \text{ (Kcal)} = 3.886 \, O_2 + 1.200 \, CO_2 - 0.518 \, CH_4 - 1.431 \, N \text{ (3)},$$

where O_2, CO_2 and CH_4 refer to gaseous exchange (liters) and N refers to urinary N (g). The logic of this approach to estimating H has been described in detail by Blaxter (1967). The measurements of CH_4 and N are, of course, an essential part of the determination of the ME value of feeds, and therefore RE. However, their contribution to the calculation of H from equation 3 is small and if they were neglected altogether the error in estimating H would seldom approach 2%. For short-term measurements, it is often sufficient to estimate H from O_2 consumption alone (MacLean, 1972): $H \text{ (Kcal)} = 4.890$ (4).

Indirect or respiration calorimeters are of two types, open circuit or closed circuit (Fig. 8-4). In the closed circuit system the animal is confined in a temperature controlled chamber. The air in the system is circulated continuously through silica gel and KOH to absorb H_2O and CO_2. Pressure inside the system is maintained by a supply of pure O_2. CH_4 cannot be absorbed and accumulates within the system. Respiration exchange is calculated from the gain in weight of CO_2 and the volume of O_2 admitted, both corrected for small changes in concentration of these gases within the system over the period of measurement. CH_4 production is calculated from the product of chamber volume and concentration change.

Open circuit respiration apparatus depends on the continuous analysis of the concentrations of O_2, CO_2, and CH_4 in a stream of air which moves at a precisely measured rate and includes all the air expired by the animal. This may involve the use of a mask, a hood enclosing the head, or a chamber accommodating the entire animal (Fig. 8-5). The system is flexible and easy to construct, but dangerously susceptible to error. In order to estimate O_2 consumption to an accuracy of $\pm 1\%$ when the concentration of O_2 in the sample is about 5% below that in the atmosphere, the concentrations of O_2 in ingoing and outgoing air must be measured to an accuracy of 1 part in 20,000. Good general descriptions of the techniques of indirect calorimetry are given by Blaxter (1967) and Flatt (1969).

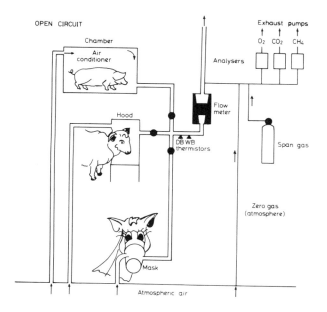

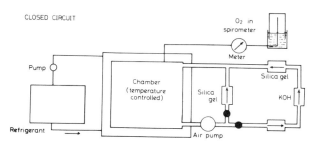

Fig. 8-4. Indirect calorimetry: principles of open and closed circuit measurement of respiratory exchange. **Open circuit.** Exhaust air from the animal passes over thermistors to record dry bulb (DB) and wet bulb (WB) temperature and a meter to record total flow. Gas analyzers record concentrations of O_2, CO_2, and CH_4 in the sample line. They are calibrated using atmospheric air and a span gas of known composition. **Closed circuit.** Chamber air is circulated over silica gel to remove water vapor and over KOH and silica gel to remove CO_2. Pure O_2 enters the system to maintain atmospheric pressure.

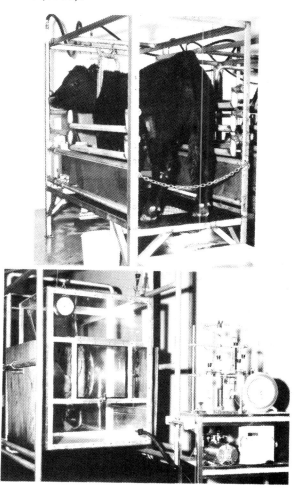

Fig. 8-5. Upper. Metabolism stalls for digestibility studies with cattle. Lower. Head chamber for collecting radioactive CO_2 and CH_4. Courtesy of T.S. Rumsey, USDA Beef Cattle Research Center, Beltsville, Md.

Measurement of Energy Retention

Energy retention (RE) is, of course, calculated from ME-H. The most obvious way to measure RE directly is the comparative slaughter technique; kill half of a group of animals at the beginning of an experiment, the other half at the end and determine the energy value of the bodies of both groups (Blaxter, 1967). Where this is not practicable it is possible to estimate RE from gains in body protein and fat, estimated from specific gravity measurements (Lofgreen and Garrett, 1968) or the use of markers for specific body constituents. For further details of these approaches see Blaxter (1967) and Webster (1978).

THE HEAT PRODUCTION OF RUMINANTS

The four principal factors that determine the heat production of a ruminant are body size, a function of body weight (W); the heat increment of feeding, a function of ME intake; activity; and the work of thermoregulation.

In confined and thermally comfortable conditions similar to those existing in a calorimeter or in a good intensive production unit, activity is minimal and the work of thermoregulation is nil. In these circumstances H is determined by the amount of food eaten (ME) and the weight of the animal that eats it. These two factors are not independent, but there are certain effects on H which can be attributed chiefly to the quantity and quality of the food and others which can be attributed chiefly to the size and physiological state of the animal. These will be considered in order.

Food Intake and Heat Production

When adult ruminants are given ME in excess of maintenance, the resulting HIF has clearly been shown to be proportional to the amount of fiber in the diet (inversely proportional to ME/GE). The relative yields of the volatile fatty acids (VFA acetate, propionate and butyrate) from rumen fermentation are also related to the fiber in the diet since the molar ratio of non-glucogenic acetate and butyrate to glucogenic propionate also increases as ME/GE declines. Armstrong and Blaxter (see Blaxter, 1967; Annison and Armstrong, 1970) infused different mixtures of VFA's into the rumen of sheep, obtained different heat increments and concluded that HIF was proportional to the molar proportion of acetate in the infusate or, in more normal circumstances, in the end products of digestion. Ørskov (1975) has criticized this work on theoretical grounds and concluded that HIF should not vary much over a wide range of VFA mixtures. If Ørskov is correct, then some other explanations must be found to account for the fact that HIF for normal feeds does vary and varies in a way that is proportional to the fiber in the diet. The measurable factors which contribute to HIF in adult ruminants are as follows (Webster, 1978): energy cost of eating; energy cost of ruminating; heat of fermentation; work of digestion; and the work of nutrient metabolism.

The energy cost of eating is less related to the amount of food eaten than to the length of time spent eating. On average it amounts to about 7-9 cal/kg body wt/min. The contribution of eating to HIF ranges from only about 3 Kcal/Mcal ME for concentrate feeds eaten very quickly to about 35 for grazed herbage (Osuji, 1974). These costs do not include the energy costs of standing to eat or walking to graze. Rumination, curiously, is a much less expensive process and the total energy cost of rumination even for about 8 h/day is only about 20 Kcal/Mcal ME. Hungate (1966) predicted from molar relationships that the heat of fermentation would be about 65 Kcal/Mcal of fermented energy irrespective of the nature of the other end products of fermentation. This has been confirmed by direct experimental evidence (Webster et al, 1975).

The work of nutrient metabolism in the body tissues should correspond to the HI produced when a ruminant is given no food and supported entirely by the intraruminal infusion of VFA's, casein and other essential nutrients which are not allowed to ferment. The evidence that exists suggests that the work of nutrient metabolism accounts for about 65-70% of total HIF. The energy costs of eating, rumination and fermentation account for about 20-25%, which suggests that the work of digestion—the muscular and secretory processes arising from the presence of food in the gut, accounts for about 10%. At this stage, the work of nutrient metabolism refers only to the case of the adult ruminant using nutrients for maintenance and energy retention almost entirely as fat. This is a convenient way to compare differences between feeds in HIF, but it says nothing about the relative efficiencies of utilization of energy for fat deposition,

Table 8-2. Analysis of the heat increment of feeding for a 50 kg sheep getting 4000 Kcal ME/day (about twice maintenance).

Item	Chopped hay, Kcal	Fresh grass, Kcal
Total heat increment of feeding	1812	1888
Work of ingestion and digestion,		
eating	53	129
rumination	31	31
fermentation	318	318
digestion	84	84
% total HIF	27	30
Work of nutrient metabolism	1326	1326

protein deposition and milk production. These will be considered later.

Table 8-2 presents an analysis of HIF for an adult sheep getting either chopped hay or grazing fresh herbage. The magnitude and variability of factors other than the work of nutrient metabolism cannot possibly account for the fact that, for normal feeds, HIF can vary from 400-750 Kcal/Mcal and in a way that is predictable from the physical form and metabolizability (q) of the diet (Blaxter, 1973). These differences must relate somehow to the work of nutrient metabolism but how far they can be explained simply in terms of VFA rations is still uncertain.

BODY SIZE AND HEAT PRODUCTION

Fasting Metabolism. The obvious way to measure the effect on H of body size, uncomplicated by ME intake, is to measure H in a fasting animal. To get a reasonably stable measurement of fasting heat production (F) in a ruminant it is necessary to measure H on the third and fourth days of a period of starvation. This is not a reasonable proposition for very young animals. Brody (1945) and Kleiber (1961) have shown that fasting metabolism in different species of adult mammals is, in general, about 70 Kcal/ kg $W^{0.75}$/day. The exponent 0.75 was used by them to confer proportionality on measurements made of F in species differing considerably in mature body weight. Body weight to the power 0.75 is often called metabolic body size. It has been adopted, with varying degrees of success, to confer proportionality on measurements made of H and food energy requirements in animals within a species changing in W by virtue of growth.

In fact, F, even in adult ruminants, does not correspond very closely to the Brody/ Kleiber mean value of 70 Kcal/kg $^{0.75}$/day. In sheep it is about 60 and in cattle about 80 (Blaxter, 1967). In wild ruminants, such as the red deer, F appears to vary markedly from about 80 in winter to 100 in summer.

One problem with F is that it is not an absolute property of the animal itself but depends to a considerable degree on its prior nutrition and prior level of production. For example, a rapidly growing steer fasted for four days will have a value for F about 20% higher than that of an animal previously restricted to a maintenance ration for four weeks (Webster, 1978). While F is, in theory, a logical way of assessing the relationship between W and H uncomplicated by ME, it is not in fact a very good measure of the energy metabolism of a highly productive animal (see Webster et al, 1974).

Maintenance Requirement. Maintenance requirement is that amount of ME which exactly balances H and produces no loss or gain in RE. On average, ME requirement for maintenance in adult cattle is about 112 Kcal/kg $^{0.75}$/day, or about 1.4 times fasting metabolism. The difference between F and H at maintenance is a measure of HIF below maintenance, in this case 112-80/112 = 0.29 Kcal H/Kcal ME. Alternatively, in the conventions of the ME system for expressing the energy value of feeds, k_m = 1-0.29 = 0.71. H at maintenance in any adult animal will vary slightly due to small differences between feeds in HIF below maintenance and thus in k_m (Blaxter, 1967, 1973). However, for beef cows and breeding ewes, which spend a large proportion of their adult lives at or near maintenance, values of 112 and 84 Kcal/kg$^{0.75}$ /day, respectively, can be assumed for maintenance H in confined adult animals not subject to cold stress. In sheep, there is a decline of about 20% in H between one and six years of age (Toutain et al, 1978). Comparable measurements are not available for other ruminants.

Activity

Values given previously for maintenance requirement apply to animals kept in a calorimeter or under similarly confined conditions on the farm or ranch. The increased energy cost of activity for an animal on open range, for example, depends on the energy cost of each activity per unit of time and the

Table 8-3. The daily energy expenditure of a beef cow on range compared with that of a similar animal confined in a calorimeter. *

Activity	Energy cost of activity	Amount of activity		Additional cost of activity on range, Kcal/day
		confined	on range	
Eating	8.5 cal/kgW/min	1.5h	5-9h	880 - 1880
Standing	1.3 cal/kgW/min	5h	5-15h	0 - 380
Changing position	13 cal/kgW	20 actions	20-30	0 - 70
Walking	0.5 cal/kgW/horizontal m NIL 6.3 cal/kgW/vertical m		1- 6 km	240 - 1500

Extra energy cost of outdoor activity, Mcal/day	1.12 - 3.83
Heat production at maintenance in confinement, Mcal/day	11.84
Heat production on range, Mcal/day	12.96 - 15.67
Increase due to activity, %	9 - 32%

*Values derived from Webster (1978).

additional time spent in each activity on range above that in confinement. Table 8-3 lists the energy costs of major activities for cattle and compares the energy expenditure of a 500 kg cow on range with that of a confined animal.

Table 8-3 indicates that, for cattle kept at a high stocking intensity on good pasture, H is only about 10% above that of the confined animal. On short grass ranges, where cows have to work quite hard to harvest their food, the increment in H is about 30%. The same relative increments apply to sheep. For a more complete review see Osuji (1974).

Daily energy expenditure also depends on the state of vigilance of the animal and the length of time it spends asleep. Variations in the duration of the latter do not alter H by more than about 2%, but variations in vigilance and nervousness while awake are probably more important (Toutain et al, 1978).

Effects of Climate

There are several reviews of the effects of climate on the energy metabolism of sheep (Alexander, 1974) and cattle (Webster, 1974, 1976). Heat stress, which is a major practical hazard to cattle and sheep production in the tropics (see Hafez, 1968), has little direct effect on H. However, the invariable response of ruminants to moderate heat stress is to reduce ME intake. This has the secondary effect of reducing metabolic H which benefits the animal by reducing the work of thermoregulation but reduces RE and thus the efficiency of the animal as a production unit. It is also the most productive animal that is first to experience heat stress, by

virtue of its high H. During severe heat stress the work of thermal regulation becomes so great that H rises. This condition may often occur during hot, sunny days but cannot be sustained indefinitely.

Cold stress does affect H directly and thus ME requirements. Fig. 8-6 illustrates the balance between metabolic heat production and heat loss in relation to air temperature. An animal that is neither too cold nor too hot is said to be in a thermoneutral environment; metabolic heat production is unaffected by air temperature and the animal regulates body temperature by adjusting its pathways of heat loss at negligible energy cost. Sensible heat loss by conduction, convection and radiation is principally determined by climatic factors, air temperature, wind speed, precipitation in the form of rain or snow, and radiation exchanges. The animal is protected against sensible heat loss by two layers of thermal insulation, tissue insulation of the body shell (I_t) and external insulation (I_e), provided by the coat of hair or wool and the air trapped in it and on it. Tissue insulation is determined partly by physical factors such as the thickness of the skin and subcutaneous fat, but more by the rate of blood flow through the superficial tissues of the body. Thus, tissue insulation is maximal when vasoconstriction is maximal. Coat thickness and climatic factors such as wind and precipitation obviously have marked effects on external insulation.

Heat is also lost by evaporation of water from the surface of the skin and from the respiratory tract. In warm and hot conditions cattle regulate evaporative heat loss by sweating and thermal panting. Sheep, which

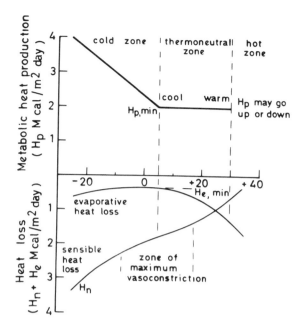

Fig. 8-6. Schematic illustration of heat exchanges in a ruminant in relation to air temperature (horizontal axis). Units of heat production and heat loss are Mcal/m surface area/day. For further explanation see text and Webster (1974).

do not sweat efficiently, depend almost entirely on a very efficient mechanism for regulating evaporative loss from the respiratory tract (Hales, 1974). In cold environments evaporative heat loss is reduced to a minimum (Fig. 8-6).

The cold tolerance of an animal is thus determined by metabolic heat production in a thermoneutral environment and by the thermal insulation terms I_t and I_e. The lower limit to the zone of thermal neutrality is called the lower critical temperature. As air temperature falls below the lower critical temperature, the animal must increase metabolic heat production in order to maintain homeothermy.

If two animals have similar thermal insulation $(I_t + I_e)$, the more productive animal, with the greater ME intake and heat production, will be the more cold tolerant. Since ME intake is a major determinant of heat production expressed per unit of metabolic body weight $(W^{0.75})$, it is a major determinant of cold tolerance.

The increase in heat production, and thus in ME requirement per °C fall in air temperature $(^dH/dTa)$ below the lower critical temperature is given by equation 5, which applies both indoors and outdoors since the chilling

Table 8-4. Some factors determining the cold tolerance of adult cattle, sheep and red deer eating ME sufficient for maintenance in a thermoneutral outdoor environment (15% activity increment).

Item	Species		
	Cow	Sheep	Red deer hind
Body weight, kg			
Thermoneutral heat production ($H_{p,min}$):	500	50	70
Kcal/kg$^{0.75}$/day	129	97	129†
Mcal/m² surface area/day‡	2.35	1.47	2.01
Thermal insulation: (°C/m²/day/Mcal)			
tissue insulation (It)	9.5	6.5	5.0
external insulation (wind 0.4 m/s)	16.0	30.0	16.0
(wind 4.5m/s)§	8.0	15.0	8.0
Lower critical temperature °C (wind 0.4 m/s)	-16	-7	+1
(wind 4.5 m/s) §	0	+11	+14

† in winter
‡ 1 m surface area = 0.09 x body weight
§ 4.5 m/sec = 10 miles/hour.

effects of wind and precipitation are accommodated within the term for external insulation (I$_e$): dH/dTa = I/C (I$_t$ + I$_é$) (5).

Table 8-4 gives examples of values for thermoneutral heat production, I$_t$, I$_e$ and lower critical temperature for adult cattle, sheep and red deer all with full winter coats and all getting ME sufficient for maintenance in thermoneutral conditions out of doors. For more detail see Alexander (1974) and Webster (1974). Both adult cattle and sheep are very resistant to cold and neither is likely to be severely stressed by low air temperatures alone in any of the livestock producing areas of the world. Red deer are rather less cold tolerant. Bison and yak, however, appear to be more tolerant to cold than domestic breeds of European cattle (Christopherson et al, 1976). Wind and precipitation can increase H although almost never, in a well-fed adult, to the point where the animal will fail to maintain body temperature and die of hypothermia. The problem of cold stress for the adult is, thus, a problem of chronic increase in H at a time when ME is scarce or expensive.

Lower critical temperatures in still air for calves and lambs in their first weeks of life are about 10° and 18°C, respectively, in both cases considerably higher than their mothers. The rate at which their tolerance to cold improves depends on how rapidly they are allowed to grow; again, the most productive animal is the one that most quickly reaches the point where the direct effects of cold on energy requirement are minimized.

FEEDING SYSTEMS

All systems of rationing feeds for ruminants seek first to match the supply of feed energy to the requirements of the animal, then adjust nitrogen supply to requirement and, finally, balance the diet with respect to minerals and vitamins. The capacity of a feed to meet the energy requirements of an animal depends, as has been shown already, on the nature of the feed and on the specific requirements of the individual.

The feeding system for ruminants traditionally used in the USA was based on TDN. This is a fair assessment of digestible energy but ignores *small* differences between feeds in the ratio ME:DE and *large* differences in HIF attributable both to the quality of the food and the metabolic use to which it was put (maintenance, growth, lactation, etc.).

Thus, while the amount of TDN required to support a given level of production could be determined empirically in feeding trials, TDN units could never be used precisely to balance energy intake to requirement.

The traditional European feeding system was based on Starch Equivalent (SE). At the end of the last century Kellner fed pure starch to steers in addition to a maintenance ration and observed that for each gram of starch digested the animals deposited 0.248 g of fat. In effect, this was a measure of the capacity of starch, fed above maintenance, to provide NE for fattening. When barley, for example, was substituted for starch, 1 kg barley promoted only 0.20 g fat deposition. The fat-promoting power of barley relative to starch was therefore 0.20/0.248 x 100 = 81%, which was said to be its SE.

There has been a tendency in Europe to consider SE as being somehow more respectable than TDN because it does take into account HIF. This respectability is hardly justified because the HIF in question refers only to one situation, that of a mature ox getting food above maintenance and retaining energy only as fat—hardly a situation of economic importance. Both TDN and SE are essentially empirical systems which have had long and successful runs in practice. They both have two major limitations. First, neither uses genuine energy units, common to feed, heat and animal product, which, in my opinion, makes them unnecessarily difficult to understand. Secondly, both assume that the interaction between feed and animal that converts feed into product can be described solely in terms of the feed. This is simply not so.

In Eastern Europe a feeding system based on NE for fattening has recently been adopted (Nehring, 1969). This is, in essence, only an SE system expressed in proper energy units, so it only meets the first of the previous two objections.

The currently accepted feed energy systems in the USA and the UK are based on NE and ME, respectively, yet there is, in fact, no fundamental difference between the two. To explain both it is necessary to describe the logic of the ME system proposed and developed by Blaxter (1967) and now adopted for use in the UK (ARC, 1965; MAFF, 1975).

To measure, for example, the capacity of a feed to support maintenance and promote energy retention (principally as fat) in a sheep, calorimetric measurements are made

Feed	GE[+]	Q	ME	k_m	k_f	NE_m	NE gain
A	4·4	0·65	2·86	0·74	0·55	2·12	1·57
B	4·4	0·45	1·98	0·68	0·37	1·34	0·73

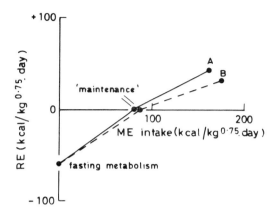

Fig. 8-7. Utilization of the metabolizable energy of two feeds A and B for maintenance and gain in a fattening sheep. Values for GE, ME, NE_m and NE_{gain} are in Mcal/kg DM.

Originally, Blaxter (1967) considered that the relationship between ME content (Mcal/kg of DM), k_m and k_f was the same for all classes of feeds for ruminants. Recently, he has revised this conclusion in the light of more evidence and shown that these relationships differ for different classes of feeds (Blaxter, 1974). Fig. 8-8 shows that k_m values for dried grasses and hays are very dependent on ME content. Recent unpublished work shows that the same applies to silages. For pelleted diets and mixtures of cereals and dried forages, k_f varies much less with changes in ME content.

A feeding system for lactating animals based on ME or NE_{milk} is complicated by the fact that the energy balance equation includes not only ME, H and energy in milk, but energy movement in and out of body stores. In early lactation, a good dairy cow will 'milk off her back,' i.e. the sum of milk energy and H will be greater than the amount of ME that she can consume, while in late lactation ME above maintenance will be used both for milk production and fat deposition

of ME and H at three levels of intake of ME: zero, or fasting metabolism; about maintenance; and about twice maintenance. This approach is illustrated in Fig. 8-7 by two examples, feeds A and B having the same GE of 4.40 Mcal/kg DM but metabolizabilities (q) of 0.65 and 0.45, thus ME contents of 2.86 and 1.98 Mcal/kg DM, respectively. The three points relating RE to ME do not fall on a straight line. In fact the relationship between RE and ME is best described by an exponential curve (Blaxter, 1974). It is simpler, however, to describe this curve by two straight lines, the first between fasting and maintenance to give k_m, the net efficiency of utilization of ME for maintenance, the second between maintenance and twice maintenance, k_f, gives the net efficiency of utilization of ME for fattening. ME intakes greater or lesser than twice maintenance would, of course, give lower or higher values for k_f, respectively, for the same feed.

As defined earlier, NE_m and NE_g correspond in theory to k_m x ME and k_f x ME respectively. However, these values as given by NRC (1976) from which the basis of the so called California Net Energy (CNE) system for beef cattle were derived from estimates of RE based on measurements of specific gravity in growing cattle (Lofgreen and Garrett, 1968) and do not, in fact, agree very closely with those on which the ME system is based.

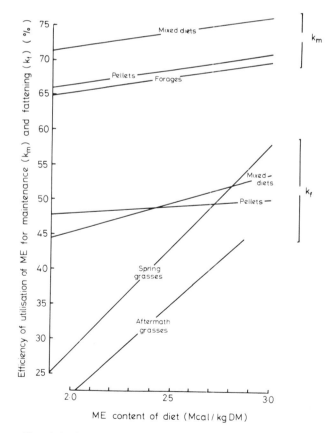

Fig. 8-8. Prediction of the efficiency of utilization of ME for maintenance (k_m) and for fattening (k_f) from the ME content of the diet (Mcal/kg DM).

(Moe and Flatt, 1969). Nevertheless, the logic of the ME system is the same, k_l is considered to be the net efficiency of utilization of ME, fed above maintenance, for lactation. The NE lactating cows (NE_{lc}) system recommended for use in the USA for the limited range of diets suitable for high-yielding dairy cows, can, in practice, be considered a linear function of DE for all purposes, maintenance, lactation and body gains; NE_{lc} (Mcal/kg DM) = 0.84 DE - 0.77 (6). The term NE_{lc} is preferred here because it does not have the same precise meaning as NE_{milk}.

ENERGY REQUIREMENTS IN PRACTICE

The purpose of this chapter is to introduce the topic of energy metabolism and to illustrate the principles which govern the different feeding systems which have been developed to assess the energy values of feeds and meet the energy requirements of ruminants. The steps which one follows to formulate a ration to meet the energy requirements for a particular ruminant enterprise according to the net energy convention adopted in the USA are clearly documented by the NRC for dairy cattle (NRC, 1971), beef cattle (NRC, 1976) and for sheep (NRC, 1975). In the UK, energy allowances and feeding systems for all groups according to the ME system are covered by MAFF Bulletin 33 (1975). These publications give worked examples of ration formulation. The last section of this chapter is intended to complement and explain these publications, not to reproduce them.

The first thing that can be said is that, in practice, it is not always necessary, or even sensible, to attempt to achieve the degree of precision that is possible in theory. There are a number of short cuts to the calculation of energy requirement, the acceptability of which depends on the precision with which one can assess the energy value of the feed inputs. Obviously, it would be futile to attempt to ration the energy intake of a beef cow on open range with the same degree of precision as that appropriate to a dairy cow receiving her entire feed in the form of a processed diet of known composition.

Maintenance

In practice, the maintenance energy requirement has two distinct meanings. First, it refers, quite correctly, to the amount of energy required to keep an adult in energy balance when not producing babies or milk. For adult cows and ewes, maintenance energy requirement for ME is most precisely measured by dividing fasting metabolism by k_m and adding appropriate increments for activity and cold thermogenesis as necessary. Since k_m differs only slightly between feeds, it is often acceptable to assume that the ratio of fasting metabolism to ME requirement for maintenance is constant at 0.71 and that for animals near their mature body size ME requirement for maintenance is a linear function of body weight.

It is then possible to calculate maintenance requirements of cattle and sheep in confinement from the following equations, which, in fact, deliberately overestimate calorimetric data by about 5% to give a margin of safety: ME for maintenance (Mcal/day) cattle = 2.6 + 0.02 W (kg) (7); sheep = 0.4 + 0.03 W (kg) (8). Values calculated from these simple formula are all within 5% of those given in detailed tables of requirements by MAFF (1975) and NRC (1971, 1975, 1976) on the assumption, in the latter case, that the ratio NE_m in the USA tables to ME maintenance is about 0.6. The fact that this is not the same thing as k_m (which is about 0.71) derives from the method of measurement. Lofgreen and Garrett (1968) extrapolated measurements made with animals in positive energy balance to zero energy intake; they did not measure fasting metabolism directly. For most purposes this does not matter. The UK and the USA systems agree reasonably well as to H and thus energy requirement for maintenance in the adult animal.

The second meaning of maintenance is quite arbitrary. In a growing or lactating animal it refers to the requirement for NE additional to that retained as NE_g or NE_{milk}. It is thus a large residual term relating requirement for NE_m or ME to some function of body weight. There is no reason to suppose that it should be the same value as the ME requirement for maintenance of a non-productive adult of the same size and it is rather unfortunate that it is given the same name.

Pregnancy

The efficiency of utilization of ME for synthesis of fetal tissue in the sheep is about 12% (Rattray et al, 1974). In both cattle and sheep the energy cost of pregnancy seems to be related to the total weight of the products of conception, irrespective of the numbers of offspring carried to term. Since the products of conception increase in weight and energy content more or less exponentially during pregnancy, the energy requirement of a pregnant animal is most appropriately calculated by adding an exponential function of the duration of pregnancy to maintenance requirement (MAFF, 1975). Thus ME requirement for maintenance and pregnancy (Mcal/day)

$$\text{for cattle} = ME_{maintenance} + 0.27e^{0.0106t} \quad (9),$$

where t = number of days pregnant and e = 2.718 the base of the natural logarithm.

Adult ewes can differ in body weight by a factor of about two and these differences are reflected in birth weight of the lambs. Moreover, the number of lambs born varies and quads are quite common.

The equations used by MAFF (1975) to calculate the energy requirement of ewes carrying single lambs or twins take these variations in ewe and lamb weight into account.

ME requirements for maintenance + pregnancy (Kcal/day) are:

$$\text{ewes carrying singles} = (290 + 12W)e^{0.0072t} \quad (10);$$

$$\text{ewes carrying twins} = (190 + 10W)e^{0.0105t} \quad (11).$$

Tables of ME allowances for pregnant ewes based on these equations are given by MAFF (1975).

The experimental evidence to support these equations is not very thorough. Some incomplete work on the energy cost of pregnancy in sheep suggests that these values may be too low to prevent losses of maternal energy during pregnancy, although not too low for successful breeding from ewes in good condition at the time of mating.

Lactation

ME System. The ME system for dairy cattle involves the separate calculation of maintenance and production allowances which are then added together. In calculating ME requirement for maintenance, it is assumed that the maintenance requirement of a productive dairy cow is the same as that of a dry cow, i.e., F/k_m. The net efficiency of utilization of ME for lactation becomes, as a first approximation, $k_l = 0.62$ for the limited range of feeds given to dairy cattle.

The NE requirement for milk production is, of course, the energy of the milk secreted which depends on yield (Y, kg) and the energy value of the milk (EV_l Kcal/kg) which is calculated from equation 12: $EV_l = 9.22$ BF + 4.88 SNF - 56.2 (12), where BF is butter fat and SNF is solids not fat in g/kg milk. For a typical Friesian or Holstein cow, EV_l would be about 685 Kcal/kg milk giving an ME requirement of 685/0.62 = 1105 Kcal/kg milk. For a Jersey cow ME requirement would be 830/0.62 = 1338 Kcal/kg milk.

In practice, the very high yielding cow in early lactation will almost inevitably lose more energy as milk and heat than she can take in as ME unless given a diet so rich in high energy cereals that it would almost inevitably cause metabolic disorders. Consider the example of a cow weighing 650 kg and producing 40 kg of milk/day having an EV_l of 685 Kcal/kg. Maintenance requirement for ME (equation 7) = 15.6 Mcal/day; ME requirement for lactation = 40 x 0.685/0.62 = 44.2 Mcal/day; total requirement for ME = 59.8 Mcal/day.

In early lactation a cow of this size could probably eat no more than about 20 kg of dry matter. To meet her ME requirements, the ration would have to be formulated to have an ME content of 3.0 Mcal/kg of DM. If the feeds available were forage and a dairy concentrate having ME contents of 2.2 and 3.0 Mcal/kg of DM, respectively, she would need to eat nothing but concentrates to maintain energy balance. If she received 50 forage: 50 concentrates by weight and managed to eat 20 kg, she would then get (10 x 2.2) + (10 x 3.0) = 52 Mcal ME/day.

52 Mcal ME/day provides for (1) maintenance = 15.6 Mcal and (2) NE_l = 0.62 x 36.4 = 22.5 Mcal. Actual milk yield, as NE_l = 40 x 0.685 = 27.4 Mcal; deficit.in NE_l = 4.9 Mcal.

The efficiency of utilization of body energy reserves for milk synthesis is high, about 0.82, thus energy loss from body reserves = 4.9/0.82 = 5.98 Mcal. How much this represents in body weight loss depends on the proportions of energy lost as fat and as protein. If it were entirely fat, the loss would be only about 5.98/9.3 = 0.64 kg/day. The energy content of body weight loss is probably nearer 5 Mcal/kg, which would imply the cow would lose about 1.2 kg/day.

Other more detailed examples of ration formulation, according to the ME system, to meet, or meet as nearly as possible, the energy requirements of the dairy cow are outside the scope of this chapter, but are well covered by MAFF (1975, Bulletin 33).

Broster (1972, 1976) has demonstrated how feeding to ensure maximum milk yield in early lactation has a markedly beneficial effect on total yield in the full lactation period. The example just given illustrates that, even at a very high concentrate intake, the high yielding cow cannot meet her energy requirement. In practice, therefore, such cows in early lactation will benefit from free access to concentrate feeds, so long as roughage is also available. In late lactation the same cows should be given ME in excess of their needs for maintenance and milk production so as to build up reserves for the next lactation. There is evidence that the efficiency of ME retention as fat in lactating cows is the same as k_l, about 0.62, which is significantly more efficient than fat deposition in a dry cow. There is an extreme, although defensible view, that says that high yielding dairy cows should always be fed to appetite. A more reasonable ration formulation pattern would attempt to balance the availability of forage and concentrate so that adult dairy cows, eating to appetite, get a progressively higher proportion of roughage as lactation proceeds and are able just to balance total ME intake to requirement over the entire lactation.

Net Energy, Lactating Cows. NRC(1971) bases the energy requirements of lactating cows on a single value, NE_{lc}, which is an acceptable simplification proposed by Moe and Flatt (1969). Energy values of all appropriate feeds are expressed as NE_{lc} and the EV_l is given for milks differing in butter fat content.

Taking the same example as before, a 650 kg Holstein cow producing 40 kg of milk having an EV_l of 0.685 = 27.4 Mcal. According to NRC (1971) her requirement for NE_{lc} would be 10.9 Mcal for maintenance + 27.4 Mcal as milk = 38.3 Mcal NE_{lc}. The same forage and concentrate diets have NE_{lc} values of 1.36 and 1.93, respectively. The cow eating 10 kg of each would get 13.6 + 19.3 = 32.9 Mcal NE_{lc} and be in deficit to the extent of 5.4 Mcal. This corresponds quite closely with the deficit of 4.9 Mcal calculated according to the ME system.

This illustrates the important point that while the two systems differ quite a lot in theory and in detail, they do tend to give much the same results in practice, results which are moreover precise and reasonably easy to calculate. Both systems must be considered a success and a marked improvement on TDN or SE.

Growth

It is inherently more difficult to predict the energy requirements of a growing steer than a lactating cow. The composition and thus the energy content of body gains is seldom known with high precision, and the effect of body weight on energy requirement (so called maintenance requirement of the growing animal) is constantly changing.

Energy is retained in the body of a growing animal principally as fat and protein which have energy contents of about 9.4 and 5.6 Kcal/g, respectively. Fat-free tissue, including muscle, also contains about 4 g H_2O/g protein and so has an energy content of only 1.1 Kcal/g. Thus, the NE_g requirement for 1 g pure fat is about 9 times greater than that for 1 g fat-free tissue! In practice the energy content of body gains does not vary quite as much as that, but it is quite common to see 4-5 fold differences in the energy content of body gains attributable to differences in maturity, sex, rate of gain and breed type. Even at the same body weight and feed intake the energy content of the body gains of a Hereford steer may be three times greater than that of a Limousin bull.

Recent evidence reviewed has also indicated differences attributable to breed, sex and rate of gain in so called 'maintenance' requirement (Webster, 1978). Neither the CNE system (Lofgreen and Garrett, 1968) approved for use in the USA by NRC (1976), nor the ME system as described by MAFF (1975) for use in the UK really came to grips with either of these two problems, simply because the necessary evidence was not available when they were published.

California Net Energy System

Values for NE_m and NE_g have been derived from experiments made with cattle fattened at different rates in conditions very similar to those which exist in a commercial feedlot. This is a major merit of the system. RE was determined from measurements of specific gravity on carcasses at slaughter (Lofgreen, 1964). Increments of RE between cattle raised at different intakes of food energy sufficient to promote gains were used to calculate NE_g (Fig. 8-9). The effect of body size on H was assumed a priori to be a constant function of $W^{0.75}$ and basal metabolic rate was predicted by extrapolation to zero energy intake of log RE against ME, both expressed as Kcal/kg$^{0.75}$/day (Lofgreen and Garrett, 1968). Basal metabolism, thus predicted, was 77 Kcal/kg$^{0.75}$/day, which is taken by NRC (1976) to be the NE$_m$ requirement of all classes of beef cattle, although Garrett (1971) has since indicated that maintenance requirements of beef steers are about 10% less than those of dairy steers.

Equations relating body weight gain (G) to RE are, for steers RE = (0.05272 G + 0.00684 G^2) W$^{0.75}$ (13); for heifers RE = (0.05603 + 0.01265 G^2) W$^{0.75}$ (14).

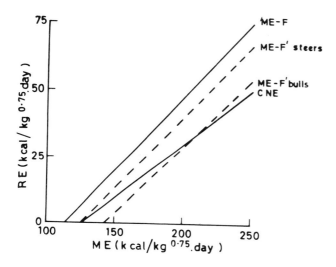

Fig. 8-9. Different predictions of energy retention (R) in growing beef cattle having an energy intake between maintenance and about twice maintenance. CNE = California Net Energy System, ME-F = ME system based on fasting metabolism, ME-F' = ME system based on predicted basal metabolism. The diet has an ME content of 2.6 Mcal/kg DM.

Equations 13 and 14 recognize differences between steers and heifers in the energy content of gains. They also recognize that the proportion of fat, and thus energy content, increases in a curvilinear fashion with increased rate of gain. The use of the 0.75 exponent of W is unfortunate since it suggests that the energy value of gains increases with increased W at a declining rate, whereas the reverse is the case.

The main disadvantage of the CNE system is the amount of work required to evaluate a single feed. Lofgreen and Garrett (1968) showed, for one set of concentrate and roughage mixtures varying from 2 to 100%, roughages, that NE$_m$ and NE$_g$ were proportional to ME content. The comprehensive list of values for NE$_m$ and NE$_g$ pulished by NRC (1976) is based on the assumption that the same relationships between NE and ME hold for all classes of feeds. Blaxter (1973) showed clearly that this is not so (see Fig. 8-8).

The CNE system is quite successful in practice if applied to a situation similar to that in which it was developed; steers and heifers of traditional British origin beef breeds confined and fattened on high intakes of concentrated feeds. It is not, at present, able to predict energy requirements for growth in entire males and in the large European breeds because of uncertainty in estimating the energy value of gains. Neither does it attempt to take into account effects of activity or of the thermal environment on NE$_m$ requirement for maintenance. Finally, it is not a system that simply lends itself to a program of direct evaluation of the NE of a wide range of different feeds and feed mixtures. However, where appropriate, it is very easy to use.

Consider the case of a 300 kg steer getting 8.30 kg/day of a typical mixture of corn and corn silage having NE$_m$ and NE$_g$ values of 1.77 and 1.11 Mcal/kg of DM, respectively. We wish to know how much feed would be required to produce a gain of 1.0 kg/day.

NE$_g$	=	RE (from equation 13)	=	0.05956 x 72.7	= 4.29 Mcal
NE$_m$	=	0.077 W$^{0.75}$	=	5.55 Mcal	
DM requirement for maintenance			=	5.55/1.77	= 3.1 kg/day
DM requirement for gain			=	4.29/1.11	= 3.86 kg/day
	Total DM requirement =	7.0 kg/day			

The ME System

To predict live weight gain from ME intake according to the ME system, one proceeds as follows. First, the ME contents (Mcal/kg of DM) of the ingredients of the diet are obtained from tables or from prediction equations based on proximate analysis or in vitro digestibility (MAFF, 1975). Maintenance requirement is obtained from equation 7, and adjusted for activity or for cold stress. The efficiency of utilization of ME for growth and fattening (k_f) is predicted from ME content as shown in Fig. 8-7, and energy retention, RE, is obtained from equation 15:
$RE = k_f (ME - E_m)$ (15).

The term E_m describes energy requirement for maintenance and is, according to the conventions of the ME system as practiced by MAFF (1975), F/k_m, with the added assumption that, for practical purposes, k_m is constant. To convert RE into live weight gain (LWG) one needs then to know the energy value of the gain (EV_g Kcal/kg). According to MAFF (1975) this is obtained from equation 16: $EV_g = 1.50 + 0.3RE + 0.0045 W$ (kg) (16). This is, obviously, a gross oversimplification in that it assumes that cattle of all types have the same composition of body gains at the same live weight. It is probably about right for Hereford sized crossbred steers. A review of published and unpublished material would suggest that the value for EV_g thus calculated should be increased by 6% for smaller breeds, like the Aberdeen Angus, and for heifers, and decreased by 6% for large breeds and for bulls. Thus the EV_g in a Charolais bull would be 24% lower than that in an Aberdeen Angus heifer at the same weight and RE. This, of course, explains why, at the same body weight, conversion of feed to weight gain is more efficient in bulls than in steers and heifers, even though the efficiency of conversion of ME to RE may be less. Even differences of 24% may not be enough to include bulls of very lean European breeds like the Limousin (see Webster, 1978).

Let us, however, for the moment, consider a Hereford crossbred steer of 300 kg. There are three questions a feeder might ask. (a) How fast will this animal grow and thus reach slaughter weight, given the ration it is getting now? (b) How could this ration be adjusted so as to bring this steer to slaughter weight at the time of my choosing (when the market is right)? (c) What combination of feeds will provide the ME necessary to bring this steer to slaughter weight at the best time and at least cost?

The first question is the most simply solved. Suppose the 300 kg steer eats 6 kg alfalfa hay per day and is given 3 kg/day of a barley based supplement.

	DM	ME content Mcal/kg DM	Intake/day DM, kg	Intake/day ME Mcal
6 kg alfalfa hay	0.87	1.9	5.22	9.91
3 kg barley supplement	0.84	3.1	2.52	7.81
		Total intake	7.74	17.72

ME content of whole diet (Mcal/kg DM) = 2.29
For mixed diets, k_f (from Fig. 8-7) = 0.48

Energy requirement for maintenance in confinement (equation 7)	= 8.60 Mcal
Energy retention = 0.48 (17.72-8.60)	= 4.38
Energy value of live weight gain (equation 16)	= 4.43 Mcal/day
Predicted live weight gain	= 0.99 kg/day

The second problem, formulation of a ration to give a desired rate of production cannot be solved in a single step but requires an iterative (trial and error) approach. Suppose the feeder wishes to get 1.0 kg LWG/day from barley and grass silage. He knows that his steers will not eat more than 20 kg/day of a silage having a DM content of 20% and an ME content of 2.1 Mcal/kg DM. He wants to know how much barley to add to achieve this rate of gain. Obviously k_f, and thus RE will depend on the proportions of silage and barley in the diet. Thus, he must first guess at the amount of barley required and proceed from there.

1st attempted solution	DM	ME content Mcal/kg DM	Intake/day DM, kg	Intake/day ME, Mcal
20 kg grass silage	0.20	2.1	4.0	8.40
3 kg barley	0.84	3.1	2.52	7.81
Total intake			6.52	16.21

ME content of whole diet, Mcal/kg DM	= 2.49
k_f (Fig. 8-7)	= 0.49
Energy requirement for maintenance	= 8.60 Mcal
Energy retention = 0.49 (16.21 - 8.60)	= 3.73
Energy required /kg LWG	= 4.43

This first solution has underestimated RE by 15%. The MAFF (1975) bulletin then suggests that he makes an intuitive guess at how much extra barley to feed and recalculates RE. In fact, one can anticipate the correct ration a little more positively than that.

Increasing the proportion of barley will increase k_f slightly, let us say to 0.51. To achieve an RE of 4.43 Mcal/day when k_f = 0.51 requires (4.43/0.51) + 8.60 (maintenance) = 17.3 Mcal ME/day, an increase of 1.1 Mcal RE over that calculated at the first attempt. If this is to be provided by barley, it will require (1.1/3.1) = 0.35 kg of DM, or 0.42 kg air-dry feed.

2nd attempted solution	DM	ME content Mcal/kg DM	Intake/day DM, kg	Intake/day ME, Mcal
20 kg grass silage	0.20	2.1	4.0	8.40
3.42 kg barley	0.84	3.1	2.87	8.90
			6.87	17.30

ME content of whole diet (Mcal/kg DM)	= 2.52
k_f	= 0.50
Energy retention = 0.5 (17.30 - 8.60)	= 4.35

In this example the increase in k_f was overestimated slightly and thus energy retention is slightly less than anticipated, but near enough to make no difference for practical purposes. With access to a computer, it is, of course, easy to seek iterative solutions to problems of ration formulation without giving the matter much thought. It is also easy, using the same approach, to devise least-cost rations to suit the economic demands of the moment.

The ME system, once grasped, is both theoretically sound and reasonably easy to operate. In practice, however, the ME system, like the CNE system, has not really been a convincing improvement on the traditional Starch Equivalent or TDN systems because it has not yet led to any obvious increase in the precision with which one can predict performance. The major area of uncertainty attached to the prediction of the energy requirements of growing cattle is the difficulty in predicting the energy content of body gains. This point has been alluded to already and is discussed at length elsewhere (Webster, 1978).

There are other fundamental objections to the ME system for growing cattle. The determination of k_m and k_f is based on energy balance trials with mature sheep retaining energy almost entirely as fat. Differences between cattle and sheep in the efficiency of utilization of ME are probably small, but all the interactions between animal and feed that make one animal different from another and that make growth different from fattening are expressed by a measurement of fasting metabolism. This is not only assumed to be the same function of W for all animals but there must be a large degree of uncertainty involved in predicting RE in growing cattle at an ME intake of about twice maintenance measurements by combining measurements made with cattle when ME = 0 with measurements made of k_m and k_f using mature sheep.

Thus, the main criticism of the ME system as a basis for predicting energy requirements for growing cattle is that it is not based on experiments with growing cattle. When calorimetric measurements were made of energy retention in rapidly growing cattle, there were differences in heat production between breeds and between bulls and steers at the same ME intake and body weight, which the ME system does not, at present, take into account (Webster, 1978). The ME system assumes, in practice, that k_m and k_f are determined entirely by feed quality (the ME content of the diet, Fig. 8-8). Thus, between animal differences in the relationship between ME intake and RE can only, within the existing system, be included within the concept of basal metabolism (Fig. 8-6). These direct measurements made of RE in continuously growing cattle were used therefore to derive values for predicted basal metabolism (F') which is an empirical term similar in concept to that used to calculate

NE_m according to the CNE system and can be defined as *the value which accurately predicts RE in growing cattle from ME, when k_m and k_f are defined according to the conventions of the ME system* (Webster et al, 1974; Webster, 1978).

Fig. 8-8 illustrates different estimates of RE in growing cattle according to the conventions of the CNE and ME systems, both of which assume that for this purpose all cattle are equal. Also illustrated are predicted RE values for bulls and steers based on the ME system using predicted basal metabolism as the intercept to derive maintenance requirement.

Fig. 8-9 shows clearly that the ME system based on measurements of fasting metabolism (ME-F) overestimates RE relative to the other approaches. The use of predicted basal metabolism (ME-F') takes into account differences of 10-15% in H between bulls and steers and also suggests (not indicated in Fig. 8-9), in common with Garrett (1971), that H is about 10% higher in dairy than in beef breeds. These and other differences between animals can easily be built into any revision of MAFF (1975) bulletin 33. At present, however, neither the ME nor the CNE systems take sufficient account of differences between animals in heat production and in the energy content of body gains so neither can yet be used with high precision for beef production. The ME system has been used with great success by nutritionists to evaluate the energy content of different feeds. The prior need now is to know more of the different energy requirements of different classes of cattle.

References Cited

Alexander, G. 1974. In: Heat Loss from Animals and Man, p 173. Butterworths, London.

Annison, E.F. and D.G. Armstrong. 1970. In: Physiology of Digestion and Metabolism in the Ruminant, p 422. Oriel Press, Newcastle Upon Tyne.

ARC. 1965. The Nutrient Requirements of Farm Livestock. No. 2. Ruminants. H.M. Stationery Office, London.

Blaxter, K.L. 1967. The Energy Metabolism of Ruminants. 2nd Ed. Hutchison and Co., London.

Blaxter, K.L. 1973. In: Nutrition Conference for Feed Manufacturers No. 7, p. 3. Butterworths, London.

Brody, S. 1945. Bioenergetics and Growth. Reinhold, New York.

Broster, W.H. 1972. Dairy Sci. Abstr. 34:265.

Broster, W.H. 1976. In: Principles of Cattle Production, p 271. Butterworths, London.

Christopherson, R.J., R.J. Hudson and R.J. Richmond. 1976. University of Alberta Feeders' Day Report 55:51.

Faichney, G.J. 1972. J. Agr. Sci. 79:493.

Feedingstuffs Evaluation Unit. 1975. 1st report. Department of Agriculture and Fisheries for Scotland.

Flatt, W. P. 1969. In: Nutrition of Animals of Agricultural Importance Vol. I, p 491. Pergamon Press, Oxford.

Garrett, W. N. 1971. J. Animal Sci. 32:451.

Hales, J.R.S. 1974. In: Environmental Physiology. MTP Int. Revs. of Science. Physiology Vol. 7, p 107. University Park Press, Baltimore.

Hafez, E.S.E. 1968. Adaptation of Domestic Animals. Lea and Febiger, Philadelphia.

Hungate, R.E. 1966. The Rumen and its Microbes. Academic Press, London.

Kleiber, M. 1961. The Fire of Life. Wiley, New York.

Lofgreen, G.P. 1964. In: 3rd Symp. Energy Metabolism of Farm Animals, p 309. Academic Press, London.

Lofgreen, G.P. and W.N. Garrett. 1968. J. Animal Sci. 27:793.

MacLean, J.A. 1972. Brit. J.Nutr. 27:597

MAFF. 1975. Tech. Bull. 33. H.M. Stationery Office, London.

Moe, P.W. and W.P.Flatt. 1969. J. Dairy Sci. 52:928.

Mount, L.E. 1968. The Climatic Physiology of the Pig. Arnold, London.

NRC. 1971. Nutrient Requirements of Domestic Animals. No. 3. Dairy Cattle. Nat. Acad. Sci. Washington, D.C.

NRC. 1975. Nutrient Requirements of Domestic Animals. No. 5. Sheep. Nat. Acad. Sci., Washington, D.C.

NRC. 1976. Nutrient Requirements of Domestic Animals. No. 4 Beef Cattle. Nat. Acad. Sci., Washington, D.C.

Nehring, K. 1969. In: 4th Symp. Energy Metabolism of Farm Animals, p 5. Pub. Eur. Ass. Anim. Prod. No. 12. Oriel Press, Newcastle Upon Tyne.

Ørskov, E.R. 1975. World Rev. Nutr. Dietet. 22:152.

Osuji, P.O. 1974. J.Range Mang. 27:437.

Pullar, J.D. 1969. In: Nutrition of Animals of Agricultural Importance Vol. I, p 471. Pergamon Press, Oxford.

Rattray, P.V., W.N. Garrett, N.E. East and N. Hinman. 1974. J. Animal Sci. 38:383.

Schneider, B.H. and W.P. Flatt. 1975. The Evaluation of Feeds through Digestibility Experiments. University of Georgia Press. Athens, Ga.

Swift, R.W. 1957. J. Animal Sci. 16:753.

Tilley, J.M.A. and R.A. Terry. 1963. J. Brit. Grassland Soc. 18:104.

Toutain, P.L., Clair Toutain, A.J.F. Webster and J.D. McDonald. 1978. Brit. J. Nutr. (in press).

Van der Honing, Y., A. Steg and A.J.H. Van Es. 1977. Livestock Prod. Sci. 4:57.

Van Soest, P.J. 1967. J. Animal Sci. 26:119.

Webster, A.J.F. 1974. In: Heat Loss from Animals and Man, p 205. Butterworths, London.

Webster, A.J.F. 1976. In: Principles of Cattle Production, p 103. Butterworths, London.

Webster, A.J.F. 1978. World Rev. Nutr. Diet. (in press).

Webster, A.J.F., J.M. Brockway and J.S. Smith. 1974. Animal Prod. 19:127.

Webster, A.J.F., P.O. Osuji, F.White and J.F. Ingram. 1975. Brit. J. Nutr. 34:125.

Chapter 9 - Vitamins

Vitamins are a group of chemically unrelated organic compounds which are essential for life and normal productive functions of animals. In the 1890's Eijkman discovered that rice hulls cured a disease of fowl and related this to beriberi in man. Thiamin, of course, was shown to be the rice hull factor. According to Silverman (1958), the first crystalline vitamin was isolated in 1926, and since then some 15 or more vitamin-like compounds have been chemically identified and demonstrated to be essential for growth or other physiological functions in certain animal species. In ruminants dietary requirements for the fat-soluble vitamins (A, D, E, K) have been rather well established for many situations and classes of animals.

The need for dietary sources of B vitamins, with the exception of vitamin B_{12}, has not been established for animals on conventional rations. In general, the preruminant calf or lamb fed a purified diet has been the basic model for B vitamin studies with ruminant species. When working with these young animals (or gnotobiotic animals) on purified diets, it can be shown that they need many of the B-complex vitamins (see Ch. 10), but the need under more typical and practical conditions is less clear.

Hungate (1966) has pointed out that the dietary concentration of B vitamins is inversely related to the amount of rumen synthesis (see Ch. 15, Vol. 1); thus, providing needed nutrients are available for microbial growth and vitamin synthesis, rumen synthesis is believed to be more than adequate in ruminating animals. As a result the NRC recommendations for sheep, dairy cattle or beef cattle do not include any specific dietary recommendations other than for preruminants or in milk replacers. Readers desiring more details on chemical formulas, structure and other aspects are referred to basic nutrition books such as Church and Pond (1974) or a good biochemistry text.

FAT-SOLUBLE VITAMINS
VITAMIN A AND CAROTENE

As the informed reader will know, there is a large quantity of research literature on the subject of vitamin A and carotene metabolism and requirements with ruminants. This is so because vitamin A is generally conceded to be the vitamin most apt to be limiting for many different classes and species of ruminant animals. Literature on the subject dates back to the 1920's. As a consequence, the literature citations in the following discussion will be selective.

For those readers interested in reviews, a very comprehensive older one was published by Moore (1957). Mitchell (1967) has published a good, although a relatively brief paper. Bauernfeind (1969) and Jensen (1969) have presented information that may be of interest to many readers, although the information is not restricted to ruminants.

Chemistry

Vitamin A, or retinol, is a complex 20 carbon cyclic alcohol which has conjugated double bonds in the side chain of the molecule. Due to the presence of the double bonds, it can exist in different isometric forms which have different biological activities. Vitamin A aldehyde (retinene) is also found in biological materials as is vitamin A acid (retinoic acid). In addition, various esters may be found or have been synthesized--vitamin A acetate or palmitate, for example. Vitamin A is found only in animal tissues, whereas its precursors; the carotenoids, are found in plant tissues.

Vitamin A was first produced synthetically in 1947. The methods were refined and developed for commercial production very rapidly with the result that vitamin A is readily available at very modest prices (Bauernfeind and DeRitter, 1972). It is sold in a dry, gelatin coated form to which antioxidants have been added or in liquid forms which are water miscible, in oil solutions or as injectable preparations.

Vitamin A has a structure somewhat similar to a drying oil; the double bonds present in the side chain are, thus, readily oxidized (Bauernfeind, 1969). Photochemical and enzymic action may also cause rapid vitamin A destruction. Conditions such as hot temperatures and excessive acidity or alkalinity may lead to hydrolysis or oxidation; consequently, both vitamin A and carotenes need to be protected from destruction in normal feed handling systems.

A wide variety of carotenoids may exist in different plant tissues. These are pigmented compounds that are present in relatively high concentrations in green plant tissues, but are found in only very small quantities in seeds, one exception being the cryptoxanthin found in yellow corn. β-carotene, primarily, and to a lesser extent α and γ carotenes serve as precursors to vitamin A, being converted to variable extents to the vitamin in the wall of the intestine. The carotenes also exist as *trans* and *cis* isomers and in different states of oxidation. Conditions that result in rapid destruction of vitamin A also apply to the carotenes. For example it has been shown in many instances that a high proportion of the carotenes are inactivated in the process of field-curing hays.

Plant tissues such as hays stored in the interior of a bale may retain some carotene for a time, but processing will speed up losses. When handled carefully, carotene losses can be minimized. For example, when forage plants were chopped, dried in hot air, and stored loose or in bags, there was very little carotene loss after 112 days and 58% remained after 224 days (Hennig and Guther, 1975).

Functions

The only specific biochemical function that can be attributed to vitamin A is its participation in vision. It has been shown that light-sensitive pigments in the photoreceptors of the retina of the eye contain visual purple (rhodopsin), which is a combination of a *cis* isomer of vitamin A aldehyde and a protein. Light bleaches this compound to *trans*-retinal + the protein, opsin and the *trans*-retinal is isomerized to 11-*cis*-retinal. In the dark the retinal recombines with opsin to yield rhodopsin which is then ready for recycling.

Jensen (1969) points out that vitamin A acid (retinoic acid) fulfills most of the biological functions of vitamin A, but will not substitute for vitamin A in the synthesis of rhodopsin. In other tissues it is well known that vitamin A is required for maintenance and normal functioning of the epithelial tissues of the animal body, thus it may affect the skin, mucosal tissues in the gut and respiratory passages, and gonadal tissues. Bone growth is also affected, possibly because of an involvement of vitamin A in the synthesis of chondroitin sulfate. However, no specific biochemical role has yet to be shown for the involvement of vitamin A other than in vision.

Rumen Metabolism

There are a number of papers which indicate that appreciable amounts of caro-

tene or vitamin A may be degraded in the forestomach (King et al, 1962; Keating et al, 1964; Mitchell et al, 1965). King et al suggested that as much as 40% of the carotene might be lost in the stomach. In studies with sheep on semipurified diets, stomach losses of carotene amounted to 23% regardless of whether starch or cellulose was the main energy ingredient (Potkanski et al, 1974); further studies with natural forages indicated recoveries of 85-90% of carotene in the abomasum (Potkanski, 1976). In vitro studies suggest that carotene was little affected when fermented with rumen liquor from steers given high roughage rations as compared to liquor from animals on high grain rations (Keating et al, 1964), but Pastrana et al (1975) found fairly high losses in carotene from grass samples suspended in the rumen. Adding molasses to the diet reduced losses relative to the control. Other research with cows, calves and sheep suggest that β-carotene losses in the entire stomach amount to 10-11% (Fernandez et al, 1976).

With regard to vitamin A, Mitchell et al (1965) estimated that only 43% of dietary vitamin A was recovered from the abomasum of steers fed primarily a forage ration. When wethers or steers were fed a diet primarily of corn and alfalfa hay, Long et al (1971) found that 62-69% of the vitamin A was lost in the forestomach. Adding some cottonseed oil increased losses somewhat (69-70%). Data from this laboratory (Mitchell et al, 1968) also demonstrated that gelatin coated vitamin A preparations were not stable in the rumen, losses ranging from 70-80% of diet vitamin A. Addition of large amounts of α-tocopherol did not prevent losses of vitamin A acetate. Other data on a ram with the pylorus ligated suggest a loss of 30% in 24 hr (Fernandez et al, 1976). In addition to these various studies mentioned, other information demonstrates that intramuscular injections of vitamin A are much more effective in maintaining or increasing liver vitamin A stores than intraruminal injections (Martin et al, 1971), thus providing indirect evidence that losses occur in the stomach or as a result of low absorption.

Data on rumen fat metabolism indicated that conjugated double bonds are less subject to hydrogenation than non-conjugated bonds. It has been suggested that this may be one reason that carotene is more resistant to hydrogenation in the rumen. In the case of vitamin A, degradation might well be due to other types of reactions that could render the molecule biologically inactive.

Absorption and Excretion

Numerous studies with ruminant species have shown that carotene and vitamin A are readily absorbed by the gut with a rapid increase in serum vitamin A. Data reported by Diven and Erwin (1958) showed that vitamin A absorption was maximal at 12 hr post treatment, while β-carotene was absorbed at a slower and more sustained rate. Vitamin A acetate was absorbed at a rate comparable to the alcohol. Tucker et al (1967) published data which indicated that carotene cannot be absorbed from the cecum or large intestine of sheep.

With regard to apparent digestibility of carotene, Wing (1969) reported that it averaged ca. 78% for various forages fed to cattle. Variables that influenced carotene digestibility were month of the year, type of forage (hay, silage, greenchop or pasture), species of plant, and DM content of the plant. Martovitskaya et al (1975) found that apparent digestibility of carotene ranged from 19 to 55%, being greatly affected by type of diet. Postabomasal absorption, as estimated with chromic oxide, indicated absorption ranging from 5 to 33% on a variety of different diets (Potkanski, 1976). Thus, it seens that a major portion of plant carotene is either degraded in the stomach or is not absorbed from the intestinal tract.

Workers at the Kentucky Experiment station have been active in studying the excretion of isotopically-labeled vitamin A and carotene after intravenous infusions. Menzies et al (1967) reported experiments in which lambs were given ^{14}C-β-carotene intravenously or intraruminally. Of that given via the rumen, they recovered 94 and 97% (2 lambs) in the feces and intestinal contents. When carotene was given by vein, little radioactivity was found in the intestines. Some radioactivity was recovered in urine and various tissues. In the case of animals given vitamin A acetate intravenously (Mitchell et al, 1967), radioactivity was not detected in urine, although subsequent data (Boling et al, 1969), showed that about 21% of injected vitamin A and 18% of the carotene was recovered in the bile during a 24-hr collection period, the majority of it being excreted during the first 12 hr. It was also shown that metabolites excreted in the bile could be absorbed when infused into the duodenum; of course, this is not to say that such metabolites would have biological activity. Data obtained on labeled vitamin A acid (Hume et al, 1971) indicated that more

than 50% of the activity was excreted in bile and 35-41% in urine within 12 hr. Total recovery of label amounted to 95-97% within 24 hr after I.V. administration.

With respect to the gut, it is interesting to note that some time ago McGillivray (1951) suggested that synthesis of carotene might occur in the gut of sheep, evidence being based on lignin:carotene ratios. Majumdar and Gupta (1960) also found this to be the case in goats and additional data were obtained on rats indicating a higher biological value than for standard carotene given in equivalent amounts. Almendinger and Hinds (1969) have also reported similar results in that more β-carotene and total carotenoids were recovered in feces than were found in the ration given to cattle. They suggest that apparent increases may have been due to a release of residual carotenoids not extracted from the feed by the usual procedure. If this is not the case, then it would seem that the increased carotene must be derived from synthesis by microorganisms in the gut or carotene excreted into the gut via the bile, as demonstrated in studies already mentioned.

Tissue Distribution and Metabolism

Information is available from many different reports which shows tissue levels of carotene and vitamin A which may be expected in different situations. Examples from different classes of cattle are shown in Table 9-1. These data illustrate several pertinent facts regarding carotene and vitamin A metabolism that have been well documented by many different studies. First, it will be noted that blood and liver concentrations in the young animal may be very low as compared to levels in adults. This is because very little vitamin A crosses the placental membranes, although the amount can be increased by large doses to the mother. For example, data with sheep showed that 0.12% retinol and 0.37% retinyl palmitate from injected doses were transferred to the liver of the lamb fetus (Mitchell et al, 1975).

Secondly, the blood and liver concentrations gradually increase with age, documentation having been published on this subject by Bayfield and Mylrea (1969) and Taylor et al (1968) as well as in many older papers. A third point is that liver reserves are apt to be relatively low in lactating cows and in fat steers, apparently because a higher rate of productivity increases the requirement for vitamin A and leaves less for storage.

Table 9-1. Blood and liver concentrations of vitamin A and carotene in cattle.

Animal	Plasma or serum		Liver		Reference
	carotene, mcg/100 ml	vitamin A, mcg/100 ml	carotene, mcg/g	vitamin A, mcg/g	
Beef cows, early gestation	150-400	25-50	15-50[a]	200-1,000[a]	Church et al, 1956
early lactation on low-	50-150				
carotene rations	50-150	20-25	5-25[a]	10-150[a]	
Beef calves at birth	0-5	5-10	--	0-5[a]	
Dairy cows early lactation on high-roughage ration and grain	320	33			Swanson et al, 1968
late lactation	460	36	5	30	
Holstein heifers	230-300	25-27	4	55-66	Miller et al, 1969
Fat steers	85-95	25-30	1-2	2-4	Jordan et al, 1963

[a] Analyses on a dry weight basis which is roughly equivalent to 4 times the concentration on a wet basis.

Carotene that is absorbed from the gut is converted to vitamin A in the intestine or in other tissues such as the lung (Kon et al, 1955). Sheep show an increase in blood vitamin A after I.V. infusions of carotene whereas much lower increases are shown by calves (Church et al, 1954; Kon et al, 1955; Schuh et al, 1959). This indicates that sheep are probably more efficient users of carotene than cattle.

In the blood vitamin A and carotene are found mainly bound to the albumin fraction (Erwin et al, 1959), a complex which serves to transport the vitamin to other tissues. However, there may be seasonal variations in the retinol-binding proteins in blood since Glover et al (1976) noted minimal levels in summer and increased levels in the autumn. Perhaps this is a mechanism designed to conserve the vitamin for times of scarcity.

In the liver and other organs (adrenals, spleen, etc.), vitamin A is found esterified to long-chain fatty acids. Liver carotene levels are very slow to change (Table 9-2) during a period in which vitamin A may increase or decrease drastically (Kirk et al, 1971). Tissue carotenoids are believed to serve no useful functions other than what value may be derived from skin pigmentation. Species and breed differences exist in blood and epidermal carotene. Sheep and goats, for example, have almost no detectable carotene in the blood or milk. In cattle there is a consider-

able difference in the amount of carotenoid compounds that are deposited in the skin, breeds such as the Guernsey and Jersey having large amounts while those such as Ayrshire and Holstein have very little.

Table 9-2. Effect of time on depletion of liver vitamin A and carotene in feedlot steers. [a]

Time, days	Liver levels*	
	Vitamin A	Carotene
Initial	105	15
28	71	12
56	43	7
84	23	6
112	12	5
140	9	5

[a] Data from Kirk et al (1971)

*mcg/g fresh liver; all animals on a deficient diet.

Studies on liver turnover rate of vitamin A labeled with tritium have shown time for loss of half of the activity ranged from 89-187 days in one experiment with lambs (Mitchell et al, 1967) and averaged 163 days in another for mature rams (Boling et al, 1969). Turnover time in the latter case was 234 days. In work with steers, average turnover time was

138 days for steers receiving a ration with 6% crude protein and 126 days for steers receiving 12% (Hayes et al, 1968). In another experiment with mature steers, mean half time of liver vitamin A was calculated to be 320 days (Fields et al, 1969). In dairy cows, Swanson et al (1968) calculated that liver vitamin A was depleted at a rate of 35%/mo. when cows were fed a deficient diet. With feedlot cattle, liver stores were higher at 35 and 65 days preslaughter after receiving injections of vitamin A, but not so at 147 days, indicating depletion of the reserves (Martin et al, 1971).

Vitamin A Deficiency

Research literature on vitamin A deficiencies in ruminants extends back to well documented reports of more than 40 years ago. Some of the early classical literature would include papers by Guilbert and Hart (1934, 1935), Moore (1939, 1941), Moore et al (1943), Schmidt (1941) and Madsen and Earle (1947).

A deficiency of vitamin A, as might be expected, is more apt to occur in young, rapidly growing animals than in feedlot animals or adults. Furthermore, the symptoms seen in young animals are generally more diverse and extensive than those reported in older animals. There are also minor differences seen in different species.

The diverse symptoms seen in vitamin A-deficient animals are a result of a deficiency acting on very different tissues. It is well known that vitamin A is involved in sight and maintenance of the integrity of epithelial tissues. Since epithelial tissues include those covering body surfaces and lining body cavities as well as some of the tissues in various endocrine glands and the gonads, it is obvious that many different body functions are likely to be affected by a severe deficiency.

Deficiencies in Cattle

Young Animals. The young calf is quite susceptible to a deficiency, particularly if born to a dam on a deficient diet (see section on mature animals). This is so because only minimal amounts of vitamin A are transferred to the liver—the main storage depot—of the fetal tissues and, when born to deficient dams, the vitamin A concentration in colostrum is much lower than normal. Even calves born to adequately-fed cows will develop deficiency symptoms within a few weeks if intake via milk or other sources is restricted (Madsen and Davis, 1949; Byers et al, 1956; Church et al, 1955, 1956.)

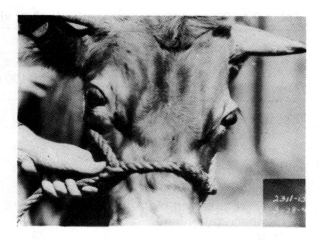

Fig. 9-1. Heifer showing exopthalmia or bulging eye condition due to high cerebrospinal fluid pressure and partial closure of the optic foramen. Courtesy of L.A. Moore, U.S.D.A.

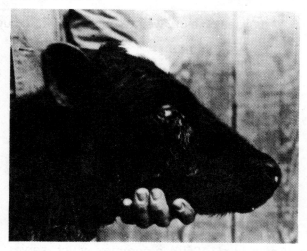

Fig. 9-2. Calf showing xeropthalmia, a dry, thickened condition of the conjunctiva with an opaque cornea. Photo by Guilbert and Hart, Calif. Agric. Expt. Sta.

It has been reported that one of the first clinical symptoms is anorexia (Abrams et al, 1969; Calhoun and Woodmansee, 1968), but other signs that develop in rapid order include night blindness, severe diarrhea, incoordination, exopthalmia (Fig. 9-1), excessive lacrimation of the eye and nasal discharges, convulsions at irregular intervals, permanent blindness and ruptured cornea of the eye (Fig. 9-2). Other signs are an unthrifty appearance characterized by a rough, dry hair coat (Fig. 9-3) and failure to gain or loss of weight (Helmboldt et al, 1953; Spratling et al, 1965). Blood vitamin A levels much below 12-15 mcg/100 ml may be considered to be deficient in calves other than newborn animals.

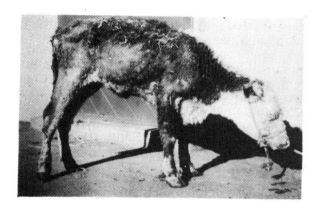

Fig. 9-3. Vitamin A deficient calf. Note the emaciated appearance and evidence of diarrhea. The calf also shows excessive lacrimation and nasal discharges characteristic of the deficiency. Courtesy of G. Patterson, Chas. Pfizer Co.

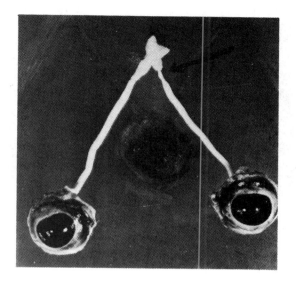

Fig. 9-4. Picture shows the effect of closure of the optic foramen. Arrow points to the pinched section. Courtesy of L.A. Moore, U.S.D.A.

The changes that occur in the eye are not all due to the same cause and are not seen to the same extent in older animals and adults. The development of night blindness is due to an insufficient amount of light-sensitive pigments (rhodopsin). Papilledema develops in the eye (Moore and Sykes, 1940; Spratling et al, 1965), probably as a result of a greatly increased cerebrospinal fluid pressure seen in deficient animals (Moore and Sykes, 1940; Helmboldt et al, 1953; Mikkilineni et al, 1973). Normal cerebrospinal pressures are on the order of 100 mm of H_2O, but may rise to as much as 400-600 mm in deficient animals. The increase in pressure is apparently due to a deficient absorption of cerebrospinal fluid (Calhoun et al, 1968). Increased cerebrospinal fluid pressure is one of the first quantitative symptoms that can be detected. In addition to these changes, the optic foramen—the hole through which the optic bundle passes—gradually gets smaller and smaller with the result that the optic bundle is severely pinched (Fig. 9-4), eventually causing permanent blindness and deterioration of the eyeball (corneal rupture). It is assumed that the high cerebrospinal fluid pressure is also responsible for the convulsions that occur in deficient animals, in this case due to pressure on the brain, although there appears to be little if any effect on brain growth (Mikkilineni et al, 1973).

In studies with young Holstein calves, Eaton et al (1970) found that 50% of the calves had ocular papilledema when blood levels of vitamin A were at 10 mcg/100 ml. At 5 mcg/100 ml, 85% of the calves had papilledema. In addition 60% of the calves had squamous metaplasia of the parotid duct at 10 mcg/ml and 93% were affected at blood levels of 5 mcg/100 ml.

Changes in the skin and other tissues are a result of replacement of normal types of epithelium with stratified, keratinized epithelium in the respiratory tract, eyes, alimentary tract and genito-urinary tract. The diarrhea that occurs is probably a reflection of metaplasia of the normal mucosal cells which line the intestines. Histological examination may show metaplastic changes in the ducts of the parotid salivary gland and necrotic hepatitis of the liver (Helmboldt et al, 1953; Rousseau et al, 1954); very rapid depletion did not result in lesions of the kidney, adrenals or pituitary which have been reported elsewhere. Calves depleted at a less rapid rate, however, have been shown to have cystic pituitary glands as well as keratinized tissues in the reticulo-rumen (Nielsen et al, 1966) and kidney function becomes less efficient in clearing some chemicals from the blood (Richards et al, 1970).

Ritzman et al (1945) have reported that deficient calves consumed more food but made 50% less gain than similar calves receiving adequate vitamin A. They also reported that protein utilization was depressed considerably and that digestion, absorption and metabolizable energy were depressed although basal metabolism and heat increment were unaffected.

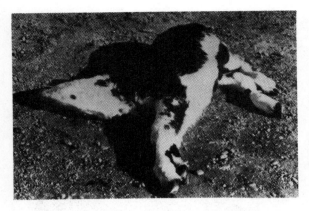

Fig. 9-5. Vitamin A deficient steer with convulsions which may be seen relatively early in the deficiency. U.S.D.A. photo, courtesy of L.L. Madsen.

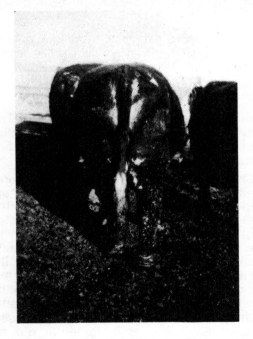

Fig. 9-6. Vitamin A deficient steer with anasarca, a relatively long-standing deficiency resulting in edema of the legs and brisket. U.S.D.A. photo, courtesy of L.L. Madsen.

Steers and Heifers. Guilbert and Hart (1934) reported that steers were apt to develop severe deficiencies of vitamin A when in the feedlot. Subsequent reports by Schmidt (1941), Madsen and Earle (1947) and others have confirmed these observations. Steers are especially prone to develop deficiencies to the point where they show night blindness and have occasional convulsions (Fig. 9-5). Schmidt indicated that nasal and eye discharges as well as some ulcerated corneas

were seen. Madsen and Earle (1947) reported that anasarca (Fig. 9-6), an edema of the legs and brisket, was apt to develop after steers had been on deficient rations for long periods of time (some time after convulsions were seen). Rations containing silage are also prone to result in deficiencies (Church, 1956; Jordan et al, 1963; Martin et al, 1971) even though apparent carotene intake may be adequate. Madsen and Earle noted that affected animals had reduced levels of plasma ascorbic acid, increased levels of plasma globulin and total N, and decreased levels of plasma albumin. Erwin et al (1957) found that total serum proteins were not changed by a deficiency, but β-globulins were higher than in normal animals and albumin was lower; administration of vitamin A or carotene caused a rise in serum albumin. Mee and Stanley (1974) reported that low blood vitamin A was related to increased packed cell volume. In heifers, Woelfel et al (1965) observed that deficient animals excreted greater volumes of urine of lower osmolality; other data indicating edema accompanied by hemodilution, hyponatremia and possibly hyperkalemia. Blood plasma vitamin A of 20 mcg/100 ml may be considered borderline to deficient in feedlot steers.

Mature Animals. Some of the available information on beef cows indicates that they are relatively resistant to the development of severe vitamin A deficiencies (Madsen and Davis, 1949; Church et al, 1955, 1956; Wheeler et al, 1957). Evidence indicates that dairy cows may, in some cases (Schmidt, 1941; Byers et al, 1956), go for extended periods of time without marked problems, but other evidence (Ronning et al, 1959; Swanson et al, 1968) indicates that deficiencies may be produced in as little as 4 mo. This difference between beef and dairy cows is probably due to the fact that a higher rate of feed intake has been shown to increase the need for vitamin A (Church et al, 1956; Hazzard et al, 1962). Deficiency studies in cows have shown that depleted animals are still fertile although breeding efficiency may be reduced. Uterine involution and appearance of first estrus are delayed. Survival of the embryo appears to be lower during implantation and placentation (Mingazov, 1975). Depleted cows tend to calve earlier than expected, and there are reports indicating a greater incidence of retained placenta. Severely deficient cows may abort several wk to 2-3 mo. preterm. They may also

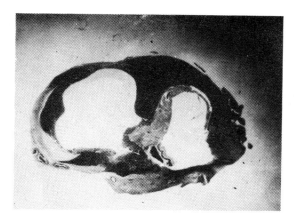

Fig. 9-7. Cystic pituitary gland from a deficient cow. Cysts are present both in the anterior and posterior parts of the gland. U.S.D.A. photo, courtesy of L.L. Madsen.

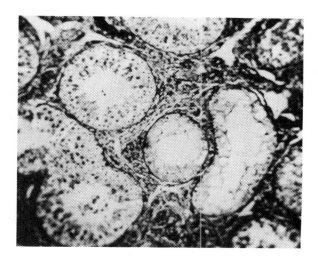

Fig. 9-8. Histological section from testis of a vitamin A deficient bull. The picture shows degeneration of the seminiferous tubules. Courtesy of J.F. Proctor, Nat. Dairy Prod. Corp.

show other typical symptoms such as anasarca, convulsions, night blindness, photophobia, incoordination, and a dry, harsh, hair coat. Exopthalmia and more progressive eye conditions are less likely to be seen in adults, although high cerebrospinal fluid pressures occur as do ocular lesions such as papilledema (Moore, 1941). Cystic pituitary glands may be seen (Fig. 9-7). Calves from depleted cows may show degeneration of the optic nerve and be hydrocephalic, and such calves often are dead or very weak at birth and do not survive very long (Byers et al, 1956).

In the case of bulls, Madsen et al (1948) found that sexual activity and ability decreased rapidly and semen samples showed a marked increase in the precentage of abnormal sperm with progressive declines in motility. Histological evidence of testicular injury was shown to persist for many months after they were returned to a diet with sufficient carotene (Fig. 9-8). In adult animals blood vitamin A levels of 20-25 mcg% are borderline to deficient. Carotene supply may also be a factor since Weiss (1977) fed a ration low in carotene but with added vitamin A and concluded that the deficient ration resulted in more abnormal sperm cells and disturbed maturation of the epididymis.

Deficiencies in Other Species

Of the domestic ruminant species, cattle are, apparently, more subject to deficiencies than sheep or goats. It is generally thought that mature sheep are more resistant to depletion. Another possibility may be that sheep utilize carotene more efficiently than

cattle (see section on metabolism). At any rate, there are relatively few research reports in the literature on vitamin A deficiencies of sheep.

Lindley et al (1949) have described deficiency symptoms in young, rapidly growing rams. Symptoms were seen as early as 7 wk after being placed on deficient rations. The animals began having attacks characterized by stiffness of the legs, cocking of the head to one side, and inability to stand. Some animals showed only anorexia until they suddenly became moribund and died. An incoordinated gait with progressive weakness was often seen. Some animals showed a swayed back (Fig. 9-9), possibly because of loss of control over the leg muscles. All animals were night-blind by the 21st wk, but none showed xeropthalmia. Other symptoms included sullenness and evidence of pain. Rate of gain was reduced and most eventually lost weight. Blood plasma vitamin C was reduced. With respect to reproductive functions, libido was evident in deficient rams, but semen quality was markedly reduced as was testicular size. Germinal epithelium was degenerated. On autopsy, it was shown that most pituitary glands had small cysts.

In other reports, Eveleth et al (1949) found that spinal fluid pressure in deficient sheep was considerably higher than in controls. Incoordination and weakness were seen, and animals had difficulty in breathing after strenuous exercise. Night blindness was common, but permanent blindness was very

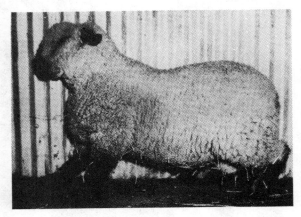

Fig. 9-9. A deficient ram showing posture said to be typical of many deficient animals. From Lindley et al, 1949.

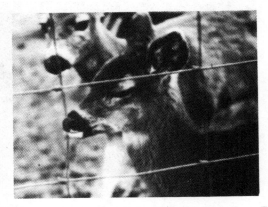

Fig. 9-10. Vitamin A deficient black-tailed deer. The deer closest the fence shows photophobia, an early symptom of vitamin A deficiency. Courtesy of D. Smith, Oregon Agric. Expt. Sta.

slow to develop. More recently, Webb et al (1968) have shown that vitamin A deficiencies in wethers resulted in a much increased excretion of urine which was lower in osmolality and specific gravity. A marked elevation of inorganic phosphate excretion and a reduced excretion of Ca were also observed. Evidence on Na indicated a greater salt retention and increased plasma urea indicated some alteration in Na metabolism. On the basis of work done elsewhere with rats, it was suggested that the deficient animals had an altered adrenal metabolism resulting in the secretion of elevated levels of glucocorticoids. Subsequent research on this subject (Webb et al, 1971) indicated some change in hormone synthesis (in vitro), but no change in excretion of urinary hormones.

With respect to goats Dutt and Majumdar (1969) have shown that adult male goats were very resistant to depletion of vitamin A. Symptoms observed included corneal ulceration, unthrifty condition, night blindness, elongated hooves, and loss of hair in patches. Histological examination indicated metaplasia and keratinization of tissues only in the trachea. Friere et al (1974) have demonstrated increased cerebrospinal fluid pressures in deficient adult goats which was confirmed by squamous metaplasia in the parotid salivary gland.

In the case of wild species there is little information available. Captive deer may be depleted to a sufficient extent to exhibit photophobia (Fig. 9-10) which responded to vitamin A therapy. However, blood sampling of Nevada mule deer during the winter suggests that blood vitamin A levels are ample to avoid deficiency problems (Hunter et al, 1973). Liver analyses on wild elk, which showed low reproduction rates, did not indicate any likelihood of vitamin A deficiency (Church, 1969).

INTERRELATIONSHIPS OF THE FAT-SOLUBLE VITAMIN

Vitamins

A limited amount of data are available in which interactions of the fat-soluble vitamins have been studied in ruminants. For example, Light et al (1952) found that a deficiency of both vitamins A and D caused a reversal of wool pigmentation in black and white wools. Vitamin A supplementation caused no response but supplementation of vitamin D in addition caused wool colors to return to their original color.

With respect to vitamins A and E, Whiting et al (1949) reported that supplementing ewes with tocopherol increased the liver stores of vitamin A in lambs born to these ewes, although little effect was seen in kids. Tocopherol had no influence on vitamin A in colostrum. In calves Dicks et al (1959) found that tocopherol resulted in an increase in the utilization of vitamin A given at relatively high levels; however, it was also noted that tocopherol concentration in tissues decreased as the vitamin A intake increased. Rousseau et al (1973) noted very little effect in calves when deficient animals were supplemented with α-tocopherol, either on various blood components or on development of deficiency lesions. In work with steers Chapman et al (1964) found that either supplemental vitamin A or E increased vitamin A and Cu in liver, but there was less growth response to vitamin A when it was fed in combination with vitamin E. In other work with steers (O'Donovan, 1967; Perry et al, 1968), vitamin E apparently had no effect on serum or liver vitamin A, nor did vitamin K.

Other Factors Affecting Vitamin A Utilization

Anderson et al (1962) have shown that protein-deficient rations fed to sheep resulted in much less efficient utilization of vitamin A given intraruminally, although there was little effect on carotene. Later work by Faruque and Walker (1970) also demonstrated that young lambs on high protein diets utilized retinyl palmitate more efficiently than those on low protein diets. Erwin et al (1963) have studied the effect of low and high energy and protein diets with or without an antioxidant (ethoxyquin) on liver vitamin A in steers. The data presented indicated that increasing dietary protein on the low energy diets tended to reduce liver vitamin A retention, whereas it had little effect on the high energy rations. Likewise, the addition of ethoxyquin to the low energy-low protein diet reduced liver losses. Rousseau et al (1956a) have also reported that antioxidants increased liver reserves in calves and Shubin and Kovalskii (1976) observed improved plasma and colostrum vitamin A in cows as well as improved breeding performance when an antioxidant was fed with vitamins A and D.

The feeding of soybean lecithin (Eaton et al, 1949) has been shown to have little effect on absorption of vitamin A, whereas fat in the diet is said to increase liver carotene but not vitamin A (Erwin et al, 1956). Thomas et

al (1953) suggested that a P deficiency might inhibit vitamin A mobilization from the liver. Page et al (1959) found that high ambient temperatures resulted in increased liver vitamin A losses as did exposure to solar radiation.

With respect to nitrates or nitrites some of the earlier work indicated that these compounds might reduce liver or blood levels or vitamin A. Hoar et al (1968) found that Na nitrate had more effect on vitamin A metabolism of lambs during a repletion phase than during a depletion phase and concluded that the greatest effect was to reduce the amount of dietary vitamin A reaching hepatic stores rather than by acceleration of depletion of existing stores. More recent studies with sheep on heavily fertilized pastures did not show any effect of forage nitrate on blood or liver vitamin A or on blood levels (Table 9-3), results similar to those reported by Cunningham et al (1968). In the latter report it was shown that in vitro fermentations with rumen liquor from nitrate- or nitrite-fed steers did not indicate any effect on carotene or vitamin A. Similar results were obtained with hydroxylamine.

Ethanol, fed at a level of 3% to heifers, has been shown to increase hepatic vitamin A (Miller et al, 1969) and aflatoxin at levels of 0.08 mg/kg of body wt caused progressive declines in serum carotene and vitamin A (Lynch et al, 1968). Chlortetracycline and stilbestrol apparently have little effect (Erwin et al, 1956), although intramuscular administration of triiodothyronine apparently increases blood carotene and blood and liver

Table 9-3. Effect of N source and K nitrate on liver and plasma vitamin A.[a]

Item	Days	Added K nitrate level, %			
		0	1	0	1
		Urea		Soybean meal	
Liver vitamin A, % depletion	33	67	59	54	63
	60	82	76	74	80
	125	88	99	88	85
	188	93	03	90	87
Plasma vitamin A, mcg/100 ml	initial	34	38	36	30
	33	34	30	37	30
	60	30	33	34	38
	125	27	22	29	28
	188	25	23	28	24

[a] Data from Lichtenwalner et al (1973)

vitamin A concentrations (Jordan et al, 1963).

It is interesting to note that Braun (1945) concluded that a variety of stresses such as parturition (shown by others also), abortion, or acute infections such as localized abscesses or gangrenous mastitis may cause a drop in blood vitamin A, and that it does not return to normal until infections subside. This is an area that would be interesting to study in terms of liver vitamin A mobilization and dietary requirements, particularly from a point of view of preventing or alleviating stress.

Availability of Different Forms of Carotene or Vitamin A

It was pointed out previously that the biological activity of carotenes is variable, being influenced by the presence of different isomers which may be present. The only way to check activity is to carry out a very careful chemical assay for the various carotenoid compounds and then to calculate vitamin A potency on the basis of known biological values, most of which are based on rat or chick work. The discrepancy in evaluation of the various carotenoids and vitamin A esters leaves much to be desired in current feeding standards, and it appears that there is a poor relationship between chemical methods and biological assays done with animals (Ullrey, 1972).

Several reports are available to indicate how the biological activity of forage carotenes may differ. For example, Rousseau et al (1956) depleted calves and then fed graded levels of carotene (as alfalfa) and vitamin A. Their results indicated that alfalfa carotene, when fed at the rate of 132 mcg/kg of live wt, had a value of ca. 15-20% of vitamin A; when fed at a rate of 397 mcg/kg, it was worth only ca. 8-10%, and had a value of only 4-5% when fed at a rate of 1,190 mcg/kg. Anderson et al (1962) found that intraruminal vitamin A injections were approximately 9 times more effective than intraruminal injections of carotene (as measured by liver storage) when given to protein-deficient lambs and more than 18 times as effective in lambs receiving adequate protein. Martin et al (1968) compared corn silage carotenes with all-*trans*-retinyl palmitate with respect to liver storage in lambs that had been depleted of vitamin A. Regression analyses of their data indicated that 1 mg of corn silage carotene was equivalent to 0.24 mg of vitamin A palmitate, or 436 IU/mg of carotene. Data reported by Little et al (1968)

indicated that carotene fed at a rate of 20 mg/day to lambs was equivalent to ca. 280 IU of vitamin A fed at a level of 10,000 IU/day. Based on relative weights of β-carotene and retinyl palmitate (Faruque and Walker, 1970), it required 5-25X as much carotene to produce equivalent blood vitamin A levels and 3-9X for comparable liver levels. Thus, these data show a tremendous difference, and have led many nutritionists to disregard forage carotenes when evaluating vitamin A needs in critical situations.

With respect to vitamin A sources, Sherman et al (1958) found that aqueous and gelatin beadlets were used more efficiently than oil solutions. Calhoun and Woodmansee (1968) have shown that retinoic acid may be used by calves, but withdrawal resulted in prompt development of deficiency symptoms—indicating little or no storage. Perry et al (1967) have compared oral vitamin A (20,000 IU/day) vs. injectible forms (one dose of 1, 4 or 6 million IU) in calves that were fed 210 days. At this rate the 4 million IU was essentially the same dose as the oral intake and produced approximately equivalent responses.

Vitamin A Requirements

It is the author's opinion that the many variables affecting carotene and vitamin A metabolism make it quite difficult to suggest minimum requirements except for rather specific situations. Fortunately, vitamin A is normally a problem only for the very young animal, in animals given poor quality feeds during the winter (or dry season in the tropics) or which have been exposed to long-term droughts, or in those confined to the drylot for extended periods of time. Since synthetic vitamin A is readily available and cheap, the practical need to define minimum requirements is less critical than for some other nutrients. There has been a reduction in research in vitamin A metabolism and requirements in ruminants, probably as a result of the low cost.

Rather than taking space to review some of the research papers on this topic, space will be utilized to review briefly the recommendations put forward by the NRC Committees on sheep, dairy cattle and beef cattle. The NRC bulletin on sheep (1975) suggests that the amount of vitamin A required to prevent night blindness is 4.3 mcg or 25 mcg of β-carotene/kg of body wt. For replacement ewe lambs the minimum value is set at 2.5X the minimum suggested above and for late pregnancy and lactation, values are suggested of 25 mcg of vitamin A/kg or about 5X the minimum to prevent night blindness. In addition to these differences, different conversion values have been used for converting plant carotenes to vitamin A equivalents, depending on the animals involved. There would not seem to be much justification for this from a practical point of view.

The NRC committee on dairy cattle (1971) has used a conversion factor of 400 IU of vitamin A activity/mg of carotene. They have suggested a practical requirement of growing cattle of 10.6 mg/100 kg of body wt (Eaton et al, 1964, 1972) or 4 mg/kg of dry ration. For dry pregnant cows and lactating cows, they suggest 8 mg/kg of dry ration or 19 mg/100 kg of body wt. Swanson et al (1968) concluded that 50,000 IU of vitamin A/day was adequate for cows receiving deficient diets and that diets sufficient to allow normal reproduction did not improve milk yield. At minimum intakes, however, concentration in milk will be much less than for animals getting green feed in abundance.

The beef committee (1976) has used the 400 IU conversion value, but they did not specify, otherwise, how carotene or vitamin A requirements were calculated. It was suggested that growing and finishing steers and heifers fed for several months require ca. 2,200 IU; pregnant heifers and cows, 2,800 IU; and lactating cows and breeding bulls about 3,900 IU/kg of dry ration. It might be presumed that some of the estimates for steers were derived from data in papers by Perry et al (1962, 1965, 1967), reports which indicated that steers required about 20,000 IU of vitamin A/day for adequate performance. For cows, data of Swanson et al (1968) were probably drawn on. Other research reports would tend to substantiate the figure for steers, but it happens to be the author's opinion (which can be substantiated with data), that the value for cows suckling calves is much too low to sustain a calf that does not have access to green feed.

Vitamin A Toxicity

Toxicity of vitamin A is not believed to be a practical problem in ruminant species, however the vitamin is toxic at high levels. Hazzard et al (1964) have described symptoms produced by feeding concentrations ranging from about 137 to about 35,000 IU/kg of live wt in young calves. The amount required to produce tissue changes varied with the different tissues, bones being affected by the least (ca. 1,300 IU/kg). They

stated that characteristic signs of hypervitaminosis were seen in all calves fed ca. 17,600 IU or more. An example of a skull section of one calf is shown in Fig. 9-11. A later report from this laboratory (Frier et al, 1970) indicated that reduced cerebrospinal fluid pressures seen in affected animals was due to a greater absorption of fluid in affected animals.

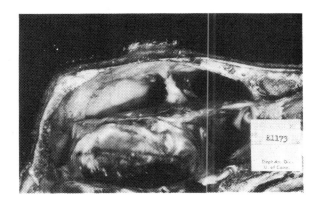

Fig. 9-11. Vitamin A toxicity. Picture of a longitudinal section of skull and frontal sinus of a calf given ca. 22,000 I.U. of vitamin A/kg of wt. Note marked enlargement of frontal sinus. Courtesy of S.W. Nielsen, Conn. Agric. Expt. Sta.

VITAMIN D

There is not much recent literature on vitamin D with respect to ruminant animals except for some studies relating vitamin D treatments and milk fever (see Ch. 12). The lack of research interest is, no doubt, a reflection of the belief by most nutritionists that vitamin D is seldom a cause for concern. For those readers interested in a brief and concise review of the older literature, the information presented by the ARC (1965) is recommended. Other more recent reviews include those of Greenbaum (1973), Dobson and Ward (1974) and Wasserman (1975).

Details of the metabolism of vitamin D have been eleaborated in recent research from Cornell and Wisconsin (summarized in Church and Pond, 1974). Briefly, the information shows that vitamin D is metabolized by the liver to an isomer, 25-hydroxycholecalciferol or 25-OH-D_3; 25-OH-D_3 is metabolized to 1,25-$(OH)_2 D_3$ by the kidney, the reaction being catalized by parathormone. This latter vitamin D isomer stimulates the formation of a Ca-binding protein in the intestines, facilitating absorption of Ca from the gut or mobilization of Ca from

242

the bone. Blood levels of both Ca and P have an effect on production of these compounds.

In animals deprived of sunlight but receiving adequate dietary amounts of Ca and P, it has been shown clearly that vitamin D is required for calcification of the bone matrix. When animals are given massive doses (see Ch. 12), bone Ca is more easily mobilized and blood levels of Ca will be maintained more readily in situations which would otherwise cause a decline in blood Ca.

Little recent information on vitamin D is available. That which is will be mentioned briefly. For example, Dalgarno et al (1962) have studied the vitamin D concentration in the blood of lambs. They found that it ranged from 3 to 30 IU/100 ml of blood. Quarterman et al (1964) have presented further information on factors affecting blood levels. They found that the blood level of shorn, grazing sheep was at a maximum of 40-90 IU/100 ml of whole blood in August or September, the level dropping to 10-30 IU in November; it was at a minimum of about 5 IU in April. Blood values were much lower in sheep that were not clipped. The administration of 1 million IU intramuscularly caused a marked rise in blood values which were maintained for over 4 mo.

A deficiency of vitamin D affects primarily the bone of young, rapidly growing animals (Fig. 9-12). Some information on this subject is mentioned in Ch. 4 and pictures of rickets are shown. In young calves a vitamin D deficiency results in reduced growth, health and feed efficiency. Nitrogen digestion and retention are reduced with no apparent effect on other common nutrients. Metabolic rate tends to be increased and blood Ca and P are reduced along with the usual bone deformities (Colovos et al, 1951). It has been shown in ruminants (Benzie et al, 1960; McRoberts et al, 1965) that low-Ca diets are not apt to cause rickets, but that diets with low-P or low-P with inadequate vitamin D are the prime causes of rickets in young ruminants. Benzie et al found that the addition of vitamin D to a D- and Ca-deficient ration stimulated growth but not mineralization of the bones; even so there was no evidence of rickets. Supplementation of the diet with both Ca and vitamin D improved bone quality, but further supplementation with P improved bone mineralization. With respect to the teeth, McRoberts et al (1965) reported that a low-P and low-vitamin D diet depressed dentine development with little effect on the enamel of the teeth of sheep. Other data from this laboratory showed that diets low in P or P and vitamin D caused a marked depression of blood inorganic P, bone of extremely poor quality (X-ray and ash analyses), and severe rickets.

Complex deficiencies (more than one vitamin) may sometimes occur in young animals. A recent example of this has been reported by Spratling (1976). One animal was diagnosed to have a severe deficiency of vitamin D and a slight to moderate deficiency of

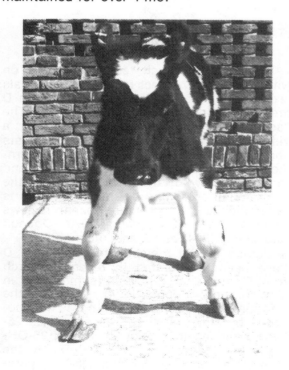

Fig. 9-12. A vitamin D deficient calf. Note the similarity to the calf with rickets shown in Ch. 4. Courtesy of F.R. Spratling, U. of Cambridge.

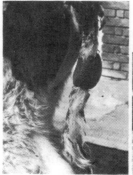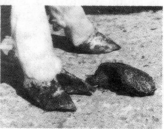

Fig. 9-13. Fecoliths on the tail and hooves of an animal shown to be deficient in both vitamin A and D. From Spratling (1976).

vitamin A. In addition to the usual bone deformations, papilloedema was observed, indicating a vitamin A deficiency. This animal, as well as some without vitamin A deficiency, had fecoliths on the tail and hind feet (Fig. 9-13). According to the author, the fecolith on the tail is the result of recumbency, not of diarrhea. The overgrown feet and the fecoliths in which they were embedded develop because of reduced walking by a rickety calf causing less than normal wear of the hooves and the misshapen feet accumulate the layers of dried feces which in turn increased the discomfort and reluctance to walk. This particular animal had very small stature when the deficiency was observed (7 mo.). Even after recovery at 22 mo. of age (Fig. 9-14), she had a small stature, short legs, a narrow masculine pelvis, and an unusually dished face more like a Jersey than an Ayrshire.

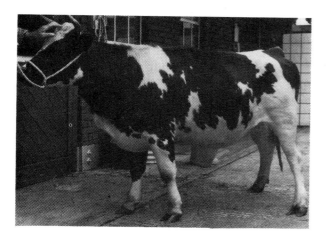

Fig. 9-14. Animal in Fig. 9-12, now recovered and 22 mo. of age. She has a small stature, short legs and a narrow pelvis. From Spratling (1976).

Rickets do not normally develop in young animals unless they are maintained on deficient diets and not given access to sunlight. Since most ruminating animals have some access to sun cured feeds in winter months, deficiencies are not as likely as for young animals with inadequate tissue reserves. Deficiencies in vitamin synthesis in the tissues following exposure to sunlight (ultraviolet light) are more likely in northern climates since the sun's rays have little antirachitic power when the sun is at an elevation of 35° or less (ARC, 1965). An unusually high incidence of rickets in young

sheep has been reported from time to time when grazing on cereal crops or good quality pastures in Australia, New Zealand or Northern Europe. This condition responds readily to vitamin D treatment. Some information has been published implicating vitamin A but other information negates this finding; further information is required to resolve the answer.

Symptoms have been produced in adult cows after feeding deficient rations for several months (Wallis, 1944). Cows exhibited lower blood Ca and P, bone breakage, decreased milk production, failure to show estrus and many of the symptoms of rachitic calves. More recent information (Hignett and Hignett, 1953; Cohen, 1962; Ward et al, 1971) shows that supplementary vitamin D has frequently resulted in earlier estrus after calving or restored fertility in anestrus cows.

In some areas relative excesses of Ca are a problem. Skeletal problems are frequently encountered in South Africa in cattle which are not entirely prevented by supplemental P. This problem can be alleviated by providing animals with additional vitamin D (Zintzen and Boyazoglu, 1973).

With respect to requirements for vitamin D, the ARC (1965) points out that vitamin D requirements are reduced when adequate dietary levels of Ca and P are present. Furthermore, as the Ca intake (and probably P) decreases, the requirement for vitamin D increases. Older work indicated that the vitamin D requirement is high only when energy intake is sufficient to promote growth in young animals. Data presented by Benzie et al (1960) confirmed this to be the case. Requirements in the short run are, of course, modified by tissue storage of vitamin D. Older papers reviewed in the ARC (1965) suggest that young lambs have a sufficient reserve for about 6 wk. Calves which received only vitamin D in milk for the first 10 days of life developed rickets within 60 days and within 30 days in calves which were deprived of vitamin D. High producing lactating cows developed symptoms in 3-4 months, although low producers (11-18 kg milk/day) did not show symptoms for 6-8 months.

The NRC recommendations for vitamin D are 5.5 IU/kg of body wt for sheep and 6.6 IU for early weaned lambs, 6.6 IU for dairy calves, and 275 IU/kg of dry ration for beef cattle. The ARC (1965) points out that data are insufficient, in most cases, to accurately suggest well defined requirements for ruminants. On the basis of published data, they have suggested 4 IU/kg of live wt for young calves, 2.5 IU for growing cattle, 10 IU for pregnant and lactating cows, and 5.0 IU for sheep.

There is little doubt that vitamin D, when given in large amounts, can be toxic. Some information on this is mentioned in Ch. 12 in the section on treatment of milk fever. Other data on calves (Blackburn, 1957) indicate that oral administration of 10 million IU resulted in a marked depression in growth, diarrhea, distress on exercise, and stiffness of the joints. The toxicity of vitamin D can be alleviated, at least partially, by providing supplementary Mg (Meyer et al, 1971).

VITAMIN E

Vitamin E, along with vitamin A, is a vitamin of primary interest in ruminant nutrition. Many research reports on this vitamin are in the literature and numerous reviews are available; one of the more complete being that found in Volume 20 of Vitamins and Hormones. An older annotated bibliography of papers relating to cattle gives a good historical coverage of the subject (Ames et al, 1957). A more recent review has been prepared by Oksanen (1973).

Vitamin E activity is present in compounds known as tocopherols, of which there are numerous isomers. The highest activity is from α-tocopherol (5,7,8-trimethyltocol) which is used as the reference base for establishing biological activity. Vitamin E is generally thought to be widely distributed in nature. However, it is relatively unstable and the biological activity of a given feed source may decrease rapidly. The naturally occurring form is an alcohol. A synthetic form, dl-α-tocopheryl acetate, is readily available commercially and has a defined biological value of 1,000 IU/g as compared to 1,360 IU for the natural form. The synthetic form is more stable than the natural form and natural isomers are more stable in dry than in wet feeds such as silage or wet corn grain (Young et al, 1975).

The functions of vitamin E have not been conclusively defined. It is well known that tocopherols have antioxidant properties being able, for example, to reduce the peroxidation of polyunsaturated fatty acids or the destruction of vitamin A in vitro. However, evidence is not clear that this is a mechanism that functions in vivo. Further work has shown enzyme aberrations in deficient animals, but there is no conclusive proof that the changes are directly related to a need for vitamin E. Some workers suggest that the change may be due to disruption of cell membranes, perhaps due to oxidation of lipid components of the cell membranes.

Metabolism by Ruminants

In ruminants it is clear that tocopherol concentrations are low in the young animal. For example, Bayfield and Mylrea (1969) reported that serum tocopherol concentrations increased from 0.22 in calves to 0.37 mg/100 ml in weaners whereas heifers and cows had levels of 0.54 to 0.90 mg/100 ml. Poukka (1968) found that vitamin E concentration was lower in the heart and skeletal muscle and liver of young calves than in older animals, data which are similar to those reported by others. The low values in the young animal are, no doubt, due to the inefficiency with which vitamin E is transferred to the fetus (Paulson et al, 1968b), which, in turn may be partly due to the rapidity of excretion (see succeeding paragraph).

In the rumen of cattle, Alderson et al (1971) have shown that preintestinal disappearance of vitamin E ranged from 8-42% as diets contained increasing amounts of corn (20-80%). Additional evidence was obtained on sheep indicating substantial loss of vitamin E in the stomach (Hidiroglou and Jenkins, 1974; Hidiroglou et al, 1970), the data showing lower absorption of labeled tocopherol when given via the rumen as compared to the duodenum, although Astrup et al (1974) found very little loss in activity when labeled vitamin E was incubated with rumen fluid from a steer consuming alfalfa and oats. Other research on this topic (Hidiroglou and Lessard, 1976; Hidiroglou, 1977) suggests that vitamin E supplementation to a purified diet resulted in an increase in rumen acetate, butyrate and valerate, and evidence has been reported to show that feeding corn silage as compared to grass silage or hay resulted in lower tissue levels of vitamin E and greater uptake of a labeled dose.

Hidiroglou et al (1969a, b) have studied the fate of radiotocopherol when administered to young lambs or to ewes. In the case of lambs data indicated greatest uptake of label in the tissues of the stomach, duodenum and liver as well as in the adrenals. The jejunum is the principal absorption site (Hidiroglou and Jenkins, 1974). In studies with pregnant ewes, labeled vitamin E was taken up most rapidly by the liver. It was taken up and released more slowly by heart, skeletal muscle, kidneys and lungs. Equilibrium between maternal and fetal tissues was achieved by 13 days after the dose was given, however the ewes excreted more than 70% of the label within 4 days, mainly in the feces. Carvaggi and Wright (1969) also found that sheep rapidly excreted an oral dose of α-tocopherol acetate, most of it by 4 days. However, an intramuscular dose resulted in apparently greater tissue deposition, only about 16% being excreted within 4 days.

Vitamin E Deficiency

There are many reports in the literature of experiments in which vitamin E has been used to prevent the development of nutritional muscular dystrophy (NMD), a disease that would appear to be due to a marked deficiency of vitamin E or Se or to inadequate intake of both nutrients. The symptoms of this disease have been discussed in detail in Ch. 5 and various illustrations are shown. Another example is shown in Fig. 9-15. Current information on Se-vitamin E interactions have also been discussed.

Ample information is available in the literature to show that the feeding of very small quantities of polyunsaturated fatty acids will produce NMD in young calves or lambs or in lambs produced from ewes which were fed fish oils (Blaxter et al, 1953; Maplesden and Loosli, 1960; Welch et al, 1960; Tollersrud and Ribe, 1967; and Boyd, 1968). Numerous other reports show that NMD can be produced by feeding young ruminants purified diets of other types (for example, see Safford et al, 1954; Thomas and Okamota, 1956; Erwin et al, 1961; and Hopkins et al, 1964). In most cases it was shown that the addition of

vitamin E either prevented or partially alleviated the symptoms of NMD that otherwise occurred.

The symptoms generally seen in NMD caused by the feeding of polyunsaturated fatty acids, low vitamin E, or by including feedstuffs such as torula yeast appear to be quite similar to those described for naturally occurring NMD in young animals born to ewes or cows on natural rations. The typical white or dystrophic muscle is characteristic. There may be considerable calcification of affected muscles; an increase in lipid content of the muscle; a reduced N content as well as reduced globulin N and increased nucleic acid content—the latter indicating leakage of cellular contents of damaged tissue. There may be increases in serum enzymes such as aspartate and alanine transaminase and glutamate and lactate dehydrogenase. Of these enzymes lactic dehydrogenase and alanine transaminase appear to the the most specific indicators of NMD. Red blood cells may be more susceptible to hemolysis by peroxide. Electrocardiograms may show abnormal activity of the heart muscles (Blaxter and Wood, 1952; Safford et al, 1954; Thomas and Okamota, 1956; Hopkins et al, 1964; Tollersrud and Ribe, 1967; Boyd, 1968; 1973; Paulson et al, 1968a,b).

Blaxter et al (1952) noted that N balance was reduced in dystrophic calves, resulting in higher urinary excretion of urea and ammonia. Oxygen consumption was increased, as well. Thus, pronounced changes occur in muscle metabolism as a result of the dystrophy that develops in affected animals. In most cases these changes are similar if not essentially identical to those

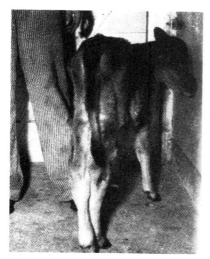
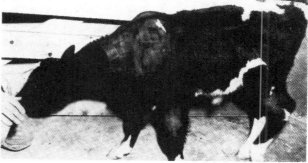

Fig. 9-15. Left. Vitamin E-deficient calf. This calf shows a stance with the hind legs crossed, said to be typical of deficient calves. Right. Calf standing with lowered, extended head and illustrating the prominent suprascapula. From Safford et al (1954).

that are produced by a Se deficiency. For that matter it seems highly likely that some might have been due to lack of Se. Blaxter et al (1953b) pointed out that the tocopherol content of muscles of both dystrophic and normal calves was approximately the same, thus indicating some effect other than tissue level of tocopherol.

Maplesden and Loosli (1960) observed that the addition of cod liver oil to a dystrophogenic diet intensified degeneration of muscles in E-deficient calves and that the addition of Se to the basal diet did not prevent NMD. When fish oil was fed to ewes (Welch et al, 1960), it was shown that Se decreased but did not eliminate the occurrence of NMD, results similar to those reported for calves by Kuttler and Marble (1960). However, Jenkins et al (1970) stated that linoleic acid did not increase the incidence of NMD in ewes or lambs. In wethers fed a dystrophogenic diet which contained cod liver oil, Hidiroglou and Barrowsky (1970) found that rumen liquor and other tissues contained less labeled vitamin E (given orally) than in those not given cod liver oil. Other reports showing the deleterious effects of vitamin E-free fish liver oils, corn oil or fish protein concentrate include those of Rochester and Carvaggi (1971), Tollersrud (1971), Michel et al (1972) and Evarts and Oksanen (1973). Thus, these as well as other experiments would tend to show that vitamin E is a vital nutrient with respect to the maintenance of normal muscle metabolism, but its effects, in many cases, must be highly related to Se metabolism.

Although antioxidants have been said to prevent NMD in lambs fed a diet containing

Table 9-4. Effect of vitamin E or ethoxyquin on prevention of NMD in lambs.[a]

Treatment	NMD lesions	LDH activity[a]
Low Se alfalfa	15/25	3600
Ethoxyquin, 250 mg/day to ewes	2/18	477
α-tocopherol acetate to lambs	1/14	432
Low Se hay + Se injections	0/20	478

[a] Data from Whanger et al (1976)
[b] LDH or lactic acid dehydrogenate enzyme activity.

coconut oil and torula yeast (Erwin et al, 1961), other data (Hogue et al, 1962) have indicated no protective effect when antioxidants were given to pregnant ewes. However, Whanger et al (1976) found that ethoxyquin, when fed to ewes or lambs, was effective in preventing NMD on natural diets low in Se (Table 9-4).

In long-term studies with dairy animals (Gullickson, 1949), results indicated that a ration low in vitamin E did not interfere with spermatogenesis or other measures of reproductive activity in bulls. In the case of breeding females, successful reproduction occurred through three successive generations of animals fed the experimental diet. The major problems seen were sudden death losses (6 of 23 cases), the cow usually dying suddenly 1 to 3 mo. before due to calve or within 3 wk after calving. The calves that were born were normal at birth. One bull died suddenly. Electrocardiograms indicated death in these animals was due to cardiac failure.

Buchanan-Smith et al (1969) have reported studies with ewes and rams fed purified diets supplemented with vitamin E (700 IU) and Se (5 mg) which were given intramuscularly once weekly. They reported that sheep receiving the basal diet died between the 80th and 230th day of the trials. Vitamin E treatment to 3 surviving ewes prevented their deaths; Se delayed but did not prevent death. Death was sudden and post mortem examination indicated muscle and myocardial necrosis. NMD was noted in all lambs from ewes not receiving the vitamin E-Se supplements; reproduction was satisfactory only in ewes receiving the combination of vitamin E and Se. No pathology was observed in the reproductive tracts of ewes or rams given the deficient diets.

There is very little information on the incidence of NMD (vitamin E related) in species other than sheep and cattle. NMD sometimes crops up in species confined in zoos (see Ch. 16, Vol. 3). NMD has also been diagnosed in camels and the authors suggested that it may be more prevalent than indicated by the literature (Finlayson et al, 1971).

Vitamin E Requirements

Current information, in the opinion of the author, is not sufficient to define minimum requirements of vitamin E. This thought is also reflected by the NRC publications. The beef report suggests 15-60 mg/kg of dry diet and the sheep report suggests that lambs do well when receiving 11 mg/kg of body wt weekly providing Se is adequate. The report on dairy animals suggests only that calves be fed 300 mg/kg of milk replacer. This information is based, primarily, on some of the early work of Blaxter and co-workers. When calves were given unsaturated fatty acids, Blaxter et al (1952, 1953a) found that 50 mg of vitamin E/day would protect calves against 15-18 ml of cod liver oil. In other work (Blaxter et al, 1953a) data indicated that 2.5 mg of vitamin E supplemented to a diet of dried skim milk did not result in NMD in calves. Thomas and Okamota (1956) found that 44 mg of vitamin E/day/100 kg of body wt was not sufficient for calves and that an additional 50 mg/day maintained blood levels.

With respect to ewes, some reports (see Muth et al, 1959, for example) indicate that vitamin E supplementation to natural rations with low levels of Se have not been effective in preventing NMD in their young. Other reports dealing with natural rations indicate a partial effectiveness when vitamin E was given at levels ranging from 700 to 1,000 IU/wk (Hogue et al, 1962; Paulson et al, 1968b). Still other reports state that vitamin E has been effective in preventing NMD when the vitamin was administered to lambs (Hidiroglou et al, 1970, 1972) or to ewes (Whanger et al, 1972); in the latter case newer preparations were used which were believed to be more available than older vitamin E preparations. Another study with natural rations plus fish oil (Welch et al, 1960) indicated that a level of 1,000 IU/wk was satisfactory. The work of Buchanan-Smith et al (1969) with purified diets indicated that 700 IU/wk given subcutaneously was adequate.

Probably the most comprehensive study with lambs is that of Ewan et al (1968). Data presented in this paper on lambs fed purified diets in the presence of adequate Se would indicate that the requirement for vitamin E was somewhat greater than 5.5 mg/kg of body wt/wk when given orally. Information presented on serum enzymes, survival of the lambs, and incidence of NMD indicated that 11 mg/kg was probably just as satisfactory as 22 mg/kg/wk.

The interrelationships between Se and vitamin E have been shown clearly in several reports—Hopkins et al (1964), Paulson et al (1966) and Ewan et al (1968) with lambs fed purified diets; Nelson et al (1964) with beef cows; Buchanan-Smith et al (1969) with ewes and rams fed purified diets and the work of Hogue et al (1962) with ewes on natural diets. These results as well as those from other experiments not cited would seem to indicate clearly that the requirements of vitamin E can only be quantitated in the presence of adequate Se.

VITAMIN K

It has been known for some time that vitamin K is involved in the blood clotting mechanism, apparently because it is needed by the liver for synthesis of prothrombin. Evidence with other species indicates that there are a variety of compounds which have vitamin K activity. The basic molecule is a napthaquinone and the various isomers differ in the nature and length of the side chain. A synthetic product, menadione, has no side chain, but has almost as much activity for chicks as the natural isomers.

Older work (McElroy and Goss, 1940) showed that vitamin K is synthesized in the rumen. Matschiner (1970) has confirmed this, his evidence showing that three different isomers of menaquinone present in the rumen were also isolated from bovine liver, thus indicating that these isomers were of bacterial origin. Vitamin K is known to be synthesized in the gut of many species.

A deficiency of vitamin K is brought about by the ingestion of dicumarol, an antagonist of vitamin K, or by the feeding of sulfonamides (monogastric species) at sufficient levels to inhibit synthesis of vitamin K in the intestine. Dicumarols are produced by molds, particularly those that attack sweet clover, thus giving rise to the term, sweet clover disease. The ingestion of large quantities of dicumarols results in severe hemorrhaging due to a deficiency in prothrombin production. The incidence of vitamin K deficiency in ruminants is believed to be very low. Goplen and Bell (1967) have shown in cattle that vitamin K_1 is much more potent as an antidote to dicumarol than vitamin K_3. Data on feedlot cattle (O'Donovan, 1967; Perry et al, 1968) indicate that supplementary vitamin K was of no value under the conditions prevailing in their experiments.

B-COMPLEX VITAMINS

The B vitamins are required as co-factors in enzyme systems of major metabolic pathways in animals. As such, the B-complex vitamins are necessary for the metabolism of carbohydrates, lipids and proteins. Details of specific chemical reactions are available in most biochemistry books.

In ruminants the rumen microbes synthesize the B-complex vitamins (see Ch. 15, Vol. 1) and most of the evidence indicates that supplementary feeding is of little value unless some unusual condition prevails. In pre-ruminants, dietary requirements have been experimentally demonstrated for thiamin, riboflavin, niacin, pyridoxine, pantothenic acid, cobalamin and biotin (see Ch. 10). Only in the case of cobalamin and thiamin have severe problems been demonstrated in animals with a functioning rumen and when consuming natural feedstuffs.

Thiamin

Dietary requirements for thiamin have been demonstrated for preruminant calves (Johnson et al, 1948; Kon and Porter, 1954; Benevenga et al, 1967) and lambs (Draper and Johnson, 1951). Deficiency symptoms were characterized as anorexia and death from dehydration. In lambs, convulsions were evident in about 4 wk. Also, opisthotonus and bradycardia were evident (see illustrations, Ch. 10). Intramuscular injections of thiamin hydrochloride were effective in promoting rapid recovery from spasms and anorexia. Benevenga et al (1967) showed that thiamin deficiency in the calf affects the route of metabolism of pyruvate, apparently diminishing the fraction metabolized through acetyl-CoA.

Research information has shown that rumen microorganisms as well as those in the gut can and do synthesize thiamin; thus, ruminating animals should not have a dietary requirement for this vitamin in ordinary circumstances. Nevertheless, animals are affected, at times, with a thiamin-responsive condition known as polioencephalomacia (PEM) in the USA or as cerebrocortical necrosis in Europe. This disease is a non-infectious condition which occurs most often in feedlot cattle and sheep, usually in animals on diets high in readily available carbohydrates. Young animals are more susceptible, presumably because tissue reserves are lower. Loew (1975) has a good review on this topic.

Jensen et al (1956) first described the syndrome which includes a high-intracranial pressure which is manifested by blindness, muscle tremors, grinding of the teeth, opisthotonus and convulsions. In sheep, acute and subacute forms are seen. In the acute form affected lambs may be found dead or prostrate. When fatal the course of the disease is 1-2 days. In the subacute form affected lambs become blind, uncoordinated and weak. In early stages some lambs isolate themselves from the flock. When disturbed they developed muscular tremors and fell. Some were blind and moved aimlessly. Characteristic stances included lowering of the head to ground level, staring above the horizon and extending the head over the back. After 6-12 hr such lambs became prostrate and developed opisthotonus. The cerebrum was often swollen with characteristic necrosis of the neurons as well as other histological signs. It frequently takes 4-6 wk for animals to develop clinical symptoms on a PEM-prone diet (Pierson and Jensen, 1975).

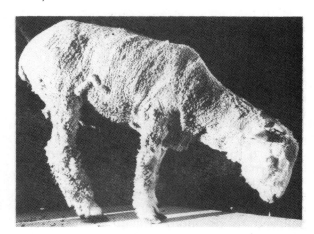

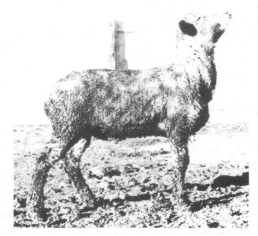

Fig. 9-16. Lambs affected with PEM. Upper. A common stance of a feedlot lamb in early stages of PEM. The head is lowered, vision is impaired and the animal is in a somnolent state. Lower. Another common stance of a lamb in early stages of PEM. The animal shows opisthotonus with the head and neck extended and vision impaired. Courtesy of Rue Jensen, Colorado State University.

The information at this time is not adequate to define the exact causes of PEM because of conflicting reports. Total blood thiamin levels are similar in normal and affected animals (Loew and Dunlop, 1972; Loew et al, 1975), although the diphosphorylated form of thiamin is greatly decreased (Loew, 1972). Brain and liver levels are lower (Edwin and Jackman, 1973) and rumen levels may or may not be lower (Sapienza and Brent, 1974; Quaghebeur et al, 1975). Some data on ruminal synthesis suggest that high starch diets may favor thiamin synthesis (Hayes et al, 1966) but other information suggests lower production, particularly when ruminal pH is low (Sapienza and Brent, 1974).

Numerous studies have shown that there is destruction of thiamin in the rumen either because of plant thiaminases such as in the bracken fern (Evans et al, 1975) or, perhaps, from rumen microorganisms (Markson et al, 1966; Edwin et al, 1968; Loew et al, 1970; Edwin and Jackman, 1973; Roberts and Boyd, 1974; Sapienza and Brent, 1974, 1975). Aerobic and anaerobic microorganisms have been isolated from the rumen and studies on thiaminase activity suggest that there is ample present in affected animals to degrade all of the dietary thiamin (Boyd and Walton, 1977). Quaghebeur et al (1975) stated that thiamin-destroying activity in their experiments was not a result of enzymic action since the compound(s) was heat stable and depended on the pH of the medium and on thiamin concentration. At this time the source of ruminal thiaminase remains uncertain (Boyd and Walton, 1977). Thiaminases are also found in abundance in the lower gut, feces, and other tissues (Roberts and Boyd, 1974). Linklater et al (1977) observed that as many as one third of the normal sheep from an affected flock might be excreting thiaminase at a given time and that over half were excreting thiaminase during an outbreak of PEM. Excretion was variable and sometimes intermittent and was unaffected by changes in diet, pasture or environment.

Symptoms apparently identical to PEM can be produced by administering amprolium, a coccidiostat which acts as an antagonist to thiamin (Pill et al, 1966; Edwin et al, 1968; Loew and Dunlop, 1972; Markson et al, 1966, 1972, 1974). Similar conditions can be produced in adult sheep by feeding dried bracken fern rhizomes (Evans et al, 1975). Bracken has long been known to be high in thiaminase activity. In one instance (Linklater et al, 1977) outbreaks of PEM

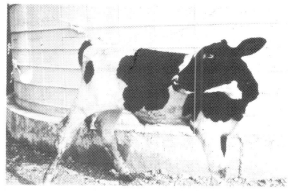
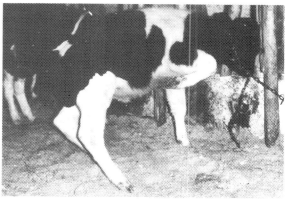

Fig. 9-17. Upper. A calf affected with PEM. This animal shows symptoms of nystagmus and opisthotonus as a result of involvement of the central nervous system. Courtesy of C.K. Whitehair, Michigan State University. Lower. A fattening bull calf showing disturbance in balance after development of acidosis and a thiamin deficiency, presumably very similar if not identical to the early stages of PEM. Courtesy of A. Hennig, U. of Leipzig.

occurred in sheep following the administration of anthelmintics.

Whatever the conditions which result in PEM, thiamin administration (IV or IM) is quite effective in bringing about a remission of the syndrome (Davies et al, 1965; Markson et al, 1966; Hentschl et al, 1966) or in preventing PEM when amprolium was asministered (Markson et al, 1972).

Sapienza and Brent (1975) suggest that the problem in PEM is caused by metabolism of thiamin to pyrithiamin, which in turn causes severe metabolic disturbances. Markson et al (1972) killed one calf by dosing with pyrithiamin (after 21 days) with only slight lesions similar to PEM. Flachowsky et al (1974) found that thiamin, when added to a mixture of starch, glucose and casein which was infused into the rumen of lambs, resulted in a fall in rumen pH, and increased heart rates.

However, intramuscular injection of thiamin (at least 2 hr before ruminal infusion) prevented the increased heart rate even though a severe acidosis developed. These results would tend to support the theory that the toxicity is a result of pyrithiamin or other metabolites of thiamin. It may be that bufffering power of the ration, particle size which affects chewing rate and saliva production, level of readily available carbohydrates in the diet and other factors such as plant and bacterial thiaminases may all be factors in the etiology of this disease. Further information is required to sort out the true facts.

Riboflavin

The requirement of calves for riboflavin has been established by Wiese et al (1947), Warner and Sutton (1948), Brisson and Sutton (1951), Draper and Johnson (1952) and Kon and Porter (1954) to be 15-45 mg/kg of body wt. Although these investigators used several different breeds of cattle and their experimental diets varied considerably, the recommended level of riboflavin is probably 20-30 mg/kg of body wt. Deficiency symptoms (examples shown in Ch. 10) are anorexia, excessive lacrimation and salivation, scouring, soreness in the corners of the mouth, shedding of hair and death (Roy, 1969). It is unlikely that acute deficiencies of riboflavin occur under practical conditions. Even on diets practically devoid of riboflavin, goats and cows produce normal levels of riboflavin in their milk (Johnson et al, 1941).

When excessive quantities of riboflavin are fed to ruminants, metabolites appear in the milk and urine (Owen and West, 1970). The primary metabolite is hydroxyethylflavine along with smaller quantities of formylmethylflavine (Owen and West, 1968).

These metabolites of riboflavin arise when rumen contents are incubated in vitro but do not occur in the urine when riboflavin is injected subcutaneously. Hobson and Summers (1969) and Owen and West (1970) have concluded that riboflavin metabolites arise in the ruminant via degradation of riboflavin by rumen microbes. Consequently, it is not surprising that Johnson et al (1941) failed to increase the riboflavin content of cows' milk very much with dietary supplements of riboflavin.

Niacin

Winegar et al (1940) and Johnson et al (1947) showed that lambs and calves fed niacin-deficient rations synthesized sufficient quantities of niacin to meet their metabolic requirements. It was later shown by Blaxter and Wood (1952) and Hopper and Johnson (1955) that a dietary deficiency of niacin could be produced in the calf (see Ch. 10 for pictures); the ability to produce a niacin deficiency was dependent on the use of a low-tryptophan milk diet. From these studies, it may be concluded that a dietary requirement of niacin for ruminants does not exist as long as the level of tryptophan is maintained near 0.2% of the diet.

More recently, Mizwicki et al (1975) supplemented high concentrate (97% corn) lamb diets with 500 ppm of niacin. Niacin appeared to reduce feed consumption but there was a trend for increased digestion and N retention. Rumen fluid in supplemented animals had higher levels of N and in vitro data suggested an increase in protein synthesis. In a second trial feed efficiency of lambs apparently increased up to 15% with niacin supplemented at 200 ppm.

Pyridoxine

Pyridoxine (vitamin B_6) has been shown to be essential for the young calf when selected experimental diets were used (Johnson et al, 1947; Kon and Porter, 1954). Some calves showed symptoms of anorexia, scouring, convulsive seizures and death in 3-4 wk; while others grew poorly to 4 mo. without showing these extreme deficiency symptoms. Kirchgessner et al (1965) found that increasing the pyridoxine level from 2.4 to 5.5 mg/kg of milk substitute did not improve weight gains or feed efficiency.

Pantothenic Acid

Johnson et al (1947) and Sheppard and Johnson (1957) have produced pantothenic acid deficiencies experimentally in calves. The major symptoms were anorexia, reduced growth, rough haircoat, dermatitis under the lower jaw and eventual death. If deficient calves were treated with calcium pantothenate, they responded with increased appetite and weight gains and subsequent losses of dermatitis. However, at the present time pantothenic acid is not considered a dietary essential for ruminants consuming conventional diets.

Biotin

Wiese et al (1947) apparently produced a biotin deficiency in calves. On the other hand, Kon and Porter (1954) failed to produce a biotin deficiency even though raw egg white was fed as a source of avidin, a biotin antagonist. At the present time, the need for biotin even in diets for preruminant calves and lambs is questioned.

Para-Aminobenzoic Acid (PABA)

A dietary requirement for PABA has not been demonstrated in higher animals. However, PABA is a growth factor for certain microorgainsims; Bentley et al (1955) found that rumen microbes needed PABA for maximum in vitro cellulose digestion. It has been suggested that the actual role of PABA is to supply this component for the synthesis of folic acid by those organisms that do not require preformed folacin.

Folic Acid

A dietary requirement of folic acid has not been demonstrated for ruminants. Ford et al (1972) found that plasma folate was low at birth (I ng/ml) but it increased rapidly and was at a level of 28 ng/ml by 2 days of age. They concluded that almost all of a folate-protein complex from colostrum was transmitted intact into the young animal's blood circulation.

Inositol

In ruminants a dietary deficiency of inositol has not been demonstrated. Inositol has a lipotropic action in experimental animals where deficiency symptoms have been produced in the chicken and the rat.

Cyanocobalamin (Cobalamin, B_{12})

In pre-ruminants cobalamin is a required nutrient whereas Co will suffice in ruminating animals. In young calves the blood levels of cobalamin are appreciably higher than for cows, but they decrease to adult levels by ca. 2 wk (Schuh and Stockl, 1975).

The production of cobalamin by rumen microbes depends on the presence of Co (see Ch. 5 or Ch. 15, Vol. 1). Absorption occurs primarily from the small intestine (Rerat et al, 1956, 1958; Smith and Marston, 1970) and most of that in the rumen appears to be bound to rumen microorganisms until released in the abomasum (Smith and Marston, 1970). Thus, Marston (1970) found that 1 mg of Co/day orally resulted in greater liver storage of cobalamin than did 25 mg/day by injection. At full feed sheep converted Co to the vitamin with an efficiency of 13% of the basal diet and 3% for supplemental Co (Smith and Marston, 1970). This finding is in agreement with an earlier report by Kercher and Smith (1955) when they estimated the oral retention of

cobalamin to be only 3% that of injected cobalamin.

Other reports (Elliot et al, 1971; Hedrich et al, 1973) show that net absorption (disappearance) ranged from slightly negative to ca. 0.5 mg/day in sheep. Absorption appears to be enhanced by greater synthesis in the rumen (higher % of true B_{12}) and by slower rates of digesta passage. Studies with isolated intestinal loops (Wootten, 1972) suggest absorption of 6-11%. In studies where ^{57}Co-labeled cobalamin was administered into the duodenum of sheep, Rickard and Elliot (1978) observed that 8-38% was absorbed (disappeared). Total recovery of label in urine and feces amounted to 87-95%.

Draper and Johnson (1952) estimated the cobalamin requirement to be 0.2 to 0.28 mg/kg of body wt daily. Smith and Loosli (1957) later estimated the requirement to be ca. 0.4 mg/kg of body wt. These estimates are probably quite satisfactory since Roy et al (1964) found that veal calves grew at a normal rate with 0.54 mg of the vitamin/kg of body wt. Marston (1970) estimated the minimum prophylactic dose of cobalamin to be 6 mg/day for sheep on a diet containing 0.03 mg Co/g of feed. The total requirement of cobalamin is probably 10-11 mg/day (Smith and Loosli, 1967; Smith and Marston, 1970).

The symptoms of Co deficiency, which resemble starvation (see Ch. 5), appear to be entirely due to the lack of cobalamin in the tissues. It is probable that some rumen microbes require the vitamin or other cobamides, but the minimum requirements for fermentation are met by levels which are too low to support the animal's tissue requirements. At the tissue level, cobalamin is required as a coenzyme in the conversion of methylmalonly-CoA to succinyl-CoA (Smith and Marston, 1971) and a deficiency results in a build up of intermediates such as propionate in the tissues. Consequently, cobalamin is a key factor in the utilization of propionic acid, the primary glucose precursor in ruminant tissues. Somers (1969) reported that a cobalamin deficiency which reduced feed intake by 40% also decreased the clearance rates of acetate and propionate from the blood. Under severe deficiency symptoms (feed intake reduced by 70%), clearance of VFA, either absorbed from the rumen or injected into the blood, was adversely affected.

Walker and Elliot (1972) have observed that synthesis of B_{12} was reduced by roughage restrictions; although serum levels were

252

higher in cows on restricted diets, they suggested that this might be due to B$_{12}$ analogues. Recently Frobish and Davis (1977) observed that daily intramuscular or intravenous injections of hydroxycobalamin increased milk fat yields in cows with low milk fat. Dosage with 150 mg/day increased fat yield to 88% of normal. Thus, they concluded that a B$_{12}$ deficiency might be one factor related to low milk fat production in lactating cows.

Choline

Although choline may not be a true vitamin, Johnson et al (1951) demonstrated a dietary requirement of choline for the young calf. It is generally assumed that microbial synthesis in the rumen is sufficient to satisfy the choline requirements of ruminants. Dyer et al (1966) have reported substantial increases in rate and efficiency of gain when choline was added to fattening rations. Dyer et al (1966) and Swingle and Dyer (1970) have suggested that supplemental choline increases the bacterial numbers indicating a possible choline or methyl group requirement of certain rumen microbes. The lack of a dose response in all of the work of Dyer et al and the fact that Wise et al (1964) and Harris et al (1966) have failed to find

performance reponses in cattle supplemented with choline are highly suggestive that practical benefits from choline supplementation are questionable.

B-Vitamin Supplementation

Several attempts have been made to stimulate animal performance in ruminating animals by providing supplementary B-complex vitamins in rations. Papers on this topic include those of Oltjen et al (1962), Thrasher et al (1964), Clifford et al (1967) and Perry and Hillier (1969). In none of these cases were vitamins found to be stimulatory to animal performance (gain, feed efficiency, digestibility of rations). One paper showing some effect with niacin was mentioned earlier. An additional report (Smith et al, 1974) suggests some effect when a mixture of lipotropic vitamins (choline, inositol, folic acid, cobalamin) was administered intraruminally or intraperitoneally at weekly or biweekly intervals to feedlot cattle. They concluded that phospholipid content of liver and liver N were increased and there was an improvement in yield grade score and a reduction in back fat when the lipotropic mixture of vitamins were administered, but differences in gain were not different.

References Cited

General References

ARC. 1965. The Nutrient Requirements of Farm Livestock, No. 2 Ruminants. Agr. Res. Council, London

Church, D.C. and W.G. Pond. 1974. Basic Animal Nutrition and Feeding. O & B Books, Corvallis, Oregon.

NRC. 1971. Nutrient Requirements of Dairy Cattle. 4th ed. Nat. Acad. Sci., Washington, D.C.

NRC. 1975. Nutrient Requirements of Sheep. 5th ed. Nat. Acad. Sci., Washington, D.C.

NRC. 1976. Nutrient Requirements of Beef Cattle. 5th ed. Nat. Acad. Sci., Washington, D.C.

Vitamin A

Abrams, J. T. et al. 1969. Inter. J. Vit. Res. 39:416.

Almendinger, R. and F.C. Hinds. 1969. J. Nutr. 97:13.

Anderson, T.A., F. Hubbert, C.B. Roubicek and R.E. Taylor. 1962. J. Nutr. 78:341.

Bauernfeind, J.C. 1969. World Rev. Animal Prod. 21:23.

Bauernfeind, J.C. and E. DeRitter. 1972. Feedstuffs 44(50):34.

Boling, J.A. et al. 1969. J. Animal Sci. 29:504; J. Nutr. 99:502.

Braun, W. 1945. J. Nutr. 29:61.

Byers, J.W., I.R. Jones and J. F. Bone. 1956. J. Dairy Sci. 29:1556.

Calhoun, M.C. et al. 1968. J. Dairy Sci. 51:1781.

Calhoun, M.C. and C.W. Woodmansee. 1968. J. Dairy Sci. 51:978 (abstr.)

Chapman, H.L. et al. 1964. J. Animal Sci. 23:669.

Church, D.C. 1956. Ph.D. Thesis, Oklahoma State University, Stillwater, Okla.

Church, D.C. 1969. Unpublished data. Oregon Agr. Expt. Sta.

Church, D.C. et al. 1954. J. Animal Sci. 13:677.

Church, D.C. et al. 1955. Oklahoma Agr. Expt. Sta. Misc. Pub. MP-43.

Church, D.C., L.S. Pope and R. MacVicar. 1956. J. Animal Sci. 15:1078.

253

Cunningham, G.N., M.B. Wise and E.R. Barrick. 1968. J. Animal Sci. 27:1067.

Dicks, M.W. et al. 1959. J. Dairy Sci. 42:501.

Diven, R.H. and E.S. Erwin. 1958. Proc. Soc. Expt. Biol. Med. 97:601.

Dutt, B. and B.N. Majundar. 1969. Indian Vet. J. 46:789.

Eaton, H.D. et al. 1949. J. Animal Sci. 8:224.

Eaton, H.D. et al. 1964. Conn. (Storrs) Agr. Expt. Sta. Bul. 383.

Eaton, H.D. et al. 1972. J. Dairy Sci. 55:232.

Eaton, H.D., J.J. Lucas, S.W. Nielsen and C.F. Helmboldt. 1970. J. Dairy Sci. 53:1775.

Erwin, E.S., I.A. Dyer and M.E. Ensminger. 1956. J. Animal Sci. 15:1147.

Erwin, E.S., C.J. Elam and I.A. Dyer. 1957. Science 126:702.

Erwin, E.S., R.S. Gordon and J.W. Algeo. 1963. J. Animal Sci. 22:341.

Erwin, E.S., T.R. Varnell and H.M. Page. 1959. Proc. Soc. Expt. Biol. Med. 100:373.

Eveleth, D.F., D.W. Bolin and A.I. Goldsby. 1949. Am. J. Vet. Res. 10:250.

Faruque, O. and D.M. Walker. 1970. Brit. J. Nutr. 24:11,23.

Fernandez, S.C. et al. 1976. Intern. J. Vit. Nutr. Res. 46:439.

Fields, C.L., G.E. Mitchell, C.O. Little and J.A. Boling. 1969. J. Animal Sci. 28:135 (abstr).

Frier, H.I. et al. 1970. J. Dairy Sci. 53:1051.

Frier, H.I. et al. 1974. Am. J. Vet. Res. 35:45.

Glover, J., C. Jay, R.C. Kershaw and P.E. B. Reilly. 1976. Brit. J. Nutr. 36:137.

Guilbert, H.R. and G.H. Hart. 1934. J. Nutr. 8:25.

Guilbert, H.R. and G.H. Hart. 1935. J. Nutr. 10:409.

Hayes, B.W., G.E. Mitchell and C.O. Little. 1968. J. Animal Sci. 27:516.

Hazzard, D.G. et al. 1962. J. Dairy Sci. 45:91.

Hazzard, D.G. et al. 1964. J. Dairy Sci. 47:391.

Helmboldt, C.F., E.L. Jungherr, H.D. Eaton and L.A. Moore. 1953. Am. J. Vet. Res. 14:343.

Hennig, A. and G. Guther. 1975. J. Animal Sci. 27:1727.

Hoar, D.W., L.B. Embry and R.J. Emerick. 1968. J. Animal Sci. 26:1727.

Horn, F.P., R.L. Reid and G.A. Jung. 1975. J. Animal Sci. 41:635.

Hume, I.D., G.E. Mitchell and R.E. Tucker. 1970. J. Animal Sci. 31:244 (abstr).

Hume, I.D., G.E. Mitchell and R.E. Tucker. 1971. J. Nutr. 101:1169.

Hunter, V.E., A.L. Lesperance and M.J. Papez. 1973. Proc. West Sec. Am. Soc. Anim. Sci. 24:213.

Jensen, L.S. 1969. In: Animal Growth and Nutrition. Lea & Febiger Pub. Co., Philadelphia.

Jones, I.R. et al. 1966. J. Dairy Sci. 49:491.

Jordan, H.A. et al. 1963. J. Animal Sci. 22:738.

Keating, E.K., W.H. Hale and F. Hubbert. 1964. J. Animal Sci. 23:111.

King, T.B., T.G. Lohman and G.S. Smith. 1962. J. Animal Sci. 21:1002 (abstr).

Kirk, W.G., R.L. Shirley, J.F. Easley and F.M. Peacock. 1971. J. Animal Sci. 33:476.

Kon, S.K., W.A. McGillivray and S.Y. Thompson. 1955. Brit. J. Nutr. 9:244.

Lichtenwalner, R.E., J.P. Fontenot and R.E. Tucker. 1973. J. Animal Sci. 37:837.

Light, M.R., E.W. Klosterman, M.L. Buchanan and D.W. Bolin. 1952. J. Animal Sci. 11:599.

Lindley, C.E., H.H. Brugman, T.J. Cunha and E.J. Warwick. 1949. J. Animal Sci. 8:590.

Long, R.D., G.E. Mitchell and C.O. Little. 1971. Internat. J. Vit. Nutr. Res. 41:327.

Lynch, G. P., R.W. Miller and D.F. Smith. 1968. J. Dairy Sci. 51:978 (abstr).

Madsen, L.L. and R.E. Davis. 1949. J. Animal Sci. 8:625.

Madsen, L.L. and I.P. Earle. 1947. J. Nutr. 34:603.

Madsen, L.L. et al. 1948. J. Animal Sci. 7:60.

Majumdar, B.N. and B.N. Gupta. 1960. Indian J. Med. Res. 48:388.

Martin, F.H., D.E. Ullrey, H.W. Newland and E.R. Miller. 1968. J. Nutr. 96:269.

Martin, F.H. et al. 1971. J. Animal Sci. 32:1233.

Martovitskaya, A.M. et al. 1975. Nutr. Abstr. Rev. 46:1155.

McGillivray, W.A. 1951. Brit. J. Nutr. 5:223.

Mee, J.L.M. and R.W. Stanley. 1974. Nutr. Rpts. Inter. 9:401.

Menzies, C.S., G.E. Mitchell and C.O. Little. 1967. Inter. Ztschr. Vitaminforsch. 37:443.

Mikkilineni. S.R. et al. J. Dairy Sci. 56:395.

Miller. R.W., R.W. Hemken, D.R. Waldo and L.A. Moore. 1969. J. Dairy Sci. 52:1998.

Mitchell, G.E. 1967. J. Am. Vet. Med. Assoc. 151:430.

Mitchell, G.E. et al. 1965. J. Animal Sci. 24:898 (abstr).

Mitchell, G.E. et al. 1968. Internat. J. Vit. Res. 38:304.

Mitchell, G.E., C.O. Little, H.B. Sewell and B.W. Hayes. 1967. J. Nutr. 91:371.

Mitchell, G.E., P.V. Rattray and J.B. Hutton. 1975. Internat. J. Vit. Nutr. Res. 46:299.

Mingazov, T.A. 1975. Nutr. Abstr. Rev. 45:654.

Moore, L.A. 1939. J. Dairy Sci. 22:803.

Moore, L.A. 1941. J. Dairy Sci. 24:893.

Moore, L.A., M.H. Berry and J.F. Sykes. 1943. J. Nutr. 26:649.

Moore, T. 1957. Vitamin A. Elsevier Publ. Co., Amsterdam.

Nielsen, S.W., J.H.L. Mills, C.G. Woelfel and H.D. Eaton. 1966. Res. Vet. Sci. 7:143.

O'Donovan, J.P. 1967. Dissert. Abstr. 27:3734B.

Page, H.M., E.S. Erwin and G.E. Nelms. 1959. Am. J. Physiol. 196:917.

Pastrana, M.T. et al. 1975. Nutr. Abstr. Rev. 45:1059.

Perry, T.W., W.M. Beeson, M.T. Mohler and W.H. Smith. 1962. J. Animal Sci. 21:333.

Perry, T.W., W.M. Beeson, W.H. Smith and M.T. Mohler. 1967. J. Animal Sci. 26:115.

Perry, T.W. et al. 1968. J. Animal Sci. 27:190.

Potkanski, A.A. et al. 1974. Internat. J. Vit. Nutr. Res. 44:147.

Richards, J.I. et al. 1970. Internat. J. Vit. Nutr. Res. 40:567.

Ritzman, E.G., N.F. Colovos, H.A. Keener and A.E. Terri. 1945. N. Hampshire Agr. Expt. Sta. Tech. Bul. 88

Ronning, M., E.R. Berousek, J.L. Griffith and W.D. Gallup. 1959. Oklahoma Agr. Expt. Sta. Tech. Bul. T-76.

Rousseau, J.E. et al. 1954. J. Dairy Sci. 37:857.

Rousseau, J.E. et al. 1956. J. Dairy Sci. 39:1565,1671.

Rousseau, J.E. et al. 1973. J. Dairy Sci. 56:246.

Schmidt, H. 1941. Am. J. Vet. Res. 2:373.

Schubin, A. and S. Kovalskii. 1976. Nutr. Abstr. Rev. 46:575.

Schuh, J.D., M. Ronning and W.D. Gallup. 1959. J. Dairy Sci. 42:159.

Sherman, W.C. et al. 1958. J. Animal Sci. 17:586.

Spratling, F.R. et al. 1965. Vet. Rec. 77:1532.

Swanson, E.W., G.G. Martin, F.E. Pardue and G.M. Gorman. 1968. J. Animal Sci. 27:541.

Taylor, R.L., O.F. Pahnish and C.B. Roubicek. 1968. J. Animal Sci. 27:1477.

Thomas, O.O., W.D. Gallup and C.K. Whitehair. 1953. J. Animal Sci. 12:372.

Tucker, R.E., G.E. Mitchell and C.O. Little. 1967. J. Animal Sci. 26:225 (abstr).

Ullrey, D.E. 1972. J. Animal Sci. 35:648.

Webb, K.E., G.E. Mitchell and C.O. Little. 1971. J. Animal Sci. 32:157.

Webb, K.E., G.E. Mitchell, C.O. Little and G.H. Schmitt. 1968. J. Animal Sci. 27:1657.

Weiss, R.R. 1977. Nutr. Abstr. Rev. 47:387.

Wheeler, R.R. et al. 1957. J. Animal Sci. 16:525.

Whiting, F., J.K. Loosli and J.P. Wellman. 1949. J. Animal Sci. 8:35.

Wing, J.M. 1969. J. Dairy Sci. 52:479.

Woelfel, C.G. et al. 1965. J. Dairy Sci. 48:1346. ·

Vitamin D

Benzie, D. et al. 1960. J. Agr. Sci. 54:202.

Blackburn, P.S., K.L. Blaxter and E.J. Castle. 1957. Proc. Nutr. Soc. 16:xvi (abstr).

Cohen, P.H. 1962. Vet. Rec. 74:399.

Colovos, N.F., H.A. Keener, A.E. Terri and H.A. Davis. 1951. J. Dairy Sci. 34:735.

Dalgarno, A.C., R. Hill and I. McDonald. 1962. Brit. J. Nutr. 16:91.

Dobson, R.C. and G. Ward. 1974. J. Dairy Sci. 57:985.

Greenbaum, S.B. 1973. Feedstuffs 45(16):30.

Hignett, S.L. and P.G. Hignett. 1953. Vet. Rec. 65:21.

McRoberts, M.R., R. Hill and A.C. Dalgarno. 1965. J. Agr. Sci. 65:1;15.

Meyer, H., J. Pohlanz, S. De Barros and R. Krebber. 1971. Nutr. Abstr. Rev. 41:1143.

Quarterman, J., A.C. Dalgarno and A. Adam. 1964. Brit. J. Nutr. 18:79.

Spratling, F.R. 1976. Brit. Vet. J. 132:557.

Wallis, G.C. 1944. S. Dakota Agr. Expt. Sta. Bul. 372.

Ward, G., R.C. Dobson and J.R. Dunham. 1972. J. Dairy Sci. 55:768.

Wasserman, R.H. 1975. Cornell Vet. 65:3.

Zintzen, H. and P.A. Boyazoglu. 1973. J.S. African Vet. Assoc. 44:25.

Vitamin E

Alderson, N.E. et al. 1971. J. Nutr. 101:655.

Ames, S.R., W.F. Kujawski, M.I. Ludwig and P.L. Harris. 1957. Annotated Bibliography of Vitamin E in Cattle Nutrition 1927 to 1956. Distillation Products Industries, Rochester, NY.

Astrup, H.N., S.C. Mills, L.J. Cook and T.W. Scott. 1974. Acta. Vet. Scand. 15:451.

Bayfield, R.F. and P.J. Mylrea. 1969. J. Dairy Res. 36:137.

Blaxter, K.L., P.S. Watts and W.A. Wood. 1952. Brit. J. Nutr. 6:124.

Blaxter, K.L. and W.A. Wood. 1952. Brit. J. Nutr. 6:144.

Blaxter, K.L., W.A. Wood and A.M. MacDonald. 1953. Brit. J. Nutr. 7:34;287.

Boyd, J.W. 1968. Brit J. Nutr. 22:411.

Boyd, J.W. 1973. Acta. Agr. Scand., Suppl. 19.

Buchanan-Smith, J.G. et al. 1969. J. Animal Sci. 29:808.

Carvaggi, C. and E. Wright. 1969. N. Z. J. Agr. Res. 12:655.

Erwin, E.S. et al. 1961. J. Nutr. 75:45.

Evarts, R.P. and A. Oksanen. 1973. Brit. J. Nutr. 29:293.

Ewan. R.C., C.A. Baumann and A.L. Pope. 1968. J. Animal Sci. 27:751.

Finlayson, R., I.F. Keymer and V.J.A. Manton. 1971. J. Comp. Path. 81:71.

Gullickson, T.W. 1949. Ann. New York Acad. Sci. 52:256.

Hidiroglou, M. 1977. Brit. J. Nutr. 37:215.

Hidiroglou, M. and E. Borrowsky. 1970. J. Animal Sci. 31:244 (abstr).

Hidiroglou, M., I. Hoffman and K.J. Jenkins. 1969a. Can. J. Physiol. Pharm. 47:953.

Hidiroglou, M. and K.J. Jenkins. 1974. Ann. Biol. Anim. Bioch. Bioph. 14:667.

Hidiroglou, M., K. Jenkins and R.B. Carson. 1969b. Ann. Biol. Anim. Bioch., Biophys. 9:161.

Hidiroglou, M., K.J. Jenkins and A.H. Corner. 1972. Can. J. Animal Sci. 52:511.

Hogue, D.E., J.F. Proctor, R.G. Warner and J.K. Loosli. 1962. J. Animal Sci. 21:25.

Hopkins, L.L., A.L. Pope and C.A. Baumann. 1964. J. Animal Sci. 23:674.

Jenkins, K.J., M. Hidiroglou, R.R. Mackay and J.G. Proulx. 1970. Can. J. Animal Sci. 50:137.

Kuttler, K.L. and D.W. Marble. 1960. Am. J. Vet. Res. 21:437.

Maplesden, D.C. and J.K. Loosli. 1960. J. Dairy Sci. 43:645.

Michel, R.L., D.D. Mackdani, J.T. Huber and A.E. Sculthorpe. 1972. J. Dairy Sci. 55:489.

Muth, O.H., J.E. Oldfield, J.R. Schubert and L.F. Remmert. 1959. Am. J. Vet. Res. 20:231.

Nelson, F.C., M. Hidiroglou and H.A. Hamilton. 1964. Can. Vet. J. 5:268.

Okansen, H.E. 1973. Acta. Agr. Scand., Suppl. 19.

Paulson, G.D., C.A. Baumann and A.L. Pope. 1968a. J. Animal Sci. 27:497.

Paulson, G.D., A.L. Pope and C.A. Bauman. 1968b. Proc. Soc. Expt. Biol. Med. 122:321.

Poukka, R. 1968. Brit. J. Nutr. 22:423.

Rochester, S. and C. Carvaggi. 1971. Res. Vet. Sci. 12:119.

Safford, J.W., K.F. Swingle and H. Marsh. 1954. Am. J. Vet. Res. 15:373.

Thomas, J.W. and M. Okamota. 1956. J. Dairy Sci. 39:928.

Tollersrud, S. 1971. Acta. Vet. Scand. 12:365.

Tollersrud, S. and O. Ribe. 1967. Acta. Vet. Scand. 8:1.

Welch, J.G., W.G. Hoekstra, A.L. Pope and P.H. Phillips. 1960. J. Animal Sci. 19:620.

Whanger, P.D. et al. 1976. Nutr. Repts. Internat. 13:159.

Young, L.G. et al. 1975. J. Animal Sci. 40:495.

Vitamin K

Goplen, B.P. and J.M. Bell. 1967. Can. J. Animal Sci. 47:91.

Matschiner, J.T. 1970. J. Nutr. 100:190.

McElroy, L.W. and H. Goss. 1940. J. Nutr. 20:527.

O'Donovan, J.P. 1967. Dissert. Abstr. 27:3734B.

Perry, T.W. et al. 1968. J. Animal Sci. 27:190.

B-Complex

Thiamin

Benevenga, N.J., R.L. Baldwin, M. Ronning and A.L. Black. 1967. J. Nutr. 91:63.

Boyd, J.W. and J.R. Walton. 1977. J. Comp. Path. 87:581.

Davies, E.T., H.H. Pill, D.F. Collings and J.A.J. Venn. 1965. Vet. Rec. 77:290.

Draper, H.H. and B.C. Johnson. 1951. J. Nutr. 43:413.
Edwin, E.E. and R. Jackman. 1973. Vet. Rec. 92:640.
Edwin, E.E., G. Lewis and R Allcroft. 1968. Vet. Rec. 83:176.
Evans, W.C. et al. 1975. J. Comp. Path. 85:253.
Flachowsky, G., H.J. Lohnert and A. Hennig. 1974. Arch. Exper. Vet. Med. Bd. 28:543.
Hayes, B.W., G.E. Mitchell, C.O. Little and N.W. Bradley. 1966. J. Animal Sci. 25:539.
Hentschl, A.F., J.F. Walton and E.W. Miller. 1966. Mod. Vet. Pract. 47(7):72.
Jensen, R., L.A. Griner and O.R. Adams. 1956. J. Am. Vet. Med. Assoc. 129:311.
Johnson, B.C., T.S. Hamilton, W.B. Nevens and L.E. Boley. 1948. J. Nutr. 35:137.
Kon, S.K. and J.W.G. Porter. 1954. Vit. and Hor. 12:53.
Linklater, K.A., D.A. Dyson and K.T. Morgan. 1977. Res. Vet. Sci. 22:308.
Loew, F.M. 1972. Rev. Cubana Cienc. Agr. 6:301.
Loew, F.M. 1975. World Rev. Nutr. Dietet. 20:168.
Loew, F.M., J.M. Bettany and C.E. Halifax. 1975. Can. J. Comp. Med. 39:291.
Loew, F.M. and R.H. Dunlop. 1972. Can. J. Comp. Med. 36:345; Am. J. Vet. Res. 33:2195.
Loew, F.M., R.H. Dunlop and R.G. Christian. 1970. Can. Vet. J. 11:57.
Markson, L.M., E.E. Edwin, G. Lewis and C. Richardson. 1974. Brit. Vet. J. 130:9.
Markson, L.M., S. Terlecki, and G. Lewis. 1966. Vet. Rec. 79:578.
Markson, L.M. et al. 1972. Brit. Vet. J. 128:488.
Pierson, R.E. and R. Jensen. 1975. J. Am. Vet. Med. Assoc. 166:257.
Pill, A.H. 1967. Vet. Rec. 81:178.
Pill, A.H., E.T. Davies, D.F. Collings and J.A.J. Venn. 1966. Vet. Rec. 78:737.
Quaghebeur, D., W. Oyaert, E. Muylle and C. Hende. 1974. Zent. Vet. Med. A. 22:296.
Roberts, G.W. and J.W. Boyd. 1974. J. Comp. Path. 84:365.
Sapienza, D.A. and B.E. Brent. 1974. J. Animal Sci. 39:251 (abstr).
Sapienza, D.A. and B.E. Brent. 1975. Kans. Agr. Expts. Rept. Progress 230.
Terlecki, S. and L.M. Markson. 1961. Vet. Rec. 73:23.

Pyridoxine

Johnson, B.C., A.C. Wiese, H.H. Mitchell and W.B. Nevens. 1947. J. Biol. Chem. 167:729.
Kirchgessner, M., H. Frieselke, J. Krippl and B. Rolle. 1965. Nutr. Abstr. Rev. 36:5103.
Kon, S.K. and J.W.G. Porter. 1954. Vit. and Hor. 12:53.

Pantothenic Acid

Johnson, B.C., A.C. Wiese, H.H. Mitchell and W.B. Nevens. 1947. J. Biol. Chem. 167:729.
Sheppard, A.J. and B.C. Johnson. 1957. J. Nutr. 61:195.

Biotin

Kon, S.K. and J.W.G. Porter. 1954. Vit. and Hor. 12:53.
Wiese, A.C., B.C. Johnson, H.H. Mitchell and W.B. Nevens. 1947. J. Nutr. 33:263.

Para-Aminobenzoic Acid

Bentley, O.G., et al. 1955. J. Nutr. 57:389.

Folic Acid

Ford, J.E., G.S. Knaggs, D.N. Salter and K.J. Scott. 1972. Brit. J. Nutr. 27:571.

Cyanocobalamin

Draper, H.H. and B.C. Johnson. 1952. J. Nutr. 46:37.
Elliot, J.M., R.N.B. Kay and E.D. Goodall. 1971. Life Sci. 10:647.
Frobish, R.A. and C.L.Davis. 1977. J. Dairy Sci. 60:268.
Hedrich, M.F., J.M. Elliot and J.E. Lowe. 1973. J. Nutr. 103:1646.
Kercher, C.J. and S.E. Smith. 1955. J. Animal Sci. 14:458.
Marston, H.R. 1970. Brit. J. Nutr. 24:615.
Rerat, A., H. LeBars and R. Jacquot. 1956. Comptes Rendus 242:679.
Rerat, A., H. LeBars and J. Molle. 1958. Comptes Rendus 246:1920,2051.
Rickard, T.R. and J.M. Elliot. 1978. J. Animal Sci. 46:304.
Roy, J.H.B. et al. 1964. Brit. J. Nutr. 18:467.
Schuh, M. and W. Stockl. 1975. Nutr. Abstr. Rev. 45:986.
Smith, R.M. and H.R. Marston. 1970. Brit. J. Nutr. 24:857,879.
Smith, R.M. and H.R. Marston. 1971. Brit. J. Nutr. 26:41.
Smith, S.E. and J.K. Loosli. 1957. J. Dairy Sci. 40:1215.
Somers, M. 1969. Aust. J. Expt. Biol. Med. Sci. 47:219.
Walker, C.K. and J.M. Elliot. 1972. J. Dairy Sci. 55:474.
Wooten, J. 1972. M.S. Thesis, Univ. Aberdeen, Aberdeen, Scotland.

Choline

Dyer, I.A., R.J. Johnson and J. Templeton. 1966. Feed Age 16:19.

Harris, R.R., H.F. Yeates and J.E. Barnett. 1966. J. Animal Sci. 25:248.

Johnson, B.C., H.H. Mitchell, J.A. Pinkos and C.C. Morrill. 1951. J. Nutr. 35:137.

Swingle, R.X. and I.A. Dyer. 1970. J. Animal Sci. 31:404.

B-Vitamin Supplementation

Clifford, A.J., R.D. Goodrich and A.D. Tillman. 1967. J. Animal Sci. 26:400.

Oltjen, R.R., R.J. Sirney and A.D. Tillman. 1962. J. Animal Sci. 21:277, 302.

Perry, T.W. and R.J. Hillier. 1969. J. Dairy Sci. 52:1786.

Smith, G.S. et al. 1974. J. Animal Sci. 38:627.

Thrasher, D.M. et al. 1964. J. Animal Sci. 23:895 (abstr).

Riboflavin

Brisson, G.J. and T.S. Sutton. 1951. J. Dairy Sci. 34:28.

Draper, H.H. and B.C. Johnson. 1952. J. Nutr. 46:37.

Hobson, P.N. and R. Summers. 1969. Proc. Nutr. Soc. 28:53A.

Johnson, P., L.A. Maynard and J.K. Loosli. 1941. J. Dairy Sci. 24:57.

Kon, S.K. and J.W.G. Porter. 1954. Vit and Hor. 12:53.

Owen, E.C. and D.W. West. 1968. J. Chem Soc. (C), p. 34.

Owen, E.C. and D.W. West. 1970. Brit. J. Nutr. 24:45.

Roy, J.H.B. 1969. In: Nutrition of Animals of Agricultural Importance. Part II. Pergamon Press.

Warner, R.G. and T.S. Sutton. 1948. J. Dairy Sci. 31:976.

Wiese, A.C., B.C. Johnson, H.H. Mitchell and W.B. Nevens. 1947. J. Nutr. 33:263.

Niacin

Blaxter, K.L. and W.A. Wood. 1952. Brit. J. Nutr. 6:56.

Hopper, J.H. and B.C. Johnson. 1955. J. Nutr. 56:303.

Johnson, B.C., A.C. Wiese, H.H. Mitchell and W.B. Nevens. 1947. J. Biol. Chem. 167:729.

Mizwicki, K.L., F.N. Owens, H.R. Isaacson and B. Schockey. 1975. J. Animal Sci. 41:411 (abstr).

Winegar, A.H., P.B. Pearson and H. Schmidt. 1940. Science 91:508.

Chapter 10 - Nutrition of Preruminants

By D.M. Walker

The preruminant stage of life is usually understood to span the interval from birth until that time when the developing animal ceases to be dependent on a liquid feed and can rely fully on the ruminant mode of digestion for its supply of nutrients. However, in considering the nutrition of preruminants it would be unwise to underestimate the importance of nutrition during fetal life. Should fetal nutrition be inadequate in late pregnancy, a train of events ensues that will, in a majority of cases, adversely affect post-natal development (NRC, 1968; Allden, 1970). The size of the newborn may be reduced, its reserves diminished, and its chances of survival endangered (Wallace, 1948; Thomson and Aitken, 1959; Alexander, 1974).

A number of excellent reviews have appeared in recent years on the nutrition of preruminants. These reviews have been mainly concerned with the calf (Porter, 1969; Radostits and Bell, 1970; Roy, 1970a, b; Roy and Stobo, 1975; Davey, 1974; Appleman and Owen, 1975), though more attention has recently been given to the artificial rearing of the lamb (Pearce, 1972; Treacher, 1973; Owen, 1974; Theriez, 1975) and the goat kid (Fehr, 1975). There is little information on the nutrition of other preruminants.

Digestion

The digestive tract of the preruminant at birth is anatomically similar to that of the newborn nonruminant (see Ch. 3, Vol 1). During the first 3-6 weeks of life the young animal depends for its nutrient requirements on liquid feed, although from a few days of age it may pick at grass and other solid feeds (Walker, 1950). The liquid feed is consumed by sucking from a teat or drinking from a bucket. In either case, if the stimulus is sufficient to activate the pattern of behaviour associated with the act of sucking, e.g. bunting the udder, tail wagging, then the majority of the liquid feed bypasses the undeveloped reticulo-rumen by means of the esophageal groove and goes direct to the abomasum (Watson and Jarrett, 1944; Titchen and Newhook, 1975). Should the stimulus be absent or insufficient in intensity, then liquid will spill over into the reticulo-rumen and, at this early stage of life,

may putrefy or lead to an undesirable fermentation. The result is poor appetite and failure to thrive (Lawlor et al, 1971).

The first feed of the preruminant after birth is invariably colostrum. This first secretion from the udder not only differs from milk in the content of major nutrients (Table 10-1) but, with its immune globulins, colostrum also enables the preruminant to acquire passive immunity against organisms that would otherwise cause disease and often death. During the first 24 hours of life a high proportion of these immune globulins can be absorbed from the small intestine unchanged. This process is assisted by a number of special properties of colostrum; (1) the high concentration of immune globulins provide an excess of substrate for the proteolytic enzymes of the stomach and pancreas; (2) the γ-globulin fraction contributes the major part of the buffering capacity of colostrum against acid and thus tends to reduce gastric proteolysis; (3) protein breakdown in the intestine is lessened by the trypsin inhibitor in colostrum; (4) factors are present, as yet unidentified, that facilitate the absorption into the blood of immune globulins which escape digestion (Hardy, 1970).

The digestion of nutrients by the preruminant differs in a number of respects from that of other young animals. The physical changes which occur in the abomasum when milk is taken as a single meal have been studied in calves with abomasal fistula (Ash, 1964; Henschel et al, 1961). The subsequent phases of digestion involving the passage of chyme from the abomasum and along the intestine has also been studied in calves with reentrant intestinal fistulas (Smith, 1964; Mylrea, 1966). The sequence of events has been summarized by Porter (1969). The preruminant which is fed by bucket is usually restricted in the number of feeds offered per day. Hill et al (1970) have pointed out that when the young animal sucks its dam or takes milk by teat from a self-feeder, there may be a difference in the pattern of flow of digesta from that observed with animals fed irregularly and usually with long intervals between feeds (Ternouth et al, 1977).

Carbohydrate Digestion

In the immediate postnatal period the

Table 10-1. Composition of colostrum (first 24 hours) of the cow and of the milks of the cow, sheep and goat. [a]

Component	Cow		Sheep	Goat
	Colostrum	Milk		
Total solids, %	21.9	12.5	18.4	13.0
Fat, %	3.6	3.7	7.5	4.5
Protein, %	14.2	3.4	5.6	3.3
Casein, %	5.2	2.6	4.2	2.5
Lactose (anhydrous), %	3.1	4.6	4.4	4.4
Ash	1.0	0.8	0.9	0.8
Calcium, %	0.26	0.13	0.19	0.14
Phosphorus, %	0.24	0.10	0.15	0.12
Magnesium, %	0.04	0.01	0.02	0.02
Sodium, %	0.07	0.06	0.04	0.04
Potassium, %	0.14	0.16	0.19	0.17
Chlorine, %	0.12	0.10	0.14	0.15
Iron, mg/100g	0.20	0.05	0.05	0.05
Copper, mg/100g	0.06	0.02	0.01	0.01
Cobalt, μg/100g	0.50	0.05	-	-
Manganese, mg/100g	0.016	0.003	0.006	0.004
Iodine, μg/100g	0.03	0.01	-	-
Carotenoids, μg/g fat	35	7	-	-
Vitamin A, μg/g fat	45	8	8	9
Vitamin D, IU/g fat	4	2	-	2
Vitamin E, μg/g fat	125	20	20	14
Thiamin, μg/100g	60	40	70	50
Riboflavin, μg/100 g	500	150	500	120
Niacin, g/100g	100	80	500	200
Pantothenic acid, μg/100g	220	350	350	350
Vitamin B_6, μg/100g	50	52	70	7
Vitamin B_{12}, μg/100g	1.0	0.3	1.0	0.1
Biotin, μg/100g	4	2	5	1.5
Folic acid, μg/100g	1	5	5	0.2
p-Aminobenzoic acid, μg/100g	-	10	-	-
Choline, mg/100g	53	13	4	13
Ascorbic acid, mg/100g	2.5	2.0	3.0	2.0

[a] Values taken from miscellaneous sources including Ling et al (1961); Roy (1970a); Underwood (1977).

young animal is dependent on milk for its nutrients. The supply of carbohydrate, which occupied such a central role in fetal life (Shelley, 1969), is suddenly reduced at birth and the preruminant has to adapt to fat as the major energy source. The carbohydrate in milk is lactose, which must be hydrolyzed before it can be absorbed. It is now established that while the preruminant can readily utilize glucose, galactose and lactose, it has only a limited ability to utilize maltose and starch and is unable to utilize sucrose (see Dollar and Porter, 1957; Walker, 1959; Huber, 1969).

The activity of the enzyme responsible for lactose hydrolysis in the small intestine (β-galactosidase) rises shortly before birth and declines with age, but even at 8 weeks (in the calf) is ten times higher than in the adult. Maltase and isomaltase activities increase during the first 1 to 4 weeks of life, but thereafter, the values are similar to those in adult animals, the activity of isomaltase being half that of maltase (Coombe and Siddons, 1973; Toofanian et al, 1973). It has been suggested that the extent of digestion of starch in the small intestine is limited by low pancreatic amylase activity. However, Mayes and Ørskov (1974) suggest that in lambs the major limitation to the digestion of starch lies not with the activity of α-amylase but with the utilization of some of the breakdown products of starch, namely glucose, maltose and maltotriose. Nevertheless, the disappearance of starch that has been observed in digestibility studies is in part the result of microbial activity in the large intestine. Excess quantities of starch will cause diarrhea, as will the excessive intake of any sugar, even lactose or glucose (Blaxter and Wood, 1953; Walker and Faichney, 1964).

There would seem to be an upper limit to the amount of glucose that can be absorbed from the small intestine of the preruminant, and the limit appears to be much lower than that of young non-ruminants. The enzyme to hydrolyze sucrose is absent from the small intestine at all ages and, while fructose can be metabolized in the tissues of the preruminant (Ballard and Oliver, 1965), it is poorly absorbed, if at all (Velu et al, 1960). The severe scouring that occurs after feeding fructose indicates that much of the sugar passes unabsorbed through the small intestine.

Thus, the digestion of carbohydrates by the preruminant differs from that in the ruminant animal in a number of respects: the carbohydrates that can be digested and absorbed in any quantity are limited to lactose, glucose and galactose; complex polysaccharides such as starch, which are converted to volatile fatty acids by microbial enzymes in the adult ruminant, are digested only to a limited extent in the small intestine of the preruminant; polysaccharides that escape digestion in the small intestine may be metabolized by microbial action in the large intestine, but the products of digestion are, in the main, unavailable to the preruminant and may lead to digestive upsets. Some values for the apparent digestibilities of carbohydrates in milk replacers for calves are given in Table 10-2.

Fat Digestion

In the young suckling lamb, calf and probably other preruminants, the digestion of lipids appears to be similar to that of monogastric animals, in that large amounts of

Table 10-2. Apparent digestibilities of carbohydrates in milk replacers for calves.

Carbohydrate	Apparent Digestibility %
Lactose	94[a]
Maltose	97[a]
Sucrose	57[a]
Amylose	83[a]
Amylopectin	89[a]
Tapioca starch	80[a]
Flojel starch	80[a]
Maize starch	76[b]

[a]Huber et al (1961); [b]Raven and Robinson (1958).

monoglycerides and free fatty acids are present in the contents of the small intestine. The extent to which pancreatic lipase is responsible for this hydrolysis is in dispute, since considerable hydrolysis is also found in abomasal contents due to the action of a pregastric esterase that is secreted in the pharyngeal region in young calves (Ramsey et al, 1956). Hydrolysis has also been shown to occur in other preruminants (Grosskopf, 1965). Gooden and Lascelles (1973) suggest that there is an additive effect of pancreatic lipase and pregastric esterase activity in very young calves. At one week of age they estimated that pregastric esterase activity was sufficient to hydrolyze 65-70% of the lipid offered in a milk diet. There appears to be general agreement that both enzymes exhibit an intermolecular specificity for glycerides containing short chain fatty acids, although Grosskopf (1965) was of the opinion that pregastric esterase had an absolute specificity for butyrate linkages. Edwards-Webb and Thompson (1977) have suggested that there is a difference in the pattern of release of fatty acids from cows' milk fat by salivary and pancreatic lipases, and that the overall extent of lipolysis by salivary lipase is limited by its inability to release long-chain acids. The net result of the action of the pregastric esterase is an accumulation of free fatty acids in the abomasal contents. It has been suggested that in very young preruminants the output of pancreatic lipase may be insufficient to hydrolyze all the dietary lipid and that hydrolysis by pregastric esterase activity, which is known to be very high during the first few days of life, may be relatively more important (Gooden, 1973).

The true digestibility of butterfat by calves and lambs is almost 100%. The substitution of other fats and oils for butterfat in milk replacers will lead, in many cases, to a reduction in digestibility. Early work by Gullickson et al (1942) on the utilization by calves of various fats and oils in milk replacers indicated that such vegetable oils as cottonseed, soybean and corn oils were poorly digested. However, it seems likely that in these experiments the diets were deficient in vitamin E. Animal fats such as lard and tallow are also less well digested than butterfat. There is a need for a reassessment of the digestibilities of a wide variety of vegetable oils by calves. Some values which have been obtained, although rarely under identical dietary conditions, are given in Table 10-3, together with values for lambs.

To attain high apparent digestibilities it is necessary to use an effective emulsifying agent, such as lecithin or glyceryl mono-stearate, and preferably to homogenize the fat into the diet so that the particle size is less than $3-4\mu$ in diameter. If these precautions are not taken, diarrhea and loss of hair will occur in the younger calf less than 3 weeks of age (Roy et al, 1961). The factors responsible for the reduction in digestibility

Table 10-3. Apparent digestibilities of different fats in milk replacers for calves and lambs.

Fat	Apparent digestibility, %	
	Calf[a]	Lamb[b]
Butter	96-98	97
Lard	83-90	88
Tallow	72-87	76
Coconut	94-96	99
Coconut (hydrogenated)	83-84	-
Palm	91-95	-
Palm (hydrogenated)	87	-
Palm-kernel	87	-
Palm-kernel (hydrogenated)	91	-
Rapeseed	-	59
Groundnut	93	98
Corn	90	97
Cottonseed, soybean, olive	-	97-99

[a] Mean literature values taken from Raven (1970), Toullec and Mathieu (1969); [b] Walker and Stokes (1970).

of vegetable oils and animal fats have variously been attributed to the chain length of the constituent fatty acids, to the degree of saturation of the fatty acids, to the positioning of individual fatty acids on the glycerol molecule, and to the proportion of saturated triglycerides in the fat. It should be pointed out that much of this research has been with laboratory rats and much less of it with preruminants. However, a most useful contribution is that of Raven and Hamilton (1971), who have shown an improvement in the digestibility of tallow with calves from 88.7 to 93.1% as a result of interesterification (a random rearrangement of the constituent fatty acids on the glycerol molecule). Interesterification of butterfat was without effect on digestibility, indicating that the high digestibility of butterfat is not dependent on any specific triglyceride structure. The incorporation of 10% butyric acid into tallow by interesterification resulted in a marked increase in digestibility (cf. Hopper et al, 1954, who fed a milk replacer containing butyrated lard, with the same butyric acid content as butterfat, and obtained live-weight gains similar to those of calves fed on whole milk). Butterfat contributes about 30% of the DM in cows' milk. The substitution of vegetable oils and animal fats for butterfat to maintain a concentration of 30% generally leads to a further reduction in digestibility that is not observed if these substitutes are incorporated to provide 10 or 20% of the dry matter.

The values given in Table 10-3 would suggest that in comparable experiments there is little difference between calves and lambs in their capacity to digest a wide variety of fats. Walker and Stokes (1970) gave lambs milk replacers that contained 30% of fat in the dry matter supplied by vegetable and animal fats. Digestibilities of seven different vegetable oils were 97-99%. In further experiments the digestibility of rapeseed oil was improved (94%) when a rapeseed variety (Oro) with a low content of erucic acid was given, compared with varieties Target and Bronowski, with high erucic acid contents and fat digestibilities of 82 and 74%, respectively (Gorrill and Walker, 1974). High values for fat digestibility are dependent on the presence in milk replacers of adequate amounts of high quality protein. If the quantity or quality of protein is reduced, there is a fall in the digestibility of most fats with the exception of butterfat (Gibney and Walker, 1977).

Protein Digestion

Milk proteins have a high apparent digestibility for the preruminant, and the absorbed amino acids are efficiently utilized for protein synthesis (Blaxter and Wood, 1952; Walker and Norton, 1971a). However, the quality of the whey proteins may be adversely affected during dehydration of whole or skimmed milk. The detailed studies of Roy and co-workers (Roy, 1964), on the detrimental effects of excessive heat treatment during spray drying of milk, are now well known. Diarrhea and poor growth may be a consequence. There is evidence of a similar effect in lambs if the proportion of undenatured whey proteins is considerably reduced (Penning et al, 1978).

The replacement of milk proteins by vegetable proteins has in the past been relatively unsuccessful. There are a number of reasons for the poor performance of preruminants given milk replacers based on vegetable proteins. Soybean proteins, for example, which have been most widely studied provide some 41% of the dry weight of the soybean; the oil contributes 22% and miscellaneous carbohydrates a further 27%. In addition the soybean contains various compounds which interfere with normal digestion and growth. It is normal practice to dehull the soybean and extract the oil. The products that result from processing include: (1) defatted soymeal (about 52% protein); (2) defatted, dehulled soy flour (about 56% protein); (3) soy protein concentrate (70-72% protein) and (4) isolated soybean protein (90-96% protein). During the preparation of the concentrates and isolates, the soluble carbohydrates, raffinose, stachyose and sucrose cannot be digested in the small intestine and, if not removed, may cause diarrhea after fermentation in the large intestine. Rackis (1966) has shown that about 6% of the protein in the soybean consists of up to 10 different antitrypsins (Obara et al, 1970), destroyed by heating the soy meals. Van Adrichem and Frens (1965) and Van Leeuwen et al (1969) have shown that when calves are fed on milk replacers containing certain soy meals and isolates, they will develop antibodies in the blood against soy protein. Subsequent work by Smith and Sissons (1975) has confirmed these findings but has not established a definite relationship between the production of antibodies and poor performance in calves. Nevertheless, it is considered desirable to destroy or remove the compounds responsible by hot ethanol-water extraction.

Colvin and Ramsey (1968, 1969) have reported some success in improving the nutritive value of soy flour for calves by pretreatment of trypsin inhibitor-free soy flour with acid or alkali, but the reason for the improvement is unexplained. The residual carbohydrates in soy concentrates (about 17%) are made up of pectin-like compounds such as neutral arabinogalactans, acidic polysaccharides and arabinan (Kellor, 1974). These carbohydrates are indigestible and do not appear to have any deleterious effect in milk replacers for calves. Gorrill and Thomas (1967) have reported that a soy protein concentrate (71% protein) providing 86% of the protein of a milk replacer gave results as good as whole milk did. It is apparent that such other growth-retarding substances as phenolic compounds, hemagglutinins, and various goitrogenic factors, which are present in soybeans (Rackis, 1974) should be removed during processing.

Other milk protein substitutes, such as the flours or isolates from the peanut, field bean (*Vicia faba*) or field pea (*V. sativa*) have promise, but must be prepared free of growth-retarding substances similar to those present in the soybean before they can be used successfully in milk replacers for preruminants. Yeast and bacterial proteins, as well as fish flours, with or without defatting, are now being investigated as alternative sources of protein (Dodsworth et al, 1977).

Some values for the apparent digestibilities of various proteins by calves and lambs are given in Table 10-4. It is clear from the values given that alternative non-milk sources of protein may be highly digestible if the concentrate or isolate has been prepared in such a way as to remove the compounds discussed previously. Although the experiments with calves and lambs may not be strictly comparable, the digestion coefficients for lambs are generally higher than those for calves.

ESTIMATES OF NUTRIENT REQUIREMENTS

Nutrition and Body Composition

The term, chemical maturity, was defined by Moulton (1923) as the age at which the fat-free body of an animal attains a constancy in chemical compostion that is characteristic of the adult of the species. Moulton showed that for a diverse range of mammals the age of chemical maturity was some 4.5% of the total life span, and for

Table 10-4. Apparent digestibilities of proteins in milk replacers for calves and lambs.

Protein source	Protein, % of dry matter	Protein as % of total dietary protein	Apparent digesti- bility, %	Reference
CALVES				
Dried whole milk	28.5	100	93.3	Blaxter and Wood (1952)
Casein	29.5	100	92.3	Brisson et al (1957)
Gelatin	16.4	100	63.5	Blaxter and Wood (1952)
Soya, 71% protein	21.0	70	81.6	Gorrill and Nicholson (1969)
Soya, 71% protein	28.3	75-84	72-82	Nitsan et al (1971, 1972)
Fish, 73.4% protein	21.4	100	79.9	Huber and Slade (1967)
Fish, 80% protein	22.0	100	53.8	Huber (1975)
Fish, 90% protein	27.1	73	82-92	Paruelle et al (1974)
LAMBS				
Dried whole milk	28.5	100	96.3	Walker and Norton (1971a)
Dried skimmed milk	28.0	100	95.9	Soliman et al (1976)
Casein	25.6	100	92.6	Kirk (1973)
Soya, 71% protein	25.9	100	91.0	Maluf and Walker (1977)
Soya, 91% protein	25.6	100	92.5	Walker and Kirk (1975)
Soya, 93% protein	27.9	100	95.4	Maluf and Walker (1977)
Groundnut, 91% protein	27.5	100	95.4	Phillips and Walker (1977)
Fish protein hydrolysate	28.0	100	95.5	Soliman et al (1976)
Yeast, 60.7% protein	27.9	100	87.9	Walker (1977)

cattle the actual age was 150 days post-partum or 435 days after conception. The protein content of the mature fat-free body was taken to be 21%. The fat-free body of the newborn calf has a protein concentration of 18-19% and that of the newborn lamb about 19% (Haecker, 1920; Jagusch et al, 1970). Thus, the newborn ruminant is relatively mature at birth when compared with mice (12.8% protein in the fat-free body), rats (10.9%) and other species which are born both physically and chemically immature (see Armsby and Moulton, 1925; Widdowson, 1950; Spray and Widdowson, 1950).

At birth the lipid reserves of the ruminant are very low (e.g. calf, 3.5% of liveweight; lamb, 2-3%) when compared with other newborn mammals such as the guinea pig (10.1%) and human baby (16.1%) (for other values see Widdowson, 1950). Furthermore, as shown by Langlands and Sutherland (1968) in studies with the developing lamb fetus, over 50% of the lipid accumulates in the last 15% of pregnancy. However, much of the lipid that is present in the body of the preruminant at birth differs from normal adipose tissue, in that it is rich in mitochondria and metabolically very active. This fat is called brown fat, due to its characteristic pigmentation, and is concerned with nonshivering thermogenesis (Smith and Horwitz, 1969). Its presence has been reported in the newborn lamb (Gemmell et al, 1972), in the calf (Alexander et al, 1975); and in the goat kid (Thompson and Jenkinson, 1970) but it is rapidly replaced by white adipose tissue within the first few weeks of life.

Table 10-5. Composition of the gain in empty body weight (EBW) of lambs, pre-natal and post-natal.

Component	Pre-natal[a] Between 125 and 145 days gestation (from 2 to 4 kg EBW)	Post-natal[b,c]	
		Between 4 and 9 kg EBW	Between 9 and 14 kg EBW
Total nitrogen, g/kg EBW gain	24.7	29.1	27.8
Wool nitrogen, g/kg EBW gain	-	3.5	3.0
Fat, g/kg EBW gain	30.5	110.2	253.1
Ash, g/kg EBW gain	39.0	34.9	30.3
Energy, MJ/kg EBW gain	4.8	8.5	13.9

[a] Langlands and Sutherland (1968); [b,c] Jagusch et al (1970); Norton et al (1970).

In the period immediately after birth—the suckling period—there is a continued rapid accretion of protein, fat and minerals, which are retained from milk with a high efficiency, and result in considerable changes in body composition. The young animal gains fat more rapidly than protein. For example, during the first six weeks of life the lamb gains fat 2.5X faster than protein, so that whereas at birth the weight of protein in the body far exceeds the weight of fat, this situation is reversed within a few weeks in an animal given an unlimited supply of milk. The values shown in Table 10-5 are for the composition of the gain in empty body weight (EBW) of a preruminant lamb that increased in weight from 2 kg at 125 days after conception to 4 kg at birth (145 days), and from 4 kg at birth to 14 kg. The amounts of N retained in wool and body tissues were relatively constant/kg EBW gain in all three periods, but the amount of fat deposited increased more than eight fold. Comparable values for the protein energy gain as % of total energy gain for sheep and cattle are given in Table 10-6.

McCance and Widdowson (1964) have stated that while "it may be possible to improve upon mother's milk as a food for newborn animals, ...this has yet to be proved, and until it has been done the protein and calories provided by mother's milk may be taken to represent satisfactory amounts for her young." There is, in fact, considerable uniformity in the compositions of the milks of the common domesticated ruminants in their contents of protein, fat and carbohydrate, when expressed on an energy basis. If the components in Table 10-1 are given gross energy values of 23.0 KJ/g protein, 38.5 KJ/g fat and 15.5 KJ/g lactose, then it can be calculated that protein supplies about 25% of the total energy in the milk of the ox, sheep and goat, fat between 50-60% and lactose about 20%; ewes' milk is an exception in providing a lower proportion (ca. 14%) of the total energy as carbohydrate.

It has been observed in the growing preruminant that there is a close relationship between bodyweight and body composition (Reid et al, 1968; Norton et al, 1970). However, although this observation implies that for the preruminant the body composition can be predicted from bodyweight, this is true only for animals within a species which are reared on the same diet. Although

Table 10-6. Composition of gain in weight of sheep and cattle. Protein energy as % of total energy gain.

Species	Milk feeding period	Adult
Sheep	40[a]	16-22[b]
Cattle	32[c]	11-18[b]

[a] Graham and Searle (1972); [b] Blaxter and Wainman (1964); [c] Gonzalez-Jiminez and Blaxter (1962).

it is not known whether small changes in the proportions of carbohydrate to fat will affect body composition, it is known that if the ratio of protein to nonprotein energy is changed, the body composition at a particular bodyweight is also changed. If the protein concentration in the diet is reduced, the animal will convert excess energy into body fat. Conversely, if the protein concentration is increased, excess dietary protein will be catabolized as a source of energy to meet the needs of body protein turnover and synthesis or as a source of glucose, and the fat content at a particular bodyweight will be reduced. It is more difficult, but not impossible, to change the composition of the fat-free body by manipulation of the dietary protein concentration. Dietary amino acid deficiencies have the same effect on body composition as a reduction in protein intake, namely, an increased deposition of fat relative to protein (Walker, 1974). The fatty acid composition of body fat is readily changed and, as in other monogastric animals, largely reflects the composition of the dietary fat (Stokes and Walker, 1970).

Energy Requirements

The ARC Committee (ARC, 1965) stated in their section on growth of young ruminants that "Little work has been done on the utilization of energy by young ruminants, animals in which the proportion of protein to fat in the gains is greater than that observed in mature stock" (cf. Table 10-6). The situation has improved somewhat in the past decade but, even now, there is little information about preruminants fed on diets of different composition, for the digestibility, metabolizability and retention of energy. A summary of some of the available data on lambs for the metabolizability of GE is given in Table 10-7. The following conclusions can be drawn from the data in this table: (1) within a wide range of protein concentrations and energy intakes, the metabolizability of the energy of cows' milk is constant at about 94%; (2) losses of energy in urine are increased if the lamb is given excess dietary protein or if body tissue is metabolized as a source of energy; (3) losses of energy in feces and urine are independent of each other; (4) there is no effect of age on

Table 10-7. The metabolizability by lambs of the gross energy of milk replacers that varied in protein content and source of fat.

Protein energy, %	Fat source	Protein source	Energy loss, % Feces	Energy loss, % Urine	Metabolizable energy, %
5	Butter	Cow's milk	6.5	1.5	92.0[a]
5	Lard	Cows' milk	6.6	3.6	89.8[a]
10	Butter	Cows' milk	5.0	1.0	94.0[a]
10	Butter	Cows' milk & methionine	1.9	1.6	96.5[a]
29	Butter	Cows' milk	1.8	4.2	94.0[a]
45	Butter	Cows' milk	1.6	4.4	94.0[a]
25	Lard	Cows' milk	6.6	3.6	89.8[a]
25	Coconut	Cows' milk	1.4	2.5	96.1[a]
25	Cottonseed	Cows' milk	2.8	2.3	94.9[a]
25	Rapeseed	Cows' milk	23.2	4.2	72.6[a]
25	Groundnut	Cows' milk	2.3	2.4	95.3[a]
30	Ewes' milk		1.5	1.9	95.6[b]
30	Ewes' milk (energy intake sub-maintenance)		1.9	6.2	91.9[b]
49	Fat-free	Cows' milk	3.5	7.3	89.2[a]

[a] Values taken from miscellaneous experiments of Walker, Norton, Cook, Stokes, Faruque (1968-75).
[b] Jagusch and Mitchell (1971).

the metabolizable energy content of cows' milk. The metabolizability of cows' milk for calves is about 95% (Roy et al, 1958; Blaxter, 1962; Holmes et al, 1975). There would seem to be no information on the metabolizability of energy in milk replacers containing alternative proteins to milk protein.

Basal Heat Production and Maintenance

In the factorial method of estimating nutrient requirements of farm animals, the total energy requirement is partitioned into (a) basal (fasting) heat production; (b) maintenance (basal heat production plus an activity increment); and (c) energy required for growth. Estimates of the ME required for maintenance (zero energy retention) by the preruminant calf and lamb are summarized in Table 10-8. Estimates of basal heat production for calves, which should, of course, be less than the estimates of ME for maintenance, have varied considerably. The ARC (1965) used a preferred value of 0.58 MJ/kg$^{0.75}$/day. The estimates of Holmes et al (1975) for Jersey and Friesian calves receiving whole milk, were between D.385 and D.448 MJ/kg$^{0.75}$/day, and are more in agreement with the maintenance values for calves shown in Table 10-8. For lambs there are few estimates of basal heat production. Blaxter's recalculation (1962) of Ritzman's experiments gave values of 0.533 MJ/kg$^{0.75}$ at 1

week of age, falling to 0.473 MJ/kg$^{0.75}$ at 6 weeks. Walker & Faichney (1964) gave a value of 0.424 MJ/kg$^{0.75}$ and Graham et al (1974) a value of 0.498 MJ/kg$^{0.75}$/day for lambs at 5 weeks of age. These values are all in excess of the estimated ME requirements for maintenance. However, the estimates of basal heat production and of requirements for maintenance are often considered to be of theoretical interest only, since zero energy retention in the preruminant animal does not normally occur, and should occur only as the result of semistarvation during sickness. Nevertheless, the estimate of energy maintenance requirement is still widely used as a base value from which to calculate the partial efficiency of energy utilization for energy gain and the energy costs of protein and fat deposition.

If the term maintenance is used, then it should always be prefaced with the adjectives 'energy,' or 'liveweight,' or 'nitrogen,' whichever applies, since only in exceptional circumstances will energy maintenance coincide with zero liveweight-, zero fat- and zero N-change. Blaxter and Wood (1952), in their studies with young Ayrshire calves, showed that at liveweight maintenance growth continued in terms of the accretion of N, Ca and P. A further example is given in Table 10-9 which shows that when energy retention in the preruminant lamb is zero, fat may be retained and N lost from the body, or vice versa, according to the protein content of the diet that is being fed to maintain energy equilibrium. Again, the ME requirement for energy maintenance is different from the requirement for maintenance of N- or liveweight equilibrium.

Table 10-8. Metabolizable energy requirements for maintenance of energy equilibrium of preruminant calves and lambs.

Metabolizable energy, MJ/kg$^{0.75}$ per day	Reference
CALVES	
0.577	Blaxter (1952)
0.532	Bryant et al (1967)
0.505	Brisson et al (1957)
0.559	Roy et al (1958)
0.426	Van Es et al (1969)
0.452	Johnson (1972)
0.452	Jacobson (1969)
0.409	Holmes et al (1975)
0.431	Thorbek and Henckel (1976)
LAMBS	
0.450	Blaxter (1962)
0.418	Ørskov and McDonald (1970)
0.407	Walker and Norton (1971b)
0.361	Kielanowski (1965)

Table 10-9. The metabolizable energy intakes and the retentions of fat and protein associated with zero energy retention for lambs given diets of different protein content (values expressed per day per kg$^{0.75}$).[a]

When energy retention is zero	Protein content of diet dry matter, %		
	12.0	28.5	45.5
Metabolizable energy intake, MJ	0.510	0.403	0.480
Fat retention, g	+ 0.88	- 0.56	- 1.51
Protein retention, g	- 1.49	+ 0.94	+ 2.59

[a] Adapted from Walker and Norton (1971b).

Table 10-10. Estimates of the net efficiency of utilization of the metabolizable energy of milk diets for growth in calves and lambs.

CALVES		LAMBS	
Net efficiency, %	Reference	Net efficiency, %	Reference
85	Blaxter (1952)	69	Walker and Norton (1970)
67	Holmes et al (1975)	55	Graham and Searle (1972)
63	Johnson (1972)	65	Kielanowski and Lassota (1960)
69	Van Es (1970)	64	Graham (1970)
69	Vermorel et al (1974)	71	Walker and Jagusch (1969)
65	Kirchgessner et al (1976)		

Efficiency of Utilization of Metabolizable Energy

Estimates of the net efficiency of utilization of the ME of diets based on cows' milk are given in Table 10-10 for the preruminant calf and lamb. Jagusch and Mitchell (1971) obtained a value of 77% for the efficiency of utilization of the ME of ewes' milk by the lamb. These estimates of net efficiency were determined from the slope of the line relating ME intake to energy retention, and differ from estimates of gross efficiency in that they are independent of ME intake, provided that the relationship between ME intake and energy retention is rectilinear. Some curvilinearity in the relationship may occur around maintenance (zero energy retention). This led Kielanowski and Lassota (1960) and Walker and Jagusch (1969) to propose that for cows' milk the net efficiency of ME utilization for maintenance (K_m) in lambs was higher (84 and 81%, respectively) than that for growth (K_f = 65 and 71%, respectively). A similar conclusion has been reached with the calf, where K_m is between 80 and 85% and K_f is between 65 and 70% (Blaxter, 1952; Gonzalez-Jiminez and Blaxter, 1962). The evidence on which these differences are based is, however, slender and in practice, academic, since the normal preruminant grows rapidly.

It is common practice to state requirements for energy as though the maintenance requirement is constant/unit of bodyweight and as though each increment of bodyweight gain has the same content of energy. As shown elsewhere, both assumptions represent an oversimplification, since basal heat production (and hence the maintenance requirement) varies according to age, previous level of feeding, and to metabolic body weight (Graham and Searle, 1972), while the energy content of successive increments of bodyweight gain increases to maturity.

Some estimates of DE requirements of calves for liveweight maintenance and for different rates of liveweight gain have been given by Roy (1970b) and by the NRC (1971). Table 10-11 gives values for the DE requirements of the calf and the lamb at different liveweights with different rates of liveweight gain. The values for calves assume a constant DE requirement/unit of liveweight and constant composition of the liveweight gain at all liveweights. The values for lambs take into account the decreasing requirement for maintenance (per unit liveweight) as the lamb increases in age and liveweight, and the increase in energy cost/unit of liveweight gain as liveweight increases.

When preruminants are kept on milk diets for a prolonged period, during which time there will be considerable changes in body composition (Haecker, 1920; Butterfield et al, 1971), it might be anticipated that there will also be changes in the utilization of the dietary constituents. The experiments of Roy et al (1964), with veal calves given large volumes of whole milk for 12 weeks, showed that while there was no change in apparent digestibility of dry matter between 4 and 10 weeks, there was a reduction in the retention of N consumed from 65-50% and in the biological value of the protein from 78 at 4 weeks to 63 at 10 weeks. While the energy intake/unit of metabolic liveweight decreased only slightly between 4 and 10 weeks, there

Table 10-11. Estimated digestible energy requirements of the calf and lamb, MJ/day.

Liveweight, kg	CALF[a]		
	Maintenance	Maintenance + 0.5 kg gain/day	Maintenance + 1.0 kg gain/day
40	8.8	15.1	21.4
80	17.6	23.9	30.2
120	26.4	32.7	39.0
	LAMB[b]		
	Maintenance	Maintenance + 100 g gain/day	Maintenance + 200 g gain/day
5	1.4	2.5	3.7
10	2.4	3.9	5.4
15	3.2	4.9	6.8

[a]Constant values of 0.22MJ digestible energy/kg liveweight for maintenance; 12.55 MJ digestible energy per 1 kg gain in weight (Roy, 1970b).
[b]Calculated from equations of Norton et al (1970); Walker and Norton (1971b).

was a fall in liveweight gain from 51 to 32 g/kg$^{0.73}$/day and in feed conversion efficiency from 0.87 to 0.58. These changes in energy and N utilization reflect the increasing proportion of fat in the liveweight gain and the reduced requirement for N (as a % of total energy intake) with an increase in age.

Thus, it is evident that if calves and lambs are maintained as preruminants for an extended period, as in veal production, the energy cost of liveweight gain will increase due to the increase in the proportion of fat in the gain relative to protein. There are as yet few values for the energy costs of protein and fat deposition with preruminants given milk diets. Kirchgessner et al (1976), working with veal calves over the liveweight range of 55-155 kg, calculated that protein was deposited with an efficiency of 45% and fat, 85%. Values for lambs (Walker and Norton, 1971b) were 65% for protein and 84% for fat. These estimates assume a fixed maintenance requirement and constant partial efficiencies, regardless of age and level of energy intake, and also make the assumption that there is one common pathway for the synthesis of protein and fat, which is of course invalid. No estimates of the rates of protein and fat turnover with their respective energy costs are yet available, although

Millward et al (1974) have summarized present knowledge for protein and have calculated that in preruminant lambs whole body protein turnover represents 25% of total heat production.

Protein Requirements

Nitrogen in the form of amino acids, peptides and protein is required by the preruminant to replace endogenous losses of N in urine, feces, skin and scurf and to supply amino acids for protein synthesis. The total requirement for protein for an individual animal may be estimated by the factorial method of Blaxter and Mitchell (1948), as fully explained in the ARC publication (ARC, 1965), or on the basis of N balance and feeding trials (Roy et al, 1958; and NRC, 1971, for calves; Walker and Norton, 1971a; Black et al, 1973; Chiou and Jordan, 1973; Black and Griffiths, 1975 for lambs). A summary of the estimates of endogenous losses of N by preruminants is given in the ARC publication, together with values for the N content of the liveweight gain. Comparisons between factorial estimates and practical feeding trials are also given in the ARC publication. An example is shown in Table 10-12.

Some estimates of the requirements for apparently digestible crude protein (R_{ADP}) by

Table 10-12. Digestible crude protein requirements for growth of calves given liquid diets: comparison between data taken from Cunningham et al (1958) and factorial estimates.[a]

Live weight, kg	Gain kg/day	Dry Matter Intake, kg/day	Digestible crude protein, g/day Cunningham et al, 1958	Factorial
40	0.34	0.6	100	90
45	0.51	0.7	130	125
50	0.77	1.0	185	175
55	0.87	1.2	220	200

[a]Adapted from ARC (1965)

calves and lambs are given in Table 10-13. These estimates were calculated by the factorial method, using the equation

$$R_{ADP} = 6.25[\frac{1}{(BV)}(E + G + M.D) - M.D]$$

where M is the metabolic fecal N excretion (g/kg DM ingested), and D is the DM intake (kg/day). BV is the biological value (as a coefficient), E is the endogenous urinary N (g/day) and G is the N retention (g/day) for a particular weight gain. Values are also given in Table 10-13 (in parentheses) for the actual intake of apparently digestible protein if calves and lambs are fed on cows' milk to

meet their DE requirements (as shown in Table 10-11). In most cases the intake of ADP will be in excess of the minimum requirements as estimated by the factorial method. It is now appreciated that predictions of endogenous N losses, when determined from experiments with animals fed on N-free diets of low digestibility, generally overestimate the actual endogenous losses that occur when milk diets of high digestibility are fed. Furthermore, estimates of the N content of the liveweight gain, determined by balance methods, are generally higher than those determined by comparative slaughter

Table 10-13. Factorial estimates of the apparently digestible crude protein requirements of the calf and lamb, g/day.

Live weight, kg	CALF[a] Maintenance (of live weight)	Maintenance + 0.5 kg gain/day	Maintenance + 1.0 kg gain/day
40	25 (107)[b]	140 (184)	260 (260)
80	40 (213)	155 (290)	275 (367)
120	50 (320)	170 (397)	285 (474)

Live weight, kg	LAMB Maintenance (of energy)	Maintenance + 100 g gain/day	Maintenance + 200 g gain/day
5	8 (17)	26 (30)	48 (44)
10	15 (28)	30 (47)	52 (65)
15	22 (38)	33 (58)	56 (81)

[a]Roy (1970b).

[b]Values in parentheses were calculated from the estimates of DE requirements given in Table 10-11, assume that energy was supplied as cows' milk.

analyses (Duncan, 1966). The discrepancy between the two methods decreases as the dietary protein concentration increases (Walker and Norton, 1971a).

Cows' milk is the usual feed given to calves and lambs reared artificially. Thus, the protein intake of these young animals is controlled by their intake of energy. The ratio of digestible protein energy to total DE in cows' milk is about 0.28 (assuming a protein content of 0.285 in the DM, an apparent digestibility of protein of 0.963 and of energy, 0.982), and it is likely that, when milk intake is limited so that liveweight gains are low, protein is present in excess relative to energy and will be deaminated as a source of energy. Blaxter and Wood (1951) calculated the percentage of the total DE (in a liquid diet for a calf weighing 30 kg) that must be present as protein to avoid the necessity to deaminate dietary protein to meet energy requirements. These values are given in Table 10-14 together with a similar estimate for a lamb weighing 10 kg. It is apparent that the dietary protein requirements of the preruminant are not constant/ unit of energy intake. The requirement will, in fact, be affected by factors which include: (a) liveweight; (b) liveweight gain; (c) protein concentration of the diet and (d) the source and quality of the dietary protein. It would appear from the values given in Table 10-14 that the protein requirement/unit of energy intake increases with an increase in energy intake. Black and Griffiths (1975) suggest that for lambs this conclusion is true only for light-weight lambs, and that as lambs approach maturity the opposite situation is found, reflecting "the change in the partition of ME intake during growth between protein synthesis and lipogenesis as animals become heavier." The same situation may apply to calves reared on milk for veal production.

Table 10-15 gives an example of the effect of variation in the dietary protein concentration on the utilization of energy and protein and on liveweight gain. This table illustrates the important effect of the dietary protein concentration on the composition of the liveweight gain, an aspect that was discussed previously in the section on body composition.

Amino Acid Requirements and Supplementation

When preruminants are fed on milk, the true digestibility of protein is nearly 100%. When the GE intake is 2-3X the maintenance requirement (for energy equilibrium), the absorbed N has a biological value of 70-80 (Blaxter and Wood, 1952; Walker and Norton, 1971a). Nevertheless, it can be shown that the utilization of cows' milk proteins can be improved in both calves (Robert, 1971) and lambs (Walker and Kirk, 1975) by the addition of methionine and, in some cases,

Table 10-14. Estimates of the percentage of the total digestible dietary energy that must be present as protein in order to avoid deamination of dietary protein to meet energy requirements (uncorrected for losses in digestion and metabolism).

CALF, 30 kg live weight		LAMB, 10 kg live weight	
Gain in weight, g/day	Estimate[a]	Gain in weight, g/day	Estimate[b]
0	6.9	0	9.1
100	10.7	50	11.6
200	13.5	100	14.4
400	17.1	150	16.1
800	21.1	200	17.7
1000	22.2	300	19.3

[a] Blaxter and Wood (1951b); [b] Calculated from Norton et al (1970); Walker and Norton (1971a).

Table 10-15. The effect of variation in the dietary protein concentration on the daily performance of a lamb weighing 5 kg.[a]

Item	Protein, % of dry matter		
	12.0	28.5	45.5
Gross energy intake, MJ	3.39	3.39	3.39
Digestible energy intake, MJ	3.22	3.33	3.33
Metabolizable energy intake, MJ	3.20	3.20	3.20
Energy retention, MJ	1.13	1.31	1.03
Gross energy requirement for energy equilibrium, MJ	1.82	1.44	1.72
Nitrogen intake, g	2.3	6.5	10.4
Nitrogen retention (comparative slaughter), g	0.7	3.9	4.4
Nitrogen balance, g	1.2	4.4	4.6
Proportion of total N retained in wool, %	34	18	14
Liveweight gain, g	87	149	146
Empty body weight gain, g	63	135	135
Fat retention, g	27	20	10
Efficiency of gross energy retention, %	33	39	30
Efficiency of energy retention above maintenance, %	72	67	62
Energy retained, MJ/100 g live weight gain	1.30	0.88	0.71
Energy retained, MJ/100 g empty bodyweight gain	1.79	0.97	0.76

[a] Adapted from Walker and Norton (1970).

by lysine, also. The importance of the balance of amino acids in the diets of pigs, poultry and other monogastric animals is well recognized, and estimates of requirements for individual essential amino acids have been made. There is as yet little comparable information for preruminants. Downes (1961) has suggested that the tissues of sheep probably require the same amino acids as those regarded as essential for growing rats, with the exception of arginine which can be synthesized by sheep. In the adult ruminant these tissue requirements for amino acids may be largely satisfied by microbial synthesis in the rumen, whereas the preruminant animal is as dependent on the quality of dietary protein as any other monogastric animal (Blaxter and Wood, 1952). It is only within recent years that attempts have been made to assess the requirements of preruminants for selected amino acids (Patureau-Mirand et al, 1973; Tzeng, 1974; Williams and Smith, 1975; Walker and Kirk, 1975b; Foldager et al, 1977). The techniques used have been those developed with monogastric species, but as yet these studies are in their infancy and no estimates of requirements for a wide range of amino acids can be given. Carpenter (1971) has summarized some of the problems in formulating simple recommended allowances of amino acids for farm animals. He points out that requirements for amino acids are most safely tied to energy intake. The importance of nutrient-to-energy ratios has long been recognized and, although frequently discussed, as for example by Hegsted (1959) and Crampton (1964) is, even now, not fully implemented in statements of dietary requirements.

A further aspect of importance in considering amino acid requirements has been explored by Young and Zamora (1968), who have drawn attention to the importance of the ratio of essential to dispensable amino acids in the diets of rats. Dove et al (1977) have recently studied this aspect of amino acid nutrition with preruminant lambs. They showed that if the ratio differs from that found in milk proteins (approximately 1:1) then liveweight gain is adversely affected. Rogers and Egan (1975) have also shown that preruminant lambs are sensitive to a dietary amino acid imbalance, in a manner analagous to that found in other simple-stomached animals, and that deletion of a specific amino acid from the diet is associated with a depression in food intake.

Utilization of Non-Protein Nitrogen

The classical experiments of Rose and his colleagues (Rose et al, 1949; Rose and Dekker, 1956) on the utilization of non-protein nitrogen (NPN) with rats, showed conclusively that the monogastric animal can utilize NPN to synthesize dispensible amino acids under certain clearly defined conditions. These conditions can be summarized as follows: (1) the diet must supply adequate nonprotein energy and should contain the essential amino acids in amounts sufficient to satisfy the minimum requirements of the animal, or a minimum amount of protein balanced in its content of essential amino acids; (2) the source of NPN is not of great importance and simple ammonium compounds can be utilized. However, excess amounts of single amino acids will unbalance the ration, and the requirement for essential amino acids may change when NPN is added to a low-protein diet; (3) the utilization of some sources of NPN, such as urea, is dependent upon microbial breakdown in the alimentary tract, since it is generally assumed that urease is not present in the body tissues. However, Fitzgerald (1950) has reported that there is some urease activity in the liver and kidney, but there are considerable species differences in activity; (4) the ratio between essential and dispensible N is of paramount importance.

Paduceva et al (1967) have provided evidence with preruminant lambs that NPN may be incorporated into body tissues in some circumstances. At the present time NPN is not used in the diet of preruminants for the following reasons: (1) to demonstrate the utilization of NPN the diet must contain the minimum requirements for essential amino acids (and these are not known), and the diet must be deficient in dispensible amino acids; (2) milk proteins, and most other sources of proteins that could be used in milk replacers, are imbalanced with respect to the essential amino acids, but the balance between essential and dispensible amino acids would seem to be near the optimum; (3) many sources of NPN, e.g. diammonium citrate, ammonium chloride, glycine, are not well accepted in any quantity in milk replacers, while glutamic acid is of low solubility. Urea is well tolerated in a liquid diet by lambs but, up to the present time, it has not been possible to demonstrate its utilization in diets containing high quality protein (author's unpublished observations).

Water Requirements

Cow and goat milks contain about 87% water and ewes' milk about 81%; under normal circumstances it is not necessary to provide extra water for preruminants obtaining all their nutrients from milk. However, when milk replacers are given that contain different concentrations of energy and protein in the DM, with different intakes of salt, and when the preruminants are reared in high environmental temperatures, then extra water should be provided (Roy, 1970b). Cow and ewe milks provide 7.0 and 4.4 kg water/kg DM, respectively, or on an energy basis, 30 and 17g water/100 KJ. Pettyjohn et al (1963) fed calves on milk replacers that contained 5, 10, 15, 20 or 25% dry matter, with water available free choice. The total intakes of water were 18.7, 9.4, 6.4, 5.0 and 4.6 kg/kg DM (100, 50, 34, 26 and 24 g water/100 KJ GE; or 1.06, 0.67, 0.53, 0.43 and 0.42 kg water/kg $^{0.75}$/day). Although the GE intakes increased with an increase in milk DM concentration (1.06, 1.33, 1.56, 1.60 and 1.71 MJ/kg$^{0.75}$ /day), the liveweight gains did not increase in proportion (29, 37, 44, 33 and 37 g/kg$^{0.75}$ /day). It was not possible to conclude that the reduction in liveweight gain at the higher milk DM concentrations was attributable to the reduction in total water intake. There were no data on energy retention, gut fill or body composition at the end of the experiment. N retention values were of no value in determining whether the composition of the liveweight gain differed between groups.

Large (1965) fed lambs on cows' milk, reconstituted to contain 10, 15, 20 or 25% DM, and measured total water intakes of 0.52, 0.36, 0.27 and 0.28 kg/kg $^{0.75}$/day. There were no significant differences in liveweight gain between groups or in DM intake, though a linear trend was observed towards higher DM intakes with increasing DM concentration. Molenat and Theriez (1974) observed a reduction in DM intake if lambs were given a milk replacer with a DM concentration of 10%, compared with diets containing 16, 22 or 28%.

It would seem that preruminants consume milk replacers of widely varying DM concentrations in amounts sufficient to meet their energy requirements. The consumption of additional water may be appreciable if the

DM concentration of the milk replacer is increased. In the experiments of Pettyjohn et al (1963) with calves, the additional water contributed 1.9, 9.0, 17.0, 34.9 and 52.4% to the total water consumption, as the DM concentration of the milk replacer increased from 5 to 25%. Comparable values for the lambs in the experiments of Large (1965) were 0, 0.6, 4.4 and 21.8% for milk replacers with DM concentrations of 10, 15, 20 and 25%. On the basis of these two experiments the water requirement of calves is about 0.5 kg/kg$^{0.75}$/day and of lambs, about 0.3 kg/kg$^{0.75}$/day.

NUTRIENT DEFICIENCIES

The preruminant animal is vulnerable to nutrient deficiencies both pre- and postnatally. In the prenatal period the nutrient supply to the fetus is controlled, not only by the concentration of nutrients in the maternal circulation but also by the selective permeability of the placenta. Any imperfections in the nutrient supply will be reflected in the impaired development of the fetus, leading to an increase in abortions and stillbirths and in the number of abnormal and weak animals born at full term.

Postnatally, the preruminant is dependent on colostrum, and subsequently on milk to supply nearly all the nutrients required for normal growth and development during the first 2-3 weeks of life. Energy reserves at birth are small and, in the absence of food, give only a temporary reprieve from death by starvation. Other nutrient reserves may also be small and, in some cases, inadequate. Thus, colostrum and milk must meet not only the day to day requirements but must also permit a reserve to be built up to protect against future inadequacies in nutrient supply.

There is a high correlation between the intake of milk and liveweight gains for all preruminants. Thus, if the supply of milk to the young animal is limited in early postnatal life, growth rate is reduced. Although undernutrition leads to retardation of development, the period of underfeeding may be as long as 13 months in the sheep without having a permanent stunting effect (Allden, 1968). If the intake of energy from milk is sufficient for normal liveweight gains, then deficiencies of protein, carbohydrate and the major minerals (Ca, P) cannot occur. However, if milk replacers are fed, then diets that are deficient in protein or carbohydrate may be prepared inadvertently.

A protein deficiency reduces the rate of liveweight gain and can lead to changes in body composition (cf. Table 10-15). A diet low in protein and devoid of carbohydrate leads to death (Gibney and Walker, 1978). However, it has been shown experimentally with preruminant goats that carbohydrate-free diets can be tolerated and that growth is normal if the protein content of the diet is similar to that of ruminant milk (Tanabe and Kameoka, 1976).

An adequate intake of Ca and P without sufficient vitamin D leads to bone disorders (see Ch. 4). Conversely, a diet containing adequate vitamin D, but with insufficient Ca or P can also lead to abnormal skeletal development (Benzie et al, 1960). Milk itself has a low content of vitamin D that may need supplementing, especially during winter in the longer latitudes or in those circumstances where preruminants are reared without access to sunlight. Milk also has a low content of Mg that may be insufficient to prevent the onset of a true Mg deficiency (Blaxter et al, 1954). In calves this is recognized by convulsions, frothing at the mouth, profuse salivation, and by a retraction of the head (see Ch. 4) in many ways reminiscent of a thiamin deficiency. Na and K deficiencies are unlikely to occur unless the losses of these elements are severe, as in animals with diarrhea (Blaxter and Wood, 1953).

The concentrations in milk of trace element cations such as Fe, Mn, Cu and Co are under physiological control and are little affected by variation in dietary intake (Ashton et al, 1977). The concentrations of I and F, on the other hand, are more easily affected (Ling et al, 1961). While the concentrations of these minor elements in milk may be insufficient for normal growth when milk is the sole source of nutrients, supplementation with the salts of copper must proceed with caution, since lambs in particular are most easily poisoned by excess copper (see Ch. 5).

The concentrations of vitamins A and E in milk are related to the concentrations in the diet of the dam, whereas the amount of vitamin D is proportional to the fat content of the milk, to the concentration in the diet and to the exposure of the dam to sunlight. Milk is a relatively poor source of vitamin K and the concentration is unaffected by the dietary supply.

The vitamins of the B complex that are present in ruminant milk are mainly synthesized in the rumen. Their concentrations in

274

milk show little variation and are relatively unaffected by fluctuations in dietary supply. Ruminant colostrum is generally much richer in the fat-soluble vitamins than milk, but the relationship between the content of the water-soluble vitamins in colostrum and milk is more variable. Although the reserves of the water-soluble vitamins in the newborn are small, the content in milk is normally adequate to meet the requirements for growth. Nevertheless, since microbial activity in the rumen is absent in the preruminant, a deficiency of vitamins of the B complex can occur if milk replacers are given that are inadequately supplemented. Examples of deficient animals are shown in Fig. 10-1, 2, 3.

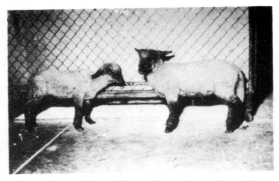

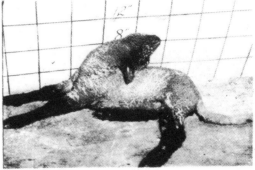

Fig. 10-2. B-complex vitamin deficiencies in lambs. Top, lamb which is deficient in folic acid. Note lack of growth compared to control. Bottom, lamb deficient in thiamin. Note the retracted head, a symptom typical of thiamin deficiency in other species. U. of Illinois photos.

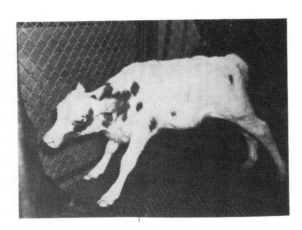

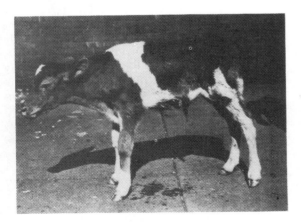

Fig. 10-1. B complex vitamin deficiencies in calves. Top. Thiamin deficiency. Calf shows incoordination and was unable to stand unless its feet were supported. Bottom. Riboflavin deficient calf showing excessive lacrimation and a moist condition of the naval area. University of Illinois photos courtesy of B.C. Johnson.

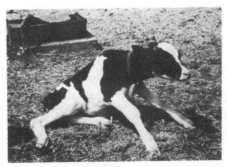

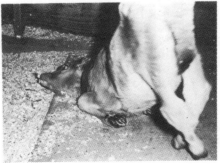

Fig. 10-3. Calves with multiple vitamin deficiencies. The calf at the top has ataxia of the rear legs while the lower one has ataxia of the forelegs. Courtesy of M. Ronning, U. of California.

Vitamin C is synthesized in the body tissues and need not be added as a dietary supplement (Wiese et al, 1947), while there is no evidence that the content of vitamin K in milk is insufficient to meet the requirements of the preruminant, or that supplements of inositol or p-aminobenzoic acid are required. An increased requirement for vitamin E has been reported in calves given liquid diets containing small amounts of highly unsaturated fatty acids as, for example, in cod liver oil (Blaxter et al, 1952). Muscular dystrophy, or white muscle disease, in calves and lambs is scarcely distinguishable from the congenital conditions caused by a maternal selenium deficiency, but may also result from a vitamin E deficiency (see Ch. 5).

Table 10-16 shows a comparison between the suggested dietary allowance of vitamins in a milk replacer given to a calf weighing 40 kg and the amounts supplied by whole milk when fed to give a gain of 1 kg/day. It is apparent that milk supplies the requirements of the calf with the exception of vitamin B_{12}, where the level in milk may be marginal, and vitamin E, where the presence of unsaturated fat in a milk replacer may increase the requirement. The supply of niacin in whole milk will be adequate, since there is sufficient tryptophan in the dietary protein to allow some conversion to niacin.

Table 10-16. Comparison between suggested dietary allowances for vitamins in a synthetic diet for a calf weighing 40 kg and the amounts of vitamins supplied by whole milk when liveweight gain is 1 kg per day.

Vitamin	Suggested dietary allowance/ day[a]	Intake[b] when given 7.5 l whole milk to gain 1 kg/day
Vitamin A, IU	1680	7500-11,250
Vitamin D, IU	160	135-173
Vitamin E, mg	2.8-2.4	5.3
Thiamin, mg	2.6	3.0
Riboflavin, mg	1.4-1.8	11.3
Niacin, mg	10.4	6
Pyridoxine, mg	2.6	3.9
Biotin, mg	0.08	0.15
Pantothenic acid, mg	7.8	26.3
Choline, mg	1038	975
Vitamin B_{12}, μg	17.6-35.2	22.5

[a] Huber and Thomas (1967). [b] Calculated from digestible energy requirement (Table 10-11) and milk composition values (Table 10-1).

There is no doubt that preruminants require a dietary supply of B complex vitamins. Experiments with calves and lambs using synthetic milk diets have demonstrated the need for thiamin, riboflavin, niacin, pyridoxine, biotin, pantothenic acid, choline and vitamin B_{12}. Some illustrations of the effects of deficiencies of vitamins of the B complex on preruminants are shown in Figs. 10-1, 2, 3.

COMPARATIVE NUTRITION OF PRERUMINANTS

The quantitative data on which to base a comparison of the efficiencies of utilization of nutrients by different preruminant species are sparse and, for the majority of species, totally absent. Thus, any discussion of differences and similarities in nutrient utilization between species must be based on isolated observations from different laboratories, rather than on direct comparisons made in the same laboratory. Hodge (1974) has recently compared the relative efficiencies of baby pigs and lambs given the same diet. No similar comparisons are available for the common preruminants, with the exception of those observations based on feeding cows' milk to calves and lambs in different laboratories. When comparisons are made on the basis of equal metabolic body weight, the similarities between the species outweigh the differences (cf. Table 10-17).

The milks of the ox, sheep and goat are similar in composition when compared on the basis of the relative contributions of protein, fat and carbohydrate to total milk energy. Nevertheless, minor differences in composition do exist, though at present it is not known whether the differences have any nutritional significance. A few examples are given without any attempt to speculate on their importance to individual species.

The first example is concerned with the composition of the main protein in milk, namely casein. This protein contributes some 80% to the total protein in the milks of the ox, sheep and goat. Casein is made up of a number of components that can be separated electrophoretically. The components are designated α, β, γ, etc., in order of decreasing mobility. In cows' milk the distribution is 75% α, 22% β, and 3% γ (Hipp et al, 1952), whereas Dovey and Campbell (1952) report that in goats' milk casein, there are equal parts of α and β with a small amount of γ. There are also differences in the amino acid compositions of the main casein fractions, in their isoelectric points, and in their content of P. Since these differences in composition may affect the quality of the curd formed in the abomasum, they may, in turn, affect the rate of digestion.

A second example of a species difference relates to the pigmentation of the fat depots by the carotenoids. This pigmentation is found only in the fatty tissues of the calf and not in those of the lamb or goat. The explanation lies either in the ability of the calf to absorb carotenoids unchanged or in the more efficient conversion of carotene to vitamin A by sheep and goats. In all three preruminant species a proportion of the dietary carotene is converted to vitamin A in the wall of the small intestine, though it should be pointed out that carotenoids do not represent a normal dietary ingredient for preruminant lambs and goats, since the milk fats of the sheep and goat are almost devoid of carotenoids. Once again, the significance of this difference between species is not known.

Goats' milk is a very poor source of folates when compared with cows' milk, and the circulating plasma levels of folate in the young goat are much smaller than those of the calf (Ford et al, 1972). However, there is at present no evidence of a higher incidence of folate deficiency in the goat kid than in the calf.

In conclusion, it would seem that there is as yet too little evidence to indicate whether the nutrient requirements of the various preruminant species are different, once adjustment has been made to a common base of comparison, such as metabolic body size (Kleiber, 1975).

The preruminant animal can adapt to a wide variety of proteins and fats as alternatives to milk protein and butter fat, but is limited to glucose, galactose and lactose as major sources of carbohydrate. The body composition of the growing animal can be manipulated by changes in the protein content of the diet but, on any one diet and within the same species and breed, body composition is mainly dependent on body weight. Energy requirements for maintenance and liveweight gain of calves and lambs are similar when expressed per unit of metabolic weight ($kg^{0.75}$), while the protein and energy components of cows' milk are digested and utilized with the same efficiency by both species. There is little quantitative information on the requirements for amino acids; the utilization of nonprotein nitrogen (e.g. urea) is negligible under practical conditions. Water requirements of calves and lambs appear to range between 0.3-0.5 $kg/kg^{0.75}$/day. Although the preruminant animal is as susceptible to deficiencies of amino acids, vitamins and minerals as the young non-ruminant, a diet of cows' milk, when given in amounts near to *ad libitum*, will provide sufficient of the majority of nutrients required for rapid growth with certain well-documented exceptions. There is as yet too little evidence to support the contention that the nutrient requirements of the common preruminant species are different, once an adjustment has been made to a common base of comparison, e.g. metabolic body weight.

Table 10-17. A comparison of the performance of preruminant calves and lambs fed on cows' milk.[a]

Item	Calf	Lamb
Liveweight, kg	40	10
Gross energy intake, MJ/$kg^{0.75}$/day	1.26	1.26
Metabolizable energy intake, MJ/$kg^{0.75}$/day	1.19	1.19
Liveweight gain, g/$kg^{0.75}$/day	47	56
Apparent digestibility coefficients:		
Dry matter	0.983	0.980
Crude protein	0.963	0.963
Fat	0.989	0.973
Endogenous urinary nitrogen, mg/$kg^{0.75}$/day	194	178
Metabolic fecal nitrogen, g/100 g dry matter intake	0.19	0.20
Apparently digested nitrogen retained, %	69.2	69.1
Net efficiency of metabolizable energy utilization, %	66	65
Basal heat production, MJ/$kg^{0.75}$/day	0.43	0.43

[a] Values determined from data of Blaxter and Wood (1951); Roy et al (1964); Roy (1970b); Table 10-10; Walker and Faichney, (1964); Walker and Norton (1971a).

REFERENCES CITED

ARC. 1965. The Nutrient Requirements of Farm Livestock. No. 2. Ruminants. London, H.M. Stationery Office.

Alexander, G. 1974. Ciba Foundation Symposium. No. 27. Size at birth. Elsevier.

Alexander, G., J.W. Bennett and R.T. Gemmell. 1975. J. Physiol. 244:223.

Allden, W.G. 1968. Aust. J. Agr. Res. 19:621.

Allden, W.G. 1970. Nutr. Abstr. Rev. 40:1167.

Appleman, R.D. and F.G. Owen. 1975. J. Dairy Sci. 58:447.

Armsby, H.P. and C.R. Moulton. 1925. The Animal as a Converter of Matter and Energy. A Study of the Role of Livestock in Food Production. Chemical Catalog Company.

Ash, R.W. 1964. J. Physiol. 172:425.

Ashton, W.M., M. Williams and J. Ingleton. 1977. J.Agr. Sci. 88:529.

Ballard, F.J. and I.T. Oliver. 1965. Biochem. J. 95:191.

Benzie, D., et al. 1960. J. Agr. Sci. 54:202.

Black, J.L. and D.A. Griffiths. 1975. Brit. J. Nutr. 33:399.

Black, J.L., G.R. Pearce and D.E. Tribe. 1973. Brit. J. Nutr. 30:45.

Blaxter, K.L. 1952. Brit J. Nutr. 6:12.

Blaxter, K.L. 1962. The Energy Metabolism of Ruminants. Hutchinson Pub. Co., London.

Blaxter, K.L. and H.H. Mitchell. 1948. J. Animal Sci. 7:351.

Blaxter, K.L. and F.W. Wainman. 1964. J. Agr. Sci. 63:113.

Blaxter, K.L. and W.A. Wood. 1951. Brit. J. Nutr. 5:11,55.

Blaxter, K.L. and W.A. Wood. 1952. Brit. J. Nutr. 6:1,56.

Blaxter, K.L. and W.A. Wood. 1953. Vet. Rec. 65:889.

Blaxter, K.L., J.A.F. Rook and A.M. MacDonald. 1954. J. Comp. Pathol. Therap. 64:157.

Blaxter, K.L., P.S. Watts and W.A. Wood. 1952. Brit. J. Nutr. 6:125.

Brisson, G.J., H.M. Cunningham and S.R. Haskell. 1957. Can. J. Animal Sci. 37:157.

Bryant, J.M., C.F. Foreman, N.L. Jacobson and A.D. Mc Gilliard. 1967. J. Dairy Sci. 50:1645.

Butterfield, R.M., E.R. Johnson and W.J. Pryor. 1971. J. Agr. Sci. 76:453.

Carpenter, K.J. 1971. Proc. Nutr. Soc. 30:73.

Chiou, P.W.S. and R.M. Jordan. 1973. J. Animal Sci. 36:597.

Church, D.C. 1975. Digestive Physiology and Nutrition of Ruminants, Vol. 1, 2nd ed. O & B Books, Corvallis, Oregon.

Colvin, B.M. and H.A. Ramsey. 1968. J. Dairy Sci. 51:898.

Colvin, B.M. and H.A. Ramsey. 1969. J. Dairy Sci. 52:270.

Cook, L.J. 1968. M.Sc. Thesis. University of Sydney, Sydney.

Coombe, N.B. and R.C. Siddons. 1973. Brit. J. Nutr. 30:269.

Crampton, E.W. 1964. J. Nutr. 82:353.

Cunningham, H.M., et al. 1958. Can. J. Animal Sci. 38:33.

Davey, A.W.F. 1974. Proc. N.Z. Soc. Anim. Prod. 34:133.

Dodsworth, T.L., et al, 1977. Animal Prod. 25:19.

Dollar, A.M. and J.W.G. Porter. 1957. Nature 179:1299.

Dove, H., G.R. Pearce and D.E. Tribe. 1977. Aust. J. Agr. Res. 28:917.

Dovey, A. and P.N. Campbell. 1952. Nature 169:1014.

Downes, A.M. 1961. Aust. J. Biol. Sci. 14:254.

Duncan, D.L. 1966. In: Recent Advances in Animal Nutrition. Churchill.

Edwards-Webb, J.D. and S.Y. Thompson. 1977. Brit. J. Nutr. 37:431.

Faruque, O. 1968. Ph.D. Thesis. University of Sydney, Sydney.

Fehr, P.M. 1975. In: L'allaitement Artificiel des Agneaux et des Chevreaux. Institut National de la Recherche Agronomique.

Fitzgerald, O. 1950. Biochem. J. 47:ix.

Foldager, J., J.T. Huber and W.G. Bergen. 1977. J. Dairy Sci. 60:1095.

Ford, J.E., G.S. Knaggs, D.N. Salter and K.J. Scott. 1972. Brit. J. Nutr. 27:571.

Gemmell, R.T., A.W. Bell and G. Alexander. 1972. Amer. J. Anat. 133:143.

Gibney, M.J. and D.M. Walker. 1977. Aust. J. Agr. Res. 28:703.

Gibney, M.J. and D.M. Walker. 1978. Aust. J. Agr. Res. 29:133.

Gonzalez-Jimenez, E. and K.L. Blaxter. 1962. Brit. J. Nutr. 16:199.

Gooden, J.M. 1973. Aust. J. Biol. Sci. 26:1189.

Gooden, J.M. and A.K. Lascelles. 1973. Aust. J. Biol. Sci. 26:625.

Gorrill, A.D.L. and J.W.G. Nicholson. 1969. Can. J. Animal Sci. 49:315.

Gorrill, A.D.L. and J.W. Thomas. 1967. J. Nutr. 92:215.

Gorrill, A.D.L. and D.M. Walker. 1974. Can. J. Animal Sci. 54:411.

Graham, N.McC. 1970. In: Fifth Symposium on Energy Metabolism. Juris Druck and Verlag, Zurich.

Graham, N. McC., and T.W. Searle. 1972. J. Agr. Sci. 79:383.

Graham, N. McC., T.W. Searle and D.A. Griffiths. 1974. Aust. J. Agr. Res. 25:957.

Grosskopf, J.F.W. 1965. Onderstepoort J. Vet. Res. 32:153.

Gullickson, T.W., F.C. Fountaine and J.B. Fitch. 1942. J. Dairy Sci. 25:117.

Haecker, T.L. 1920. Minnesota Agr. Expt. Sta. Bul. 193.

Hardy, R.N. 1970. In: Physiology of Digestion and Metabolism in the Ruminant. Oriel Press Limited.

Hegsted, D.M. 1959. Fed. Proc. 18:1130.

Henschel, M.J., W.B. Hill and J.W.G. Porter. 1961. Proc. Nutr. Soc. 20:xl.

Hill, K.J., D.E. Noakes and R.A. Lowe. 1970. In: Physiology of Digestion and Metabolism in the Ruminant. Oriel Press Limited.

Hipp, N.J., M.L. Groves, J.H. Custer and T.L. McMeekin. 1952. J. Dairy Sci. 35:272.

Hodge, R.W. 1974. Brit. J. Nutr. 32:113.

Holmes, C.W., A.W.F. Davey, N.A. McLean and G.C. Jukes. 1975. Proc. N.Z. Soc. Animal Prod. 35:36.

Hopper, J.H., K.E. Gardner and B.C. Johnson. 1954. J. Dairy Sci. 37:431.

Huber, J.T. 1969. J. Dairy Sci. 52:1303.

Huber, J.T. 1975. J. Dairy Sci. 58:441.

Huber, J.T., et al. 1961. J. Dairy Sci. 44:1484.

Huber, J.T. and L.M. Slade. 1967. J. Dairy Sci. 50:1296.

Huber, J.T. and J.W. Thomas. 1967. Symposium on "Digestive Physiology in the young Ruminant with Special Consideration to the Forestomach Bypass Calf" Univ. of Maryland.

Jacobson, N.L. 1969. J. Dairy Sci. 52:1316.

Jagusch, K.T. and R.M. Mitchell. 1971. N.Z. J. Agr. Res. 14:434.

Jagusch, K.T., B.W. Norton and D.M. Walker. 1970. J. Agr. Sci. 75:273.

Johnson, P.T.C. 1972. S.Afr. J. Animal Sci. 2:177.

Kellor, R.L. 1974. J. Amer. Oil Chem. Soc. 51:77A.

Kielanowski, J. 1965. In: Third Symposium on Energy Metabolism. Academic Press, New York.

Kielanowski, J. and L. Lassota. 1960. Zesz. probl. Postep Nauk roln. 22:173.

Kirchgessner, M., H.L. Muller and K.R. Neesse. 1976. In: Seventh Symposium on Energy Metabolism. G. de Bussac, Clermont-Ferrand, France.

Kirk, R.D. 1973. Ph.D. Thesis. University of Sydney, Sydney.

Kleiber, M. 1975. The Fire of Life - An Introduction to Animal Energetics. Robert E. Kreiger Publ. Co.

Langlands, J.P. and H.A. M. Sutherland. 1968. Brit. J. Nutr. 22:217.

Large, R.V. 1965. Animal Prod. 7:325.

Lawlor, M.J., S.P. Hopkins and J.K. Kealy. 1971. Brit. J. Nutr. 26:439.

Ling, E.R., S.K. Kon and J.W.G. Porter. 1961. In: Milk: the Mammary Gland and its Secretion, Vol. 2. Academic Press.

Maluf, N. and D.M. Walker. 1977. Unpublished observations.

Mayes, R.W. and E.R. Ørskov. 1974. Brit. J. Nutr. 32:143.

McCance, R.A. and E.M. Widdowson. 1964. In: Mammalian Protein Metabolism, Vol. 2. Academic Press.

Millward, D.J., P.J. Garlick and P.J. Reeds. 1976. Proc. Nutr. Soc. 35:339.

Molenat, G. and M. Theriez. 1974. Annales de Zootech. 23:491.

Moulton, C.R. 1923. J. Biol. Chem. 57:79.

Mylrea, P.J. 1966. Res. Vet. Sci. 7:333.

Nitsan, Z., R. Volcani, S. Gordin and A. Hasdai. 1971. J. Dairy Sci. 54:1294.

Nitsan, Z., R. Volcani, A. Hasdai and S. Gordin. 1972. J. Dairy Sci. 55:811.

Norton, B.W. 1968. Ph.D. Thesis. University of Sydney, Sydney.

Norton, B.W., K.T. Jagusch and D.M. Walker. 1970. J. Agr. Sci. 75:287.

NRC 1968. Prenatal and Postnatal Mortality in Cattle. Publ. 1685. Nat. Res. Coun., Washington, D.C.

NRC 1971. Nutrient Requirements of Dairy Cattle. Nat. Acad. Sci., Washington, D.C.

Obara, T., M. Kimura-Kobayashi, T. Kobayashi and Y. Watanabe. 1970. Cereal Chem. 47:597.

Ørskov, E.R. and I. McDonald. 1970. In: Fifth Symposium on Energy Metabolism. Juris Druck and Verlag, Zurich.

Owen, J.B. 1974. Roche Information Service.

Paduceva, A.L., T.M. Karatun and V.S. Lekarev. 1967. Dokl. vses. Akad. sel'-khoz Nauk, No. 6:25.

Paruelle, J.L., R. Toullec, P. Patureau-Mirand and C.M. Mathien. 1974. Ann. Zootech. 23:519.

Patureau-Mirand, P., J. Prugnaud and R. Pion. 1973. Ann. Biol. Animale Biochim. Biophys. 13:225.

Pearce, G.R. 1972. Aust. Meat Res. Comm. Rev. No. 6:1.

Penning, P.D., I.M. Penning and T.T. Treacher. 1978. J. Agr. Sci. 90:221.

Pettyjohn, J.D., J.P. Everett and R.D. Mochrie. 1963. J. Dairy Sci. 46:710.

Phillips, D.D. and D. M. Walker. 1977. Unpublished observations.

Porter, J.W.G. 1969. Proc. Nutr. Soc. 28:115.

Rackis, J.J. 1966. Food Tech. 20:1482.

Rackis, J.J. 1974. J. Amer. Oil Chem. Soc. 51:161A.

Radostits, O.M. and J.M. Bell. 1970. Can. J. Animal Sci. 50:405.

Ramsey, H.A., G.H. Wise and S.B. Tove. 1956. J. Dairy Sci. 39:1312.

Raven, A.M. 1970. J. Sci. Food Agr. 21:352.

Raven, A.M. and R.K. Hamilton. 1971. In: Proc. International Milk Replacer Symposium. National Renderers Association.

Raven, A.M. and K.L. Robinson. 1958. Brit. J. Nutr. 12:469

Reid, J.T. et al. 1968. In: Body Composition in Animals and Man. Nat. Res. Coun., Washington, D.C.

Robert, J.C. 1971. In: Proc. International Milk Replacer Symposium. National Renderers Association.

Rogers, Q.R. and A.R. Egan. 1975. Aust. J. Biol. Sci. 28:169.

Rose, W.C. and E.E. Dekker. 1956. J. Biol. Chem. 223:107.

Rose, W.C., L.C. Smith, Womack and M. Shane. 1949. J. Biol. Chem. 181:307.

Roy, J.H.B. 1964. Vet. Rec. 76:511.

Roy, J.H.B. 1970a. The calf; management and feeding, 3d ed. The Pennsylvania State Univ. Press.

Roy, J.H.B. 1970b. The calf; nutrition and health, 3d ed. The Pennsylvania State Univ. Press.

Roy, J.H.B., et al. 1964. Brit. J. Nutr. 18:467.

Roy, J.H.B., K.W.G. Shillam, G.M. Hawkins and J.M. Lang. 1958. Brit. J. Nutr. 12:123.

Roy, J.H.B., K.W.G. Shillam, S.Y. Thompson and D.A. Dawson. 1961. Brit. J. Nutr. 15:541.

Roy, J.H.B. and I.J.F. Stobo. 1975. In: Digestion and Metabolism in the Ruminant. Univ. New England, Armidale

Shelley, H.J. 1969. Proc. Nutr. Soc. 28:42.

Smith, R.E. and B.A. Horwitz. 1969. Physiol. Rev. 49:330.

Smith, R.H. 1964. J. Physiol. 172:305.

Smith, R.H. and J.W. Sissons. 1975. Brit. J. Nutr. 33:329.

Soliman, H.S., E.R. Ørskov, I.M. Mackie and T.L. Dodsworth. 1976. Proc. Nutr. Soc. 35:91A.

Spray, C.M. and E.M. Widdowson. 1950. Brit. J. Nutr. 4:332.

Stokes, G.B. 1968. M.Sc. Thesis. University of Sydney, Sydney.

Stokes, G.B. and D.M. Walker. 1970. Brit. J. Nutr. 24:435.

Tanabe, S. and K. Kameoka. 1976. Brit. J. Nutr. 36:47.

Ternouth, J.H., et al. 1977. Brit. J. Nutr. 37:237.

Theriez, M. 1975. In: L'allaitement Artificiel des Agneaux et des Chevraux. Institut National de la Recherche Agronomique.

Thompson, G.E. and D. McE. Jenkinson. 1970. Res. Vet. Sci. 11:102.

Thomson, W. and F.C. Aitken. 1959. Diet in Relation to Reproduction and the Viability of the Young. Tech. Comm. No. 20. Commonwealth Agricultural Bureaux.

Thorbek, G. and S. Henckel. 1976. In: Seventh Symposium on Energy Metabolism. G. de Bussac, Clermont-Ferrand, France.

Titchen, D.A. and J.C. Newhook. 1975. In: Digestion and Metabolism in the Ruminant. Univ. New England, Armidale.

Toofanian, F., F.W.G. Hill and D.E. Kidder. 1973. Ann. Rech. Vet. 4:57.

Toullec, R. and C.M. Mathieu. 1969. Ann. Biol. Animale Biochim. Biophys. 9:139.

Treacher, T.T. 1973. Vet. Rec. 92:311.

280

Tzeng, D. 1974. Ph.D. Thesis. Univ. Illinois, Urbana-Champaign.

Underwood, E.J. 1977. Trace Elements in Human and Animal Nutrition, 4th ed. Academic Press, New York.

Van Adrichem, P.W.M. and A.M. Frens. 1965. Tijdschr. Diergeneesk. 90:525.

Van Es, A.J.H. 1970. In: Fifth Symposium on Energy Metabolism. Juris Druck and Verlag,Zurich.

Van Es, A.J.H., H.J. Nijkamp, E.J. Van Weerden and K.K. Van Hellemond. 1969. In: Fourth Symposium on Energy Metabolism. Oriel Press, Newcastle Upon Tyne, England.

Van Leeuwen, J.M., H.J. Weide and C.C. Braas. 1969. Versl. landbouwk. Onderz. Ned. No. 732.

Velu, J.G., K.A. Kendall and K.E. Gardner. 1960. J. Dairy Sci. 43:546.

Vermorel, M., J.C. Bouvier, P. Thivend and R. Toullec. 1974. In: Sixth Symposium on Energy Metabolism. Universitat Hohenheim, Germany.

Walker, D.M. 1950. Bul. Animal Behav. No. 8:5.

Walker, D.M. 1959. J. Agr. Sci. 53:374.

Walker, D.M. 1974. In: Sixth Symposium on Energy Metabolism. Universitat Hohenheim, Germany.

Walker, D.M. and G.J. Faichney. 1964. Brit. J. Nutr. 18:187,209.

Walker, D.M. and K.T. Jagusch. 1969. In: Fourth Symposium on Energy Metabolism. Oriel Press, Newcastle Upon Tyne, England.

Walker, D.M. and R.D. Kirk. 1975. Aust. J. Agr. Res. 26:673,1025.

Walker, D.M. and B.W. Norton. 1970. In: Fifth Symposium on Energy Metabolism. Juris Druck and Verlag, Zurich.

Walker, D.M. and B.W. Norton. 1971a. Brit. J. Nutr. 26:15.

Walker, D.M. and B.W. Norton. 1971b. J. Agr. Sci. 77:363.

Walker, D.M. and G.B. Stokes. 1970. Brit. J. Nutr. 24:425.

Wallace, L.R. 1948. J. Agr. Sci. 38:368.

Watson, R.H. and I.G. Jarrett. 1944. Bul. No. 180. CSIRO, Melbourne.

Widdowson, E.M. 1950. Nature 166:626.

Wiese, A.C., B.C. Johnson, H.H. Mitchell and W.B. Nevens. 1947. J. Dairy Sci. 30:87.

Williams, A.P. and R.H. Smith. 1975. Brit. J. Nutr. 33:149.

Young, V.R. and Zamora, J. 1968. J. Nutr. 96:21.

Chapter 11 - Taste, Appetite and Regulation of Energy Balance and Control of Food Intake

PART I. APPETITE: TASTE AND PALATABILITY
By D.C. Church

There has been a great deal of interest in recent years in the various factors affecting feed consumption of ruminants. This is understandable in view of the economic aspects related to feed intake. Since there is a great mass of evidence to show that the gross efficiency of production can be increased considerably in animals producing milk or by those in the feedlot if their consumption can be maintained at a high level without developing problems as a consequence. Secondly, the need for greater economy and efficiency as evidenced by the utilization of more and more by-products and waste products, non-nutritive additives and synthetic nutrients has a bearing because of the need to attain a relatively high level of feed intake with rations which may not always be the most palatable or of the best quality. Thirdly, there is a need for materials to restrict feed consumption, particularly for range animals being fed protein and energy supplements, but also in other situations.

There are numerous research papers and reviews on this subject. One of the better reviews strictly on ruminants is that of Balch and Campling (1962) which also cites a number of earlier reviews. More recently, Longhurst et al (1968), Baumgardt (1969), Baile and Forbes (1974), Baile (1975), Bines (1976) and Journet and Remond (1976) have published reviews. A series of papers were presented in the book edited by Phillipson (1970), and Goatcher and Church (1970c) have presented a review on taste in ruminants. For those interested in information dealing with the physiological mechanisms and chemical senses as related to food intake by animals (most on monogastric species), the author would suggest the books edited by Zotterman (1963) or Kare and Maller (1967).

PALATABILITY AND TASTE

Palatability has been defined as dietary characteristics or conditions which stimulate a selective response by animals. This is,

obviously, not a quantitative measure unless one measures feed intake over a given time span. Palatability is, essentially, a summation of many different factors sensed by the animal, representing stimulation derived from sight, smell, touch and taste as affected by physical and chemical factors, all of which may be modified by physiological or psychological differences in individual animals (Goatcher and Church, 1970c). The effect of these various senses on feed selection or total intake in ruminants has had relatively little attention by scientists interested in feed intake and appetite.

Effect of Sight, Smell and Touch

The effect of sight has not been completely elucidated, although there is some information on it with respect to feed selection. Tribe and Gordon (1949) found that sheep were unable to distinguish between blue and red colors and Smythe (1955) concluded that cattle and sheep are color blind. Wallace and Riggs (1967) found no difference in feed intake by calves when given feed with natural color or when dyed blue, green or red, and Putnam and Richardson (1968) observed that red, green or blue light did not influence eating patterns of steers. Similar results were found by Ivos and Marjanovic (1972) who noted that calves did no better in natural light than in darkness or in alternating periods of darkness and white, red, orange or blue light.

Arnold (1966) has studied grazing habits of sheep wearing "blinkers" over their eyes. The blinkers allowed long distance vision but restricted vision at the point of forage selection. After a number of experiments, he concluded that sight was of importance mainly for orientation of the animal to space. When grazing clover and grass, sheep without blinkers took more clover than grass while sheep with blinkers took more grass than clover. The main differences observed were on tall forage when the blinkered sheep tended to consume more of the tall grass than unblinkered sheep.

Arnold (1966) has also studied the effect of smell, taste and touch in sheep which had the olfactory lobes of the brain removed surgically or the appropriate nerves sectioned. Sheep with all combinations of impaired senses were studied, also. In sheep deprived of smell, Arnold observed that the flowering stems of grasses were not eaten whereas sheep with unimpaired sense of smell readily ate the flowering heads. Impairment of smell reduced intake on 2 plant species and did not increase it statistically on any. The reduced intake of flowering heads applied to a lesser extent when touch was impaired. Impairment of taste alone or touch alone increased intake in some instances and in others decreased intake. Arnold concluded that sense impairment might alter the acceptability ranking of strains or species of plants, but rarely to the extent where regularly acceptable species became highly acceptable. Some of his data are shown in Table 11-1. These data show clearly that the effect of a given sense on intake varies with the plant in question. It would be difficult to predict the effect of any given sense in animals exposed to an unknown plant with the knowledge presently at hand. Krueger et al (1974) have carried out similar studies with sheep in which the sheep were blindfolded or the other senses inhibited with chemicals. They concluded that taste was the most influential sense and that smell was of minor importance. Touch and sight were thought to be related to plant conditions such as succulence and growth form. Simultaneous impairment of these four senses resulted in increased consumption of unpalatable plants, but not in completely random selection.

Table 11-1. Calculated relative digestible organic matter intake by sheep with various senses impaired.[a]

Plant species	Senses Impaired			
	None	Smell	Taste	Touch
P. tuberosa (dry)	100	84	91	78
D. glomerata	100	65	123	118
M. sativa	100	108	80	103
T. repens	100	94	118	91
E. curvula	100	86	161	78

[a] From Arnold (1966)

Table 11-2. Effect of odor contamination on feed intake of sheep.[a]

Compound Added	Change in feed intake, %	
	No choice	Free choice
Butyric acid	10.6	19.9
Amyl acetate	8.0	-13.4
Coumarin	-9.3	16.9
Glycine	-18.8	-15.3
Butanol	0.0	-12.7
Glutamic acid	0.0	11.3

[a] From Arnold (1970)

Arnold (1970) has presented other data showing the effect on feed intake when various odoriferous compounds were added to feed in a no choice situation or in a situation with a choice of a control feed or feed with the additives. His data (Table 11-2) show that odor may have a substantial effect, but the effect may be different if there is a choice of feedstuffs available. On the basis of observation of feeding deer, Longhurst et al (1968) state that smell is the first sense used in selection followed by taste. Willms (1977) agrees with this and points out that deer may initially bite off herbage and then reject it after tasting it; that smell appears to be responsible for initial selection while taste determines the duration and ingestion rate for a particular plant.

Most livestock feeders will have observed different reactions to odors by animals. Some feedstuffs, such as feather meal or dried poultry waste, are objectional to cattle. However, they eventually will eat rations containing these ingredients with no problems and cows can be conditioned to eat forage sprayed with a slurry of manure (Smith, 1973).

Goatcher and Church (1970a) and Crawford and Church (1971) have reported indirect evidence of the effect of smell when comparing the intake of solutions of acetic and butyric acid by sheep and deer. Both deer and sheep reject butyric acid solutions at much lower concentrations than is the case with acetic acid, thus giving some indication that odor may have inhibited intake; there was no indication that pH of the solutions was a factor in this comparison.

In another example where olfactory bulbectomy was performed on sheep, McLaughlin et al (1974) found that bulbectomized sheep, in contrast to control sheep, did not avoid feed adulterated with acetic acid or feed in containers smeared at the top with camphor or iodobenzene. Operated sheep tended to eat more frequently and to eat smaller meals but total energy intake was similar to control sheep.

Taste Studies with Ruminants

Only a moderate amount of research has been done to evaluate taste responses in ruminant species. Most of that published has been carried out using the two-choice preference technique with test chemicals in water. With this procedure animals are offered water and water plus the test compound which is gradually increased or decreased in concentration (Fig. 11-1). While the same procedure can be used with test chemicals in dry feeds, few comparisons are available.

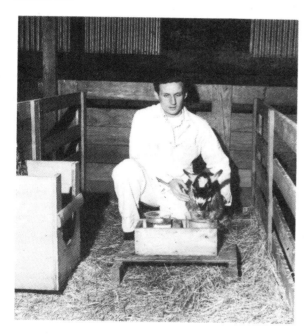

Fig. 11-1. Facilities and equipment used for two-choice preference studies with ruminant species. Former graduate student W.D. Goatcher is shown with a pygmy goat which was used in preference experiments in the author's laboratory.

Animal responses in taste research are notable for the variation between and within animals. Generally, an intake of the test solution between ca. 40 and 60% of total fluid consumed may be described as a zone of non-discrimination. An intake above 60% indicates a preference for the test solution and an intake below 40% indicates rejection. One of the major disadvantages of this tech-

nique is that an animal may be able to detect low concentrations of the test chemical but may not prefer or reject it.

Other reports are available in which the response has been determined by measuring the electrochemical response of nerves when test chemicals have been placed on the tongue of experimental animals (Bernard and Kare, 1961; Bernard, 1964; Bell and Kitchell, 1966). This method is much more sensitive in determining if the taste buds can detect the presence of a test chemical, but it provides no information as to whether the animal likes or dislikes the material.

Published literature on taste response of ruminant species includes the following: goats (Bell, 1959; Goatcher and Church, 1970b; Baile and Martin, 1972; Mehren and Church, 1976, 1977); sheep (Goatcher and Church, 1970a,b; Arnold, 1970; Randall and Church, 1973); cattle (Stubbs and Kare, 1958; Bell and Williams, 1959; Goatcher and Church, 1970b; Weeth and Digesti, 1972; Weeth and Green, 1974; Randall and Church, 1973; Mehren and Church, 1977); and black-tailed deer (Goatcher et al, 1970; Crawford and Church, 1971; Rice and Church, 1974).

Comparative responses for different species (cattle, sheep, normal goats, pygmy goats and black-tailed deer) are shown in Fig. 11-2 through 11-5 for sucrose, acetic acid, NaCl and quinine hydrochloride. This information was derived from papers by Goatcher and Church (1970a,b) and Crawford and Church (1971). The responses of the different species can be summed up as follows.

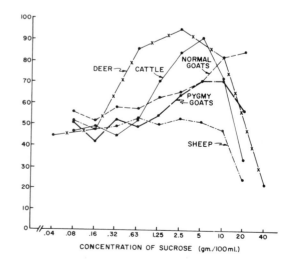

Fig. 11-2. The response of different ruminant species to increasing concentrations of sucrose.

284

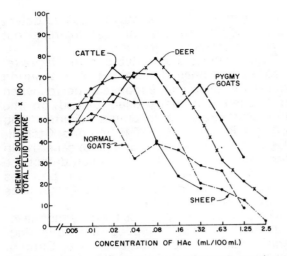

Fig. 11-3. Response of different ruminant species to increasing concentrations of acetic acid.

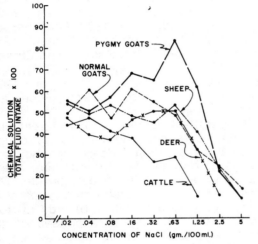

Fig. 11-4. Response of different ruminant species to increasing concentrations of NaCl.

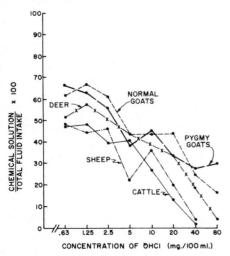

Fig. 11-5. Response of different ruminant species to increasing concentrations of quinine hydrochloride.

Sheep. Sheep generally show only a weak preference for some sweet-tasting compounds (not indicated in Fig. 11-2); some animals show a response to glucose, fructose, sucrose, lactose and maltose but the average response is indifference or rejection. When given a choice of maltose or sucrose, the preference may go either way, depending on the individual; the same applies to a choice of sucrose or glucose. Only a very slight preference is apt to be shown for saccharin solutions. Of all other compounds tested, sheep on the average show no preference for any of them (NaCl, Na acetate, propionate and butyrate; acetic, propionic, butyric, lactic and hydrochloric acids; quinine hydrochloride, urea, ethanol or NaOH). Individual animals may, however, show a weak to moderate preference for a variety of these compounds at relatively low concentrations, particularly for Na acetate, propionate and butyrate (see Goatcher, 1969).

Cattle. Cattle generally show a moderate to strong preference for sucrose or molasses solutions, a moderate response to low concentrations of acetic acid, and reject solutions of NaCl and quinine. An example of the nature of variability sometimes (usually) observed in taste research is shown in Table 11-3. Note the tremendous variation in consumption at a given concentration.

Goats. Normal goats show a moderate to strong preference for sucrose, reject acetic acid at low concentrations, show no preference or a weak preference for NaCl, and a weak preference for low concentrations of quinine hydrochloride.

Table 11-3. Consumption of NaCl solutions by cattle.[a]

Animal No.	NaCl concentration, g/l.			
	0.2	0.8	3.2	12.5
1	49.5	53.5	2.5	2.0
2	42.0	58.0	56.5	2.0
3	49.0	1.5	72.0	10.0
4	22.0	11.5	7.5	12.5
5	65.0	47.5	1.0	2.5
6	66.0	62.5	17.5	6.0
7	10.5	51.5	50.0	43.5
8	51.0	48.0	8.0	1.0
Mean	44.4	41.8	26.8	9.9

[a] From Goatcher (1970); values are expressed as % of test solution of total fluid consumed.

Pygmy Goats. Pygmies show a weak preference for sucrose and acetic acid over a wide range of concentrations, a moderate to strong preference for NaCl and a weak preference for quinine. They are the only species tested which showed a preference for all major taste categories (sweet, salt, sour and bitter).

Deer. Deer show the most pronounced preference for sucrose of any of the species tested; their reaction being moderate to strong over a wide concentration. They also showed a moderate preference for acetic acid over a wide concentration. NaCl was not preferred at any concentration, nor was quinine, on the average.

Other data on deer indicate that deer showed a weak to moderate preference for Na acetate, and little response to butyric or HCl acids. Sex differences were seen in several instances. Buck deer showed a stronger preference for Na acetate than does and bucks showed a weak preference for low concentrations of quinine sulfate and hydrochloride. Sex differences are also quite pronounced for extracts of some browse plants and organic acids common to some plant species (Rice and Church, 1974). Presumably, sex differences would be evidenced in domestic species but very little information is available on this topic. Mehren and Church (1977) have demonstrated differences between immature male and female calves when given a variety of mineral solutions.

The results mentioned on goats compare quite favorably with those of Bell (1959) whose goats showed preferences for quinine, glucose, NaCl and acetic acid. Results of Bell and Williams (1959) on cattle are similar, also (see Goatcher and Church, 1970c, for literature comparisons).

If we wish to compare the response of these various species, one way to do it is to rank them on the basis of the lowest concentration of the test material that will be discriminated (i.e., they show either preference or rejection) and on the basis of tolerance (i.e., greatest concentration taken). Comparisons of this sort are shown in Table 11-4.

To briefly sum up these results, the data indicate that sheep show only a weak preference for sweet, cattle show a preference for sweet and sour (acid), deer show preference for sweet, sour and bitter, and goats or pygmy goats show a preference for sweet, salt, sour and bitter. If an over all ranking were to be made on sensitivity, the order would be: cattle, deer, pygmy goats, normal goats and sheep.

It should be pointed out that the reaction of sheep and cattle to sugar solutions may be affected by the nature of the remaining part of the diet. In the example shown in Table 11-5, lambs and calves were given a choice of 5% sucrose or water and, later, a choice of 20% sucrose or water. The 5% solution is a level usually preferred whereas the 20% solution is usually adverse to both species. In this example, note that sucrose consumption was considerably higher by both lambs and calves when they were fed the alfalfa pellet.

Table 11-4. Relative sensitivity and tolerance of different ruminant species for the major taste categories.

Compound	Rank
Sucrose	
Sensitivity	Deer > cattle > normal goats > pygmy goats > sheep
NaCl	
Sensitivity	Cattle = pygmy goats > sheep = normal goats = deer
Tolerance	Sheep = normal goats = pygmy goats > deer > cattle
Acetic acid	
Sensitivity	Deer = cattle > pygmy goats = normal goats > sheep
Tolerance	Pygmy goats > deer > normal goats > sheep = cattle
Quinine HCl	
Sensitivity	Pygmy goats = normal goats > deer > sheep = cattle
Tolerance	Pygmy goats > normal goats > deer > sheep = cattle

Table 11-5. Effect of ration and sucrose concentration on consumption of sucrose solutions by lambs and calves.[a]

Ration	Sucrose concentration, %[b]			
	5%		20%	
	Lambs	Calves	Lambs	Calves
Alfalfa pellet	98.0	98.4	57.1	73.8
Complete diet pellet[c]	62.3	67.2	21.0	50.5

[a] Data from Randall (1974)
[b] Data expressed as % of total fluid consumption.
[c] Pellet made up of alfalfa, barley, mill run and soybean meal.

Preference for Herbage

Ruminant animals grazing any mixture of plant species always exhibit some preferential selection. If given a choice, they will select their food from a wide variety of plants. Selectivity tends to change from day to day and season to season as the available herbage changes. When there is an abundance of feed, the grazing animal is free to express its preference. As food supply decreases, then animals must eat less acceptable plant material, the result being that animals appear to compromise and eat species neglected previously but they will still spend a high proportion of total grazing time on favored species of low accessibility (Arnold, 1970; Buchanan et al, 1972).

The environment of the grazing animal is complex and many different factors have been identified which may alter preference in a given situation. Essentially, the factors known to affect preference may be animal related or plant related. Since many different things are involved, it is not surprising that there is no single factor which can be used to establish a high correlation with animal preference in variable circumstances. Good, although older reviews on this topic include those of Heady (1964), Arnold (1964, 1970) and Marten (1970).

Plant Factors

Animals may be attracted to one plant because of its acceptable smell, another because of its taste or to another because of its physical characteristics, but the extent to which a given plant is preferred is a reflection of the overall response to favorable and unfavorable chemical and physical characteristics. Since plant tissues are complex,

the primary taste modalities are not adequate to evaluate preference.

Physical characteristics of plants such as spines, awns, hairiness, position of leaves, stickiness, succulence and texture affect palatability and preference. Leaves are generally preferred to stems or flowers. When dried plant material was separated into material primarily leaf or stem and fed singly, Laredo and Minson (1975) found that the leaf fraction was consumed by sheep in larger quantities despite small differences in digestibility (sheep did not have a choice of leaf or stem), but the rate of consumption may have been related to more rapid rumen fermentation as shown by in vitro studies. Plant height affects rate of ingestion and, presumably, preference (Allden and Wittaker, 1970).

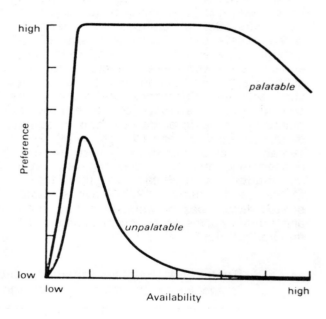

Fig. 11-6. Relationship of preference to availability for palatable and unpalatable plants. Courtesy of W. Willms, Agr. Res. Station, Kamloops, B.C., Canada.

Many studies show that green or young plant material is preferred to dry or old material. Freezing may alter preference as will the amount of dead plant material present in the herbage (Cowlishaw and Alder, 1960).

In addition, preference for a given herbage species depends on the availability of other choices (Fig. 11-6). Observations suggest that some species are grazed heavily when they occur in small quantities throughout a "better" forage, whereas in dense stands the use is light (Heady, 1964).

Most chemical analyses indicate that preferred herbage is usually higher in N, digestible energy, sometimes in P and usually in water-soluble dry matter and water-soluble carbohydrate, characteristics typical of young or immature herbage. Conversely, high fiber and lignin and low crude protein are associated with low preference and these characteristics are typical of mature herbage. The older literature suggests that tannin, coumarins and nitrates probably decrease forage palatability. In studies with plants with decreased palatability associated with manure, Plice (1952) found that the affected plants were higher in protein, Ca, K, Fe, fat, nitrates and vitamins. Unaffected plants were higher in Si, Al, P, tannin, Cl and sugars. When sugar was added to the affected plants, they were eaten readily. However, Marten and Donker (1964) observed that heavy P fertilization did not overcome unpalatability of brome grass treated with manure nor did heavy applications of N affect palatability.

In other studies Jones and Barnes (1967) found correlations between the concentration of non-volatile organic acids found in ryegrass and cocksfoot to preference rankings by cattle and sheep to be: shikimic, 0.81; quinic, 0.84; and citric, 0.78. Arnold (1970) mentions data from his laboratory, stating that solutions of succinic acid were acceptable to sheep over a wide range of concentration (0.01-0.5%) and that acotinic acid was acceptable over a narrow range (0.01-0.04%), but he did not define what was meant by acceptable.

In other work Rabas et al (1970) found that grazing preferences of both cattle and sheep for Sudan grass varieties were negatively correlated with HCN concentration but total sugar concentration was never directly associated with palatability. With Reed canary grass Marten et al (1976) found a high negative correlation between alkaloid content and palatability for sheep.

In studies with acid solutions in water, Rice and Church (1974) noted that buck black-tailed deer showed preferences for weak solutions of citric, malic, quinic and succinic acids. Does did not show preferences for any of these acids. With extracts from various woody plants utilized by deer, high preferences were shown by bucks for extracts of Douglas fir, Western hemlock, red alder and bitterbrush; does showed high preference for Douglas fir, Cascara and Western hemlock. Other information shows that palatability for deer of various browse species is negatively related to inhibitory effect of volatiles on rumen fermentation—the least palatable are the most inhibitory (Longhurst et al, 1968).

Coppock et al (1974) have published data on dairy cows given choices of corn silage and hay crop silage, hay and hay crop silage or corn silage and hay. They found that cows were relatively consistent in their choice of forage after the first week, but selection by different animals varied considerably. When permitted to consume hay, cows consume slightly larger amounts of total forage although hay was not the preferred forage. In other studies with silages, preference was related to low levels of amines, particularly tyramine and histamine, and aldehydes but higher levels of keto acids (Neumark et al, 1964).

Many studies show that fertilization may increase palatability. Fertilization with N often increases size of cells without proportionate increase in cell wall material so that the plants are more succulent. Fertilization that increases the plant content of K or P may result in more acceptable plants (Heady, 1964). In cafeteria feeding trials with hay fertilized with N, P or K, Reid and Jung (1965) observed that the first preference was for hay fertilized with P and the second was for hay with a low level of N while hay fertilized with higher N levels was often rejected. Correlations between preference and carbohydrates, N and mineral content were low. Other observations show that climate, soil type and fertility, and topography may result in altered preferences.

Numerous studies have shown high correlations between voluntary consumption of herbage and in vitro or in vivo digestion or various measures of quality such as high protein and low lignin, neutral detergent fiber, acid detergent fiber and to a high content of pepsin-soluble dry matter and to a reduction in energy required to grind dry samples in the laboratory (Laredo and Minson, 1975). However, in most instances, these studies are not a measure of preference as much as a reflection of rapid digestion in the reticulo-rumen and an increased passage rate, which, in turn, allow the animal to eat more.

Animal Factors

Numerous animal factors have been related to preference and palatability. Langlands (1969) has reported differences in the N content of the diet of grazing sheep for breed, age and previous history and Heady (1964) points out that differences have been observed in selection for preferred foods from location to location, season to season, over a few days and within the same day. The tremendous individual differences observed in taste have been mentioned previously as have sex differences in deer and bovines.

Forage preferences have also been related to pregnancy, fatness, lactation and hunger (Heady, 1964), although McManus et al (1968) did not find any differences in grazing, dry, pregnant and lactating ewes. Hunger causes animals to eat more rapidly and, no doubt, to be less selective. Certainly, there is ample evidence to show increased consumption as need is increased (i.e., lactating vs dry animals), but quantitative data are very scarce which show true differences in preference.

Previous experience (exposure) of grazing animals is certainly a factor in selectivity. In one study using sheep with different experiences, Arnold (1964) found that differences in selection of generally liked species disappeared after a short period of time but differences in acceptability of generally disliked species persisted until the sheep were forced to graze exclusively on the species for at least a month. He also noted that this type of animal reaction might occur in sheep that were 3 mo. of age. Krueger (1974) observed that yearling sheep, which had never been on a summer range, consumed more grass as well as plants unpalatable to older sheep during the first day. As adaptation occurred, they consumed more leaves but less stems and flowers. On the other hand, Longhurst et al (1968) state that young deer, without previous access to range forage, consumed the same proportions of plants in a cafeteria trial as older wild deer.

Effect of Acids on Palatability

It has been known for some time that consumption of dry matter is usually less when forage is given as silage as compared to hay. When acetic acid was added to grass silage, Hutchinson and Wilkins (1971) found some changes in feeding patterns of sheep but total consumption was not altered. McLeod et al (1970) demonstrated that the addition of $NaHCO_3$ to grass silage increased silage consumption (10-20%) when the pH was increased from ca. 4 to 5.4. If lactic acid was added and pH reduced from 5.4 to 3.8, dry matter consumption was reduced 22%. In other work with mineral acids, L'Estrange and Murphy (1972) fed 320 mequiv/kg of HCl, HCl-H_2SO_4. The HCl or the mixture reduced feed consumption by 19% and the H_2SO_4 by 30%. In another study (L'Estrange and McNamara, 1975) HCl was mixed with grass pellets with or without an equivalent amount of $NaHCO_3$ given intraruminally or when HCl was given intraruminally with untreated pellets. At a low level of HCl, food intake was reduced by 17% and this was not altered by giving $NaHCO_3$ intraruminally, but HCl given intraruminally did not reduce feed intake. At a high level of HCl supplementation (560 mmol/kg DM), feed consumption was reduced ca. 40% by each method and $NaHCO_3$ did not appreciably affect food intake although it prevented metabolic acidosis. Thus, they concluded that the adverse effects were due to a reduction in palatability associated with low dietary pH. In further work from this laboratory (Morgan and L'Estrange, 1976), cattle and sheep were fed pelleted grass meal with two levels of lactic or HCl acids. Dietary pH was reduced to 4.2 and 4.0 with the lactic acid and 4.4 and 3.8 with HCl. Feed intake by cattle was reduced 3.4 and 6.6% with the lactic acid and 22.4 and 33.8% with HCl. With sheep, corresponding values were 15.8 and 13.3% for lactic and 13 and 28.6% for HCl.

Table 11-6. Molar concentrations and pH at which sheep rejected different acids given in water solutions.[a]

Acid	Concentration, mmol.	pH
Acetic	28	3.4
Butyric	5.7	4.7
Propionic	3.9	4.2
Lactic	9.7	3.0
HCl	2.2	2.9

[a] From Goatcher and Church (1970a).

Studies with acids in water solutions indicate that pH is not the only factor causing rejection by sheep (Goatcher and Church, 1970a). Data in Table 11-6 show substantial differences between different acids. Smell may be a factor in addition to taste and pH.

Effect of Minerals on Palatability

The older literature shows little relationship between mineral composition and palatability (Ivins, 1952). More recently, Reid and Jung (1965) have shown some preference by sheep when fed fescue hay fertilized with P, and Ozanne and Howes (1971) found that sheep preferentially grazed dry clover residues fertilized with P. Less difference was noted during the grazing season. Gordon et al (1954) could not demonstrate a preference by P-deficient cattle for a Ca-P supplement as compared to limestone. Sodium-deficient animals, however, tend to select herbage species high in sodium (Arnold, 1964). Rees and Minson (1976) have demonstrated that Ca fertilization increased the Ca content of Pangola grass and voluntary intake was increased as was digestibility, but feeding a Ca supplement had no effect on either.

When comparing preference of different mineral supplements, Kercher (1968) found that cows preferred bonemeal-salt over any other mixture. Sodium tripoly phosphate was rated as 18% and dicalcium phosphate-salt as 7% of the relative palatability of the bonemeal-salt mixture. In other studies Coppock et al (1972, 1976) found that lactating dairy cows did not appear to have a specific appetite for Ca or P when fed a diet low in Ca and P and given a chance to eat dicalcium phosphate. Similarly, Crawford et al (1977) found that bulls did not consume enough of either $CaCO_3$ or $CaSO_4$ to meet Ca needs when fed a Ca-deficient diet.

In studies with minerals in solution, Weeth and Digesti (1972) observed that the sulfate ion is less palatable to cattle than the Cl ion. Boron water was also shown to be relatively unpalatable by Weeth and Green (1974). In studies with Na salts in water solution, Mehren and Church (1977) found that male calves showed weak preferences for the Cl, CO_3, HCO_3 and HPO_4 ions. Female calves showed a preference for only the HCO_3 and SO_4. With different Cl salts, male calves showed a very weak preference for NH_4 and female calves showed a preference for Na and Mn. When given a choice of NaCl or $NaHCO_3$, males preferred the Cl at 0.32% and females at 0.32 and 1.25%. Given a choice of NaCl or Na_2SO_4, no preference

was shown for the sulfate. With a choice of NaCl or Na_2HPO_4, the Cl was preferred by males and the phosphate was preferred by females at higher concentrations (0.64-1.25%). These studies show that preferences depend on the choices available and on the sex of the animal. No doubt differences in dry rations also affect choice of chemicals in water solution.

Flavoring Ingredients

With respect to published data dealing with addition of flavoring components to feedstuffs or rations, several older papers are available which show that consumption may be improved by the addition of molasses or sugars although the effect may be slight or transitory (Balch and Campling, 1962). Miller et al (1958) found that the addition of anise or imitation anise oils depressed intake of starter feeds by calves. Wing (1961) found that a commercial flavoring mixture increased the intake of a starter feed by most calves from 0-90 days of age but Thomas et al (1961) did not observe any effect on silage consumption. More recently Craplet and Merlu (1970) have reported that fenugreek stimulated greater consumption of phosphate supplements by dairy cows, but Dash et al (1972) concluded that leptaden (extract of *Leptadenia reticulata* and *Breynia patens*) did not stimulate feed consumption when added to standard rations nor did a commercial feed flavor product when added to a dairy ration containing rapeseed meal (Ingalls and Sharma, 1975). In studies with sheep, Clapperton (1969) observed that sheep were eager to eat a ration with linseed oil fatty acids added (consumption increased 40%) but they were reluctant to eat the basal ration when branched-chain fatty acids were added (consumption reduced 20%). It might be noted that numerous materials have been promoted to stimulate intake over the years but very little unbiased research information is available to substantiate the claims.

Taste Modifiers

Threre is little doubt that taste sensations of humans can be modified by some compounds (see Goatcher and Church, 1970c) or preferences can be changed in experimental animals. Three of these compounds include monosodium glutamate, gynemic acid and inosinic acid. Studies with pygmy goats (Mehren and Church, 1976) demonstrated that monosodium glutamate reduced the response to high levels (adversive) of sucrose, had no effect on low levels and reduced the response to quinine (adversive). Gynemic acid also reduced the response to adversive levels of glucose (tastes less sweet?) as well as to a low level of quinine and inosinic acid enhanced the response to a low level of quinine (more bitter?). Perhaps other organic or inorganic chemicals may be effective in altering taste in ruminants as they do in humans (Goatcher and Church, 1970b). Baile and Martin (1972) have demonstrated that a local anesthetic (carbocaine) increased the taste threshold for quinine and acetic acid but had no apparent effect on salt.

Preferences for Concentrates

There is quite a bit of literature dealing with grazing studies which show preferences for one or the other forage or forages at different stages of maturity, etc. However, there are only a few scattered reports illustrating preferences for concentrate feeds, other than information relating to feed processing methods.

Table 11-7. Diet preferences of artificially reared lambs.[a]

Feed	Age of lambs, days		
	28-32	40-44	52-56
	Consumption, % of total		
Soybean meal	34.3	26.5	23.4
Commercial pellet, LE*	19.3	19.2	21.5
Commercial pellet, HE*	15.8	16.7	18.2
Barley, rolled	5.3	19.0	14.4
Beet pulp	7.9	8.3	7.0
Fish meal	13.4	2.9	1.5
Corn, flaked	1.3	3.6	9.5
Oats, whole	2.7	3.7	4.5

[a]From Davies et al (1974); * Low and high energy, respectively.

With regard to sheep, Davies et al (1974) gave young lambs a choice of 8 different feed ingredients at different ages (Table 11-7). In this study the young lambs showed a decreasing preference for soybean meal and fish meal and an increasing preference for rolled barley and flaked corn with minor changes in other ingredients. In another study with older lambs fed a variety of different pelleted feed ingredients, it was determined that the relative preferences were: alfalfa > soybean meal = beet pulp > corn > cull peas = barley = wheat = wheat mill run (Goatcher and Church, 1969).

In studies with cattle, Ray and Drake (1959) fed corn, milo or oats as whole, coarse grind, fine grind, pelleted and reground pellets along with hay. No direct comparison was made between the grains,

Table 11-8. Effect of feed preparation on selection of cereal grains by calves.[a]

Preparation	Grain[b]		
	Corn	Milo	Oats
Whole	25	30	32
Coarse grind	26	23	31
Fine grind	25	11	17
Pelleted	17	26	15
Ground pellet	7	10	5

[a]Data from Ray and Drake (1959). Calves given a choice of test grain and hay.
[b]% of total grain consumption.

Table 11-9. Effect of feed preparation method on selection of cereal grains by black-tailed deer.[a]

Preparation	Grain[b]		
	Corn	Barley	Oats
Pelleted	63.0	63.4	79.5
Rolled	17.8	16.3	---
Whole	---	---	---
Alfalfa pellets	20.3	20.3	20.5

[a]Data from Dean and Church (1972).
[b]% of total diet.

only between methods of feed preparation. As the results show (Table 11-8), the type of feed preparation had more influence on some grains than on others. In another study, Ray et al (1975) gave inexperienced cattle a choice of alfalfa or Bermuda grass hay, rolled milo or barley and cottonseed meal pellets. Consumption ranged as follows: alfalfa hay, 10-18%; Bermudagrass hay, 5-7%; milo, 16-26%, barley 48-65%, and cottonseed meal, 1-4% of total feed.

In studies with captive black-tailed deer, it has been demonstrated that feed preparation has a more marked effect than with sheep or cattle (Dean and Church, 1972). Note in Table 11-9 that the deer highly preferred pelleted corn, barley or oats; they ate some rolled corn and barley, but refused rolled oats or whole seeds of any of these three grains. When given choices of different feed ingredients, data indicated that the deer preferred corn, wheat and soybean meal; barley and oats were selected in limited amounts, but beet pulp, cottonseed meal, linseed meal and cull peas were rejected if the deer were not forced to consume them.

PART II. REGULATION OF ENERGY BALANCE AND CONTROL OF FOOD INTAKE

By Clifton A. Baile

Introduction

Feeding behavior has been studied intensively partly because the important health problem of obesity in people has long been associated with improper control of eating behavior (Bray, 1976). While this work has generated many hypotheses, there remain many unanswered questions on the control of feeding and the incidence of obesity by and large remains unchecked as a result of the high proportion of therapeutic failures—presumably due to inadequate understanding of the basic control systems. The following includes discussion of the regulation of energy balance and the control of feed intake. Other reviews of this area include ones by Campling (1970), Baumgardt (1970), Baile and Forbes (1974) and Baile (1975; in press).

Many characteristics must be considered in studying control of feed intake of ruminants. For example, domesticated ruminants for generations have been selected for various characteristics, and much of their anatomy and many of their physiological functions may have been altered. One must ask how selection for enhanced mammary gland function of dairy cows has affected a basic regulatory function such as energy balance. Again, the genetic selection for beef production and early fattening conceivably may depend on changes in hypothalamic control of behavior and energy utilization. Therefore, results of experiments on the control of feed intake of domesticated ruminants may not be applicable to ruminants in a natural state.

In this discussion *roughage* is used to identify a feed, usually consisting of plant stems and leaves, with at least 20% fibrous materials. *Concentrate* feeds are usually plant seeds having a fiber content of <10%. *Energy balance* is the difference between energy of feed eaten and metabolizable total energy output (Blaxter, 1962). Energy balance is taken to be a condition that possibly is regulated so that a certain balance is preserved. Feed intake, on the other hand, is assumed to be a controlled function having the nature of an "on" or "off" response.

Hunger is a physiological and psychological state resulting in the initiation of feeding; *satiety*, the opposite state, results in the termination of feeding. *Appetite* is used to describe a specific hunger drive and is not used here in the more general sense.

Because the central nervous system (CNS) or psychic control of complex behaviors, gastrointestinal physiology, and the metabolic state of animals all play critical roles in the regulation of energy balance, the area is difficult to study and many questions remain unanswered. The following describes some of the present thinking about the control systems and the interrelationships of the regulator for energy balance and the controller of feeding behavior and finally some means for chemical modification of the basic systems.

ENERGY BALANCE REGULATION

Many species of mature animals, including man, maintain a relatively constant body weight and energy content even with large energy expenditure changes due to increased or decreased physiological and/or environmental demands. Other species, including hibernators, have physiological mechanisms which permit large increased energy storage followed by complete dependence on tissue mobilization for support of vital functions for sustained periods (Mrosovsky and Powley, 1977; Le Maho, 1977). Ruminants generally eat regularly through all seasons of the year, where possible, and although many dietary changes may occur, a ruminal microbial population is maintained; ruminants are not well suited to the sustained fasts that true hibernators exhibit due to the problems of maintenance of an appropriate microbial population and the re-inoculation required upon refeeding.

In general, mature domesticated ruminants have the physiological mechanisms for defending an energy balance. Growing animals also adjust their nutrient intake resulting in a constant rate of growth even though many conditions are changed. Even small but sustained errors in this apparent regulatory system can result in detrimental obesity, inefficient production, or emaciation. All of these conditions may compromise the animal's defense against metabolic disorders and infectious diseases. The concept of energy balance regulation is not supported in a number of situations in ruminants. Because the nutrient supply is dependent on feeding behavior and associated drives, various factors, e.g. sensory cues, can override apparent inhibitors resulting in fat deposition above the norm. In contrast, nutritional imbalances or deficiencies, pathological conditions, metabolic disorders, or digestible energy dilute diets can all result in sustained tissue mobilization and subsequent apparent maintenance of partially depleted fat stores. Therefore, the apparent energy balance regulator has limitations, but a preponderance of evidence supports the concept of energy balance regulation as illustrated in the following discussion.

Responses to Changes of Heat Exchange with Environment

Heat stress causes reduced feed intake and general performance. Continuous heat stress may reduce feed intake to such an extent that a negative energy balance results and ruminants may not eat at all when a climatic temperature of 40°C is maintained (Ragsdale et al, 1950; Appleman and Delouche, 1958). Although the critical temperatures or environmental conditions at which growth or lactation are reduced by heat stress vary with species and breeds within a species, animals have a relatively uniform production rate and efficiency over a range of conditions. Under severe cold conditions, which cause increased heat loss, feed intake increases and efficiency of production is reduced (Moose et al, 1969; Aimes and Brink, 1977). Deer, on the other hand, are known to adapt to cold environmental stress by reducing physical activity and thus reducing energy expenditure (see Ch. 15, Vol. 3).

The animal's covering of hair or wool provides insulation, reducing changes in rate of heat loss to the environment (see Ch. 8 and 16). When sheep are shorn, heat loss increases under some environmental conditions, and an increase in metabolic rate occurs in order to maintain body temperature. An increase in feed intake follows, and energy balance is maintained. The greater the heat loss, the greater the increase in feed intake after shearing.

Another way of showing the influence of heat balance on feeding is by direct heating or cooling of internal organs. Increasing the temperature of rumen contents in cattle from the normal 38.0° to 41.3°C with heating coils in the rumen depressed intake by 15% (Gengler et al, 1970). Decreasing the temperature of the rumen by adding sufficient cold water (5°C) resulted in a decrease in body temperature and increased intake by 24%, although addition of warm water (49°C) did not depress intake in the same experiment (Bhattacharya and Warner, 1968). Heat-stressed cattle eat more when given cold water to drink.

Effects of Lactation

Lactating ruminants increase their energy intake in response to the demands for milk synthesis, but this increase typically lags behind the increase in milk yield. Energy expenditure in high-producing dairy cows may rise to 3X the maintenance requirement. In some species several weeks may be required for the correction, i.e., feed intake adjustments for increased or decreased demands on energy pools. Lactating cows eat more than their non-lactating controls and feed intake and rate of milk production are positively correlated. Ewes also increase feed intake during lactation. While the increased intake can occur in ruminants, it is not always apparent unless their feed is calorically concentrated to a sufficient degree (Bull et al, 1976).

Effects of Diet Dilution

Several species of animals tested (e.g., rodents, dogs, pigs and chickens) have been shown to compensate for dilution of diet with indigestible materials. A variety of diluents can be used: water, which is easily absorbed; kaolin, which is indigestible and not absorbed; or materials like straw, which contain some digestible material but lower overall digestibility of the diet. The diluent changes not only the DE density of the diet but usually also the taste, texture, odor, and quite likely the fermentation process.

Dry matter intakes of sheep, calves, and heifers are not affected by the addition of water unless the dilutions are extreme. Sheep compensated for adjustments in digestibility ranging from 54 to 80% when ground straw or hay was used as a diluent of concentrate feeds (Montgomery and Baumgardt, 1965; Owen et al, 1969). Sheep compensated for the addition of sawdust, kaolin or verxite to concentrate feeds when the DE

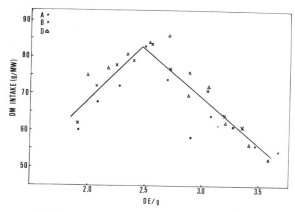

Fig. 11-7. Dry matter intake (g/body wt^0.75) of sheep fed a basal concentrate mixture diluted from 5 to 50% at 5% increments with each of 3 diluents: A, oak sawdust; B, oak sawdust with constant 3% kaolin clay; D, same as A, except N was kept constant at 17.4% crude protein. Dry matter intake increased as DE of rations increased to 2.47 Kcal/g and then declined. From Dinius and Baumgardt (1970).

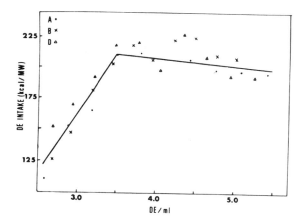

Fig. 11-8. DE intake (Kcal/body wt^0.75) of sheep fed rations varying in energy content as described in fig. 11-7. DE intake increased as DE of rations increased to 2.49 Kcal/g and remained nearly constant. From Dinius and Baumgardt (1970).

concentration was greater than approximately 2.5 Kcal/g in adults or 4.0 Kcal/g in young growing sheep (Fig. 11-7, 11-8; Dinius and Baumgardt, 1970). In other experiments responses of growing wethers were compared with those of lactating ewes fed diets of different alfalfa-concentrate ratios with a range of 2.2 to 3.5 Kcal/g of DE. The plateau for the average DE intake/unit of metabolic mass (kg^0.75) per day of the diets was 255 Kcal for growing wethers and 416 Kcal for lactating ewes (Clancy et al, 1976). The relationship of the bulk caloric density and

DE intake for the two groups of sheep in these studies is shown in Fig. 11-9. These data show that sheep can compensate for caloric dilution over a wide range and still maintain a relatively constant DE intake. In other experiments sheep did not adjust for caloric dilution; this may be related to form and composition of the diets (Andrews and Ørskov, 1970).

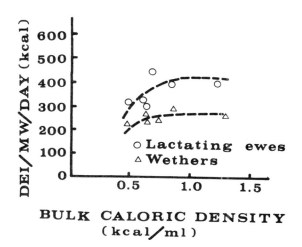

BULK CALORIC DENSITY
(kcal/ml)

Fig. 11-9. Relationship between DE intake (Kcal DE intake/mw/day) and bulk caloric density (Kcal/ml) of six forage-concentrate diets fed to sheep in two physiological states. From Clancy et al (1976).

Another illustration of the energy balance regulatory capabilities of sheep is the response to a nutrient solution injected intra-abomasally in growing lambs (Fig. 11-10; Weston, 1971). Sheep receiving the nutrient solution ate less, but growth rate remained nearly the same. Thus, addition of the nutrient supply which bypassed the fermentation processes lowered voluntary intake, but total ME supply and growth remained equal to that of sheep injected with a water solution containing no nutrients.

Growing cattle maintained a relatively constant DE intake and growth rate when roughages were used as dilutents in concentrate feed (Baile and Forbes, 1974). While this compensation for the dilutions was greater when ground roughages were fed, when diets with >30% of unground roughages were fed, cattle generally adjusted to a lower DE intake and growth rate, even though feed intakes were increased.

Cattle also maintained a relatively constant ME intake and growth rate when protein encapsulated tallow or vegetable oil was

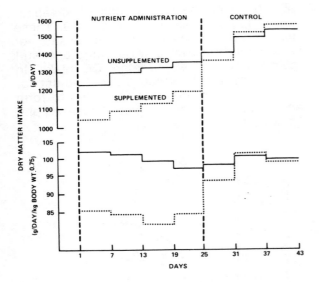

Fig. 11-10. Mean daily dry matter intakes of 2 groups of lambs during (1) a period of nutrient administration when one group (supplemented) received nutrient solution per abomasum and the other (unsupplemented) received water per abomasum and (2) a control period when no solutions were administered (n = 16 for each group). From Weston (1971).

added to a basal diet even though the estimated NE$_m$and NE$_g$ were increased up to 15 and 30%, respectively (Garrett et al, 1976). The feed additive monensin results in a more efficient rumen fermentation of dietary substrates (Richardson et al, 1976) and a more efficiently used intermediate metabolite composite for maintenance and tissue synthesis. Although initial adjustment to monensin frequently involves substantially reduced feed intakes, with concentrate rations over sustained feeding periods cattle maintain a relatively constant average daily gain and reduced average daily feed intake, resulting in improved feed efficiency (Fig. 11-11; Raun et al, 1976). The sustained reduced feed intake which occurs when monensin is added to a concentrate ration may very well be the result of a regulatory system for the maintenance of energy balance in growing cattle.

The most comprehensive set of observations on the relationship between the availability of energy from feeds and intake by dairy cows was reported by Conrad et al (1964). They analyzed data from 114 digestion trials which included rations varying from all roughage (50% dry matter digestibility) to all concentrate (80% dry matter digestibility). Although a number of assumptions were made in accounting for between-

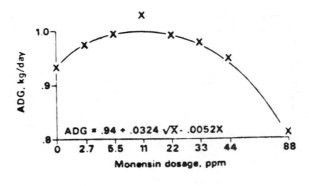

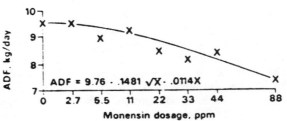

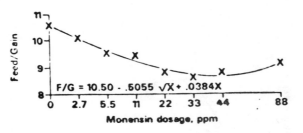

Fig. 11-11. Effect of monensin on average daily gain, feed intake, and feed efficiency of cattle. Data are plotted against the square root of monensin dosage in ppm. From Raun et al (1976).

cow variation, it was demonstrated clearly that lactating cows compensated for dilution of DE if the digestibility of dry matter of the feed was above ca. 67% (Fig. 11-12). Below this level of digestibility, DE intake declined as digestibility declined. This value (67%) has sometimes been given undue significance as an exact point above which energy balance can be maintained by ruminants. Conrad et al (1964) pointed out that this was applicable only for their conditions; they calculated that for higher yielding cows (28 kg fat-corrected milk/day) feed intake would not be controlled by nutrient requirements except when dry matter digestibility was several percentage points higher than the 67% calculated for cows of moderate yield (17 kg fat-corrected milk/day).

The relationship between level of milk production and minimum caloric density of diets fed to dairy cows shows that the greater the production the more dense the

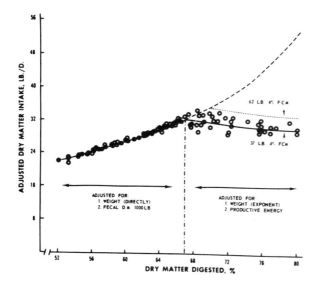

Fig. 11-12. Relationship of dry matter digestibility to adjusted feed intake at 2 levels of milk production of lactating dairy cows based on 114 trials. In a multiple regression analysis, digestibility, fecal dry matter/454 kg body weight/day and body weight accounted for variation in feed intake of mostly roughage diets between 52 and 66% digestibility, r = 0.997 (P < 0.1), while digestibility, metabolic mass and productive energy accounted for most variation in feed intake of diets between 67 and 80%. From Conrad et al (1964).

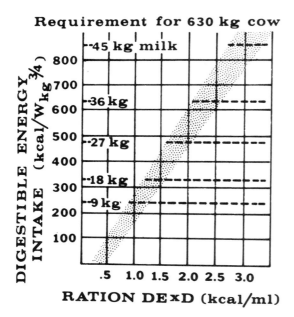

Fig. 11-13. Relationship in lactating dairy cows between caloric density (Kcal DE/ml) and DE intake (Kcal/day/kg$^{0.75}$ body weight) and the rate of milk production. From Bull et al (1976).

required diet (Fig. 11-13; Bull et al, 1976). These examples show that lactating cows, like sheep and growing cattle, can control intake to maintain constant DE intake as long as the diet has a DE concentration above the "critical" point, which is variable depending on the physiological demands for substrate.

Additional Evidence of Energy Balance Regulation

Dietary record, prestudy-period adjustments in body weight and production rates and either tissue or milk synthesis must be considered in assessing the evidence for energy balance regulation. An analysis of the pattern of energy expenditure and feed intake of dairy cows by Montiero (1972) illustrates these relationships. With application of several control theory concepts, the following equation was developed for predicting feed intake on a specific day of the lactation period:

$$F_t = \beta W_t + \alpha M_t + \gamma \sum_{i=1}^{t} (B_{t-i+1} - B_{t-i})$$
$$(1 - \omega^i) - \rho \sum_{i=1}^{t} (M_{t-i+1} - M_{t-i}) \Theta^i.$$

The feed intake of day "t", for example day 100 of a lactation period, is the sum of the partial function of; present body weight (W_t) where β is the maintenance requirement per unit weight; milk production for the day (M_t) corrected for the conversion factor for feed to milk (α); changes in daily body weight following parturition corrected for the conversion factor of feed into gain (γ) and the delay parameter for gain or loss (ω); and the negative of changes in daily milk production following parturition corrected for the effect of change of milk yield on feed intake (ρ) and the delay in time of a response in feed intake to a given change in milk yield (Θ). Thus, feed intake is dependent both upon the relationships at time "t" of milk yield, maintenance requirement (a function of body weight), rate of gain or loss, and on delays in response to previous changes in both milk yield and gain. Basic to Montiero's closed-loop system is the concept of time delays in the response of the animal to correct a disturbance in energy balance. This dampens the responses of an imprecise control of meal size to yield a more precise regulation of body energy content over a period of time. Therefore, to predict energy intake of an organism on any one day, knowledge of energy demands of the past as well as the present are required. Montiero's equation does not attempt to account for

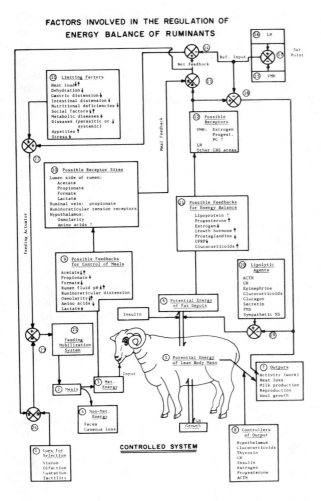

FACTORS INVOLVED IN THE REGULATION OF
ENERGY BALANCE OF RUMINANTS

and the effects of varying the concentration of available energy in the diet show that, in general, ruminants tend to maintain a constant energy balance by changing feed intake in proportion to their altered physiological and environmental circumstances. Figure 11-14 illustrates a number of the interrelationships between factors involved in control of feeding behavior and regulation of energy balance. Although increases in energy losses cause increased feed intake, this may not be the result of a direct action on feeding but of an indirect effect on the energy balance regulator. In the next sections factors involved in this control of feeding behavior are discussed. There are, however, some factors which prevent the animal from achieving energy equilibrium such as dilution of the diet with indigestible material (see Fig. 11-14, Box 21), and these also are discussed later.

FEEDBACKS FOR ENERGY BALANCE REGULATION

Although ruminants, like other mammals, regulate energy balance under certain conditions, it is not clear what component(s) of the energy content of the body is regulated. Body heat represents a very small part of the total body energy and is controlled to maintain a fairly constant body temperature by a system that acts, in many ways, independently of the energy balance regulating system. Changes in body temperature or heat flux may affect feed intake, but it is unlikely that feed intake is regulated primarily in order to maintain a constant body temperature. Long-term exposure to cold environmental temperatures may well affect feeding through changes in body depots, i.e. fat. A great part of the energy stored in the body of normal animals is in the form of fat, and there is circumstantial evidence that energy intake is controlled so as to maintain a constant body fat content (Kennedy, 1953). As discussed in previous reviews, a number of experiments indicate that some "norm" of fat depot is maintained in rodents (Baile, 1971; Mrosovsky and Powley, 1977).

Lipostasis

The possible influence of fat deposition on energy balance regulation in ruminants is not well understood. Because of genetic selection for certain traits, the "finish" that is at least in part related to fatness varies between

Fig. 11-14. Scheme illustrating some interrelationships of a regulatory system of energy balance with special emphasis on control of feed intake. Although the scheme is especially applicable to ruminants, many of the interrelationships are applicable to energy balance regulation of monogastric animals. Factors for a hunger-satiety system probably differ greatly between species and within species under various environmental, physiological and nutritional conditions. Arrows in box # 9, 11 and 21 indicate each factor's probable effect on feeding behavior. Symbols ⊗ denote comparators of signal inputs. Abbreviations used are FMS, fat-mobilizing substance; LH, lateral hypothalamus; VMH, ventromedial hypothalamus; UFRP, unidentified factor in ruminant plasma. From Baile and Forbes (1974).

environmental or nutritional stresses on the animal's regulated system which could limit availability of energy for the demands for milk yield and body gain.

The effects of varying energy requirements of the animal by changing its output of heat, deposition of body tissue, or yield of milk species and breeds of ruminants. These differences may be the result of changes in the level at which fat depots are regulated. There is evidence that fat ruminants, like rodents, eat less than thin ones and are perhaps regulating their fat depots (Baile and Forbes, 1974). One explanation given for this reduced intake by fat ruminants is that the enlarged fat depots physically limit gastrointestinal capacity (Forbes, 1970). This explanation implies that the physical outward expansion of the abdominal cavity is limited. However, Bines et al (1969) showed that fat cows fed hay and concentrate ate less than thin cows, although the observation that the ruminal digesta load was similar in the two groups both before and after their daily feeding period implies that intake was not limited by the physical capacity of the rumen. Apparently fat cows and sheep can increase their intake during lactation so that milk production is at least equal to that of lean cows. Therefore, at least with concentrated feeds, some factor(s) other than physical volume of fat must be acting to regulate energy balance.

Humoral Factors Involved in Energy Balance Regulation

If one accepts the concept that a CNS center controls energy balance and feed intake, then information on the state of body energy reserves must be transmitted to this central controlling area either by way of blood-borne substances or by the nervous system. The blood from hungry donor rats has elicited increased feed intake of satiated recipient rats. The active "satiety factor" first appears in blood of rats about 6 hr after feeding has been resumed following a fast and may be at maximal titre only after 18 to 24 hr of ad lib feeding (Davis et al, 1971). More recent work supports the contention that an energy balance regulator component and not just a hunger-satiety factor may be involved; blood exchange with obese and lean pairs caused intake of the deprived member of the pair to decrease or increase, respectively (King, 1976).

Experiments by Seoane et al (1972) lend support for a humoral factor. In sheep, as with rats, intake of a hungry member of a pair could be reduced by blood exchanges with a satiated member. In addition and perhaps more notably, satiated sheep began feeding during blood exchange with hungry sheep. In these studies, blood of the pairs was nearly equally mixed by the end of a one-hour exchange when a pump rate of 50 to 75 ml/min was used.

The sites of the receptors that are affected by these apparent hunger and satiety factors are unknown. The possibility certainly exists that the receptors are in the CNS, and furthermore, it is conceivable that a humoral factor acting on the CNS could involve the cerebrospinal fluid (CSF) as a transfer medium. CSF apparently plays an important role in various animal behaviors and physiological responses. In fact, CSF from sheep fasted 24 hr increased feed intake of satiated sheep when either 1.0 or 0.5 ml of CSF was injected into a lateral or third ventricle, respectively (Martin et al, 1973).

Certainly there must be a link between the lipid depots and the central nervous system, and quite likely it is a humoral factor. However, the nature of the factor remains nearly as obscure as when Kennedy (1953) first proposed the lipostatic mechanism.

CONTROL OF FEEDING BEHAVIOR

Although the smallest units of feeding are individual bites, a more easily studied unit of feeding behavior is the meal. Some sensory and metabolic stimuli affect feeding by changing meal frequency, while others affect feeding by changing meal size. Factors affecting meal size in animals fed ad lib may not be the same as those in animals adapted to a feeding schedule. While meals are obviously of different sizes, the amount eaten in some continuum of meals must be controlled to maintain energy balance. Signals of satiety which control meal size must change during the course of a meal and must have short time constants compared with the signals that regulate long-term energy balance. Although many physiological functions change as a consequence of feeding and may be considered possible satiety factors, only a few appear to have an influence in controlling meal size.

Analysis of Feeding Behavior

In most mammals studied, feeding is a composite of meals. Meals are not always discrete entities but must be defined in such a way as to account for most feeding behavior. Generally, three criteria are used to define meals: minimum amount eaten, maximum time during which the minimum amount must be eaten, and the minimum interval during which no feed is eaten; these criteria determine the initiation and termination of meals and intermeal intervals. Eating that occurs between meals is designated as nibbling.

A variety of systems has been used to study meals and feeding behavior of sheep, goats, beef cattle and dairy cattle (Baile, in press). Examples are given of some of the observations made with these systems.

To describe characteristics of feeding behavior in sheep, computer programs were developed for analyzing feeding behavior using data collected for several weeks for individuals and groups of sheep (Baile, 1975; Baldwin et al, 1977). Almost no correlation was found between meal size and either pre- or post-meal interval of sheep eating a 60% concentrate meal ration. In other analyses of feeding behavior (Table 11-10), most meals for sheep are from 50 to 200 g, meal duration and the time the sheep's muzzle is in the feeder are highly correlated with meal size, rate of eating is quite variable, and the frequency of raising the muzzle away from the feed for more than 2 seconds (feeding bouts) is also closely related to the meal size. There is some correlation between pre-meal interval and meal size for meals up to 300 g. But there is no correlation between post-meal

interval and meal size. If sheep ate each meal to satisfy a deficit and the degree of deficit were highly correlated to time, duration (min) of pre-meal interval divided by meal size, referred to as a hunger ratio would be nearly constant. Because the hunger ratio (Table 11-10) decreases as meal size increases, it is not apparent that sheep, under laboratory conditions, are eating meals as a result of some deficit, e.g. metabolite change. If sheep were initiating meals because of a return of some set of signals to a level that triggered feeding, then minutes of post-meal interval divided by meal size (satiety ratio) would be nearly constant for different meal sizes. Sheep, under these conditions, had post-meal intervals in proportion to weight eaten. From this work it is not apparent that meal size or intermeal intervals for sheep consuming a 60% concentrate meal diet are controlled with any degree of precision.

Comparisons were made between the feeding behavior of sheep adapted first to a 60% concentrate diet and then to a 76% roughage diet. Since with the concentrate diet meal size was not correlated with either pre-meal or post-meal interval, apparently the sheep would eat any sized meal within the normal range once feeding was initiated.

Table 11-10. Meal analysis of data from 4 days for 8 sheep. Means are shown with SEM. Average daily intake was 1319 ± 69 g of which 1088 ± 58 g was eaten in meals and 230 ± 36 g was eaten in nibbling bouts between meals. From Baile (1975).

	Meal Size range				
	43-99	100-199	200-299	300-399	400
% of total meals[a]	42	34	14	4	5
Meal size (g)	69 ± 1	143 ± 3	240 ± 5	345 ± 11	501 ± 23
Meal length (min)	13 ± 1	29 ± 2	47 ± 4	52 ± 7	61 ± 7
Pre-meal interval (min)	105 ± 20	165 ± 16	218 ± 25	133 ± 35	106 ± 0
Post-meal interval (min)	126 ± 20	150 ± 13	147 ± 17	137 ± 39	199 ± 48
Hunger ratio (min/g)[b]	$1.52 \pm .25$	$1.15 \pm .12$	$.95 \pm .12$	$.39 \pm .0$	$.23 \pm .0$
Satiety ratio (min/g)[c]	$1.92 \pm .50$	$1.04 \pm .10$	$.61 \pm .08$	$.40 \pm .0$	$.40 \pm .09$
No. of feeding pauses	11 ± 2	19 ± 2	30 ± 3	45 ± 9	54 ± 9
Min of actual eating	$5.3 \pm .6$	15.5 ± 1.7	23.5 ± 2.5	28.6 ± 6.0	35.1 ± 4.4
Rate of eating (g/min)	12.1 ± 9.0	9.3 ± 9.4	10.2 ± 1.6	12.1 ± 10.6	14.3 ± 12.6
(Min of actual eating) $\div$ (Meal length)	$.43 \pm .05$	$.52 \pm .03$	$.50 \pm .04$	$.55 \pm .07$	$.57 \pm .06$

[a]Total number of meals analyzed = 202 or an average of 6.1 meals/day/sheep.

[b]Hunger ratio = Pre-meal interval/meal size.

[c]Satiety ratio = Post-meal interval/meal size.

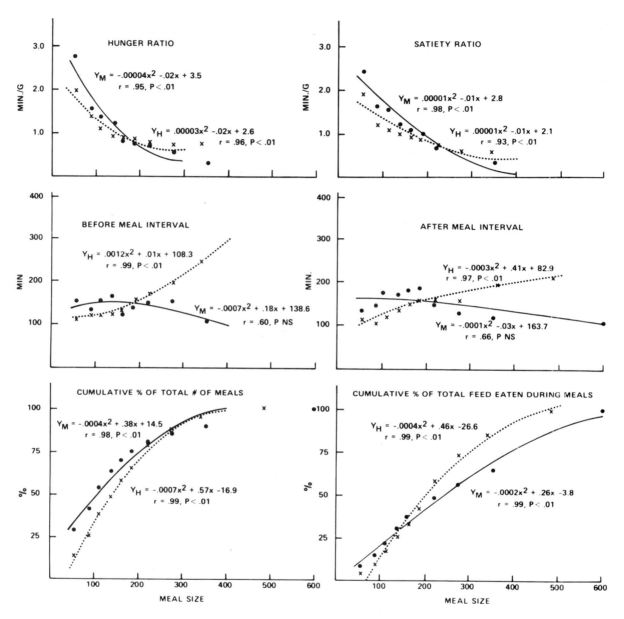

Fig. 11-15. Comparison of analyses of meals for sheep adapted to a 76% ground hay ration (H), n = 9, total of 899 meals or a 60% concentrate ground ration (M), n = 8, total of 714 meals. Per day the sheep ate a mean of 1346 + 91 g of M (1158 ± 99 g in meals and 184 ± 20 g nibbling) and 1487 ± 57 g of H (1327 ± 63 g in meals and 161 ± 15 g as nibbling). The meals were grouped into 10 meal-size intervals, i.e., 40-75 g, 76-100 g, etc.; the regression equations and correlation coefficients represent only the mean responses for the groups of sheep. They ate a greater proportion of smaller meals of M than H as shown by the cumulative % of total numbers of meals and the cumulative % of total feed eaten during meals. The relationship of before-meal intervals and meal size showed that sheep normally had waited 100-150 min before initiating a meal of M and ate meals of any size independent of before-meal interval while sheep fed H normally ate large meals only after greater before-meal intervals. The after meal interval was longer after large meals of H compared with small meals of H. In contrast there was no relationship between meal size and after-meal interval for the M ration. The lack of a constant hunger ratio (before-meal interval ÷ meal size) over the range of meal sizes shows that sheep do not initiate a meal and determine its size by eating to replete some metabolizable energy store. The satiety ratio (after-meal interval ÷ meal size) shows that a gram of feed in a small meal delays the reoccurence of feeding ca. 2 min/g while a large meal only delays reoccurence of feeding 0.5 min/g. From Baile (1975).

In contrast, with the hay diet there was a high correlation between meal size and pre-meal and post-meal interval (Fig. 11-15), indicating that the sheep were restricted from eating a large meal unless substantial time had passed since the last meal; this seems likely to be a restriction associated with a correlate of the bulk of the diet. Neither the hunger ratio nor the satiety ratio was constant over the range of meal sizes for either type of diet (Fig. 11-15). Thus there is no constant relationship between the amount of feed eaten within a meal and the time the animal will wait to eat again. In Table 11-11 are feeding behavior indices of Holstein steers fed a complete 72% concentrate diet (Chase et al, 1976). In a similar study with sheep fed an 80% concentrate diet, the number of meals per day were comparable but the smaller species ate at proportionately slower rates (Wangsness et al, 1976).

Putnam and collaborators found that in lot-fed ruminants about 75% of the time spent in feeding was between 6 am and 6 pm (Putnam et al, 1968). When light cycles were reversed or length of light periods was varied, cattle were at the feeder more during light periods irrespective of time of day. Continuous lighting eliminated most of the diurnal pattern. However, light is probably not essential since cattle adapted to partial

Table 11-11. Feeding behavior of steers fed a complete mixed ration.[a]

Parameter	Mean ± SEM[b]
Number of meals/day	10.0 ± .2
Consumption/day, g	6031 ± 178
Consumption/day/kg BW, g	30.9 ± .6
Consumption/day/kg$^{.75}$ BW, g	114.4 ± 2.3
Overall duration/day, min	221 ± 4
Actual duration/day, min	156 ± 3
Overall eating rates	
g/min	28 ± 1
g/min/kg BW	.14 ± .01
g/min/kg$^{.75}$ BW	.53 ± .01
Actual eating rates	
g/min	38.7 ± 1.0
g/min/kg BW	.20 ± .01
g/min/kg$^{.75}$ BW	.74 ± .01

[a] From Chase et al (1976).

[b] Data within a given day were pooled to give a daily value for that animal. Means represent average of 142 steer days.

or nearly complete darkness maintained similar rates of gain (Bergstrom et al, 1963).

The feeding behavior of grazing animals is not necessarily under the influence of the same stimuli that affect animals under feedlot conditions. Grazing domesticated ruminants, like many wild ruminants (Littlejohn, 1968), show diurnal patterns of feeding which differ depending on the quantity and species of herbage available.

Grazing time can vary widely from a few hours to 15 hr/day. In 24 hr beef cows may graze for 42% of the time during three separate periods and ruminate 37% of the time (Furr, 1963); most of the grazing is during daylight hours. Although sensory stimuli play an important role in grazing behavior, it is not clear if these types of stimuli play a major role in the control of feeding and energy balance (Furr, 1963; Arnold, 1970).

Grazing must be considered to be the natural form of feeding behavior of ruminants and certainly involves behavioral patterns not required of animals in a feedlot or laboratory. Grazing animals have been shown to be capable of selecting a nutritionally adequate diet. By contrast, lot-fed sheep given a choice of dietary components selected an inadequate diet. The diet of grazing animals will vary depending on type of vegetation available, fertility of land, and stage of development of the plants. That green herbage is usually selected in preference to dry is normally nutritionally advantageous. In certain cases, however, animals will selectively graze toxic plants (Arnold, 1970).

FACTORS INFLUENCING FEEDING BEHAVIOR

Sensory Cues

It appears that ruminants use the same sensory cues as other mammals for the selection of feed. It is also quite likely that these cues play a role in initiating a meal, and they are therefore shown in Fig. 11-14, No. 1 as an input influencing meals. It has been postulated that animals are more sensitive to these cues when energy is depleted and less sensitive when they are in a positive energy balance (Jacobs and Sharma, 1969). However, sheep may be most fastidious when nearly satiated and eat almost all plants and all parts of plants when hungry (Tribe, 1952). Whichever response may be important, there is very likely an interaction between sensory inputs and state of energy balance. Therefore, an input to the sensory system is shown from the energy balance and hunger-satiety feedback system in Fig. 11-14.

Although the sensory aspects of feeding are very important in feed selection and under some conditions may influence the quantity eaten, other oropharyngeal factors are probably not very important. Ruminants in which the boli are removed from the rumen continue to eat for much longer periods of time and consume larger quantities of feed than during normal feeding (Campling, 1970). It is unlikely therefore that exhaustion of the salivary glands or fatigue of the jaw muscles limits or acts as a control for feed intake. Also, there is no evidence that a monitoring of the volume of feed swallowed might influence feeding.

Ruminal Distention

There is an increase in the volume of ruminal contents during feeding despite the prandial increase in rate of emptying of the rumen. Campling (1970) has discussed the possibility that the amount eaten at a meal might be limited by the capacity of the rumen. When cattle were offered feed for ca. 6 hr/day, the increase in total weight of digesta in the rumen during this period was 48% (Table 11-12), and the increase in weight of dry matter in the rumen was 96%. The consistency of these results, considering the range of feeds and types of cattle included, supports the concept that, with roughages at least, cattle eat until a certain level of ruminal distention is achieved. This

Table 11-12. Percent increase of digesta and dry matter of ruminal contents of cattle during a daily 6-hr feeding.[a]

Type of food	% Increase of Prefeed		Reference
	Digesta	Dry matter	
Silage	60	93	Campling, 1966
	48	86	Campling, 1966
Hay	107	227	Campling, 1966
	50	116	Campling, 1966
	42	93	Bines et al, 1969
	51	89	Campling et al, 1961
	36	70	Balch and Campling, 1969
	38	76	Campling et al, 1963
Ground hay	34	73	Campling et al, 1963
Dried grass	71	184	Balch and Campling, 1969
Long dried grass	60	152	Campling and Freer, 1966
Ground dried grass	41	127	Campling and Freer, 1966
Concentrate	53	114	Balch and Campling, 1969
Hay and concentrate	51	99	Campling, 1970
Straw	30	52	Bines et al, 1969
	44	49	Campling et al, 1961
	38	49	Campling et al, 1962
Straw and urea	38	65	Campling et al, 1962
Long oat straw	32	61	Campling and Freer, 1966
Ground oat straw	36	58	Campling and Freer, 1966
Ground oat straw and urea	43	81	Campling and Freer, 1966
n	21	21	
Mean ± SEM	48 ± 3.7	96 ± 10.0	

[a] From Baile and Forbes (1974)

level of distention must be considered to be variable, however, and may be acting as a safety valve to prevent distress. In the ruminant stomach there is evidence for tension receptors with various neural adaptation times. These receptors have not yet been identified histologically.

In many experiments the change in feed intake in response to changes in the volume of rumen contents has been investigated. Transfer of ruminal digesta from a donor, intraruminal addition of feed or indigestible material and removal of digesta from the rumen have all resulted in some compensation in feed intake. Campling and Balch (1961) infused 45 kg of water intraruminally during the first 30 min of the 3-4-hr feeding period of cows fed hay. Although this rate of infusion exceeded the probable rate of absorption of water from the rumen, there was no effect on feed intake. Similar results have been obtained with heifers and sheep.

Baile et al (1969), using a system in which water was automatically pumped into the rumen of goats during spontaneous meals, found that intake of concentrate feed was not reduced until the ratio of water injected to feed eaten approached 10:1. In some experiments water was also injected into balloons in the rumen; 45 kg in cows depressed hay intake by 2.4 kg/day (Campling and Balch, 1961), although somewhat smaller quantities had no effect on intake of a pelleted feed. Air-filled balloons left in the rumen for several weeks were at least as effective as those filled with water in depressing intake; thus it appears to be their volume rather than their mass that is important. When water was pumped into balloons in the rumen while goats were eating a concentrate feed and pumped out again when the animals stopped eating, up to 1290 ml/meal had no effect on feeding behavior (Baile et al, 1969). These experiments tested the short-term effect of mass of ruminal digesta and were not designed to measure whether the animals could adapt to even larger changes. Experiments concerned with ruminal adaptation to fill are discussed in a later section.

Rumen Fluid and Body Fluid Osmolarity

Changes in osmolarity of body fluids can influence feeding behavior in monogastric animals, and there is evidence that extreme osmolarity changes can influence feeding of ruminants. Increases in rumen fluid osmolarity from about 250 to 300-350 mOsm that have been observed during the rapid eating of large meals may lead to hypertonicity of body fluids and cause dramatic renal and circulatory changes. For example, Blair-West and Brook (1969) showed that within 15 min of the initiation of rapid feeding sheep suffered from a reduced plasma volume and a rise in systolic blood pressure, probably due to the transfer of Na^+ and water from body fluid to rumen fluid; this change activated the renin-angiotensin system. When even greater increases in rumen fluid osmolarity (to 700 mOsm) were caused by intraruminal injection of NaCl, feed intake was depressed to less than half of normal. It is also well known that dehydration inhibits feeding of mammals, including ruminants (Utley et al, 1970). Despite these effects on feeding, it is not likely that changes in rumen or body fluid tonicity are large enough to limit feed intake when feeding is slow or feed is taken in small meals, e.g. when access to feed is continuous.

Rumen Fluid pH

Feeding can influence rumen fluid pH, and the importance of pH on fermentation in the rumen is well known. A depression in rumen pH is particularly marked after the ingestion of a large amount of rapidly fermented feed, such as would occur with animals offered a concentrate fed for a few hours per day. Feeding roughage in ground form also depresses rumen pH more than unground roughage. The effects of these rumen pH changes on feed intake are unclear. Addition of buffers to the feed to prevent fall in pH during and after feeding has resulted in variable effects on feed intakes.

It is likely that feed intake is depressed when rumen fluid pH falls below 5.0-5.5 because of the resulting ruminal stasis. Receptors sensitive to changes in pH in the rumen epithelium have been described (Iggo and Leak, 1970). The evidence argues against the likelihood of rumen pH as a physiological controller of intake, although under pathological conditions it may be a principal cause of an accompanying hypophagia.

Volatile Fatty Acids

Acetate, propionate and butyrate are produced in large quantities by rumen microbes, absorbed through the rumen wall, and used as energy substrates in most tissues of the ruminant; they thus supplant glucose and long-chain fatty acids used as major sources of energy by non-ruminants. Because of the importance of the volatile fatty acids (VFA) in ruminant energy metabolism, in many experiments their effects on feed intake have been investigated.

During and after feeding concentrations of VFA in rumen fluid and in blood increase (Chase et al, 1977). Most of this information comes from cattle and sheep adapted to restricted access to feed. There is some evidence that increases, albeit smaller, also occur during and after spontaneous meals. Large differences in VFA concentrations are found in different parts of the rumen for several hours after large meals because of the relatively slow mixing in the rumen. β-hydroxybutyrate concentrations in the portal blood of steers increased within 15 min after the initiation of a twice-daily feeding (Chase et al, 1977).

Acetate plays a dominant role in energy metabolism of ruminants because, of all the VFA, it is produced and absorbed in greatest quantities; it may also play a central role in the control of meal size. Intraruminal injections of acetate solutions of various concentrations before or during a scheduled meal depressed intake in cattle, sheep and goats (Baile and Mayer, 1970; Baile and Forbes, 1974). Intraruminal injections of acetate into goats or sheep during spontaneous meals of a concentrate diet decreased intake much more than could be accounted for by the caloric value of the injection, as shown in Fig. 11-16.

In a number of studies attempts have been made to identify receptor sites for the effect of acetate on feeding. Injections into the dorsal area of the rumen had a greater effect on intake than injections into the ventral rumen, reticulum, or abomasum (Baile and McLaughlin, 1970). Exposure of as little as 5% of the total rumen to high concentrations of acetate was sufficient to decrease feeding (Martin and Baile, 1972). In goats amounts of sodium acetate that depress intake when administered into the rumen, when injected into the jugular vein, resulted in much smaller depression in intake (Baile and Mayer, 1968a). This suggests that on the lumen side of the rumen there are receptors sensitive to acetate that are not activated by blood acetate levels. That ruminal receptors mediate the feeding response to acetate injected intraruminally is supported by the observation that the depression can be blocked by addition of local anesthetic to the acetate solution injected (Martin and Baile,

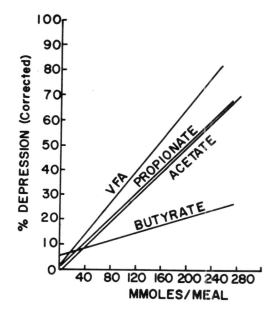

Fig. 11-16. Regression equation of data from experiments with goats injected intraruminally during spontaneous meals of a grain diet. Percent depression of feed intake was corrected for energy solution injected and mmol injected/meal were calculated. Molar proportions of the VFA mixture were 55-30-15 for acetate, propionate and butyrate, respectively. All solutions were adjusted to pH 6.5. From Baile and Mayer (1970).

1972); this may indicate that the acetate response is neurally rather than hormonally transmitted.

A second major metabolite, propionate, may also have a role in controlling meal size. Intraruminally injected propionate depressed the feed intake of cattle, sheep and goats and, as with acetate, intravenous injections in cattle decreased intake (Baile and Mayer, 1970; Baile and Forbes, 1974). Intraruminal injections of sodium propionate into goats during spontaneous meals decreased feed intakes even though changes in rumen fluid concentration remained within the limits of normal postprandial fluctuations.

Despite these similarities between the effects of acetate and propionate on feeding, the receptors involved are probably different because similar depression in intake occurred whether propionate was injected into the dorsal rumen, ventral rumen, reticulum, or abomasum (Baile and McLaughlin, 1970). In addition, injections of propionate into the ruminal vein were more effective in depressing intake than were injections into the lumen of the rumen, mesenteric, or portal veins or carotid artery. This suggests that propionate receptors may be in the ruminal vein walls and possibly also on the luminal side of the rumen, but are not in the liver or in the brain.

The rate of production of butyrate is lower than that of acetate or propionate and butyrate probably has a less important role in controlling meal size. Intraruminal injections of butyrate into goats resulted in little more than caloric compensation in feed intake (Baile and Mayer, 1969), in contrast to the effects of injections of acetate and propionate (Fig. 11-16). When injected into the jugular vein, on the other hand, butyrate depressed feed intake as much as or more than any other metabolite tested in sheep or goats. This may not be of much physiological importance, however, because much of the butyrate produced in the rumen is metabolized to β-hydroxybutyrate by the ruminal epithelium, and butyrate is not normally present in the blood of ruminants. Only after normal rumen fluid concentrations were doubled or tripled was the butyrate concentration of the ruminal vein blood affected, and even then very little reached extrahepatic tissue. The cause of the decreased feed intake in the experiments with goats and sheep may be in part the result of the ketogenicity of butyrate, its depressing effect on ruminal motility at the injection rates of this study, or its effects on the CNS which include behavioral and electroencephalogram changes similar to sleep.

Manning et al (1959) suggested that acetate has a number of qualities required for a metabolic satiety factor in ruminants, but considered it unsatisfactory because of its dependence on glucose metabolism. Propionate has some qualities acetate lacks; however, it was felt to be of limited use for a signal since very little reached the extrahepatic tissues, and the receptors were assumed to be only in the CNS. The experiments reviewed above indicate that Manning et al may have been partially correct in their reasoning. As discussed previously, receptors sensitive to concentrate changes of acetate and probably propionate may exist on the blood side of the ruminal epithelium (perhaps on the ruminal vein walls) and may play a role in the control of meal size of ruminants. There is evidence that acetate receptors in the ruminal epithelium act in the control of ruminal motility and that, although the mechanism is not clear, VFA influence ruminal blood flow. Ruminal blood circula-

tion is known to be under CNS control at least in part. In monogastric animals there is substantial evidence for various types of gastric and intestinal receptors which may influence feeding by their action on the hypothalamus (Sharma, 1967).

While an animal is eating, even when on a spontaneous meal schedule, it is possible that due to increased rate of fermentation, stratification of digesta, and slow mixing in the rumen the concentration of rumen fluid around the papilli may change substantially more than the average of the whole ingesta; thus VFA action on receptors, either at the surface or after absorption, would be enhanced. Apparently acetate and propionate are effective in ruminants because of receptors in the ruminal area.

Rates of production of one or more VFA might influence the size of individual meals by the peripheral mechanisms discussed, but are unlikely to play a major role in the regulation of energy balance. The proposed receptor system may adapt relatively quickly to sustained changes in absolute concentration but remain sensitive to changes in concentration.

Glucose

Glucose has long been regarded as a part of the controlling system for feeding in monogastric animals. Although severely reduced rates of utilization of glucose due to insulin-induced hypoglycemia or glucose analogues like 2-deoxyglucose do cause hunger and feeding, hyperglycemia and increased glucose utilization rates have had little effect on feeding (Baile and Mayer, 1969). In ruminants blood glucose levels, arteriovenous differences of glucose, and thus probably glucose utilization rates have generally been shown to decrease rather than increase with feeding diets even with ruminants adapted to a single daily meal of concentrate diets (Baile and Forbes, 1974).

The lesion that goldthioglucose produces in the medial hypothalamus of certain strains of mice and some rats has been used as evidence for glucoreceptors in this area, since other goldthio compounds are ineffective and since the lesioning action appears to depend on the presence of insulin and a high glucose utilization rate. Attempts to produce medial hypothalmic lesions in sheep or goats were unsuccessful even though glucose utilization was maintained at a very high level and nearly lethal doses of goldthioglucose were injected into a carotid artery to maximize its action (Baile et al, 1970).

Despite these wide differences between ruminants and monogastric animals in the relationship of glucose metabolism and feeding, there are, nevertheless, some similarities. (1) Insulin injections into cattle sometimes increase rate of weight gain. (2) Deoxyglucose causes feeding in ruminants when injected systematically (Houpt, 1974) or intracerebroventricularly in hypertonic solution (Seoane and Baile, 1972). (3) Injection of glucose into the carotid artery of sheep during spontaneous feeding has resulted in decreased intake, although greater molar amounts of sodium propionate had no effect; these latter two types of experiments created very unphysiological blood glucose conditions.

There is little evidence that glucose level or utilization rate has a significant role in controlling feeding in ruminants; in fact there is much evidence to the contrary. Whether this means that the hunger-satiety system of ruminants is basically different from that of monogastric animals remains to be shown conclusively.

Fatty Acids

It has been suggested that the increase in plasma free fatty acids (FFA) that occurs with starvation might act as a signal to induce feeding even though FFA levels increase not only with energy depot mobilization but also with feeding in animals adapted to a daily feeding schedule (Chase et al, 1977). Stress and several hormones (epinephrine, norepinephrine, cortisol, growth hormone) elevate FFA levels without inducing hyperphagia. Intraduodenal injections of long-chain fatty acids or fats in sheep depressed intake, but it was not clear whether this was due to the observed depression in ruminoreticulum movements or to changes in blood fat composition (Titchen et al, 1966). Therefore little information is available to show that FFA are a cause rather than an effect of changes in feeding.

Amino Acids and Their Metabolites

Since a diet with amino acid imbalance as a result of either excess or deficiency of one or more amino acids caused decreased feeding in rats within a few hours, amino acids have been considered as a possible component for the control of feeding (Harper

et al, 1970). Plasma amino acid levels in sheep decline for a few hours after a single daily feeding and then increase to a maximum about 24 hr after feeding. The suckling preruminant lamb was shown to decrease its intake about 50% in response to the dietary deletion of either threonine or isoleucine and when a low total protein level was fed (8% of GE as protein and amino acids) (Rogers and Egan, 1975). It is unlikely that meal size of ruminants is controlled by absorbed amino acids since amino acids are absorbed mainly from the small intestine several hours after ingestion. Diets containing excessive levels of protein (eg. 40%) were tolerated by cattle although blood ammonia levels exceeded 100 mg/100 ml and feed intake was near normal (Fenderson and Bergen, 1976).

Histamine is present in silages and has been considered a factor limiting intake. However, neither intraruminal, intraomasal, or intravenous injections of histamine nor its presence in feed has an effect on intake. Ruminal motility and eructation may be inhibited by histamine being injected intravenously, but not by being included in the feed. On both theoretical bases and experimental data available, it seems unlikely that the feed intake of ruminants is directly affected by plasma amino acid changes.

Hormones

Plasma concentrations of some hormones, e.g. ADH, insulin, renin, change during feeding, but it is not yet known whether one or more of these changes affect feeding. When injected into sheep during spontaneous feeding, neither insulin nor growth hormone affected daily intake. Epinephrine and norepinephrine depressed intake only when injected at near lethal doses.

Glucocorticoids caused feed intake in sheep when injected intramuscularly over periods of several weeks, but hydrocortisone injected intravenously during spontaneous meals did not affect feed intake of sheep, although during the short injection periods the rate of hormone administration was 1000 times the rate at which 17 OH-corticosteroids are normally secreted in sheep (Baile and Martin, 1971). It is likely that corticosteroids act indirectly on feed intake via their effect on energy metabolism.

Body Temperature (heat load)

A relationship between feeding and heat load suggested by Brobeck (1948) has become known as the "thermostatic" theory for the control of feeding. According to later formulations of the theory, feeding increases heat production in three ways: specific dynamic action; increase in metabolic rate as a function of the level of feeding; and increase in metabolic rate as a function of body mass (Brobeck, 1960). Presumably only the first source of heat needs to be considered as a feedback for short-term control. The other two would be more related to energy balance regulation, since they would act in maintaining a sustained heat load and heat flux but would not necessarily change during feeding.

The kinetic energy of the body is largely heat and usually represents <1% of total body energy content. Brobeck (1960) suggested that heat acts on feeding by causing temperature changes in the heat-loss center of the anterior hypothalamus or preoptic area. However, in more recent discussions of temperature regulation, importance has been given to peripheral temperature receptors, especially in the skin. Therefore, one may suppose that the hunger-satiety system is influenced by a change in heat load affecting rate of heat loss (peripheral temperature) and/or hypothalamic temperature.

Large experimentally induced changes in hypothalamic temperature can affect feeding. Andersson and Larsson (1961) showed that heating of the preoptic area via implanted thermodes caused decreased feeding in hungry goats. If the thermodes were cooled, the goats ate even though body temperature increased greatly. When thermodes were cooled for as long as 7 days, goats increased intake an average of 40% although water intake was not affected. The site of thermode placement was important; in some areas decreased thermode temperature caused near adipsia (lack of drinking) for up to three days, but feed intake remained normal. A change of 9-10°C in the thermode resulted in changes in brain temperature of similar magnitude 1.5 mm away and of 1-1.5°C 6 mm away. Because the temperature changes caused in these experiments were extreme, it cannot be concluded that there is a physiological role for hypothalamic temperature in the control of feeding.

Ruminants have, relative to carnivores, a high specific dynamic action, and a substantial proportion is due to ruminal fermentation. The heat production of steers under at least some conditions increases markedly during an hour of feeding. More specifically,

it was found that blood and skin temperatures rose during feeding in cattle and sheep and fell when feed was removed; consistent changes could be detected in skin temperatures of goats during spontaneous meals (Baile and Mayer, 1968b). Hypothalamic temperature increased when goats and sheep became active at the time of day at which feed was normally offered, even when feed was withheld. Conversely, intraruminal force-feeding has no effect on hypothalamic temperature. It appears, therefore, that feeding is not causally related to increased hypothalamic or peripheral temperature in ruminants.

Because the changes of hypothalamic and surface temperatures that occur during feeding are related more to non-specific activity than to feeding, there seems to be little evidence that temperature changes per se act under most conditions as a signal for the hunger-satiety system. Although temperature changes during a meal do not apparently have a role in hunger-satiety systems, changes of environmental temperature may affect feeding. Hot or cold environmental conditions greatly influence feeding but may only indirectly involve control of feeding through the energy balance regulatory system. Severe heat loads can limit or inhibit feeding, but this response may be related to stress rather than to a normal signal for satiety.

FACTORS LIMITING FEEDING

Many factors are known to limit feed intake and thus alter energy balance. Some are thought to play a role in normal energy balance regulation and others may assume more importance depending on the physiological condition of the animal and amount of stress present. Some of these factors may be similar in ruminants and monogastric animals.

The feeding drive is suppressed not unexpectedly, by apparent restrictions related to the state of the ruminoreticulum (Campling, 1966), palatability (Greenhalgh and Reid, 1971), nutritional deficiencies (Egan and Moir, 1965; Weston, 1971), and metabolic disorders (Baile and Forbes, 1974). Monogastric animals respond similarly to the last three factors and also restrict their intake when gastrointestinal fill limits are reached. Pregnancy places restrictions on the energy regulatory system as a result of a very significant physiological stress including severe hormonal shifts and the fetal displacement of the ruminoreticulum (Forbes, 1970; Jordan et al, 1973).

An analog computer program was developed to describe the many components controlling intake of cattle grazing on a range where the climate plays a major role in the availability of forage (Rice et al, 1974). Ruminoreticular distension in this model limits intake if forage is at a surplus. In predicting the limitations of a ration due to volume, the concept of energy density has become a useful measure (the unit KJ/ml for a diet is probably the best of these empirical relationships; Baumgardt and Peterson, 1971); however, the physiological state of the animal has an important bearing on the predictions. For example, to obtain the energy required for normal maximum growth, young growing lambs required 1110 $KJ/W^{0.75}$ and older lambs required 890 $KJ/W^{0.75}$, where W is the body weight in kg. However, the minimum caloric densities were 16.8 and 14.6 KJ/ml, respectively. It would be expected that lactating ewes or cows would demand an even greater minimum energy density than growing animals to prevent depot mobilization (Baumgardt, 1970).

Many reports are available on the effects of roughage, digestibility and rate of passage on feed intake, but because several variables are changing with each ration, several interpretations of the cause and effect relationship may be possible. Greenhalgh and Reid (1971) have shown that apparent oropharyngeal cues have a large influence on intake of forages having equal digestibilities.

There is limited work on the physiological basis for gastrointestinal restrictions of feed intake. Laplace (1970) concluded from a series of experiments that feeding in sheep is associated with an increase in reticuloomasal output and a speeding up of continuous abomasal emptying, thus causing a sustained abomasal hypermotility and consecutive gastrointestinal emptying episodes. A physiological signal that limits intake due to volume may not only be distention of stretch receptors but may involve changes in abomasal function and gastrin release (Baile, 1975). Distension of the intestine in sheep apparently does not limit forage intake (Grovum and Phillips, 1974). Many more carefully controlled studies are required to determine the interaction of the several factors that must be considered in the control of forage intake where ruminoreticular distension is apparently limiting intake.

Fill

Energy balance is maintained in some animals apparently independently of a feedback system related to energy content. For example in the blowfly energy balance is maintained by a simple hunger-satiety system in which the cue for feeding is provided by sweet receptors on the proboscis (Gelpherin and Dethier, 1967) and in which the satiety signal is provided by stretch receptors in the foregut (Gelpherin, 1967). Many writers have concluded that the ruminant also controls its intake independently of DE or ME intake.

The assumption that an animal will not eat more feed than that which would exceed the limit of rumen distention has led to a number of studies on the volume of rumen contents at the voluntary termination of a meal. Marker-dilution techniques and emptying the rumen via a fistula or after slaughter have been widely used. Earlier experiments involving inflation of the rumen with water at a standard pressure were grossly unphysiological. None of these methods allow estimation of the volume of gas present in the dorsal rumen. The use of these methods has shown that meals of various roughages are often terminated when the volume of rumen contents reaches a certain critical level, and the filling effect of roughage feeds is generally considered to be exerted in the rumen rather than in the intestines.

Campling and coworkers (1961) found that the volume of rumen contents was the same at the end of meals of various types of roughage and considered this as evidence that rumen volume limits feed intake. When ground roughages were fed, eating stopped before this critical level of rumen fill had been reached; it was postulated that the rapid rate of passage of the fine feed particles from the rumen resulted in the filling of some more distal part of the digestive tract before the rumen became full (Campling et al, 1963; Campling and Freer, 1966).

Decrease in intake of roughages by pregnant and fat ruminants has been ascribed to the compression of the rumen by the uterus and/or abdominal fat; with concentrates it is more likely the decrease in intake is due to metabolic and endocrine factors. Perhaps roughage intake is limited more by total abdominal volume than by ruminal distention.

Limitation of intake by abdominal or ruminal stretch depends on the physiological and nutritional status of the animal (Egan, 1970) and the threshold may be increased

308

during lactation, after placement of artificial bulk in the rumen and in young ruminants with higher levels of feeding. Rumen distention depends on level of intake and ruminoreticular rate of passage which is related largely to digestibility and particle size (see Vol. 1) and to motor function of the stomachs. Pressure in the reticulum, ruminoreticular fold, rumen, omasum and abomasum, sensed by vagal afferents, can stimulate motility via the efferent vagal motor pathway from the dorsal nucleus; however, gross distention in the stomachs and the duodenum can inhibit contractions. The omasum may play a regulatory role in digesta flow rate from the ruminoreticulum since, in sheep, feeding is associated with increased omasal canal motor activity, decreased reticulo-omasal transit time and interlaminary filling of the omasal body, while rumination is associated with decreased motor activity in the greater omasal curvature and thus decreased reticuloomasal output (LaPlace, 1970).

It is not clear that roughage intake is limited by digestibility. For example intake of roughage increases when nutrient requirements increase. The common observation that ruminants often eat a preferred feed even immediately after a satiating meal is evidence that oropharyngeal factors influence regulation of intake of roughages (Greenhalgh and Reid, 1971). A possibly more reliable long-term regulatory system limiting energy balance than ruminal capacity, which is adaptable and affected by feeding, drinking and salivation, would be intestinal fill; contents of the intestines flow relatively constantly and may be a composite of numerous feedings.

Nutritional and Metabolic Deficiencies

Some nutritional deficiencies affect feeding behavior although the mechanisms involved may not be known. The effects of protein deficiencies, amino acid imbalance, or amino acid deficiencies have been studied extensively in monogastric animals (Harper et al, 1970). The receptor site for the plasma amino acid balance appears to be in the CNS, perhaps in the prepyriform cortex. Sheep and cattle ate less of diets deficient in protein than of diets with added protein or urea. This decrease may have been due partly to the decreased ruminal fermentation and partly to the metabolic effect on the animal. Ruminants can also develop an aversion to urea even though no clinical signs of urea toxicity are discernible (Wilson et al, 1975).

In ruminants feed intake was decreased with diets deficient in Ca, Mn, K, P, NaCl, Co, Cu, Zn, vitamin A, vitamin D, riboflavin (calves, lambs), and vitamin B_{12}. Feed intake of ruminants was also decreased with excess amounts of As, F, Mo, Se, and Zn.

Ruminants show preferences for certain feeds such as specific species of grasses, but specific hungers are mainly evident during deficiencies. The Na^+ appetite of ruminants is well established (Denton, 1967). P-deficient cattle and sheep are known to eat bones although they may not select a mineral supplement containing phosphate.

Feed intake is quickly reduced during most metabolic diseases such as pregnancy toxemia (Blaxter, 1957), acetonemia (Kronfeld, 1970), D-lactic acidosis (Dunlop and Hammond, 1965; Uhart and Carroll, 1967), ketosis (Krebs, 1966), or bloat (Clarke and Reid, 1970). Most gastrointestinal disorders of either infectious or parasitic origin as well as many systemic diseases result in decreased feed intake. The mechanisms for the feeding response to these diseases are probably varied and not necessarily restricted to signals normally regulating feed intake. Some feeds such as tall fescue contain intake depressing components under certain conditions (Julien et al, 1974).

Many forms of stress decrease feed intake, probably for a number of reasons. Heat stress (and its effect on feed intake) is probably one of the most easily studied and documented forms. Stress caused by dehydration results in decreased feeding in ruminants (Calder et al, 1964).

ROLE OF THE CENTRAL NERVOUS SYSTEM

The brain has more than 10^{10} cells and may be the most highly organized form of matter. Experiments on how the brain works at a cellular level and especially on how it controls behavior are difficult. Because the brain is a primary controller of most of the metabolic, physiological and behavioral activities of higher animals, understanding of their interactions depends on the understanding of brain mechanisms.

Experiments on the control of feeding are usually concerned with effects of changes within the animal in relation to its feeding behavior. A receptor system has often been postulated as a component in describing behavioral responses; there is little understanding yet of the parameters monitored,

OPERATIONS of CONTROLLER of FEEDING BEHAVIOR

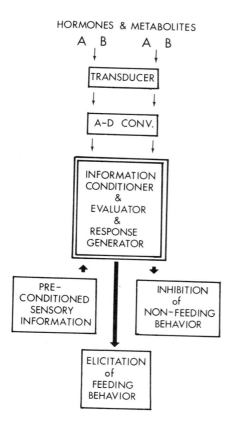

Fig. 11-17. A flow scheme illustrating proposed functions for the nervous system in the control of feeding and maintenance of energy balance. Absolute concentrations or concentration changes via specific detectors are converted from the analog signals to message units analagous to digital outputs (individual neuron firing rate changes times number of neurons affected). An information scanner and conditioner (signal conditioning meaning the matching of various types of logic systems, e.g., different neurotransmitters and inhibitory and excitatory synaptic types), an evaluator which must compare new information on the state of the system with stored references, and a response generator for the behavioral response at least in part are components in the hypothalamus. This information collection must also evaluate various types of probably preconditioned sensory information, e.g., olfactory cues, which can in some cases provide acceptable or unacceptable (YES or NO) type information for feeding. The output of the response generator can initiate or suppress several species-dependent types of food capture and feeding behaviors and probably override or suppress some types of non-feeding behaviors. From Baile (1974).

the nature of the detection systems, the anatomical sites of detectors, and the nature of the detector interfaces with the CNS.

Within the animal the transfer of information that affects feeding behavior may follow a flow scheme as illustrated in Fig. 11-17. The metabolites, hormones or gastrointestinal conditions that may be monitored act on receptor systems which, in effect, transduce analog information, e.g., concentration into neuronal units. The change in output of a single type of detector system may be the result of the changes of firing of individual neurons which interface with a detector cell (or more likely an interneuronal interface of a detector) and spike potential generator and the number of detector-neuron units which are influenced. The result of such systems is the conversion of analog information to digital information (firing rate x cells influenced).

The various types of analog information which play a role must be scanned and evaluated, as are also other factors including sensory inputs (perhaps primarily conditioned by other CNS centers). Of the various CNS structures involved, the hypothalamus plays an important role in integrating these various inputs and generating feeding behavior. The type of feeding behavior reflects the sensory information, perhaps some digital inputs which either permit or restrict feeding, and information on the state of the metabolic pools.

Lesions and Electrical Stimulation of the Hypothalamus

There is evidence that rodents have the reference system required to stabilize an energy balance feedback system (Bray and York, 1971; Mrosovsky and Powley, 1977). After prolonged fast and weight loss, rats will increase initial intake until initial weight is nearly attained. Furthermore, after prolonged force feeding and weight gain rats will decrease intake until initial weight is nearly attained. Evidence exists for presence of this memory system in the CNS but not adipose tissue (Baile, 1971).

The ventromedial hypothalamus (VMH) generally has an inhibitory effect on feeding and partial ablation of the VMH is said to raise the set point for the energy balance regulator, indicated by the negative input to the reference signal comparator, No. 17 in Fig. 11-14. Electrolytic lesions in the VMH of most laboratory animals cause hyperphagia and obesity which occur in two phases, dynamic and static. During the static phase increased weight is maintained at a nearly constant level and is regulated under fasting and overfeeding conditions (Hoebel and Teitelbaum, 1966). In mice the size of lesions caused by goldthioglucose was related to degree of obesity (Baile et al, 1971). Rats with lesions in the VMH do regulate intake, but meals are larger, less frequent and more evenly distributed during light and dark cycles than those of normal rats. Other effects of VMH lesions are decreased spontaneous activity, mating behavior, estrous cycling, releasing factor for growth hormones and gastric contractions and increased gastric acid release and plasma insulin levels.

The lateral hypothalamus (LH) generally initiates feeding and partial ablation of the LH is said to lower the set point for the energy balance regulator, indicated by the positive input to the reference signal comparator, No. 17 in Fig. 11-14. Electrolytic lesions in several species of laboratory animals (Teitelbaum, 1961) causes sustained aphagia and adipsia and eventual return to feeding but to maintain a lower body weight; in addition, there is permanent loss of several other functions related to feeding and drinking (Epstein and Teitelbaum, 1967). The duration of aphagia has been shown to be inversely related to amount of weight loss before lesioning (Powley and Keesey, 1970).

The energy balance regulating system described for rodents may not be assumed a priori to exist or operate as efficiently in domesticated ruminants which are the result of genetic selection for certain traits some of which may be related to hypothalamic-hypophyseal function. However lesions in the VMH and LH of pigs and chickens, both selected for many generations for maximum growth rate and probably thus feed intake, produce similar effects as in rodents.

Evidence that a similar system for regulating energy balance exists for ruminants as for rodents is that electrolytic lesions of the VMH but not other areas of the hypothalamus of goats caused hyperphagia (Baile et al, 1969). As for rodents there were dynamic and static phases and changes in glucose metabolism and insulin levels. However, in sheep VMH lesions have not produced hyperphagia (Holmes and Fraser, 1965; Tarttelin and Bell, 1968). Goldthioglucose did not cause VMH lesions in sheep probably because of differences in permeability of the VMH of these animals compared with mice. Electrolytic lesions in the LH of goats (Baile

et al, 1968) and sheep (Tarttelin and Bell, 1968) have caused sustained aphagia or adipsia. As in other animals electrical stimulation of the LH causes feeding in satiated goats and sheep (Larsson, 1954) and rats (Steinbaum and Miller, 1965) while stimulation of the VMH reduces feeding activity of goats (Wyrwicka and Dobrzecka, 1960).

Further evidence for existence of an energy balance regulating system for ruminants similar to one for rats has been obtained with injections of neural depressants into the CSF in an attempt to suppress the inhibitory action of the medial hypothalamus on the feeding system. Feeding responses with short latency times would indicate an effect on periventricular tissue, possibly of hypothalamic origin. Satiated goats, sheep and calves eat voraciously during perfusion of the CSF with pentobarbital as do rats. Barbiturates with anesthetic properties which were long-acting were more effective in producing feeding in sheep than those which were ultrashort-acting when injected into the 3rd ventricle (Seoane et al, 1973; Fig. 11-18). Neural depressants also cause feeding when injected directly into the medial hypothalamus of goats and sheep as in rats. It seems likely the VMH has an inhibitory action on feeding in ruminants similar to that in other mammals.

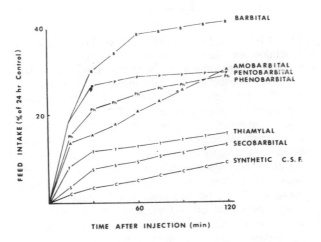

Fig. 11-18. Feed intake of sheep following 0.5 ml injections of barbiturates into the 3rd ventricle. The doses tested were based on their hypnotic activity; barbital, 100μmol; phenobarbital, 40μmol; amobarbital, 50μmol; pentobarbital, 40μmol; secobarbital, 40 μ mol; thiamylal, 40μ mol. The meal intakes following injection of the first 4 drugs listed above at 120 min were different from the control (P<0.1; n= 8). From Seoane et al (1973).

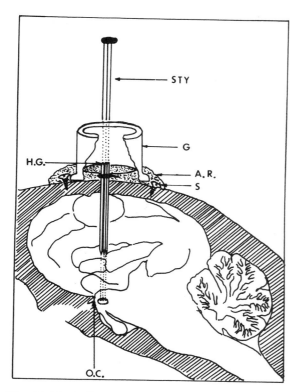

Fig. 11-19. A diagram illustrating the technique and approximate placement of cannulas into the brain of a sheep. Abbreviations are STY, stylet; G, guard (syringe barrel); HG, hypothalamic guides; AR, acrylic resin; S, stainless steel screw; OC, optic chiasm. From Baile et al (1974).

Neural Transmitters

Putative intraneuoronal transmitters are a critical link in the transfer of information related to control of feeding behavior. The specificity of post-synaptic receptors for transmitters makes chemical coding possible. Specific neuro-hormonal transmitters either increase or decrease post-synaptic firing rate; this polarity of response adds another dimension to the logic of the inter-neuronal information transmission.

L-norepinephrine, an α-adrenoceptor agonist, was the first putative neurotransmitter to be associated with feeding in rats (Grossman, 1962). From a series of experiments designed to characterize transmitter systems for feeding in cattle and sheep, several general conclusions were drawn (Baile, 1974). Intraventricular injection of α- and β-adrenoceptor agonists (pharmacological classification described by Ahlquist, 1948) elicit feeding in sheep and cattle. Sheep are more responsive to α-adrenergic agonists than cattle. The doses of β-adreno-

ceptor agonists which elicit feeding are relatively much smaller than those which decrease feeding in rats. β-adrenoceptors could not be characterized pharmacologically as β_1 or β_2 in sheep. Injection into distinct loci of the hypothalamus of sheep with either α or β_2 adrenoceptor agonists produces feeding (Fig. 11-19); however, specific loci were not located in specific areas. Feeding elicited by carbachol (Fig. 11-20), a cholinergic agonist, in sheep is greater than that elicited by adrenoceptor agonists and is blocked by atropine, a cholinergic blocker, but not by α- or β-adrenergic blockers (Forbes and Baile, 1974).

Feeding elicited in sheep by intraventricular injections of a variety of agents, e.g. 2-deoxyglucose (Seoane and Baile, 1972), Ca^{++} and Mg^{++} (Fig. 11-21, Seoane and Baile, 1975) and barbiturates (Seoane et al, 1973) is postulated to be a result of activity of neural tracts. Intrahypothalamic injection Ca^{++} and Mg^{++} also elicit feeding (Seoane and Baile, 1975).

Feeding in cattle and sheep can be elicited by injection of a variety of agents into the brain. However no series of neurotransmitters forming a feeding circuit has been

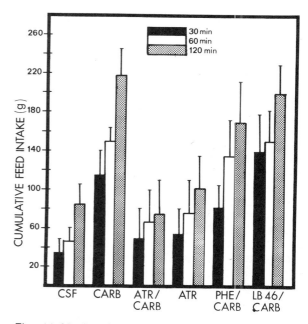

Fig. 11-20. Intrahypothalamic injections (1 μl) into sheep of synthetic cerebrospinal fluid (CSF), 28 nmol of carabachol (CARB), 28 nmol atropine sulfate (ATR), 120 nmol phenoxbenzamine HCl (PHE), an α-adrenoceptor antagonist, and 120 nmol LB-46, a β-adrenoceptor antagonist. In combination injections the second drug was given 3 min after the first. SEM's are shown. From Forbes and Baile (1974).

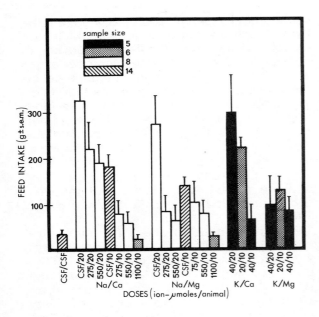

Fig. 11-21. Feed intakes of sheep 30 min after combined injections into the 3rd cerebroventricle of Na+ with Ca++ or Mg++ From Seoane and Baile (1973).

delineated. Specific agents may elicit feeding via a set of parallel systems, but some agents may act on combinations of these systems.

PREDICTION OF FEED INTAKE

If the environmental temperature, age, weight, and DE intake of an animal in various physiological conditions are known, a relatively accurate estimate of basal metabolic rate, maintenance requirements, and productive energy is possible. By contrast, it is difficult to predict with much precision the consumption of total mass, dry matter or DE of a ruminant fed any of the many possible types of diets. Examples of some proposed prediction systems and how they relate to the control system described in Fig. 11-14 are discussed.

For roughage feeds, the digestibility of the diet and animal mass have been considered by most workers to be important in predicting intake. For example, Lehmann (1941) found that dairy cows need approximately 4.3 kg of indigestible organic matter (ballast) per 500 kg body wt/day. Conrad et al (1964) included digestibility as well as indigestible dry matter and body weight in their equation, which is applicable to intake of dairy cows for roughages of up to 67%

digestibility (See Fig. 11-12). The prediction scheme of Kruger and Schultz (1956) was probably more realistic in that it attempted to include the sensory qualities and particle size of the feed; however, they did not take into account the available energy content of the diet or the energy requirement of animals.

Prediction equations for non-lactating ruminants have been derived by Crampton (1957) and Blaxter (1962). Baumgardt (1970) expressed nutrient value as DE per unit of volume and gave the minimum caloric density required of a feed to support a given level of metabolic demands. For example, lactating cows require a more calorically dense feed than do non-lactating cows if loss of body weight is to be avoided. This system, like most others, does not include the sensory effects of the feed nor does it take directly into account the particle size. The inclusion of an artificial mastication index, as developed by Troelson and Bigsby (1964), could result in improved predications from Baumgardt's system. Baumgardt et al (1977) found that for growing wethers fed 24 rations the variables per cent dry matter, bulk density, solid density, in vitro dry matter digestibility, per cent non-detergent fiber, digestion coefficient for non-detergent fiber, and a function expressing rate of digestion in vitro of non-detergent fiber accounted for 83% of the variation in feed intake. Taking a different approach, Forbes (1977) has developed computer analog models describing the variations in feed intake of fattening, pregnant, and lactating sheep and lactating cows using metabolic, physical and endocrine factors. Variables of the control of feed intake and regulation of energy balance reviewed here are most consistent with the concepts considered by Montiero (1972) and presented previously.

The intake of concentrate feeds is more closely related to energy requirements and therefore is more predictable. However, there are important exceptions in which intake is not closely related to energy expenditure.

In feeding ruminant animals it is common practice to feed concentrates with a roughage feed, the intake of which is itself insufficient to support the desired level of production. Because roughages are usually less expensive than concentrates, it is important to know whether, and to what extent, concentrate supplementation results in depressed roughage intake. The general conclusions from the results of many experiments are the lower the digestibility of the roughage, the less is its intake affected by concentrate feeding; if the roughage is low in protein the addition of small amounts of concentrate, particularly one high in protein, will stimulate intake.

Because of the complexity of the control of feed intake and its interrelationship with energy balance regulation, it is not surprising that prediction equations of feed intake are only poor guides when applied to a specific situation. Environmental, managerial, and social factors as well as previous feeding experience, physiological conditions, e.g. lactation, fat deposition, growth, many physical and nutritional qualities of the feed, and various sensory inputs can all have a marked effect on feed intake. It is difficult to imagine that one or two factors can encompass all these variables to describe feed intake of ruminants even under a limited set of conditions. For satisfactory prediction of feed intake much more information on the interrelationships of the many factors controlling feeding is required.

CHEMICALLY-INDUCED FEEDING IN RUMINANTS

Those groups of animals which eat more of a specific ration gain more rapidly and efficiently. From the previous discussion it seems likely that the feed intakes of animals are often not limited by either their digestive or their metabolic capabilities but rather by a hypothalamic regulator. Chicks selected for rapid growth provide a good example when they were force-fed for 15 days so that their intake was 170% of the control group, grew 50% faster and retained nearly 40% more of the feed energy in their carcass than did the controls (Nir et al, 1974). Therefore, the control chicks were eating at a level that did not approach their physiological capabilities.

Because animals under most conditions establish a rate of intake which may be substantially below physiological and metabolic limitations, ways have been investigated to make animals eat more to improve efficiency. As a result of this effort, methods have been developed to make cattle and sheep eat more; some of these may lead to practical applications.

In adult humans, the resistance toward eating more, resulting in weight gain in the normal subject, may be as great as the resistance toward eating less, resulting in weight loss in normal or obese subjects (Jordan, 1973). Even with substantial re-

wards, people gain weight over their norm only with difficulty and soon return to the initial weight when the test is over. The termination of sustained overfeeding in growing animals probably does not result in mobilization of the resulting extra body mass, especially lean body mass.

A sustained increase in feed intake, which is not associated with increased activity, decreased efficiency of anabolic metabolism or decreased digestibility will increase rate of gain in growing animals. This means that energy balance is being maintained at a higher level than normal which is usually the result of an adjustment at the CNS level. A variety of chemical classes has been found to stimulate feeding in ruminants when given systematically. These include barbiturates, benzodiazepines, cannabinol-like chemicals, phenylalkylsulfamide, tertiary alcohols, β-adrenergic agonists, and tropine benzohydryl ethers and 3-quinuclidinyl benzohydryl ethers (Baile and McLaughlin, 1978).

Some of the reported responses to the benzodiazepines will be discussed to illustrate the potential use of chemical feed intake stimulants. Benzodiazepines are known to elicit feeding (apparent hunger) in man, rats, chicks, dogs, pigs, sheep, cattle and horses (Baile and McLaughlin, 1978). These chemicals are potent stimulants and selectively elicit feeding. In sheep benzodiazepines override the inhibitors of feeding associated with apparent metabolic

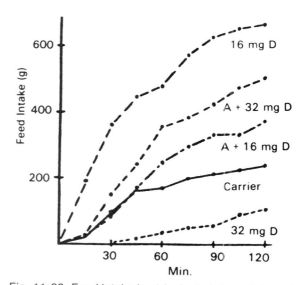

Fig. 11-22. Feed intake by 4-hr fasted sheep injected intravenously with 32 mg amphetamine and/or 16 or 32 mg Elfazepam. Based on data from Baile et al (1976).

Table 11-13. Results of three cattle trials using Elfazepam, a feed intake stimulant. [a]

Item	Feed intake, kg/day	Weight gain, kg/day	Feed efficiency
High concentrate, 16 weeks			
Control	9.45	.87	11.06
.5 ppm	9.12	.87	10.62
1.0 ppm	9.79	.96**	10.28*
2.0 ppm	9.61	.91	10.66
1.0 + 2.0 ppm	9.70	.94*	10.47*
improvement, %	3	8	6
Medium quality roughage, 17 weeks			
Control	8.16	.41	20.7
.5 ppm	8.81	.52	17.3
1.0 ppm	8.59	.50	17.9
2.0 ppm	8.89	.55	16.8
1.0 + 2.0 ppm	8.74*	.52*	17.3*
improvement, %	7.5	28	19
Low quality roughage and grain, 8 weeks			
Control	4.18	.29	21.82
.5 ppm	4.47	.38	13.26
1.0 ppm	4.61*	.43	11.98
2.0 ppm	4.81**	.48	10.89
1.0 + 2.0 ppm	4.71**	.45*	11.44*
improvement, %	11	88	76

* Different from control, p < .05.
** Different from control, p < .01.
[a] From Baile and McLaughlin (1978)

products, gastric distension, protein deficiency anorexia, heat stress, amphetamine-induced anorexia (Fig. 11-22), and, in clinical cases, pathologically associated anorexia.

These chemicals have a sustained effect in performance studies with sheep and cattle (Table 11-13). A note of caution should be added that different responses have been obtained under a variety of conditions. Although both high concentrate and high roughage rations were used, the all-roughage treatments have shown the most dramatic responses. In another experiment the feed intake depressing effect of monensin was overridden and more efficient gains resulted (Dinius and Baile, 1977).

The objective of this line of investigation has been to find ways of making animals "require" a higher energy balance so that a greater proportion of their net energy will be avilable for growth as illustrated in Fig. 11-23. Presumably, there are conditions in which increased intake may be detrimental, but it is also apparent that in most cases animals establish an energy balance with substantial safety margins. Although making animals in feedlots eat more of high concentrate feeds has been an obvious appli-

cation, now it may be even more important to make ruminants eat more roughages and by-products. For example, if cattle can be induced to eat greater quantities of 50% grain diets so that their rates of gain approach those of cattle fed 80% grain diets, the use of cheaper ingredients may become more economical. It also seems feasible that grazing animals may be stimulated to eat more, resulting in more efficient and faster growth and better carcass grades. The results of these experiments show that sheep and cattle can be induced to eat more of even unpalatable, bulky, and protein-deficient diets; this provides support for the contention that animals may utilize various types of by-products where hypophagia restricts their use presently.

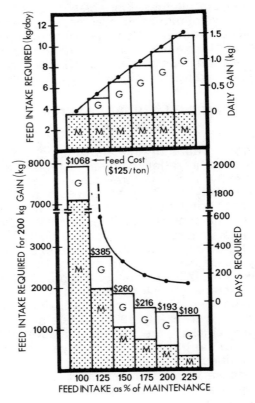

Fig. 11-23. Top. An illustration of the dependence of rate of gain on the proportion of the NE available for growth (G). These relationships assume a 400 kg steer is receiving the same diet but in increasing amounts relative to that required for maintenance (M). Bottom. The cost of growing a steer from 300 to 500 kg when increasing feed intakes relative to maintenance are maintained. The requirement for NE for the gain (G) of the 200 kg remains constant but the NE required for maintenance is reduced as the number of days required for the gain is reduced. From Baile and McLaughlin (1978).

SUMMARY

The control of feed intake of ruminants, like that of other mammals, is still only poorly understood. Because ruminants are in some ways anatomically and physiologically different from other mammals, such as the usual laboratory rodents, it is not surprising that some factors not usually important in monogastric animals probably play a role in the control of feed intake in ruminants. Fig. 11-14 illustrates some of the interrelationships of various systems playing a role in the control of feed intake, as discussed in this chapter. Sensory cues play an important part for most animals in the selection of feed where a choice is either required or possible, and may also play an important role in triggering initiation of feeding. Ruminants also appear to regulate energy balance under many different environmental and nutritional conditions; however, a number of factors can limit feed intake and thus energy balance. It is not clear what energy depot or depots are being regulated but fat depots may well be the most important of the energy stores playing a role in energy balance regulation, as is thought to be the case in other mammals. Possible factors playing feedback roles from depot fat are listed in No. 11 of Fig. 11-14, while possible receptor sites are shown in No. 12. Of the various aspects of control of feed intake of ruminants, the control of meal size may be the most different from that of other mammals. There is much evidence that neither glucostasis nor thermostasis plays a role in controlling meal size or frequency in ruminants. Most of the factors thought to play a major role in the control of feeding involve changes in the ruminoreticular contents and proposed receptors of various types in either the epithelium or serosa of these stomachs. Fig. 11-14, No. 9, lists factors that may change with feeding and play a role in controlling meal size under various feeding conditions.

It is proposed in Fig. 11-14 that the integrated feedback signals for energy balance regulation and hunger-satiety are via a comparator, No. 13. This concept includes the observed interrelationship between feed intake and energy balance. The net feedback signal for the control of feeding can stimulate or terminate feeding, but is also dependent on an animal's energy balance potential, illustrated by No. 14. This memory or reference signal is generated in part probably by positive feeding input (hunger) from the lateral hypothalamus and negative feeding input (satiety) from the ventromedial hypothalamus. Less positive input for either inherent or experimentally induced reasons (e.g. partial ablation of the lateral hypothalamus) results in lower energy balance and feed intake (hypophagia) in ruminants. For the same reasons, a decrease in the ventromedial contribution (e.g. ventromedial hypothalamic lesions) results in increased energy balance and feed intake (hyperphagia) until a new norm is reached and body weight is again stable. These proposed hypothalamic functions in the control of feed intake have many of the same experimental bases as those proposed for monogastric animals.

In Fig. 11-14, No. 21, are a number of factors that can limit or override energy balance regulation and that are shown acting on the feeding actuator signal. In particular, gastrointestinal fill or ballast quality of the feed for ruminants has been the basis for many experiments and hypotheses on both the control of feed intake and regulation of energy balance. As discussed in this chapter, it is not always clear whether the apparent relationships shown between fill characteristics and feed intake are cause and effect or whether they result from a number of other feed qualities (e.g. palatability) associated with changes in fill quality.

Even though there are many nutritional and physiological experiments in the literature on the feeding behavior of ruminants, it still remains difficult to predict the feed intake of any one diet by a group of animals. Although a number of experimenters have tried to develop a system to predict intake, most have considered only one or two qualities of the feed and one or two characteristics of the animals being fed. Because of the complexity of the control of feed intake and its interrelationship with energy balance, consideration of more aspects of the control system will probably be required to predict feed intake with much precision, which, of course will demand more complete understanding of the system itself.

Of even greater economic consequence than predicting feed intake, which may come with greater understanding of its control, will be the development of ways of either decreasing the input of certain feedback signals or increasing the set point for energy balance regulation. The resulting increased feed intake, if associated with proper

316

hormonal control of metabolic processes so that the extra metabolite supply is partitioned into the desired pools, will markedly improve potential food production from these very important groups of domesticated animals.

REFERENCES CITED

General References
Baile, C.A. 1975. In: Digestion and Metabolism in the Ruminant. Univ. of New England Pub. Unit, Armidale, N.S.W., Australia.
Baile, C.A. and J.M. Forbes. 1974. Physiol. Rev. 54:160.
Balch, C.C. and R.C. Campling. 1962. Nutr. Abstr. Rev. 32:669.
Baumgardt, B.R. 1969. In: Animal Growth and Nutrition. Lea & Febiger.
Bines, J.A. 1976. Livestock Prod. Sci. 3:115.
Goatcher, W.D. and D.C. Church. 1970c. J. Animal Sci. 31:973.
Journet, M. and B. Remond. 1976. Livestock Prod. Sci. 3:129.
Kare, M.R. and O. Maller (eds.). 1967. The Chemical Senses and Nutrition. The John's Hopkins Press.
Phillipson, A.T. (ed.). 1970. Physiology of Digestion and Metabolism in the Ruminant. Oriel Press, Newcastle Upon Tyne, England.
Zotterman, Y. (ed.). 1963. Olfaction and Taste. Pergamon Press.

Taste and Palatability
Part I
Allden, W.G. and I.A. McD. Wittaker. 1970. Aust. J. Agr. Res. 21:755.
Arnold, G.W. 1964. Proc. Aust. Soc. Animal Prod. 5:258.
Arnold, G.W. 1966. Aust. J. Agr. Res. 17:521,531.
Arnold, G.W. 1970. In: Physiology of Digestion and Metabolism in the Ruminant. Oriel Press, Newcastle Upon Tyne, England.
Baile, C.A. and F.H. Martin. 1972. J. Dairy Sci. 55:1461.
Bell, F.R. 1959. J. Agr. Sci. 52:125.
Bell, F.R. and R.L. Kitchell. 1966. J. Physiol. 183:145.
Bell, F.A. and H.L. Williams. 1959. Nature 183:345.
Bernard, R.A. 1964. Amer. J. Physiol. 206:827.
Bernard, R.A. and M.R. Kare. 1961. J. Animal Sci. 20:965 (abstr).
Buchanan, H., W.A. Laycock and D.A. Price. 1972. J. Animal Sci. 35:423.
Clapperton, J.L. 1969. Proc. Nutr. Soc. 28:57A.
Coppock, C.E. et al. 1974. J. Animal Sci. 39:1170.
Coppock, C.E., R.W. Everett and R.L. Belyea. 1976. J. Dairy Sci. 59:571.
Coppock, C.E, R.W. Everett and W.G. Merrill. 1972. J. Dairy Sci. 55:245.
Craplet, C. and J. Merlu. 1970. Nutr. Abstr. Rev. 40:1067.
Crawford, D.W., R.D. Goodrich and J.C. Meiske. 1977. Feedstuffs 49(5):20.
Crawford, J.C. and D.C. Church. 1971. J. Wildl. Mgmt. 35:210.
Dash, S.K., M.J. Owens and H.H. Voelker. 1972. J. Dairy Sci. 55:102.
Davies, D.A.R., P.M. Lerman and M.M. Crosse. 1974. J. Agr. Sci. 82:469.
Dean, R.E. and D.C. Church. 1972. Feedstuffs 44(51):37.
Goatcher, W.D. 1969. M.S. Thesis, Oregon State University, Corvallis.
Goatcher, W.D. 1970. Ph.D. Thesis, Oregon State University, Corvallis.
Goatcher, W.D. and D.C. Church. 1969. Proc. West. Sec. Am. Soc. An. Sci. 20:151.
Goatcher, W.D. and D.C. Church. 1970a. J. Animal Sci. 30:777;784.
Goatcher, W.D. and D.C. Church. 1970b. J. Animal Sci. 31:364;373.
Goatcher, W.D., D.C. Church and J. Crawford. 1970. Feedstuffs 42(47):16.
Gordon, J.G., D.E. Tribe and T.C. Graham. 1954. Brit. J. Anim. Behav. 2:72.
Hutchinson, K.J. and R.J. Wilkins. 1971. J. Agr. Sci. 77:539.
Ingalls, J.R. and H.R. Sharma. 1975. Can. J. Animal Sci. 55:721.
Ivins, J.D. 1952. J. Brit. Grassld. Soc. 7:43.
Ivos, J. and L. Marjanovic. 1972. Nutr. Abstr. Rev. 42:1183.
Jones, E.C. and R.J. Barnes. 1967. J. Sci. Food Agr. 18:321.
Kercher, C.J. 1968. Proc. West. Sec. Am. Soc. An. Sci. 19:175.
Krueger, W.C. 1974. Proc. Soc. Range Mgmt., Tucson, Arizona.

Krueger, W.C., W.A. Laycock and D.A. Price. 1974. J. Range Mgmt. 27:258.

Langlands, J.P. 1969. Animal Prod. 11:369.

Laredo, M.A. and D.J. Minson. 1975. J. Brit. Grassld. Soc. 30:73.

L'Estrange, J.L. and T.McNamara. 1975. Brit. J. Nutr. 34:221.

L'Estrange, J.L. and F. Murphy. 1972. Brit. J. Nutr. 28:1.

Longhurst, W.M., H.K. Oh, M.B. Jones and R.E. Kepner. 1968. Trans. 33rd N. Amer. Wildl. Conf., p. 181.

Marten, G.C. 1970. Proc. Nat. Conf. Forage Quality. Nebr. Center Cont. Ed., Lincoln, Nebr.

Marten, G.C. and J.D. Donker. 1964. J. Dairy Sci. 47:871.

Marten, G.C., R.M. Jordan and A.W. Hoven. 1976. Agron. J. 68:909.

McLaughlin, C.L., B.A. Baldwin and C.A. Baile. 1974. J. Animal Sci. 39:136 (abstr).

McLeod, D.S., R.J. Wilkins and W.F. Raymond. 1970. J. Agr. Sci. 75:311.

McManus, W.R., G.W. Arnold and J. Ball. 1968. J. Brit. Grassld. Soc. 23:223.

Mehren, M.J. and D.C. Church. 1976. Animal Prod. 22:255.

Mehren, M.J. and D.C. Church. 1977. Animal Prod. 25:11.

Miller, W.J., J.L. Carmon and H.L. Dalton. 1958. J. Dairy Sci. 41:1262.

Morgan, D.J. and J.L. L'Estrange. 1976. Ir. J. Agr. Res. 15:55.

Neumark, H., A. Bondi and R. Volcani. 1964. J. Sci. Food Agr. 15:487.

Ozanne, P.G. and K.M.W. Howes. 1971. Aust. J. Agr. Res. 22:941.

Plice, M.J. 1952. J. Range Mgmt. 5:69.

Putnam, P.A. and G.V. Richardson. 1968. J. Animal Sci. 27:1135 (abstr).

Rabas, D.L., A.R. Schmid and G.C. Marten. 1970. Agron. J. 62:762.

Randall, R.P. 1974. Ph.D. Thesis, Oregon State University, Corvallis.

Randall, R.P. and D.C. Church. 1973. Proc. West. Sec. Am. Soc. An. Sci. 24:384.

Ray, D.E., C.B. Roubicek and J. Kuhn. 1975. Arizona Cattle Feeders Day Series, p. 36.

Ray, M.L. and C.L. Drake. 1959. J. Animal Sci. 18:1333.

Rees, M.C. and D.J. Minson. 1976. Brit. J. Nutr. 36:179.

Reid, R.L. and G.A. Jung. 1965. J. Animal Sci. 24:615.

Rice, P.R. and D.C. Church. 1974. J. Wildl. Mgmt. 38:830.

Smith, P. 1973. Expt. Husb. 23:37.

Smythe, R.H. 1955. Veterinary Opthamology. Bailliere, Tindall and Cox Pub. Co.

Stubbs, O.J. and M.R. Kare. 1958. J. Animal Sci. 17:1162 (abstr).

Thomas, J.W., L.A. Moore, M. Okamoto and J.F. Sykes. 1961. J. Dairy Sci. 44:1471.

Tribe, D.C. and J.G. Gordon. 1949. J. Agr. Sci. 39:313.

Wallace, J.D. and J.K. Riggs. 1967. J. Animal Sci. 26:209 (abstr).

Weeth, H.J. and R.D. Digesti. 1972. Proc. West. Sec. Am. Soc. An. Sci. 23:377.

Weeth, H.J. and G.H. Green. 1974. J. Animal Sci. 39:137 (abstr).

Wing, J.M. 1961. J. Dairy Sci. 44:725.

Part II

Ahlquist, R.P. 1948. Am. J. Physiol. 153:586.

Ames, D.R. and D.R. Brink. 1977. Behav. Biol. 20:205.

Andersson, B. and B. Larsson. 1961. Acta Physiol. Scand. 52:75.

Andrews, R.P. and E.R. Orskov. 1970. Animal Prod. 12:335.

Appleman, R. and J.C. Delouche. 1958. J. Animal Sci. 17:326.

Arnold, G.W. 1970. In: Physiology of Digestion and Metabolism in the Ruminant. Oriel Press, Newcastle Upon Tyne, England.

Baile, C.A. 1971. J. Dairy Sci. 54:564.

Baile, C.A. 1974. Fed. Proc. 33:1166.

Baile, C.A. 1975. In: Digestion and Metabolism in the Ruminant. Univ. New England Pub. Unit, Armidale, N.S.W., Australia.

Baile, C.A. In press. In: CRC Handbook of Nutrition and Food, CRC Press, Inc.

Baile, C.A. et al. 1974. J. Dairy Sci. 57:68.

Baile, C.A. and M.J. Forbes. 1974. Physiol. Rev. 54:160.

Baile, C.A., M.G. Herrera and J. Mayer. 1970. Am. J. Physiol. 218:857.

Baile, C.A., L.F. Krabill, C.L. McLaughlin and J.S. Beyea. 1976. Fed. Proc. 35:579.

Baile, C.A., A.W. Mahoney and J. Mayer. 1968. J. Dairy Sci. 51:1474.

Baile, C.A. and H.F. Martin. 1971. J. Dairy Sci. 54:897.

Baile, C.A. and J. Mayer. 1968a. J. Dairy Sci. 51:1490, 1495.

318

Baile, C.A. and J. Mayer. 1968b. Am. J. Physiol. 214:677.

Baile, C.A. and J. Mayer. 1969. Am. J. Physiol. 217:1830.

Baile, C.A. and J. Mayer. 1970. In: Physiology of Digestion and Metabolism in the Ruminant, Oriel Press, Newcastle Upon Tyne, England.

Baile, C.A., J. Mayer, A.W. Mahoney and C. McLaughlin. 1969. J. Dairy Sci. 52:101.

Baile, C.A., J. Mayer and C. McLaughlin. 1969. Am. J. Pysiol. 217:397.

Baile, C.A., J. Mayer, B.R. Baumgardt and A. Peterson. 1970. J. Dairy Sci. 53:801.

Baile, C.A. and C.L. McLaughlin. 1970. J. Dairy Sci. 53:1058.

Baile, C.A. and C.L. McLaughlin. 1978. Cereal Foods World. 23:290.

Balch, C.C. and R.C. Campling. 1969. In: Handbach der Tierenahrung, Vol. 1. W. Paul Parey, Hamburg, Germany.

Baldwin, B.A., C.L. McLaughlin and C.A. Baile. 1977. Appl. Animal Ethology 3:151.

Baumgardt, B.R., L.F. Krabill, J.L. Gobble and P.J. Wangsness. 1977. Feed Composition, Animal Nutrient Requirements and Computerization of Diets. Fonnesbeck, P.V., L.E. Harris and L.E. Kearl (eds), Utah Agr. Exp. Sta., Utah State Univ., Logan, Utah.

Baumgardt, B.R. 1970. In: Physiology of Digestion and Metabolism in the Ruminant. Oriel Press, Newcastle Upon Tyne, England.

Baumgardt, B.R. and A.D. Peterson. 1971. J. Dairy Sci. 54:1191.

Bergstrom, P.L., P.C. Hart and H.E. van der Veen. 1963. Tijdschr. Diergeneesk. 88:1002.

Bhattacharya, A.N. and R.G. Warner. 1968. J. Dairy Sci. 51:1481.

Bines, J.A., S. Suzuki and C.C. Balch. 1969. Brit. J. Nutr. 23:695.

Blair-West, J.R. and A.H. Brook. 1969. J. Physiol. 204:15.

Blaxter, K.L. 1957. Proc. Nutr. Soc. 16:52.

Blaxter, K.L. 1962. The Energy Metabolism of Ruminants. Hutchinson, London.

Bray, G. 1976. The Obese Patient. W.B. Saunders Company.

Bray, G.A. and D.A. York. 1971. Physiol. Rev. 51:598.

Brobeck, J.R. 1948. Yale J. Biol. Med. 20:545.

Brobeck, J.R. 1960. Recent Prog. Hormone Res. 16:439.

Bull, L.S., B.R. Baumgardt and M. Clancy. 1976. J. Dairy Sci. 59:1078.

Calder, F.W., J.W.G. Nicholson and H.M. Cunningham. 1964. Can. J. Animal Sci. 44:266.

Campling, R.C. 1966. Brit. J. Nutr. 20:25.

Campling, R.C. 1970. In: Physiology of Digestion and Metabolism in the Ruminant. Oriel Press, Newcastle Upon Tyne, England.

Campling, R.C. and C.C. Balch. 1961. Brit. J. Nutr. 15:523.

Campling, R.C. and M. Freer. 1966. Brit. J. Nutr. 20:229.

Campling, R.C., M. Freer and C.C. Balch. 1961. Brit. J. Nutr. 15:531.

Campling, R.C., M. Freer and C.C. Balch. 1962. Brit. J. Nutr. 16:115.

Campling, R.C., M. Freer and C.C. Balch. 1963. Brit. J. Nutr. 17:263.

Chase, L.E., P.J. Wangsness and B.R. Baumgardt. 1976. J. Dairy Sci. 59:1923.

Chase, L.E. et al. 1977. J. Dairy Sci. 60:403;410.

Clancy, M., L.S. Bull, P.J. Wangsness and B.R. Baumgardt. 1976. J. Animal Sci. 42:960.

Clarke, R.T.J. and C.S.W. Reid. 1970. In: Physiology of Digestion and Metabolism in the Ruminant, Oriel Press, Newcastle Upon Tyne, England.

Conrad, H.R., A.D. Pratt and J.W. Hibbs. 1964. J. Dairy Sci. 47:54.

Crampton, E.W. 1957. J. Animal Sci. 16:546.

Davis, J.D.. C.S. Campbell, R.J. Gallagher and M.A. Zurakov. 1971. J. Comp. Physiol. Psychol. 75:476.

Denton, D.A. 1967. In: Handbook of Physiology. Alimentary Canal. Am. Physiol. Soc.

Dinius, D.A. and B.R. Baumgardt. 1970. J. Dairy Sci. 53:311.

Dinius, D.A. and C.A. Baile. 1977. J. Animal Sci. 45:147.

Dunlop, R.H. and P.B. Hammond. 1965. Ann. N.Y. Acad. Sci. 119:1109.

Egan, A.R. 1970. Aust. J. Agr. Res. 21:735.

Egan, A.R. and R.J. Moir. 1965. Aust. J. Agr. Res. 16:437.

Epstein, A.N. and P. Teitelbaum. 1967. Am. J. Physiol. 213:1159.

Fenderson, C.L. and W.G. Bergen. 1976. J. Animal Sci. 42:1323.

Forbes, J.M. 1970. Brit. Vet. J. 126:1.

Forbes, J.M. and C.A. Baile. 1974. J. Dairy Sci. 57:878.

Forbes, J.M. 1977. Animal Prod. 24:91,209.

Furr, R.D. 1963. Dissert. Abstr. 24:6.

Garrett, W.N., Y.T. Yang, W.L. Dunkley and L.M. Smith. 1976. J. Animal Sci. 42:1522.

Gelperin, A. 1967. Science 157:208.

Gelperin, A. and V.G. Dethier. 1967. Physiol. Zool. 40:218.

Gengler, W.R. et al. 1970. J. Dairy Sci. 53:434.

Greenhalgh, J.F.D. and G.W. Reid. 1971. Brit. J. Nutr. 26:107.

Grossman, S.P. 1962. Am. J. Physiol. 202:872.

Grovum, W.L. and G.D. Phillips. 1974. Fed. Proc. 33:707.

Harper, A.E., N.J. Benevenga and R.M. Wohleuter. 1970. Physiol. Rev. 50:428.

Hoebel, B.G. and P. Teitelbaum. 1966. J. Comp. Physiol. Psychol. 61:189.

Holmes, E.G. and F.J. Fraser. 1965. Aust. J. Biol. Sci. 18:345.

Houpt, T.R. 1974. Am. J. Physiol. 227:161.

Iggo, A. and B.F. Leek. 1970. In: Physiology of Digestion and Metabolism in the Ruminant. Oreil Press, Newcastle Upon Tyne, England.

Jacobs, H.L. and K.N. Sharma. 1969. N.Y. Acad. Sci. 157:1084.

Jordan, H.A. 1973. Amer. Diabetic Assoc. 62:17.

Jordon, W.A., E.E. Lister, J.M. Woulhy and J.E. Comeau. 1973. Can. J. Animal Sci. 53:733.

Julien, W.E., F.A. Martz, M. Williams and G.B. Garner. 1974. J. Dairy Sci. 57:1385.

Kennedy, G.C. 1953. Proc. Roy. Soc., London, Ser. B 140:578.

King, K.R. 1976. Physiol. Psychol. 4:405.

Krebs, H.A. 1966. Vet. Record 78:187.

Kronfeld, D.S. 1970. In: Physiology of Digestion and Metabolism in the Ruminant. Oriel Press, Newcastle Upon Tyne, England.

Kruger, L. and G. Schulze. 1956. Zuchtugskunde 28:438.

LaPlace, J.P. 1970. Physiol. Behav. 5:61.

Larsson, S. 1954. Acta Physiol. Scand. 32, Suppl. 294:1.

Lehmann, F. 1941. Z. Tierphysiol. Tiernahr. Futtermittelk 5:155.

Le Maho, Y. 1977. Amer. Sci. 65:680.

Littlejohn, A. 1968. Brit. Vet. J. 124:335.

Manning, R., G.I. Alexander, H.M. Krueger and R. Bogart. 1959. Am. J. Vet. Res. 20:242.

Martin, H.F. and C.A. Baile. 1972. J. Dairy Sci. 55:606.

Martin, H.F., J.R. Seoane and C.A. Baile. 1973. Life Sci. 13:177.

Monteiro, L.S. 1972. Animal Prod. 14:263.

Montgomery, M.J. and B.R. Baumgardt. 1965. J. Dairy Sci. 48:569.

Moose, M.G., C.V. Ross and W.H. Pfander. 1969. J. Animal Sci. 29:619.

Mrosovsky, N. and T.L. Powley. 1977. Behav. Biol. 20:205.

Nir, I., N. Shapiro, Z. Nitsan and Y. Dror. 1974. Brit. J. Nutr. 32:229.

Owen, J.B., D.A.R. Davies and W.J. Ridgman. 1969. Animal Prod. 11:511.

Powley, T.L. and R.E. Keesey. 1970. J. Comp. Physiol. Psychol. 70:25.

Putnam, P.A., R. Lehmann and W. Luber. 1968. J. Animal Sci. 27:1494.

Ragsdale, A.C., H.J. Thompson, D.M. Worstell and S. Brody. 1950. Missouri Univ. Agr. Expt. Sta. Res. Bul. 460.

Raun, A.P. et al. 1976. J. Animal Sci. 43:670.

Rice, R.W., J.G. Morris, B.T. Maeda and R.L. Baldwin. 1974. Fed. Proc. 33:188.

Richardson, L.F. et al. 1976. J. Animal Sci. 43:65.

Rodgers, Q.R. and A.R. Egan. 1975. Aust. J. Biol. Sci. 28:169.

Seoane, J.R. and C.A. Baile. 1972. Physiol. Behav. 9:423.

Seoane, J.R. and C.A. Baile. 1973. Physiol. Behav. 10:915.

Seoane, J.R. and C.A. Baile. 1975. J. Dairy Sci. 58:349,515.

Seoane, J.R., C.A. Baile and H.F. Martin. 1972. Physiol. Behav. 8:993.

Seoane, J.R., C.A. Baile and R.L.Webb. 1973. Pharmacol. Biochem. Behavior 1:47.

Sharma, K.N. 1967. In: Handbook of Physiology. Alimentary Canal. Am. Physiol. Soc., Washington, D.C.

Steinbaum, E.A. and N.E. Miller. 1965. Am. J. Physiol. 208:1.

Tarttelin, M.F. and F.R. Bell. 1968. In: 3rd Intern. Conf. Regulation of Food and Water Intake, Haverford College, Sept. 1-3.

Teitelbaum, F. 1961. Nebraska Symp. on Motivation. Univ. of Nebraska Press, Lincoln.

Titchen, D.A., C.S.W. Reid and P. Vleig. 1966. Proc. N.Z. Soc. Animal Prod. 26:36.

Tribe, D.E. 1952. In: Proc. 6th Intern. Grassland Congr., Penn., Vol. II

Troelson, J.E. and F.W. Bigsby. 1964. J. Animal Sci. 23:1139.

Uhart, B.A. and F.D. Carroll. 1967. J. Animal Sci. 26:1195.

Utley, P.R., N.W. Bradley and J.A. Boling. 1970. J. Animal Sci. 31:130.

Wangsness, P.J. et al. 1976. J. Animal Sci. 42:1544.

Weston, R.H. 1971. Aust. J. Agr. Res. 22:307;469.

Wilson, G., F.A. Martz, J.A. Campbell and B.A. Becker. 1975. J. Animal Sci. 41:1431.

Wyrwicka, W. and C. Dobrzecka. 1960. Science 132:805.

Chapter 12 - Milk Fever and Ketosis

By L.H. Schultz

The high producing dairy cow is forced to make major metabolic adjustments following calving. She goes from a dry and pregnant period during which there is need only for maintenance and fetal growth to a sudden demand for a large supply of all the nutrients needed to make a large volume of milk. Although she has remarkable ability to mobilize body reserves and eventually to increase intake to reach homeostasis, intake lags behind requirements and usually does not reach maximum for about 8 weeks. During this period it is not surprising that metabolic disorders occur. The most common are milk fever and ketosis. Others which often complicate these two primary diseases are retained placenta, metritis, fat cow syndrome (where all problems are accentuated by overconditioning when dry), and displaced abomasum (where problems of adjustment of the digestive tract to the space vacated by the fetus are accentuated by high concentrate feeding; see Vol. 1). The discussion of milk fever and ketosis will stress the role of nutrition, but it is obvious that other factors, particularly hormonal changes involved in metabolic adjustment, are also important and will be considered.

MILK FEVER

Milk fever was first reported in Germany in 1793 and many theories regarding its etiology have developed over the years. A review by Hibbs (1950) is an excellent summary of research up to that time. Other more recent discussions include Payne (1970), Kronfeld (1971), Littledike (1974), and Jorgenson (1974).

Occurrence

Data on the over all incidence of milk fever in the USA are lacking. The statistical reporting service in Wisconsin indicated in 1976 that 8% of the dairy cows were affected and 67% of all herds had the problem. Reports from England give an incidence of 3.54% with 5% mortality in those affected. It was also suggested that the productive life of affected animals was reduced 3.4 years. A number of reports suggest breed differences, with the Jersey and Swedish Red breeds having a higher incidence. There is no obvious explanation for this difference.

Incidence is also related to age. It occurs rarely, if at all, in first-calf heifers, seldom at second calving, with progressively higher incidence with increased age. Incidence is greater in cows with a previous history of milk fever. Canadian studies showed that about half of the field cases were in cows with a previous history.

Milk fever has been commonly associated with high production and Scandinavian reports support this suggestion. The problem is rare in the beef breeds where milk production is lower than in dairy breeds. Although there appears to be a general relationship to high production, many cows which are not outstanding producers develop milk fever. It is also a common belief there may be a greater incidence at times of low barometric pressure and at certain seasons of the year, but conclusive evidence for these relationships is lacking. Milk fever also occurs in lactating goats, but apparently it is less of a problem than in cattle (Payne, 1966). Hypocalcemia also occurs in sheep, but it may be precipitated by many factors other than parturition (Jensen, 1974).

The timing of the problem in relation to parturition is well known and documented. Canadian studies found that 75% of the cases of milk fever occurred between 1 and 24 hr after calving (Willoughby et al, 1970). Only 3% occurred before calving, 6% at the time of calving, 12% between 25 and 48 hr after calving, and 4% later. Although some cows go down with symptoms resembling milk fever at other stages of lactation, the etiology of these cases appears to be different.

Symptoms

One of the earliest general symptoms is lack of appetite. The digestive tract is inactive. Defecation often occurs following treatment, indicating a return to more normal activity. Most commonly the cow is dull and listless. Cold ears and a dry muzzle are characteristic. The first specific symptom is incoordination when walking. Hind legs may be spraddled in an attempt to brace herself. If made to turn, she may stagger and fall. In later stages of paralysis, the cow lies down and is unable to rise. She may struggle in attempting to stand. It is not uncommon for muscle injury and hemorrhage to occur as a result of struggling. This may result in failure to rise after treatment, even though she is alert and blood minerals are normal. It is common for the head to be turned to the side in the sternal recumbency position. Canadian workers (Willoughby et al, 1970) have divided the progress of the disease into three stages: 1. Standing, but hypersensitive and wobbly; 2. Down on chest, drowsy, muscles flaccid; 3. On side, comatose, advanced muscle flaccidity. Field cases appeared in these stages in a 1:2:1 ratio.

Physiological Changes

Contrary to the common name, milk fever, body temperature is not elevated. In fact, a decrease in body temperature is very common (Littledike, 1974). The lower the body temperature the higher was the incidence of "downers" and deaths in one study. The decrease in muscle activity, decreased appetite, and possibly a decreased metabolic rate are suggested as likely causes of the decreased temperature.

Decreased gut mobility is commonly suggested as a contributing factor to milk fever. Moodie and Robertson (1962) found that feed intake, fecal output, rumen sounds, and the frequency and strength of rumen contractions were reduced at calving. However, studies do not seem to be available comparing normal to cows prone to milk fever. Depression of neuromuscular transmission was concluded to be the major cause of the paresis associated with the hypocalcemia of milk fever by Bowen et al (1970).

Although some changes in urine constituents have been noted by some workers, Blosser and Smith (1950) found that 24 hr urine Ca excretion was similar, both prepartum and postpartum, in normal and milk fever cows. Very little P was excreted in the urine prepartum by any of the cows.

Blood Changes

The major changes in the blood of milk fever cows are a decrease in Ca and P with an increase in Mg. The characteristic low blood Ca and excellent response to Ca therapy suggest that a more appropriate name for this condition would be parturient hypocalcemia (Anderson, 1970). Table 12-1 shows the changes in blood components of normal and milk fever cows.

In addition to these blood mineral changes, a number of other changes occur in blood components. These represent changes that occur, to some degree, in all cows at parturition as a response to homeostatic mechanisms. Because of inappetence and other accentuated changes in the milk fever cow, the magnitude of the changes is greater. For example, plasma free fatty acids (FFA) are elevated at parturition in non-paretic cows but elevated still more in paretic cows. Because of the significant negative correlation between FFA and Ca, it was postulated that there was an increased uptake of Ca by adipose tissue as a result of increased lipolysis and that this may be a causative factor in milk fever. However, Horst et al (1976) were unable to demonstrate increase in Ca in subcutaneous fat at parturition in either paretic or non-paretic cows. In fact, there was a positive correlation between plasma Ca and Ca in subcutaneous fat along with a highly significant negative correlation (-.66) between plasma Ca and

Table 12-1. Blood serum concentration of cows in various metabolic states.[a]

State	Blood serum, mg/100 ml		
	Calcium	Phosphorus	Magnesium
Normal	9.4	4.6	1.7
Normal at parturition	7.7 ± .9	3.9	3.0 ± .5
Milk fever			
Stage 1	6.2 ± 1.3	2.4 ± 1.4	3.2 ± .7
Stage 2	5.5 ± 1.3	1.8 ± 1.2	3.1 ± .8
Stage 3	4.6 ± 1.1	1.6 ± 1.0	3.3 ± .8

[a] Values taken from Jorgensen (1974), Willoughby et al (1970) and Horst et al (1976).

plasma FFA. It is likely that the elevated FFA levels at calving are simply a reflection of stress plus inappetence. Elevated glucocorticoids cause an increase in FFA and lack of adequate feed intake accentuates the FFA response.

The glucose and insulin situation also changes in the parturient cow, with an accentuated response in the cow with milk fever. The usual positive relationship between glucose and insulin when the cow is in a stable condition is reversed at parturition and accentuated in milk fever. Blood glucose is high at parturition due to increased stress and the resulting elevation in glucocorticoids. The cow does not respond with elevated insulin levels, presumably because the low Ca level inhibits insulin secretion by the pancreas. This also reverses the usual inverse relationship between blood glucose and plasma FFA, with the low insulin tending to accelerate mobilization of FFA from adipose tissue. The significance of other blood changes in the paretic cow, such as decreased K, decreased citric acid, increased lactic and pyruvic acids, and increased chloride have not been clarified (Littledike, 1974).

Hormone Changes

The elevated glucocorticoid levels in the blood at parturition and increased levels in milk fever cows have already been mentioned. An explanation for the low insulin levels has also been given.

The two hormones associated with Ca homeostasis have been widely studied in relation to milk fever. When it was found in the early work of Boda and Cole (1954) that a high Ca diet during the dry period increased the incidence of milk fever, it was postulated that the parathyroid gland responsible for secreting parathyroid hormone (PTH) to increase Ca mobilization became "lazy" and failed to secrete adequate PTH at parturition. However, the availability of radioimmunoassay procedures to measure circulating PTH has resulted in considerable data showing an increase in PTH levels in milk fever cows, with very high levels when the blood Ca was very low (Mayer, 1970). There was no apparent increase in resistance to development of hypocalcemia with higher concentrations of PTH. A likely explanation of this apparent paradox is that there is a significant lag time involved in developing the capacity to mobilize large quantities of Ca from bone and gut.

Calcitonin produced by the thyroid gland is involved in reducing blood Ca in response to elevated Ca levels. Littledike (1970) and others have reported elevated levels of calcitonin in the plasma of some cows prior to parturition. However, as hypocalcemia developed, calcitonin levels decreased to levels as low as or lower than during the dry period. In most cows, however, calcitonin increase before parturition was small or non-existent. No relationship could be found between increased calcitonin levels prior to calving and the development of parturient hypocalcemia. Thus, the role of calcitonin in the development of milk fever is not well understood at this time.

Because there is a marked increase in circulating estrogens a few days before calving along with a marked decrease in progesterone, it has been tempting to associate elevated estrogens with milk fever. Some workers have reported hypocalcemia after estrogen administration (Littledike, 1970). However, no reports have been seen by this writer showing that cows prone to milk fever have a greater degree of estrogen elevation than other cows and proof is lacking that estrogens have a causative relationship to milk fever.

Interrelationship of Vitamin D to Milk Fever

It has long been known that vitamin D is involved in Ca and P balance. The preventive effects of vitamin D on milk fever have been investigated for over 40 years (Littledike, 1970). Ohio workers (Hibbs and Conrad, 1960) found that feeding massive doses of vitamin D (20 million IU/day) for 3-5 days before calving gave about 80% protection from milk fever, if calving date was predicted accurately. However, there was difficulty in predicting calving date and concern over toxic effects when these levels were fed longer than 7 days. Later work (Hibbs and Conrad, 1966) with continuous feeding of high levels of vitamin D (100,000-500,000 IU/day) showed some protection in cows with a previous history of milk fever but none in cows without a previous history. Research on the mechanism of action of vitamin D suggests that the sites of action of pharmacological amounts of vitamin D are both the GI tract and the bone. Manston and Payne (1964) concluded that vitamin D increased the net absorption of Ca and P from the GI tract of pregnant cows. Rowland et al (1972) found that feeding 30 million IU of vitamin D daily increased bone resorption with no hypercalcemia in cows fed a Ca-deficient diet, but hypercalcemia in cows fed a diet with normal amounts of Ca and P. Also, evidence of toxicity has been presented by Capen et al (1968) when cows were fed 30 million IU of vitamin D daily for extended periods of time.

In research to determine whether milk fever was the result of insufficient synthesis or secretion of $1,25\text{-}(OH)_2D_3$, Horst et al (1977) studied the levels of this metabolite in the blood of paretic and non-paretic cows. Plasma $1,25\text{-}(OH)_2D_3$ increased sharply in the paretic cows during the day preceding calving, reached a maximum of 200 pico-grams/ml at parturition, and maintained this level for 2.5 days. The non-paretic cows showed a slight depression the day before calving, and then a gradual increase up to a maximum of about 100 picograms/ml of plasma two days post calving. These results suggest that milk fever is not the result of insufficient synthesis or secretion of $1,25\text{-}(OH)_2D_3$. It does suggest that the target organs of this compound as well as para-thyroid hormone are resistant at calving time in paretic cows. This does not negate the possibility of use of vitamin D metabolites in milk fever control, since administration earlier than one day before calving may avoid this resistance or override it.

With the isolation of the vitamin D meta-bolites (see Ch. 9), it was logical to test their efficacy in the control of milk fever. The first metabolite, $25\text{-}OHD_3$, is the one on which most work has been done. It can be used at low dosage levels without dangers of accumulation or toxicity. Preliminary results using 1 mg orally every other day prior to calving or 4 mg intramuscularly once weekly showed a reduced incidence of milk fever (Jorgensen, 1974). Variable field results appear to be related to body condition and to P levels fed immediately prepartum (Frank et al, 1977). Excessive P or excessive body con-dition reduce the effectiveness. Adequate Ca in the diet is also needed, but excessive Ca is usually present. These products are still under test and are not commercially available at this writing.

Prepartum Feeding Effects

Considerable evidence has accumulated suggesting that dry period feeding has a sig-nificant effect on the incidence of milk fever. Excessive Ca was implicated as a result of the work of Boda and Cole (1954). Stott (1965) suggested that inadequate dietary P

was involved and Gardner (1973) suggested that Ca:P ratio was important and that a ratio of 2.3:1 was ideal. However, most workers now seem to agree that absolute amounts of Ca and P are more important than the ratio (Jorgensen, 1974). Iowa workers demon-strated rather clearly that milk fever could be prevented with a prepartum Ca-deficient diet (Goings et al, 1974). They fed less than 15 g of Ca/day. One problem with this proccedure is to find a practical ration which will supply this low Ca intake. The diet used (dry basis) was 50% corn silage and 50% shelled corn plus a low Ca supplement. It was also necessary to limit daily intake to 14 lb of dry matter for a 1000 lb cow. There is also some concern regarding the effect of the Ca deficiency on subsequent milk production.

Evidence is accumulating that milk fever can be kept under reasonable control by con-trolling Ca and P intake during the dry period at levels near NRC requirements. Jorgensen (1974) concluded that feeding less than 100 g of Ca/cow/day and keeping the Ca:P ratio<2 to 2.5 to 1 appeared to give the best results. It would appear that, if adequate P is fed during the dry period (18-35 g/day), Ca intake may vary from near requirements (23-40 g) to 100 g/day without markedly in-fluencing the incidence of milk fever. Jor-gensen (1974) reviewed a number of experi-ments with varying intakes and ratios of Ca and P and concluded that intake was more important than ratio. High Ca intake (over 100-125 g/day) in most instances was accompanied by a high incidence of milk fever. Attempts to counteract an excess of Ca with an excess of P have generally been unsuccessful. Ohio workers have demon-strated that an excess of P as well as Ca in-creased the incidence of milk fever (Julien et al, 1977). They conducted a field experiment and divided the cows into three groups on the basis of their Ca and P intake during the dry period. Cows in Group 1 with normal intake (about .5% Ca and .25% P) had a milk fever incidence of 9.5% (4 of 42). Cows in Group 2 with a high Ca and high P intake (>.5% Ca and >.25% P) had an incidence of 35.2% (38 of 108). In cows with a previous milk fever history the incidence was 60%. In Group 3, cows were fed low Ca and high P (<.5% Ca and >.25% P). Milk fever incidence was 18.8% (6 of 32). Again the incidence was higher in cows with a previous milk fever his-tory. Regression equations relating milk fever incidence to dietary Ca and P, blood P, and age of animals were calculated. For each increase of 0.1% of dietary Ca over .59%, incidence of milk fever increased by 14%. For every increase in dietary P of .1% above .37%, incidence of milk fever increased by 19%. Increases in dietary P were reflected in blood P and for every increase in blood P of 1 mg/100 ml above 5.80, incidence of milk fever increased by 20%. These data all suggest the rather critical importance of both Ca and P intake during the dry period in the control of milk fever. The daily requirements of a 1430 lb pregnant cow are about 36 g of Ca and 28 g of P. These can be met by feeding about 21 lb (DM) of mixed hay or 30 lb (DM) of corn silage provided absorption remains at 40% and 50% for Ca and P.

Other dietary factors may also have some influence on milk fever. Scandinavian workers (Ender et al, 1962) suggested that a high proportion of alkaline components (Na + K + Ca + Mg) in the diet in relation to acid components (Cl + P + S) was conducive to milk fever and that feeding of silage preserved with mineral acids reduced the incidence. The feeding of ammonium chloride has also been reported to increase acidity of the ration and Ca absorption (Payne, 1967). Neither of these procedures seems to have practical potential for milk fever control. Palatability of ammonium chloride apparently is a problem.

Grain feeding levels during the dry period have also been studied in relation to milk fever with conflicting results. Kendall et al (1966) suggested that increased grain feeding reduced milk fever while Emery et al (1968) found that high prepartum grain feeding increased the incidence. Possibly the difference may have been due to condition of the cows. Theoretically, heavier grain feeding should tend to increase absorption of Ca because of a depressing effect on rumen pH. However, if cows become too fat, increased stress at calving and reduced feed intake tend to increase milk fever.

Prevention

In order to recommend a control program, a rationale regarding the cause of the problem is needed, with preventive measures designed to counteract causative factors. Although there is neither complete agreement on optimum control procedures nor complete success on their adoption, enough information and consensus seems to be available to develop a rationale and make suggestions for prevention.

There seems to be reasonable agreement that the sudden Ca drain, imposed by initiation of lactation at parturition, is the basic underlying cause of milk fever. There is a drain of about 5-8 g of Ca daily for the fetus compared to 15-30 g of Ca secreted in colostrum on day 1 after calving. This difference can be greater than the total amount of Ca in the plasma and tissue fluids, the readily available body stores. The difference must be offset by an increased flow of Ca from absorption of dietary Ca from the gut or mobilization from bone. The fact that the amount of Ca excreted in the colostrum of paretic and non-paretic cows was not different (Hibbs et al, 1970) suggest variation in the ability of cows to compensate for the Ca drain. Mastectomy of milk fever prone cows did prevent milk fever at the subsequent calving (Niedermeier, 1949). Figure 12-1 illustrates possible changes in Ca balance at calving.

If the cow is relying heavily on the alimentary tract as a source of Ca to supply the demands imposed by initiation of lactation, any change in dietary supply caused by decreased appetite or a switch to a low Ca or high P diet would lead to hypocalcemia. If

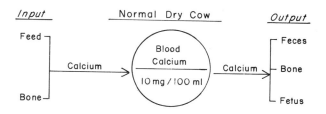

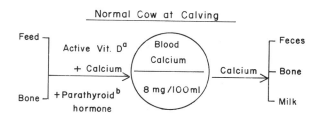

Fig. 12-1. Changes in calcium balance at calving. In the milk fever cow (a) and (b) are elevated but the response in the target tissues (gut and bone) appears to be delayed so that blood calcium drops to about 5 mg/100 ml. A high calcium diet while dry appears to delay responsiveness to (b) while a high phosphorus diet may inhibit formation of (a) as well as delay response.

the cow is relying primarily on bone mobilization (as when underfed on Ca prior to calving), inappetence would have been a lesser effect, but factors influencing bone mobilization would become more important. There is apparently a significant lag time in creating the capacity to mobilize large quantities of Ca from bone and gut, particularly bone. When cows were underfed Ca prior to calving, a severe hypocalcemia developed within 24 hr of the dietary change, but it was corrected rapidly (1-2 days) and resulted in the cows being able to meet the entire lactational Ca demand from bone sources of Ca without developing milk fever at calving (Goings, 1974). Ramberg et al (1970) suggested that in the normal cow the initial response to the lactational Ca drain is an increase in absorption from the digestive tract and that appreciable levels of bone resorption are not apparent until about 10 days after the onset of lactation. This presumably occurs in spite of elevated levels of both parathyroid hormone and $1,25\text{-}(OH)_2D_3$, both of which stimulate bone mobilization.

Specific Preventive Procedures

Milking techniques. The common practice of incomplete milking after calving has not been effective in milk fever control. The likely reason is that once the demand for Ca occurs and it moves into the udder, it is out of the system, whether it is removed from the gland or not. Prepartum milking has also been ineffective. The apparent reason is that, although the Ca drain is more gradual, there is still a large drain at parturition when target issues involved in Ca mobilization lag in responsiveness.

Vitamin D. Use of pharmacological doses of vitamin D_3 (10-30 million IU/day for 2-7 days prior to calving) has been beneficial in prevention of milk fever, but timing and toxicity problems are great enough to eliminate this as a practical approach. Year around feeding of high levels of vitamin D (100,000-500,000 IU/day) has some beneficial effect in cows with a previous history of milk fever, but again the practicality is questionable. Julien et al (1977) also found that 10 million IU of vitamin D_3 injected prior to calving reduced milk fever in cows with a previous history, but the risks of these massive doses seem to outweigh the gain.

Use of vitamin D_3 metabolites shows promise of being effective and practical,

particularly in herds where excessive Ca is being fed during the dry period and Ca intake is difficult to reduce because of the feeding of legume forage, but they are not yet available commercially. It does appear that control of P intake (adequate but not excessive) is important for maximum effectiveness.

Dietary approaches. Feeding dietary Ca according to NRC during the dry period, particularly, seems the most effective and practical way to keep the incidence of milk fever at a reasonable level. Excesses of either Ca or P have been shown to increase the incidence. Although feeding a Ca-deficient diet prior to calving may be the surest way of minimizing milk fever, it is difficult to manage and effects on the subsequent lactation have not been clarified. Assuring that adequate vitamin D is fed according to or slightly exceeding normal requirements would also be desirable to assure formulation of adequate amounts of the active metabolites. Avoiding excessive fatness at calving would aid in milk fever prevention by tending to avoid excess stress and inappetence during the calving period. All management factors which tend to keep the cow on feed at calving, such as avoidance of stress, clean comfortable calving quarters, and provision for exercise should be helpful.

Treatment

Regardless of preventive procedures, 100% freedom from milk fever is unlikely. Fortunately, treatment is very effective if initiated in time and response is rather spectacular. A cow that is down may be up and eating within an hour or two. The method of choice for treating milk fever still remains the intravenous administration of Ca gluconate (25-100 g). Usually, 500 ml of a 20% solution is given. Slow administration is needed to prevent a heart block. Figure 12-2 shows treatment of a cow in stage 2 of milk fever with calcium gluconate. Her heart is being monitored, also. Response is rapid but relapses are common (ca. 30% of cases). Presumably this is due to an elevation of blood Ca above normal, triggering mechanisms to reduce it, such as calcitonin release, along with a continued lag in the ability of the cow to mobilize adequate gut and bone Ca.

Inflating the udder with air is also effective, but generally is not used because of danger of udder infection or injury. Prior

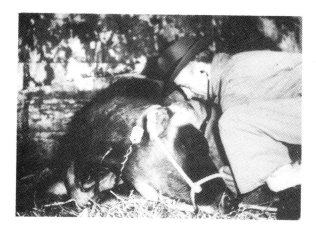

Fig. 12-2. Treating a cow with milk fever.

intramammary infusion of antibiotics and use of a pressure gauge to control pressure tends to prevent these problems. There is also evidence that relapses are reduced with udder insufflation compared to Ca gluconate treatment (Mayer et al, 1967). The insufflation technique has been shown to have a definite inhibitory effect on milk production with a 35-50% reduction during the 24-hr period after insufflation. In addition, there is 3-6 hr delay in response, so it does not work fast enough for the cow in a coma.

KETOSIS

Ketosis of varying degrees can occur in all animal species with many different causes. In farm animals it is a practical problem primarily in the lactating dairy cow, the ewe in late pregnancy, and the goat in either late pregnancy or early lactation and is associated with the glucose drain imposed by advanced pregnancy (multiple fetuses in sheep and goats) or high milk production in early lactation. Ketosis which occurs in the diabetic human is similar in certain respects but the cause—rather than a glucose drain for productive purposes—is the inability to utilize glucose due to a lack of insulin. Diabetes mellitus has been reported only rarely in sheep and cattle (Phillips et al, 1971) so true diabetes is not considered a practical problem in ruminants. Because young animals with diabetes would likely be eliminated without diagnosis, the incidence may be higher than the scattered reports indicate.

Although the hypoglycemia of lactation ketosis in dairy cattle and of pregnancy keto-

sis in sheep seems to be the factor that initiates most of the other metabolic changes, the disorders in the two species are by no means identical. The lactating cow can partially adjust to the problem by reducing milk production. But the fetuses continue to grow in the case of the ewe, resulting in less favorable response to treatment and more fatal cases.

Lactation ketosis will be discussed first along with the general metabolic relationships in ketotic ruminants, followed by a separate section on pregnancy ketosis and the fat-cow syndrome. Recent reviews on ketosis include Bergman (1970), Kronfeld (1970) and Schultz (1971, 1974).

LACTATION KETOSIS

Definitions

Ketosis is defined as a metabolic disorder in which the level of ketone bodies in body fluids is elevated. These ketone bodies are β-hydroxybutyric acid (βHBA), acetoacetic acid (AA), and acetone. The term, acetonemia, was first used to characterize this disorder and is still used in the field. Technically, it is a less correct term then ketosis since it indicates that only acetone increases in the blood. Acetone is of minor importance unless the ketosis is severe and prolonged, but it does cause the peculiar acetone odor of the breath, urine and milk of ketotic animals. Acetone is formed from AA at a rate of 5%/hr in the animal (Krebs, 1961).

Low blood ketone concentrations are found in normal animals and the ratio of βHBA to AA plus acetone is about 7:1. As the animal becomes ketotic, the ratio decreases to as low as 1:1 (Menahan et al, 1967). It is not clear whether ketone bodies are responsible for the symptoms of ketosis, but high levels of AA and acetone can depress the central nervous system (Bergman, 1971).

Occurrence

Shaw (1956) estimated the incidence of ketosis in dairy cows in the USA at a million cases per year. Payne (1966) reported an incidence of 2% in the United Kingdom. A more recent New York study reported a 12% incidence. Incidence in individual herds may be much higher. These figures would obviously be influenced by diagnostic criteria and the extent to which subclinical cases and cases complicated by other disorders were included. It is estimated that in approximately one-third of cows showing

328

elevated ketone bodies, the ketosis is secondary to other problems such as retained placenta, metritis, hardware, etc.

The incidence is higher in older cows and certain cows tend to repeat, but the problem occurs at first calving. In northern climates the incidence is higher in the winter and early spring, but this is likely due to more calvings during this period rather than a seasonal effect. Although problems can occur on pasture, recovery has often been observed when barn-fed cows with ketosis were turned out to pasture.

Primary ketosis in dairy cows almost always occurs during the first 8 weeks after calving, when there is peak lactation drain and energy intake has not caught up with output. About 3 weeks after calving is the most critical period. Complicating factors are common when problems occur within a few days of calving.

Symptoms

Visible symptoms of ketosis are not very specific and could indicate a number of different ailments. Fig. 12-3 shows a ketotic cow and Fig. 12-4 shows the same cow after recovery. The ketotic cow shows the typical gaunt and dull appearance. Occasionally cows may be highly excitable and nervous, but this is not common. Usually, rumen contractions are not as regular; the rumen contents are firmer; and the feces are rather dry. There is inappentence, with grain usually being refused at first, then silage, while the cow may continue to eat some hay. Sometimes there may be incoordination, particularly of the hind legs. Some cases

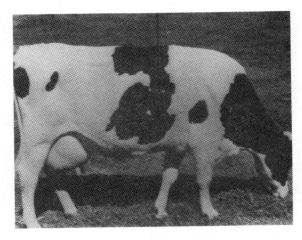

Fig. 12-4. Cow in Fig. 12-3 after recovery from ketosis.

exhibit a curvature of the spine. Decreased milk production and loss of weight are obvious consequences of the reduced feed intake. There is a distinctive acetone-like odor of the breath and fresh milk. Milk fat percentage is increased, even in subclinical ketosis. Usually, the cow progresses into this condition gradually. Very seldom does a cow die from ketosis and, when death occurs, the only obvious finding on postmortem is a fatty liver. Although an acidosis develops in diabetic ketosis in humans due to the acid ketone bodies, this seldom occurs in the ketotic cow since the alkali reserve usually remains adequate (Kronfeld, 1970).

Blood, Urine and Tissue Changes

Table 12-2 illustrates the typical changes occurring in the blood of cows with ketosis. The elevation of ketone bodies is characteristic. Normal levels could be considered anything <10 mg/100 ml. The ketone level of milk is about half the blood level, whereas the urine level exceeds the blood level by about 4X. This makes the urine test somewhat overly sensitive for diagnosis, with most high producing cows showing positive urine tests in early lactation, often without need for treatment. The milk test (Ketotest, Denver Chemical Company, Stamford, Connecticut) is more conservative but more accurate than the urine test in indicating when there may be a problem (Schultz and Myers, 1959). The test starts to become positive at about 10 mg/100 ml total blood ketones. Since the mammary gland utilizes βHBA for milk fat synthesis, the level of this component in milk is markedly lower than in

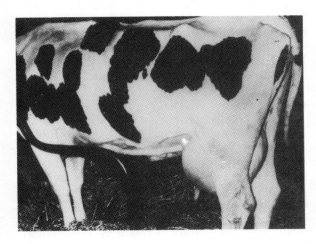

Figure 12-3. Cow with ketosis. Note gaunt appearance and dullness.

blood. It appears at a rather constant level in milk of 2 mg/100 ml. Levels of AA and acetone in blood and milk tend to be similar. The qualitative tests for ketone bodies based on the development of a purple color with sodium nitroprusside do not measure βHBA.

Table 12-2. Blood changes in clinical ketosis.[a]

Component	Normal	Ketosis
	- - mg/100 ml - -	
Blood		
Glucose	52	28
Ketones (total)	3	41
Plasma		
Free fatty acids	3	33
Triglycerides	14	8
Free cholesterol	29	15
Cholesterol esters	226	150
Phospholipids	174	82

[a]From Yamdagni and Schultz (1970)

The second major change in the blood accompanying elevated ketones is a decrease in glucose (Tables 12-2 and 12-3). Normal levels in ruminants are about 50 mg/100 ml. Values <40 can be considered subnormal. Ketotic animals may have levels as low as 25.

The depressed blood glucose is the initial change likely responsible for subsequent changes in other components. Under unusual conditions—thyroxin administration, fat cow syndrome, certain infections, diabetes, etc.—it is possible to have normal or elevated glucose along with elevated ketones, but this is not typical of primary ketosis. The causative factor(s) are different and the animals do not respond to the usual treatments.

The third blood change is an increase in free fatty acids (FFA) which are a measure of the extent of lipolysis of adipose tissue or mobilization of body fat. They are transported as an FFA-albumin complex. The sequence of events involves reduced glucose (and reduced insulin), which triggers increased lipid mobilization and elevated blood FFA. These are in turn converted to ketone bodies in the liver. In the normal cow about 40% of the ketones come from FFA while in clinical ketosis, when a cow is not eating, 100% may come from FFA. Under ketotic conditions within-cow correlations between blood glucose and ketones were negative (-.68) while there was a significant positive correlation (+.85) between FFA and ketones (Radloff and Schultz, 1967).

The other blood lipids (Table 12-2; triglycerides, cholesterols, and phospholipids) all decrease. The reason for this is not completely understood. Less lipids are consumed so there is a reduced need for transportation of absorbed lipids. In nonruminants elevated FFA result in increased production and secretion of lipoproteins into the plasma. This does not appear to be the case in ruminants. Either less triglycerides are formed in the liver because of reduced glycerophosphate resulting from low blood glucose, or there is some problem in lipoprotein release from the liver. The latter seems possible because in advanced ketosis a fatty liver may develop. Some writers have suggested that inadequate protein nutrition may result in reduced availability of the protein moiety of the lipoprotein, reducing lipoprotein release (McCarthy et al, 1968). Attempts to produce experimental fatty livers in ruminants by the author have generally been unsuccessful. Only under conditions where glucose availability is markedly reduced, such as alloxan diabetes or fasting of lactating or pregnant animals, has significant fat accumulated in the liver (Schwalm and Schultz, 1976).

Table 12-3. Comparison of blood and milk ketones.[a]

Qualitative milk test	Blood, mg/100 ml			Milk, mg/100 ml	
	Glucose	βHBA	AA + A	βHBA	AA + A
Negative	44	4.3	1.1	1.7	0.8
Trace	40	8.8	2.8	2.3	1.7
One plus	30	11.0	4.0	3.1	2.5
Two plus	35	14.7	7.0	2.8	5.5

[a]From Schultz and Myers (1959). βHBA, β-hydroxybutyric acid; AA, acetoacetic acid; A, acetone (all expressed as acetone).

Other blood components also change in ketosis, probably as a consequence of the reduced glucose. Blood acetate is usually elevated (Schwalm et al, 1969; Kronfeld, 1970). Normal levels are about 6-10 mg/100 ml in the ruminant, the primary source being rumen fermentation, with absorption through the portal system and little or no metabolism in the liver. Acetate is non-ketogenic in the ruminant and may be beneficial to the ketotic cow through a glucose-sparing action. It is likely that there are two reasons for its elevation in the ketotic cow. One is increased endogenous acetate production, although some difference of opinion exists on the extent and importance of endogenous acetate in the ruminant. The other more likely reason is a decrease in acetate utilization as a result of low glucose and insulin levels. Fed alloxan diabetic goats showed increases in blood acetate to as high as 40 mg/100 ml, while fasted diabetic goats stayed at about 5 mg/100 ml (Schwalm and Schultz, 1976). This suggests that a reduction in utilization is the major cause of the elevation. Acetate levels in subclinically ketotic cows rose to about 20 mg/100 ml by the time of peak ketones and minimum glucose about 3 weeks after calving (Schwalm and Schultz, 1976). The latter work also showed a decrease in insulin levels corresponding with decreases in glucose and increases in FFA and ketones.

Figures 12-5 and 12-6 show changes following parturition in the blood components of normal cows and cows with subclinical ketosis. No treatment was required in the subclinical animals. The marked drop in triglycerides at calving in both groups likely reflects the use of triglycerides for milk fat synthesis. The increases in cholesterol in both groups likely reflects increased lipid intake with increased grain feeding.

Diagnosis

The symptoms of ketosis are not very specific, so care in diagnosis is needed. A distinction should be made between primary or spontaneous ketosis, where no apparent pathological condition other than the true ketotic syndrome exists, and secondary ketosis, in which other factors are involved. Since primary ketosis is a metabolic disorder, there is no elevation of body temperature, so elevated temperature immediately indicates other factors. An elevated blood glucose level accompanying elevated ketones also suggests other complications.

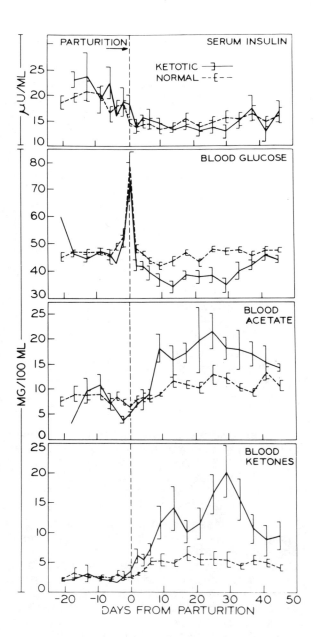

Fig. 12-5. Changes in serum insulin, blood glucose, acetate and ketones in normal and ketotic cows before and after calving.

The best field diagnostic procedure would involve a measurement of body temperature along with both a urine and milk test. A negative urine test rules out ketosis. A positive urine test and negative milk test (a common finding) suggest some body fat mobilization but, without other symptoms, no need for treatment. When the milk test becomes positive, even though the cow has not gone off feed, use of an oral glucose precursor such as propylene glycol, fed daily, is indicated. With more severe

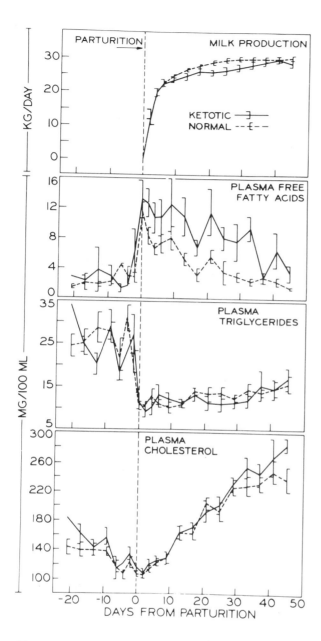

Fig. 12-6. Changes in milk production and free fatty acids, triglyceride, and cholesterol in plasma of normal and ketotic cows before and after parturition.

reactions and/or other symptoms, treatment is indicated. Radloff and Schultz (1967) tested 300 cows with a commercial powder designed for diabetics (Ketotest) which becomes positive (trace) at 4-6 mg/100 ml milk ketones representing 10-15 mg/100 ml blood ketones. During the first 8 weeks after calving, 14% were positive. Of 42 positive cows, 22, or about half, were considered to require treatment by the herdsman or veterinarian.

In problem herds a simple weekly milk test for the first 6 weeks after calving would identify cows with beginning ketosis. Corrective action could be taken with oral materials before the cases became severe.

Relationship to Glucose Metabolism

Importance of Glucose. Glucose is a critical metabolite in the high-producing dairy cow. Not only is it absorbed in much smaller proportions from the digestive tract than in the non-ruminant, but it is needed in larger amounts for the synthesis of lactose in milk. Blood glucose levels are about half those of non-ruminants and must be maintained at 40-60 mg/100 ml to maintain normal function in many body tissues. All of the glycerol for lipid synthesis in adipose tissue and most of that for milk fat synthesis apparently comes from glucose. The lactating mammary gland of the fed goat obtains 30-50% of its energy from the oxidation of glucose and 20-30% from blood acetate (Linzell, 1968).

Synthesis of lactose by the mammary gland imposes the greatest drain on blood glucose. Both the glucose and galactose of the lactose molecule are largely derived from blood glucose in both cows and goats. This suggests that slightly more glucose on a weight basis than there is lactose in milk would need to be removed by the gland daily just to make the lactose. Thus, a cow producing 40 kg of milk containing 5% lactose would need over 2 kg of glucose daily just for lactose synthesis in addition to that needed for oxidation for energy and for synthesis of glycerol. Thus, it is not surprising that milk production drops when blood glucose drops. Since the cow needs to rely primarily on gluconeogenesis for her glucose supply, optimum metabolism is necessary for the maintenance of normal blood glucose in the high producing cow.

Origin of Glucose. The pathways of gluconeogenesis and intermediary metabolism have been discussed elsewhere. It will suffice to comment here that the main source of glucose for the ketosis susceptible ruminant is propionic acid produced in the rumen. Propionate production in the rumen tends to increase with rations higher in grain. In general, such rations are beneficial to cows prone to ketosis, but care needs to be taken, when using such rations, to feed enough roughage to keep the cow on feed.

A second source of glucose is hydrolysis in the lower tract of starch which bypassed the rumen. Estimates of this contribution vary from none to a considerable amount on rations high in corn grain. Increased starch by-pass would be helpful to the ketosis prone cow.

Another source of glucose is protein. Although some amino acids are ketogenic (tyrosine, isoleucine, leucine and phenylalanine), most are glucogenic. The ketogenic effects of leucine and the glucogenic effects of valine have been demonstrated (Menahan and Schultz, 1964). Estimates of the extent of contribution of protein to glucose are variable, but most fall in the range of about 8-18% in producing animals. In experiments with normal sheep, Bergman et al (1966) estimated that metabolized protein could account for as much as two-thirds of the glucose turnover and that propionate and protein together could account for ca. 90% of the glucose.

Lactate is also a source of glucose, but when normal reactions are fed it is doubtful if there is significant absorption of lactate from the rumen. It is found in the rumen for short periods of time after normal feeding (Waldo and Schulz, 1956, 1960). Glycerol is another source of glucose. Bergman et al (1968) estimated that about 5% of the glucose is derived from glycerol in fed sheep and 23% in fasted sheep. Under normal conditions it would not be a very important source. Thus, it appears that the major dietary sources would be propionate, protein and adsorbed glucose from bypassed starch. During fasting, after liver glycogen is depleted, the major precursors would be amino acids from tissue protein and glycerol from mobilized body fat.

Since oxalacetate plays such a central role in the synthesis of glucose from propionate and many amino acids and, since adequate oxalacetate would favor fatty acid oxidation through the TCA cycle rather than formation of ketone bodies, some writers have suggested oxalacetate deficiency as a cause of ketosis (Johnson, 1953). Krebs (1966) suggested that a high rate of gluconeogenesis and an increase of the enzyme phosphoenolpyruvate carboxykinase might cause a shortage of oxalacetate, based on information from alloxan diabetic rats. A lack of precursors such as propionate may also deplete oxalacetate in the ruminant. Ballard et al (1969) were unable to find any alterations from normal in total oxalacetate in the livers of ketotic or starved cows, but suggested that there could still be a change in mitochondrial oxalacetate. It is also possible that there could be a relative shortage of oxalacetate in relation to the FFA levels, which might not show up as an absolute difference among animals.

Cause of Hypoglycemia. It is tempting to use the simple explanation that hypoglycemia and ensuing ketosis in dairy cows is due to the glucose drain imposed by high milk production coupled with an inadequate supply of glucose precursors. It is likely that these are the major predisposing causes. However, if these were the only factors, it should be possible to produce the condition experimentally by simply reducing the feed of the high-producing cow. This has not been the case. Attempts to produce in cows an experimental ketosis resembling spontaneous ketosis have been relatively unsuccessful. Fasting produces similar blood changes of lesser magnitude and milk production is reduced, but resumption of feeding brings about prompt recovery. It appears that the homeostatic mechanisms are able to prevent typical ketosis. However, further work needs to be done using high-producing cows heavily fed during the dry period, followed by prolonged feed restriction after calving. It appears that in certain cows or under certain conditions at calving, such as excessive fatness, the homeostatic mechanisms do not function properly.

Lipid Metabolism

Rumen Acids. Radloff and Schultz (1967) showed that in ketosis the concentration of VFA in the rumen was decreased and there was an increase in the proportion of acetate and a decrease in propionate. Since the same results were obtained with fasting, it was concluded that these results were simply a reflection of reduced feed intake rather than any upset in rumen fermentation.

Administration of the major rumen acids— acetic, propionic, and butyric, followed by monitoring of blood metabolites, gives a good picture of their role in ketosis (Schultz and Smith, 1951). Propionic caused increases in blood glucose and decreased ketones as expected. Acetic caused little change in either, suggesting that it was neither glucogenic nor ketogenic. It can be considered a glucose sparer, however, so could have some beneficial effect in ketosis. Butyric acid, on the other hand, was definitely ketogenic. The possible ketogenic effects of the normal rumen butyrate production are counteracted by the antiketogenic effects of propionic acid, so it is unlikely that blood ketones will be elevated above normal from butyrate produced in the rumen, except for unusual circumstances. However, cows could consume extra butyric acid when certain high moisture hay crop silages are fed and consumption of such silages could accentuate the ketosis problem (Schultz, 1971). The fact that such silages are often bad-smelling and consumed at a lower level accentuates the problem. Fortunately, corn silage and most good quality wilted hay crop silages contain little butyric acid.

Lipolysis in Adipose Tissue. When blood glucose and insulin are reduced, adipose tissue lipolysis is increased and FFA are released into the bloodstream to become the major source of ketones in the ketotic cow. The FFA appear to be taken up by the liver on a rather constant percentage, regardless of level, so lipolysis is an important aspect of ketosis. The importance of glucose in control of lipolysis is emphasized by the high negative correlation between glucose and FFA (-.92) (Schwalm et al, 1969). A large number of agents influence lipolysis as follows: rapid increase—catecholamines, ACTH, TSH, glucogen, LH, secretin, vasopressin, seratonin; slow increase—growth hormone, glucocorticoids, thyroid hormones; decrease—insulin, nicotinic acid, and α and β-adrenergic blockers. No doubt some of these are involved in the increased lipolysis in ketosis, but decreases in glucose and insulin appear to be the most important.

Recent work attempting to reduce ketosis through control of lipolysis with nicotinic acid illustrates that its action is much more complicated than simply inhibition of lipolysis (Waterman and Schultz, 1972). Pharmacological doses of nicotinic acid to ketotic cows markedly inhibited lipolysis and ketogenesis for a period of about 36 hr, but this was followed by a rebound to initial or higher levels of FFA and ketones in about 48 hr and then a gradual return to normal in symptoms and blood picture in about a week. Subsequent work suggests that nicotinic acid may have not only a direct effect on lipolysis but also specific effects on carbohydrate metabolism, including elevation of insulin levels and extended glucose tolerance curves. Any use of nicotinic acid in ketosis control should await further research on dosage level and mechanism of action.

Lipid Transport and Utilization. Chapter 6 on lipids covers normal transport and utilization of lipids. Alteration from the normal in ketosis will be stressed here. The sequence of events occurring in ketosis could be outlined as follows: (1) Blood glucose level decreases. (2) Hormone sensitive lipase activity in adipose tissue increases, presumably in response to decreased insulin and possibly other hormonal changes, resulting in elevated tissue levels of cyclic AMP. (3) Free fatty acids (FFA) are released in increased amounts into the blood stream, where they are carried as an FFA albumin complex. (4) Liver uptake of FFA is increased. About 25% of the total FFA release is taken up by the liver (Bergman et al, 1970) so elevated levels mean increased uptake. (5) Mammary gland uptake of FFA increases. Under normal conditions there is no net uptake of FFA by the mammary gland, but appreciable uptake occurs in the ketotic cow. These FFA contribute to the FFA pool for milk fat synthesis. Triglyceride uptake by the mammary gland is reduced in ketosis, but the decreased triglyceride contribution to the FFA pool is more than compensated for by the increase from FFA. A negative A-V difference for acetoacetate and acetone across the mammary gland also appears in the ketotic cow. This makes it tempting to speculate that the mammary gland is producing ketones as a result of the increased FFA uptake. However, the enzymes necessary for conversion of FFA to ketones appear to be absent. Thus, it seems that the increased AA results from an increased conversion from βHBA rather than production of ketones in the mammary gland. (6) The pathways of FFA metabolism in the liver change. Possible pathways are: (a) esterification to triglycerides and some phospholipids; (b) oxidation to CO_2, and (c) partial oxidation to ketone bodies. Bergman (1971) suggests that ca. 30% of the FFA uptake by the liver of normal fed sheep is converted to ketone bodies, but this increases to 81% in ketotic animals. This means a reduction in percentage esterification and oxidation to CO_2. (7) The lipid content of the liver increases. Although the percentage of FFA esterified is reduced, it is likely that total esterification is increased because total FFA uptake by the liver may be increased 5-10X. Lipid accumulation would be expected unless release was accelerated. (8) Blood triglyceride levels decline. Although it appears that hepatic triglyceride release in non-ruminants increases with increased FFA, Table 12-2 shows decreases in triglyceride, phospholipid, and the cholesterols in the blood of ketotic ruminants. The fact that the lipid content of the liver is higher and that of the blood is lower supports the idea of an abnormality in release from the liver.

Table 12-4 illustrates the utilization of FFA in a normal, fed, lactating ruminant compared to one with experimental ketosis. Phlorizin was used to decrease the renal threshold for glucose and increase the glucose drain in the experimental animals and labeled palmitate was the FFA source. This table shows the extremely rapid turnover of FFA and the increased pool size and turnover rate as well as the increased contribution of FFA to ketones. Essentially all of the ketones in the experimentally ketotic animals were coming from FFA.

The mechanisms responsible for the shift in FFA pathways in the liver are not well understood. The increased FFA levels present more to the liver for processing and a relative oxalacetate deficiency would tend to decrease oxidation, forcing more into ketogenesis and esterification.

Fatty Livers. The usual observation regarding the liver of cows with advanced ketosis or cows that die from ketosis is an increase in fat content. Saarinen and Shaw (1950) reported total liver fat levels in cows in the early stages of ketosis were 7.4% and in the later stages 21.5%. The author has found levels as high as 30% (68% on a dry basis) in advanced ketosis. Saarinen and Shaw (1950) were able to produce fatty livers in cows by fasting and they concluded that the fatty liver was a result of reduced feed intake and was not present in the early stages of ketosis, so should not be considered a predisposing factor. It appears that there is gradual accumulation of lipid in the liver, thus making treatment increasingly difficult as the case progresses. The gradual recovery occurring with agents that reduce FFA would suggest, however, that the fatty degeneration is not irreversible, except in older, chronic, repeater cases.

Ketone Body Metabolism

Origin of Ketone Bodies. The principal precursors of ketone bodies in the ruminant are FFA from mobilized body fat and butyric acid produced in the rumen or ingested in silage. Table 12-4 suggests that 41% of ketones came from FFA in fed animals and essentially all came from FFA in the ketotic animal. Other studies with labeled butyrate in fed goats show 47% of the βHBA and 26% of the AA coming from butyrate. Other minor sources include ketogenic amino acids, acetate, and dietary short chain fatty acids with an even number of carbons (chain length 4-10). It is suggested that these acids are absorbed from the rumen with resulting ketone body formation in the rumen wall. None of these sources appear to be significant precursors of ketones under normal circumstances.

Table 12-4. Metabolism of [1-^{14}C] palmitic acid in goats.[a]

Measurement	Normal, fed lactating	Fasted, phlorizinized, lactating
Blood, mg/100 ml		
plasma FFA	15	49
plasma TG	21	23
ketones	6	18
Liver lipids, mg/g		
triglycerides	32	135
phospholipids	16	16
Free fatty acid pool		
pool size, mg	405	1325
turnover rate, mg/kg/min.	4.7	7.9
turnover time, min.	1.8	3.1
ketones from FFA, %	41	103

[a] Constant intravenous infusion of palmitate-albumin complex for 4 hr. Taken from Yamdagui and Schultz (1969).

The major sites of ketone body formation in the ruminant are the liver and ruminal and abomasal epithelium (Bergman, 1971). Both βHBA and AA are produced by these tissues but βHBA appears to be the predominant one produced in the rumen wall. Other tissues such as lung, kidney and, sometimes, muscle, can interconvert ketone bodies and increase one or the other (βHBA or AA) but this does one not represent net production. The over all effect in these tissues is utilization. As indicated previously, the mammary gland of the ketotic cow tends to convert βHBA to AA without net production of ketones. Although βHBA may be a more desirable transport form because it is more stable, it has to be converted to AA before it is utilized in the tissues.

Utilization of Ketone Bodies. Most tissues can utilize ketone bodies. The brain and nervous tissue of normal animals presumably do not utilize ketone bodies, but there is evidence of an adaptation in humans so that after a week or so of starvation, the brain begins to use considerable amounts of ketones. Whether a similar adaptation occurs in ruminants is not known. Such adaptation might explain the 'nervous' cases of ketosis in that rapidly developing cases would exhibit nervous symptoms because adaptation for ketone utilization by the brain had not occurred.

Over the years there has been a change of view as to whether ketosis is a result of overproduction of ketone bodies in the liver or underutilization by extrahepatic tissues. The present prevailing idea is that ketone body utilization is not significantly impaired in ketosis but production increases and, as the case becomes more advanced, production exceeds utilization. Maximum utilization of ketones apparently occurs at a blood level of about 20 mg/100 ml. Beyond this point utilization cannot keep up with production, and large increases in blood levels occur.

Excretion of ketone bodies occurs in urine and milk of lactating cows, with urine excretion by far exceeding that in milk. Although excretion represents a loss of energy, it is unlikely that excretion would ever exceed 10% of the amount produced.

Regulation of Ketogenesis. The important blood components related to blood ketones are glucose and FFA. Reid and Hinks (1962), when working with sheep, showed that the positive relationship between FFA and ketones in the blood was linear up to about 1.5 meq/l. of FFA, after which ketones increased rapidly. This is likely the point at which utilization of ketones can no longer keep up with production, and the point at which the ketosis changes from what might be considered a physiological form to a pathological form.

The influence of blood glucose on ketones has been demonstrated clearly when insulin secretion was not impaired. Administration of intravenous glucose quickly decreases FFA and ketones. The glucose influence could occur through a direct effect, for example on pathways of FFA metabolism in the liver, or indirectly through reducing FFA release from adipose tissue. A path analysis of changes in these components suggested that about 75% of the variation associated with blood ketone level could be accounted for by these two effects of blood glucose level, with the indirect effect, via FFA levels, being relatively much greater than the direct effect (Radloff and Schultz, 1967).

Studies on factors influencing the ketogenecity of butyrate have shown that intravenous glucose or propionate, or oral propionate are equally effective in suppressing ketogenesis from butyrate. Since circulating FFA did not change, it is unlikely that the effect was one of reducing FFA levels. More likely, there is an antiketogenic effect of glucose at the rumen wall as well as the liver.

Hormonal Relationships

One of the early concepts (Shaw, 1956) was that bovine ketosis was due to an adrenocortical insufficiency. This was based on the observation that glucocorticoids were beneficial for treatment and the presence of histological abnormalities in the adrenals of ketotic cows. However, the fact that responses were also obtained with ACTH suggested that the adrenal gland was still responsive since the action of ACTH was to stimulate glucocorticoid release. Response to glucose or glucose precursors would also argue against degenerative changes in the adrenal as a primary cause.

Thyroxine has been used in the experimental production of ketosis (Hibbitt, 1966; Kellogg et al, 1971) but the unphysiological conditions used make it doubtful if thyroxine excess is a cause of spontaneous ketosis. Glucose is usually elevated along with ketones in fed animals. Emery and Williams (1964) showed that implants of triodothyronine at calving time increased either the severity or the incidence of ketosis.

A number of hormones have been shown to influence glucose, ketones, and FFA (Radloff and Schultz, 1966). Growth hormone, ACTH, and the catecholanines increased FFA, with glucocorticoids causing a slight increase. Glucagon caused a biphasic response in FFA, a decrease followed by an increase above normal, with opposite responses in blood glucose. In fed animals ketones did not change despite rather large increases in FFA. Insulin caused an initial depression of FFA, along with decreases in glucose, presumably reflecting increased glucose utilization. Other data on insulin which fit the concept of a low glucose supply suggest a reduced circulating level of insulin in ketotic cows (Schwalm and Schultz, 1976) and show that insulin administration to ruminants causes hypoglycemia but not ketosis (Schultz and Smith, 1951; Kronfeld, 1971). Convincing evidence of abnormal secretion of any of these hormones as a direct cause of ketosis is lacking.

Nutritional Aspects

Energy Intake. Since there is good evidence that ketosis is accentuated by excessive fatness at calving and by a negative energy balance after calving, the ideal feeding program for ketosis control from an energy standpoint would be low to moderate feeding before calving with a high level after calving. There are some practical limitations in this program, however. Although feed can be offered, maximum intake is delayed until about the 7th week after calving because of unknown physiological factors. This is after the peak ketosis problem. In addition, one-third of the diet needs to be coarse roughage in order to keep cows on feed and maintain a normal fat test. This limits the amount of energy that can be fed. The feeding of fat would increase energy concentration, but levels above ca. 5% of the total diet tend to reduce nutrient utilization. However, feeding liberal quantities of high quality feeds within these limitations should definitely aid in ketosis control. Gardner (1969), using various concentrations of energy levels designated as low and high before and after calving, found the optimum combination from the standpoint of both production and freedom from ketosis was low prepartum (115% of requirements) and high postpartum (fed to maintain body wt).

Protein. Shaw (1956) concluded that there was little evidence that feeding either high or low protein was conducive to ketosis. Euro-

pean workers have suggested that high protein rations create problems similar to ketosis, but evidence for this is lacking in the USA. McCarthy et al (1968) proposed that a shortage of methionine may be an important cause of ketosis, possibly because it played a special role in the formation of lipoproteins in the liver. However, administration of methionine analogue at a level of 40 g daily for 7 days to cows with subclinical ketosis had limited beneficial effect (Schultz, 1971). It is concluded that although adequate protein nutrition is desirable, there is a lack of specific evidence that either a deficiency or excess of protein is a primary cause of field ketosis in the USA.

Minerals and Vitamins. There is a lack of convincing evidence of the direct involvement of mineral or vitamin deficiencies in the development of primary ketosis. Control by supplementation would be easy if such were the case. Blood levels of K, P, Cl, Ca and Mg are not altered in ketosis (Shaw, 1956). Negative results have been obtained with treatment using physiological levels of B vitamins.

Since vitamin B_{12} is required as an essential cofactor in the conversion of propionate to glucose, it might be suspected that a deficiency of this Co-containing vitamin might be involved as a consequence of a Co deficiency. There is evidence that blood and liver levels of vitamin B_{12} are lower in early than in late lactation. However, there is no evidence that added Co beyond that in trace mineral salt is beneficial. Most herds with ketosis problems appear to have adequate Co in the ration.

Therapy

Many treatments have been suggested for ketosis, but only a few have stood the test of time. The following are the most commonly used and most effective (Fox, 1971).

Intravenous Glucose. Commonly 500 ml of a 40% glucose solution is given. This is the most rapid way to provide an outside source of glucose. One disadvantage is that some may spill over in the urine and be lost. Presumably the added glucose triggers insulin release and it is used up rather rapidly and blood glucose falls below normal levels within 2 hr. Therefore, the animal has to make rather rapid homeostatic adjustments to return to normal. Slow, continuous intravenous drips of glucose (2000 ml) represent a rather ideal type of therapy, but this is too cumbersome under field conditions.

Hormones. Glucocorticoids or ACTH have been used for ketosis treatment for many years (Shaw, 1956). The beneficial effect of glucocorticoids appears to be due to increases in blood glucose through stimulation of glucogenesis from amino acids. ACTH stimulates release of glucocorticoids from the adrenal cortex. The effect lasts several days. The glucocorticoids cause decreased peripheral utilization of glucose in muscle and adipose tissue, which may initially cause some increased mobilization of body fat and elevation of ketones. The major disadvantages appear to be possible changes in hormonal balance and depletion of body protein through use as a glucose source. Repeated treatment with glucocorticoids may reduce adrenal activity and disease resistance. ACTH may be indicated in cases that have been repeatedly treated with glucocorticoids in order to stimulate the bypassed adrenals. Fox (1971) suggests dosage levels for glucocorticoids equivalent to 1 g of cortisone intramuscularly or intravenously, or 200-800 units of ACTH intramuscularly.

Oral Glucose Precursors. Two oral materials have been commonly used. Sodium propionate was used initially but has gradually been replaced by propylene glycol because of advantages in cost, handling, palatability, and absence of sodium. The usual dosage level of these materials is 250-500 g/day, preferably in two administrations/day. It is usually continued for 5-10 days. Drenching may be needed in cows that are not eating. Propylene glycol is converted to glucose in the liver.

The advantage of the oral materials is that an exogenous source of glucose is provided at a modest level over a prolonged period. Often the oral materials are used as a follow-up of glucose or hormone treatments. Sugar or molasses fed or given as a drench is not an effective treatment because it is not absorbed as glucose but converted to VFA in the rumen.

Miscellaneous Treatments. Cobalt (at least 100 mg/day) may be added to propylene glycol if a Co deficiency is suspected. Chloral hydrate (28 g twice daily for 3-5 days) is sometimes used to quiet nervous cases and occasionally in other special circumstances.

Prevention

It is not possible to give a set of recommendations which will prevent all ketosis. However, procedures which will maximize energy intake, provide adequate glucose precursors, and minimize body fat mobilization have made it possible to keep this metabolic disorder under reasonable control. Specific recommendations include the following: (1) Avoid excessive fatness at calving. It is recommended that cows be in reasonable condition at drying off and that they be fed only enough to maintain that condition while dry. (2) Either eliminate or limit concentrate feeding while dry, but increase concentrates to modest levels in the late dry period, and then rapidly after calving, using care to prevent the cow from going off feed. Feed recommended levels of energy, protein, minerals and vitamins to meet current standards. (3) Feed high quality forage at a minimum of one-third of total dry matter intake after calving to keep the cows on feed and avoid a drop in fat test. (4) Do not make abrupt changes in the ration after freshening, particularly to low quality feeds. Avoid feeding high-moisture hay crop silage with elevated levels of butyric acid. (5) Maximize intake by providing palatable feeds fed at reasonable frequency along with optimum comfort, exercise, and freedom from stress. Production being equal, select for cows with good capacity and appetite. (6) In problem herds monitor the ketotic state with weekly milk tests for 6 weeks after calving. Feed propylene glycol at a level of 125-250 g daily to problem cows.

FAT-COW SYNDROME

In recent years the term, fat-cow syndrome, has been coined to desribe a condition occurring within a few days of calving in dairy cows that are excessively fat at calving time (Morrow, 1976). It is characterized by depression, lack of appetite, and general weakness. Although it has some characteristics similar to ketosis, it is a somewhat different phenomenon. Almost invariably it is associated with other problems at calving, such as milk fever, displaced abomasum, retained placenta, metritis or mastitis. Often there is an elevated temperature due to the associated infection. Although the blood ketones and FFA are usually high, the ketosis is almost always secondary to another problem. Blood glucose may be high or low. These cows often die and have fatty livers and much internal fat. Treatment is not very effective, usually consisting of intravenous glucose and antibiotics to combat the infections.

The cause appears to be grossly excessive energy intake in the dry period, possibly extending back into the latter part of lactation, followed by stress at calving time. It is often a herd problem. All-corn-silage diets and failure to separate dry cows from lactating cows in group handling situations are common predisposing factors. Current trials suggest that if these excessively fat cows can get through the calving period without complications, they may be able to adjust to the mobilization of large amounts of fat, but they have an increased susceptibility to these problems and a reduced capacity to adjust. When the animal does not eat, the liver is flooded with mobilized FFA, a fatty liver develops, and recovery is difficult. Optimum management at calving is more critical for the fat cow.

PREGNANCY TOXEMIA IN SHEEP

This condition is sometimes called lambing sickness or twin lamb disease (Jensen, 1974). It is pregnancy ketosis in late gestation in ewes carrying multiple fetuses. Increased emphasis on multiple births would tend to increase the potential for this problem.

Occurrence

Pregnancy toxemia (PT) occurs in all breeds of sheep in the second and subsequent pregnancies. Both thin and obese ewes carrying multiple fetuses develop the disease during the last month of pregnancy. The cause is a combination of rapid growth of multiple fetuses and inadequate nutrition, particularly low energy intake. Special stresses at this time may be an accentuating factor. Experimental PT cannot always be produced by fasting alone, but superimposing a stress condition on fasting is quite effective. Transport, fasting, change of feed, inclement weather, and disease can all initiate the problem. The hypoglycemia resulting from the above appears to be the primary initiating factor, as in lactation ketosis.

Symptoms

The affected ewe usually isolates from the flock and shows inappetence, weakness and incoordination; she may elevate her head. Eventually she lies down and rises only with assistance, often showing accelerated breathing and discharges from the nose. In the advanced stages there is progression to neurologic signs such as blindness, muscular tremors, convulsions, coma and finally, death. These are usually attributed to the hypoglycemia. Blood analyses will show the same changes as in lacatation ketosis, namely low glucose and high ketones. The ketones are excreted in the urine and result in positive qualitative tests. Post-mortem examination shows a fatty liver.

Treatment and Prevention

Treatment is not as effective as in lactation ketosis because the glucose drain continues to accelerate with growth of fetuses. Mortality rate of affected ewes may reach 80%. Recovery often follows parturition, either from natural birth or by surgery. The course may vary from about 2-10 days. The treatment of choice appears to be about 100 ml daily of propylene glycol by drench. Intravenous glucose in a single administration would give temporary benefit but a prolonged glucose source is needed to keep pace with the fetal glucose drain. Reports vary on the ACTH and glucocorticoid relationships in pregnancy toxemia, some indicating low and others high glucocorticoid levels. In addition the abortive effects of these hormones complicate their use for treatment (Patterson and Cunningham, 1969).

Prevention involves proper nutrition and management during pregnancy. Extremes of condition (either too thin or too fat) should be avoided. Dietary energy and protein should be increased during the last 2 months of pregnancy. An 11% protein ration and about ½ lb of grain daily is usually suggested. In special problem situations additions of about 50 ml daily of propylene glycol to the ration may be a useful preventative. Management practices which stimulate appetite, such as mild exercise, and which avoid stress are important parts of an overall control program.

REFERENCES CITED

Milk Fever

Anderson, J.J.B., ed. 1970. Parturient Hypocalcemia. Academic Press, New York.

Blosser, T.H. and V.R. Smith. 1950. J. Dairy Sci. 33:329.

Boda, J.M. and H.H. Cole. 1954. J. Dairy Sci. 37:360.

Bowen, J.M., D.M. Blackmen, J.E. Heavner. 1970. Amer. J. Vet. Res. 31:831.

Capen, C.C., C.R. Cole and J.W. Hibbs. 1968. Fed. Proc. 27:142.

DeLuca, H.F. 1973. Proc. Georgia Nutr. Conf. Feb. 14-16.

DeLuca, H.F. 1974. Fed. Proc. 33:2211.

Ender, F., I.W. Dishington and A. Helgebostad. 1962. Acta. Vet. Scand. 3:Suppl. 1.

Emery, R.S., H.D. Hafs, D. Armstrong and W.W. Snyder. 1968. J. Dairy Sci. 52:345.

Frank, F.R., M.L. Ogilvie, T.J. Kalsuk and N.A. Jorgensen. 1977. Workshop on Vitamin D. Asilomar, CA.

Gardner, R.W. and R.L. Peck. 1973. J. Dairy Sci. 56:385.

Hibbs, J.W. 1950. J. Dairy Sci. 33:758.

Goings, R.L. et al. 1974. J. Dairy Sci. 57:1184.

Hibbs, J.W. and H.R. Conrad. 1960. J. Dairy Sci. 43:1124.

Hibbs, J.W. and H.R. Conrad. 1966. J. Dairy Sci. 49:243.

Hibbs, J.W., L.A. Muir, and H.R. Conrad. 1970. In: Parturient Hypocalcemia. Academic Press.

Horst, R.L., J.H. Thornton, N.A. Jorgensen and L.H. Schultz. 1976. J. Dairy Sci. 59:88.

Horst, R.L., J.A. Eisman, N.A. Jorgensen and H.F. DeLuca. 1977. Science 196:662.

Jensen, R. 1974. Diseases of Sheep. Lea and Febiger, Philadelphia.

Jorgensen, N.A. 1974. J. Dairy Sci. 57:933.

Julien, W.E., H.R. Conrad, J.W. Hibbs and W.L. Crest. 1977. J. Dairy Sci. 60:431.

Kendall, K.A., K.E. Harshbarger, R.L. Hays, and E.E. Ormston. 1966. J. Dairy Sci. 49:720.

Kronfeld, D.S. 1971. Advan. Vet. Sci. Comp. Med. 15:133.

Littledike, E.T. 1974. Lactation, Vol. II. Academic Press, New York.

Manston, R. and J.S. Payne. 1964. Brit. Vet. J. 120:167.

Mayer, G.P., C.K. Kamberg and D.S. Kronfeld. 1967. J. Amer. Vet. 'Med. Assoc. 151:1673.

Mayer, G.P. 1970. In: Parturient Hypocalcemia. Academic Press.

Moodie, E.W. and A. Robertson. 1962. Res. Vet. Sci. 3:470.

Niedermeier, R.P., V.R. Smith and C.K. Whitehair. 1949. J. Dairy Sci. 32:927.

Payne, J.M. 1966. Vet. Rec. 78:31.

Payne, J.M. 1967. Vet. Rec. Clin. Suppl. 12, 81: I, II.

Payne, J.M. 1970. Int. Rev. Exp. Pathol. 9:191.

Ramberg, C.F., J.M. Phang and D.S. Kronfeld. 1970. In: Parturient Hypocalcemia. Academic Press.

Rowland, G.W., C.C. Capen, D.M. Young and H.E. Black. 1972. Calcif. Tissue. Res. 9:179.

Stott, G.H. 1965. J. Dairy Sci. 48:1485.

Willoughby, R.A., D.G. Butler, C.F. Cote and R.A. Curtes. 1970. In: Parturient Hypocalcemia. Academic Press.

Ketosis

Ballard, F.J., R.W. Hanson and D.S. Kronfeld. 1969. Fed. Proc. Fed. Amer. Soc. Exp. Biol. 28:218.

Bergman, E.N. 1970. In: Dukes Physiology of Domestic Animals. Cornell Univ. Press, Ithaca, New York.

Bergman, E.N. 1971. J. Dairy Sci. 54:936.

Bergman, E.N., R.J. Havel, B.M. Wolfe and T. Bohmer. 1970. Fed. Proc. Fed. Soc. Exp. Biol. 29:327.

Bergman, E.N., W.E. Rowe and K.Kon. 1966. Amer. J. Physiol. 211:793.

Bergman, E.N., D.G. Starr and S.S. Reulein. 1968. Amer. J. Physiol. 215:874.

Emery, R.S. and J.H. Williams. 1964. J. Dairy Sci. 47:879.

Fox, F.H. 1971. J. Dairy Sci. 54:974.

Gardner, R.W. 1969. J. Dairy Sci. 52:1973.

Hibbitt, K.D. 1966. J. Dairy Res. 38:291.

Jensen, R. 1974. Diseases of Sheep. Lea and Febiger, Philadelphia.

Johnson, R.B. 1953. Amer. J. Vet. Res. 14:366.

Kellogg, D.W., C.J. Balock and D.D. Miller. 1971. J. Dairy Sci. 54:1499.

Krebs, H.A. 1961. Biochem. J. 80:225.

Krebs, H.A. 1966. Vet. Rec. 78:187.

Kronfeld, D.D. 1970. In: Physiology of Digestion and Metabolism in the Ruminant. Oriel Press, Newcastle upon Tyne, England.

Kronfeld, D.S. 1971. J. Dairy Sci. 54:949.

Linzell, J.L. 1968. Proc. Nutr. Soc. 27:44.

McCarthy, R.D., G.A. Porter and L.C. Griel, Jr. 1968. J. Dairy Sci. 51:459.

Menahan, L.A. and L.H. Schultz. 1964. J. Dairy Sci. 47:1086.

Menahan, L.A., W.B. Holtman, L.H. Schultz and W.G. Hoekstra. 1967. J. Dairy Sci. 50:1409.

Morrow, D.A. 1976. J. Dairy Sci. 59:1625.

Patterson, D.S.P. and N.F. Cunningham. 1969. Proc. Nutr. Soc. 171.

Payne, J.M. 1966. Brit. Vet. J. 122:183.

Phillips, R.W., K.L. Knox, R.E. Pleason and J.B. Tasker. 1971. Cornell Vet. 61:114.

Radloff, H.D. and L.H. Schultz. 1966. J. Dairy Sci. 49:971.

Radloff, H.D. and L.H. Schultz. 1967. J. Dairy Sci. 50:68.

Reid, R.L. and N.T. Hinks. 1962. Aust. J. Agr. Res. 13:1124.

Robertson, W.G., H.D. Lennon, W.W. Bailey and J.P. Mixner. 1957. J. Dairy Sci. 40:732.

Saarinen, P. and J.C. Shaw. 1950. J. Dairy Sci. 33:515.

Satter, L.D. and W.J. Esdale. 1968. J. Appl. Microbiol. 16:680.

Schultz, L.H. 1971. J. Dairy Sci. 54:962.

Schultz, L.H. 1974. In: Lactation, Vol. II. Academic Press, New York.

Schultz, L.H. and M. Myers. 1959. J. Dairy Sci. 42:705.

Schultz, L.H. and V.R. Smith. 1951. J. Dairy Sci. 34:1191.

Schwalm, J.W. and L.H. Schultz. 1976. J. Dairy Sci. 59:255;262.

Schwalm, J.W., R. Waterman, G.E. Shook and L.H. Schultz. 1969. J. Dairy Sci. 52:915.

Shaw, J.C. 1956. J. Dairy Sci. 39:402.

Waldo, D.R. and L.H. Schultz. 1956. J. Dairy Sci. 39:1956.

Waldo, D.R. and L.H. Schultz. 1960. J. Dairy Sci. 43:496.

Waterman, R. and L.H. Schultz. 1972. J. Dairy Sci. 55:1447.

Yamdagni, S. and L.H. Schultz. 1969. J. Dairy Sci. 52:1278.

Yamdagni, S. and L.H. Schultz. 1970. J. Dairy Sci. 53:1046.

Chapter 13 - Magnesium Tetany and Urinary Calculi

By D.C. Church and J.P. Fontenot

MAGNESIUM TETANY (GRASS TETANY)

Ruminants are susceptible to a disturbance accompanied by low blood serum Mg known as grass tetany (grass staggers, hypomagnesemic tetany, lactation tetany, winter tetany or wheat pasture poisoning). Many research studies have been conducted concerning this disturbance, but the etiology of it is not completely understood. Some of the reviews available include those of Burns and Allcroft (1967), Grunes et al (1970) and Fontenot et al (1973).

Occurrence

Grass tetany occurs in Europe, North America, Australia and New Zealand where high quality pastures are used for grazing ruminants. These are areas where the temperature range is on the order of 40-60° F (5-15°C) during the spring months. Tetany is most apt to occur during the late winter and early spring, although it may occasionally strike during autumn, when animals are grazing on regrowth pasture or even in animals that are being stall-fed during the winter (Burns and Allcroft, 1967). The latent period after turning animals on to grass is said to be 5-10 days.

Usually only female animals are affected with grass tetany, although it has been reported in calves and steers (Crookshank and Sims, 1955). In the USA beef cows are affected more commonly than dairy cows, but in Europe dairy cows are frequently affected. Perhaps the practice of feeding more concentrates to dairy animals in the USA may be related to this difference.

As in the case of milk fever, grass tetany is more common in older cows, usually during the first 2 mo. of lactation, although there are many exceptions to this. European studies indicate that the overall incidence is relatively low (1-2%), but individual herds may have a high percentage of affected animals. Thus grass tetany is often of a disastrous nature to individual ranchers, since the mortality rate is often high (30% +) in clinical cases. Burns and Allcroft (1967) indicate that there are breed differences in dairy cattle, with Ayrshires being the most susceptible of the British breeds. Lactating ewes also appear to be much more susceptible than wethers or dry ewes.

Although older animals are more commonly affected, the reason for this difference is not known. Smith (1959) observed a decrease in ability to utilize Mg with increasing age in calves. However, Garces and Evans (1971) found no significant difference in Mg absorption or retention related to age in steers ranging from 10 to 88 months of age. Perhaps the increased susceptibility of older animals may be attributable to lower labile reserves of body Mg which are found primarily in the bone.

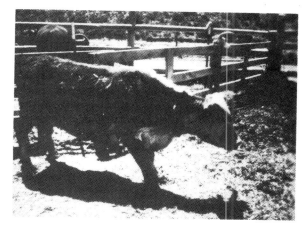

Fig. 13-1. A cow in a highly excitable stage of grass tetany. Courtesy of A. L. Lesperance, Univ. of Nevada.

Clinical Symptoms

The physical symptoms indicate that grass tetany is a nervous type of disorder (Sims and Crookshank, 1956; Blood and Henderson, 1968; Todd and Horvath, 1970). In the acute stage the animal indicates an unusual alertness and nervousness, with the ears pricked and twitching, the head held high, and with staring eyes (Fig. 13-1). Twitching of the muscles is usually evident. Slight disturbances may precipitate attacks of continuous bellowing and frenzied galloping. Incoordination of movement develops as evidenced by a staggering gait and falling and tetany of the legs followed by violent convulsions. The animal tends to lie flat on its side and the forelegs pedal periodically. There is chomping of the jaws, frothing at the mouth, and retraction of the eyelids. During convulsions the animal lies quietly, but another convulsion may be set off by touch or sudden noise. Pulse and respiratory rates are high, as is the body temperature. Heart sounds are increased and may be heard from some distance. In field cases disturbances of the ground due to leg movement indicate that tetany may last some time before death occurs. Postmortem lesions include well marked hemorrhages of the heart, at the base of the large blood vessels, and sometimes in the alimentary tract. From studies on neuromuscular irritability in hypomagnesemic calves, Todd and Horvath (1970) concluded that the main dysfunction causing tetany is not likely to be in the muscle fiber or in the central nervous systems. Rather, it is a facilitation of neuromuscular transmission involving reduction of the current required to cause contraction to about one-third of normal. Electrocardiograms were not very useful in distinguishing degree of hypomagnesemia or occurrence of tetany (Horvath et al, 1971). Histological studies show degenerative changes of vascular walls in muscular tissues and the deposition of Ca salts (Ohshima et al, 1973).

A subacute form developing over a period of several days has been described. Animals often resist being driven. Spasmodic urination and frequent defecation occur, and appetite and milk yield drop off. Muscles in the hind legs gradually develop tetany, and other symptoms of acute tetany may follow. Animals with subacute tetany may recover spontaneously. In the chronic form the condition is characterized by a stiff gait and gradual loss of body condition. It may occur over a period of several weeks, and may progress to the more acute forms or to recovery. The subacute form is not observed frequently under field conditions; instead the animals are found down in tetany or dead.

Biochemical Changes

The most characteristic change that has been observed in grass tetany is a sudden drop in blood serum Mg (Rook and Storry, 1962). The normal range in serum is 1.8 to 3.2 mg/100 ml. In cases of tetany the level may decline to 0.5 mg/100 ml or less, although clinical signs have been reported at levels just below normal. Perhaps the relatively high Mg levels found, at times, may be due to time of sampling, since Burns and Allcroft (1967) point out that serum Mg may rise temporarily at the onset of convulsions. Cows with signs of grass tetany were shown to have low cerebrospinal fluid Mg levels (Allsop and Pauli, 1975). The onset of the nervous signs of hypomagnesemia was more closely associated with low cerebrospinal fluid Mg levels than with low serum levels (Meyer, and Scholz, 1973; Pauli and Allsop, 1974). Tetany was produced in sheep by perfusion with synthetic cerebrospinal fluid solutions containing 0.6 mg Mg/100 ml (Allsop and Pauli, 1975). The signs of tetany were abolished by perfusion with a solution of normal Mg concentration. These researchers suggested that low cerebrospinal fluid Mg in hypomagnesemic tetany may result in changes in the central nervous system which would produce the nervous signs.

Hemingway et al (1965) reported a rapid fall in both plasma Ca and Mg after lactating ewes were transferred to grass. Animals with clinical cases of grass tetany were observed to have a marked hypocalcemia (6 mg/100 ml Ca), as well as hypomagnesemia (0.5 mg/100 ml). However, tetany did not occur in the high proportion of ewes which showed low plasma Mg, but which maintained normal levels of plasma Ca. Marshak (1958) found that cows with tetany had serum Ca levels which ranged from 4.5 to 7.2 mg/100 ml and Mg levels from 0.61 to 3.9 mg/100 ml. The Ca:Mg ratio was not related to the degree of tetany. A very high proportion of animals showing tetany have both low serum Ca and Mg (Burns and Allcroft, 1967; Schuster et al, 1969; Forbes, 1972). The concentrations of serum Ca and Mg were elevated 3-5 days after treatment for tetany (Hall and Reynolds, 1972).

Dobson et al (1966) observed that grazing by sheep resulted in increased K in saliva during the first 2 days, after which it fell gradually. Na fell as K rose, the result being that the sum of the two was constant. Plasma Mg fell from about 1.8 on winter feed to 1.1 mg/100 ml after 2 nights on pasture. Scott (1969) also found a marked drop in plasma Mg within 24 hr after transfer of sheep to pasture. Salivary K rose within 1 day to 1 wk, a difference being noted in two differing experiments. Field (1961) could detect no differences in availability of Mg from tetany-prone grass pastures as compared to control pastures when using wethers as experimental animals. However, Hjerpe (1968) noted that feeding clippings from tetany-prone pastures resulted in a reduced pool of body Mg which was estimated with the aid of radiomagnesium. The body Mg pool was believed to be largely in bone. Care et al (1965) have also studied Mg retention using radiomagnesium. They found that the turnover rate between two proposed body pools of Mg (total Mg in extracellular fluid vs readily exchangeable intracellular Mg of soft tissues and bone) was significantly greater on a hay diet than on a grass diet. Field (1961) observed that transfer of sheep to a spring pasture resulted in an immediate fall in urinary Mg excretion, even when the change led to an increased Mg intake. The lowest values occurred within 1-2 days after the change to pasture. Thereafter, urinary excretion tended to increase, perhaps due partly to a high intake of water in young grass (Suttle and Field, 1966). When sheep were fed a control grass or one known to cause tetany, Larvor and Violette (1970) found that blood Mg declined less with the control grass whether fresh or dried. Tetanigenic grass (when fresh) caused greater water consumption and reduced ruminal acetic acid. Urinary Mg excretion was decreased but not Mg balance and Larvor (1976) suggested that withdrawal of Mg from body reserves was reduced by the tetany-prone grass. With respect to excretion (Head and Rook, 1955), it has been observed that stall-fed cows also showed a reduction in excretion of Mg via urine when changed to spring pasture, although Mg intake was about the same. In the case of one cow excretion fell from 3-4 g/day to 1.5 g within 24 hr and then to 0.2 g by 8 days. There was a concomitant fall in blood Mg. These data on cows indicate a longer course of events than do the data of Field when working with sheep. Other research (Van't Klooster, 1965) indicates a reduced solubility of Ca and Mg in grass, which would account for some reduced absorption.

Head and Rook (1955) also observed that rumen ammonia rose from levels of about 10-30 mg/100 when on dry feed to 40-60 mg/100 ml on pasture. Jugular blood ammonia also rose. Administration of a single dose of ammonium acetate or carbonate (1,250 g to animals of varying sizes) resulted in ruminal levels comparable to those of cows on fresh grass and similar changes in urinary excretion and blood plasma Mg. Crookshank and Sims (1955) found that blood inorganic P, total diffusible Ca and Mg, and the albumin-globulin ratio decreased, while total serum protein, globulin and possibly the K level increased in affected animals.

ETIOLOGY OF GRASS TETANY

The sudden development of hypomagnesemia after a change of diet from a winter ration to that of spring grass has led to the conclusion that grass tetany cannot be a simple dietary deficiency of Mg. This conclusion is further supported by research data indicating that bone reserves are usually in the normal range in affected animals. Furthermore, the fact that treatment with Mg or Ca and Mg salts brings about such a rapid remission of symptoms leads to the conclusion that there must be some interference with Mg metabolism. This might be a result of reduced absorption or metabolism of Mg in the tissues. Some of the factors related to Mg utilization are discussed in the following sections.

Dietary Mg Requirements

Differences in dietary requirements of Mg for different ages and classes of animals may be responsible for differences in relative susceptibility of ruminant animals to grass tetany (see Ch. 4). For example, grass tetany usually occurs in cows nursing calves although it sometimes occurs in pregnant cows (Sims and Crookshank, 1956; Merchon and Custer, 1958). It appears that the dietary Mg required by cows is much lower during gestation than lactation. Research from the Virginia Experiment Station (Fig. 13-2) suggests that 7-9 g/day are required for beef cows during gestation as compared to 18-22 g/day during lactation (O'Kelley and Fontenot, 1969, 1973). Thus, this increased requirement during lactation may be a contributing factor to development of grass tetany.

Starvation and Underfeeding

Christian and Williams (1960) showed that starvation for 4 days of sheep which were exposed to cold, windy, wet weather resulted in a reduced level of serum Mg (from 2.7 to 1.9 mg/100 ml) and when sheep were allowed to graze again, serum Mg continued to fall. Ca and K levels responded to refeeding. Herd (1966) has also shown that starvation for 24-48 hr resulted in a decline in serum Mg in both cattle and lactating ewes. In the cattle serum Mg reached its lowest concentration 1-2 days after they were returned to grazing. Several of the ewes developed tetany after starvation for 24 hr. Crowley (1966) observed that tetany developed in ewes which were given restricted grazing for 10 days prior to flushing them on fall pasture. Michael (1968) maintained ewes on a high or low plane of

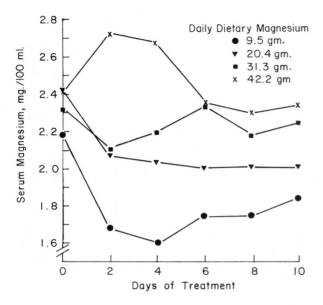

Fig. 13-2. Effect of dietary Mg level on blood serum Mg in beef cows, early lactation.

nutrition during late pregnancy and early lactation and then transferred them to grass. Results indicated that serum Ca and Mg were lower in the low plane ewes. The continuation of supplementary feed after the ewes were turned to pasture reduced the incidence of tetany. These results clearly indicate that environment and underfeeding have a very marked effect on the susceptibility of animals to hypomagnesemia.

Potassium Fertilization and Dietary Level

Incidence of grass tetany appears to be higher in animals grazing pastures which have been fertilized with K. Some workers (Hvidsten et al, 1959; Kemp, 1958, 1960) have reported that the high levels of K fertilization resulted in lowered serum Mg levels but other researchers (Smyth et al, 1958; Hemingway et al, 1963; Ritchie and Hemingway, 1963; Lomba et al, 1971) reported no substantial effect. Perhaps a change in botanical composition of the sward is necessary for K to assert an adverse effect on Mg utilization. Bartlett et al (1954) reported severe decreases in serum Mg from K fertilization in pastures in which clover was controlled, but they observed no such effect on the sward predominantly of clover. Jolley and Leaver (1974) reported that tetany-prone pastures were higher in Mg content than the tetany-free ones. Grace and Wilson (1972) observed that white clover resulted in lower blood Mg in cattle than rye-

grass, even though the clover contained more Mg. However, with sheep the opposite results were obtained.

Feeding a high level of K resulted in a depression in serum Mg in cattle and sheep (Kunkel et al, 1953; Suttle and Field, 1969; Frye et al, 1975). High dietary levels tended to accentuate the harmful effects of a low Mg intake in calves (Blaxter et al, 1960). Addition of 400 g of KCl to the ration of fresh cut grass lowered Mg availability in milking cows (Kemp et al, 1961). Administration of high levels of K via rumen cannula or by addition to the ration resulted in increased fecal excretion and decreased urinary excretion of Mg (Suttle and Field, 1967; Meyer and Stehling, 1973). However, Mudd (1970) noted that high dietary K (added as fertilizer) resulted in increased urinary excretion of K and Mg. Thus, there may be a different response if K salts are fed than when plant tissues are high in K.

A depression in Mg absorption was reported from feeding a ration containing 4% K to wether lambs (House and Van Campen, 1971). In studies with Mg administered intravenously, they found a decrease in endogenous fecal excretion of Mg from feeding the high K level. Feeding a high level of K (4.9 vs. 0.6%) to lambs during a series of 3-day balance trials resulted in a 46% depression of apparent Mg absorption (Newton et al,

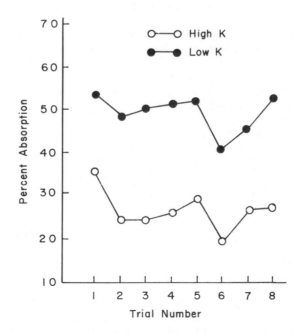

13-3. Apparent magnesium absorption. From Newton et al (1972).

1972). As shown in Fig. 13-3, the differences were established early and persisted at about the same level throughout the experiment. Average apparent absorption of Mg, expressed as percent of intake, was 49% for the sheep fed the low K ration and 26.4% for those fed the high K ration. In an experiment in which ^{28}Mg was injected intravenously, the central Mg turnover rate was lower for the sheep fed the high K rations. These results indicated that high K levels interfere with Mg absorption rather than increasing its re-excretion into the digestive tract. It appears that a depressing effect of K on Mg absorption is quantitative rather than proportional (Frye et al, 1975). The depression in Mg absorption expressed as grams/day from feeding a high K ration was similar at all dietary Mg levels, but the depression decreases with dietary Mg level, when expressed on a percentage of intake basis.

Indication was obtained that a high dietary K level may alter Mg metabolism in other ways. House and Bird (1975) found that the decrease in serum Mg levels following intravenous injection of Mg was more rapid in goats fed a 4% K diet than those fed a 0.9% K diet. They postulated that supplementary K may have advanced the disappearance of Mg from plasma and decreased urinary Mg excretion by increasing the cellular uptake and retention of Mg because of increased cellular K levels. Lentz et al (1976) reported that intravenous administration of KCl resulted in increased plasma levels of both K and immunoreactive insulin more in Mg deficient than in normal calves. They also noticed elevated plasma glucose levels in the deficient calves from administration of K. They suggested that the elevation may have resulted from stimulation of glucagon secretion by the high insulin levels.

Nitrogen Fertilization and Dietary Level
Fertilization of pastures with high levels of N has generally resulted in lowered serum Mg in ruminants grazing the pastures (Bartlett et al, 1954, 1957; Kemp, 1958, 1960; O'Kelley et al, 1969), even though Mg intake may be higher (L'Estrange et al, 1967; Lomba et al, 1971). Feeding of forage which had received high rates of N fertilization generally resulted in increased fecal and decreased urinary Mg (Stillings et al, 1964).

Fertilization with high levels of N has been shown to increase the crude protein content of forage (Bartlett et al, 1957; Kemp, 1958, 1960; O'Kelley and Fontenot, 1969). A high dietary intake of a high protein forage would result in high ruminal ammonia level which possibly could be involved in Mg utilization. Head and Rook (1955) found that administration of 1250 g of ammonium acetate or ammonium carbonate into the rumen of cows resulted in a reduction in urinary Mg excretion and lower serum levels. The premise was that the lower urinary Mg excretion was due to lower absorption. They suggested that hypomagnesemia of cows on pasture, especially in early spring, arises from an inadequate absorption of Mg and is probably associated with high ruminal ammonia production.

Moore et al (1972) found that apparent Mg absorption was similar for lambs fed rations containing 10 or 33% crude protein levels regardless of whether urea supplied 0 or 35% of the dietary N. An increase in urinary Mg excretion when the high N level was fed resulted in a marked decrease in Mg retention. The cause(s) of the differences in urinary nitrogen excretion were not apparent. Rook et al (1958) suggested that urine is the main disposal route for Mg absorbed in excess of requirements. The high correlation recorded between absorption and urinary Mg supports this hypothesis (Chicco et al, 1972). The increase in urinary excretion of Mg, resulting from the high dietary N intake (Moore et al, 1972), may indicate interference of Mg utilization within the body.

High Nitrogen and Potassium
Forages which are associated with a high incidence of grass tetany are frequently high in both N and K. The actively growing wheat plant has been shown to be quite high in these two components. Fertilization of the plants with a combination of N and K has usually produced lower serum Mg in cows than fertilizing with either alone (Smyth et al, 1958; Kemp, 1960). McIntosh et al (1973) observed that increasing K fertilizer reduced total and water-soluble Mg in grass. Increasing N fertilizer increases total and water-soluble Mg only at a low K level.

Feeding a high protein, high K ration to sheep resulted in a 41% decrease in Mg absorption (Fontenot et al, 1960). The protein and K levels were 34.4 and 4.7%, respectively, for the control ration. Other studies indicated that depression in Mg absorption was due to the high K level and not to the high N level (Moore et al, 1972). The depression in Mg absorption from feeding the high K level was of similar magnitude regardless of whether a low or high level of N was fed, and was similar to that reported when a high protein, high K ration was fed (Fontenot et al, 1960) or when only a high K level was fed (Newton et al, 1972).

Ca and P

Feeding high levels of Ca or P usually increases Mg requirements or impairs Mg utilization in non-ruminants. In ruminants apparent absorption of Mg, expressed as percent of intake, tends to be depressed by high Ca and P levels and the effect of P is more pronounced than that of Ca. (see Ch. 4). The combination appears to exert a stronger adverse effect. However, the effects are much milder than those of feeding a high K ration (Newton et al, 1972).

Plant Organic Acids

Recently, there has been a considerable interest in the relationship of plant organic acids to the incidence of grass tetany. This research was stimulated by the report of Burt and Thomas (1961) who found that Na citrate, when given orally, resulted in lower levels of plasma Mg as compared to feeding NaCl. Analytical data from the California Station (Burau and Stout, 1965; Stout et al, 1967) showed that some plants may contain very high levels of trans-aconitic acid. They examined 94 different species of plants and classed them as accumulators or non-accumulators. They found that 47% of the grasses and 17% of non-grass species could be classed as accumulators (1% or more of dry weight as trans-aconitic acid). Some species, such as crested wheatgrass (Agropyrum cristatum), are frequently associated with tetany. Seasonal collection showed that the aconitic acid content fell rapidly with the onset of increased temperatures and higher plant growth rates. They further pointed out that both aconitate and citrate form chelates with Ca and Mg and that trans-aconitate acts as a competitive metabolic inhibitor of biological activity, interfering with the conversion of citrate to cis-aconitate. Fertilization with K or N has been shown to increase organic acid concentrations in different forage species (Grunes et al, 1970).

Although Kennedy (1968) found that plasma and urinary Mg were not affected appreciably by feeding trans-aconitic or citric acids, research (Bohman et al, 1969; Scotto et al, 1971) has indicated that administration by drenching of KCl and citrate or trans-aconitate would produce a tetany in a high percentage of experimental cattle. The tetany was responsive to Ca-Mg gluconate treatment; it was, however, less prolonged than that observed in field cases. These workers observed that KCl, alone, would reduce plasma Mg over an extended period of time, whereas the KCl-citrate combination was believed to have more effect in reducing plasma Mg over an extended period of time, whereas KCl and citric acid would lower plasma Mg in 24 hr to a week. Generally, the KCl-citrate combination was believed to have more effect in reducing plasma Mg than the KCl-aconitate combination. The amount of acids given per unit of body weight varied, but data indicated that about 150-160 g/100 kg of body weight were required to produce tetany. In contrast to many field cases, blood Ca did not appear to be affected. Burt and Thomas (1961) found that high levels of citric acid depressed serum Mg in calves 4-6 mo. of age and Harmon et al (1974) have observed that a variety of di- or tri-carboxylic acids (oral) resulted in some reduction in plasma Mg. Kariya et al (1976) found that large doses of KCl or citric acid depressed serum Mg but not after simultaneous administration. Further studies (Furukawa et al, 1976) showed that simultaneous administration of KCl and citric acid resulted in elevation of serum K that caused death of sheep from heart failure.

Camp et al (1968) have studied the effect on sheep of massive doses of the free acid or the K salt of trans-aconitate. These workers observed that treated animals maintained normal levels of blood citrate (as well as lactate and pyruvate), whereas sheep given a lethal dose (4 g/kg of body wt) of K trans-aconitate had a marked increase in serum citric acid within 24 hr as well as a decline in Mg and P. When the free acid was administered, there was a decrease in serum K, but no statistical differences in Mg or P. Tetany was not observed with lethal or sub-lethal doses of either the free acid or its salt, perhaps because blood Ca levels were not affected. Wright and Wolff (1969) have also reported on the toxicity of trans-aconitate when given to sheep as a single dose via stomach tube. The dose administered was said to be equivalent to 10% of the dietary dry matter intake. With this dose they found no effect on serum Mg nor did they observe any other toxic effects. Their data, unfortunately, do not lend themselves to comparisons on treatment levels to those of the Nevada workers or Camp et al.

Higher Fatty Acids

Supplementation of diets with higher fatty acids lowered Mg absorption in dairy cows

(Kemp et al, 1964). A close relationship has been reported between higher fatty acids and crude protein content in grasses (Kemp et al, 1966). They suggested that the unfavorable effect of fertilizing grassland with N in reducing the availability of herbage Mg to the animal might be due in part to the increase in the lipid content of the herbage. A relationship between higher fatty acids and total N in herbage was also reported in New Zealand (Molloy et al, 1973). Feeding of peanut oil resulted in a depression in plasma Mg of grazing dairy cows (Wilson et al, 1969).

Readily Available Carbohydrates

Starch supplementation of grazing dairy cattle lessened the depression of plasma Mg (Wilson et al, 1969). Glucose supplementation to hay increased apparent absorption in sheep but had no effect when given with grass (Madsen et al, 1976). Inconsistent results were obtained from supplementing semipurified lamb diets with different levels of readily fermentable carbohydrates (House and Mayland, 1976). In one experiment supplementing with starch did not influence apparent absorption of Mg, but in a second experiment supplementing with sucrose tended to increase apparent absorption of Mg.

In other studies Mayland et al (1974) observed that high N and higher fatty acid content of grass coincided with the occurrence of tetany. They also noted that a rapid increase in the ratio of N to total water-soluble carbohydrates coincided with the onset of tetany and suggested that this may be an important factor.

Miscellaneous Plant Factors

It has been pointed out previously that there is an association between cool weather and grass tetany, or an association (simultaneously) with periods of reduced solar radiation. On the basis of limited experimental data Mayland and Grunes (1974) suggest that shaded forage would result in lower Mg intake than forage growing in full sunlight. Seasonal changes also occur in plant composition since McIntosh et al (1973) found that water-soluble and total Mg increased as the season progressed and L'Estrange et al (1967) noted increased utilization by sheep as the season progressed.

Geelen and others (1967) found that I.V. infusion of histamine produced some of the same symptoms seen in grass tetany (twitching, defecation, urination). When blood Mg was normal, the effects of histamine were much less severe. When

blood Mg levels were low (1.3 mg/100 ml), histamine administration killed one cow. In more recent work Henry et al (1977) concluded that histamine was without effect whereas intraruminal infusions of ammonia or ammonia plus histamine produced tetany. Ammonia also resulted in lower blood Mg.

Based on extensive analysis of small grain pasture forage, Mayland et al (1976) concluded that the estimated tetany hazard was wheat > oats = barley > rye. This ranking corresponded to blood serum Mg levels predicted from Dutch work (Fig. 13-4, Hartmans, 1973). Mayland et al concluded that wheat forage poses a greater hazard than wheatgrass because it had lower values for Ca and higher values of K, $K/(Ca + Mg)$, aconitic acid, ash alkalinity, and higher fatty acids.

The reader will probably have concluded that a variety of different factors are involved in production of grass tetany. This certainly appears to be the case at this time. Whether all of the variables affecting the incidence of tetany have been identified remains to be seen.

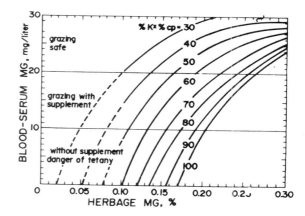

Fig. 13-4. Relation between blood serum Mg of producing dairy cows and forage Mg, K and crude protein. Isolines are products of % K and % crude protein. Taken from a paper by Hartman (1973) by permission of the Centre for Agr. Pub. & Documen., Wageningen, The Netherlands.

PREVENTING GRASS TETANY

Since the cause of grass tetany appears to be a metabolic deficiency of Mg, it has been suggested that the element would be beneficial in preventing the disturbance regardless of the cause. Recent results support this hypothesis (Frye et al, 1975). A high dietary K level (4.5%) increased fecal Mg excretion and decreased its absorption to about the same extent at widely varying Mg intakes. This relationship appears to be similar to competitive inhibition. Thus, it is assumed that depression of Mg absorption can be overcome simply by additional Mg intake.

Magnesium Fertilization

Applying Mg to the soil increases Mg content of forage (Parr and Allcroft, 1957; Birch and Wolton, 1961). Todd (1964) reported results indicating that the response to Mg fertilization depends on soil type. Results were more satisfactory on light sandy soils than on heavier soils. Form of Mg applied to the soil may be important also (Draycott et al, 1975). Fertilization with Mg has been reflected in increased serum Mg of grazing animals (Smyth et al, 1958; Campbell, 1972).

Foliar Application

Dusting herbage with supplemental Mg is helpful in preventing grass tetany (McConaghy et al, 1973; Todd, 1966; Kemp and Geurink, 1967; Rogers and Poole, 1971). A problem with this method is removal by rain or wind (Burns and Allcroft, 1967; Wilkinson et al, 1972). Satisfactory results have been obtained from using a slurry containing MgO and bentonite for foliage application (Wilkinson et al, 1972). Apparently this kind of application remains on the foliage longer than a dust.

Oral Supplementation

Serum Mg levels in cattle and sheep can be increased by oral administration of Mg (Line et al, 1958; Smith et al, 1974), so supplementation in the ration would be effective. However, grass tetany usually occurs in cows grazing or fed hay with no supplemental feed. For these animals some other form of Mg supplementation is necessary.

Mg in mineral mixtures has been helpful in preventing the drop in serum Mg in cattle. Including palatable ingredients in the mixture is often necessary to obtain satisfactory intakes of Mg during tetany-prone seasons. Mixing molasses with MgO has been shown to result in satisfactory intake of Mg. Frye et al (1977) reported satisfactory intake of supplemental Mg in cows grazing spring pasture or fed a dry ration, if a palatable ingredient was included in the mixture. The use of a 1:1:1 mixture of trace mineralized salt, MgO and palatable ingredients such as cottonseed meal, dry molasses, dehydrated alfalfa meal, ground corn grain or distillers corn grain gave similar Mg intakes. Other researchers have reported improvements in serum Mg in cows allowed access to palatable high Mg mineral mixtures (Smith et al, 1974; MacLaren et al, 1975).

Quality of Supplemental Mg

The daily Mg requirement to maintain blood serum Mg at a level of 2 mg/100 appears to be ca. 20 g/day in lactating beef cows if the Mg in the feed is highly available. In order to supply this amount of Mg the forage should contain ca. 0.2% Mg (dry basis). Frequently, forages contain much lower levels than this (Reid et al, 1970), but usually not less than 0.1% (dry basis). Thus, for cattle fed preserved forage during the winter (in which it is not likely that there will be dietary factors interfering with Mg utilization), the amount of supplemental Mg should be about 10 g from a highly utilizable source. Since certain factors in the forage may lower Mg utilization by as much as 50%, supplemental Mg for cattle grazing tetany-prone forages should be approximately 20 g/day from a highly utilizable source (see Ch. 4).

URINARY CALCULI (UROLITHIASIS)

Occurrence

Urinary calculi (urolithiasis, water belly) is an important disease in ruminant animals, since death or lower performance may result. The disease is the result of the formation of stones or calculi in the kidney or bladder with resultant obstruction of urine excretion. Although it is believed that stone formation is probably similar in both sexes, the calculi cause little trouble in females since the urethra is much larger and shorter than in males. Likewise, there tends to be more trouble in castrated animals than in intact males (Bhatt et al, 1973), probably because the urethra is larger in the latter. Calculi may be especially severe in feedlot animals, the incidence varying from an occasional case to severe outbreaks which affect a majority of the animals. Field outbreaks have also occurred in grazing cattle and sheep. Since treatment is relatively ineffective other than by surgical means, urinary calculi may result in substantial losses to the livestock industry.

Clinical Symptoms

Calculi cause severe problems due to

obstruction of the urinary tract, primarily the urethra. Obstruction of the urethra by calculi results in a typical syndrome which reflects irritation, pain or discomfort in the abdominal region. A steer may wring its tail, shift its weight back and forth from one foot to the other, and kick at the belly. The animal may also stand with hind feet stretched out behind as if to relieve pressure in the abdomen. Partial blockage may be recognized by excretion of small amounts or dribbles of blood-stained urine.

The blockage results in a build-up of urine in the bladder with eventual rupture of the bladder or urethra (in 36-48 hr). Bladder rupture results in temporary relief, but this is followed by abdominal distension, depression and death due to uremia (Blood and Henderson, 1968). Carcasses from affected animals are not acceptable for human food because of the strong urine odor.

Etiology of Calculi Formation

The composition of calculi has been shown to vary greatly. In grazing sheep and cattle, Ca, NH_4 and Mg carbonate are common constituents (Sutherland, 1958). Some are high in silica (Bailey, 1967); others have been shown to contain large amounts of phosphates. Still others have been found which were more mucoprotein in nature (Marsh, 1961).

Calculi formation may result from a wide variety of environmental situations. Studies on calculi structure suggest very rapid formation at times (Trueman and Stacy, 1969). In the feedlot the phosphatic stones are of major concern, whereas under pasture conditions, consumption of oxalates (Sutherland, 1958; Udall and Jensen, 1958), plant or exogenous estrogens (Gardiner et al, 1966; Nottle and Beck, 1974), or silicates (Bailey, 1967) have been implicated. The formation of stones in any of these situations may be affected by factors which favor development of a nucleus (i.e., nidus) around which concretions can occur. This may also be affected by factors which favor the precipitation of solutes in the urine, such as deprivation of water, loss of large amounts of water through the respiratory tract in hot climates, pH of the urine, etc. Castrated males are more susceptible to calculi than intact males (Bailey, 1975). Examples of calculi are shown in Fig. 13-5 and 13-6.

Phosphatic Calculi

A considerable amount of research has been carried out in attempts to define the

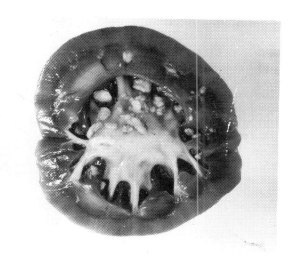

Fig. 13-5. Phosphatic urinary calculi. Sheep kidney opened bilaterally exposing phosphatic calculi. Courtesy of R.J. Emerick, S. Dakota State Univeristy.

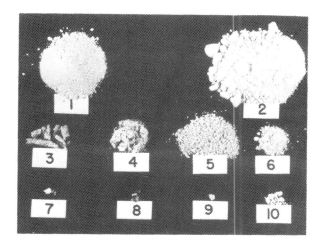

Fig. 13-6. Urinary calculi. (1) steer bladder deposit; (2) wether bladder deposit; (3) steer urethra deposit; (4) steer sheath deposit; (5) sheep bladder and urethra deposit; (6) sheep bladder deposit; (7) steer urethra deposit; (8) sheep kidney deposit; (9) steer urethra deposit; (10) sheep bladder deposit. Courtesy of R.J. Emerick, S. Dakota University.

conditions that promote development of phosphatic calculi. Packett and Hauschild (1964) developed a calculogenic diet that produced calculi in a high percentage of wether lambs. This ration is characterized by having substantial amounts of grain sorghum (45%) in addition to feedstuffs such as cottonseed hulls (27%), cottonseed meal (10%), alfalfa hay (8%) and molasses (10%) . This ration contained about 0.30% Ca, 0.22% Mg, 0.30% P, and 1.14% K.

Previous research with lambs (Lindley et al, 1953; Elam et al, 1956) showed clearly that the addition of K (as K_2HOP_4) or K and P (as K_2CO_3 and H_3PO_4) resulted in a high incidence of calculi. Subsequent research from other laboratories has shown that a high level of urinary P can be associated with the formation of calculi (Emerick et al, 1959; Packett and Hauschild, 1964; Robbins et al, 1965; Davis et al, 1969). Further data indicate that the addition of high levels of Ca to a high calculogenic diet will lower serum and urine P concentrations and reduce the incidence of calculi (Emerick and Embry, 1963, 1964; Bushman et al, 1965) or that the addition of P, alone, tends to increase calculi formation (Robbins et al, 1965). The work of Bushman et al (1965) showed that no calculi problems resulted in lambs receiving a diet with 0.25% P and either 0.31 or 0.58% Ca when the P was supplied as the dicalcium salt. However, when the P was supplied as disodium, mono-sodium or sodium tripolyphosphate salts, the incidence of calculi was high at the 0.31% Ca level, although it was reduced when 0.58% Ca was fed. Davis et al (1969) produced a high incidence of calculi in lambs fed a milo, cottonseed and sorghum silage diet which resulted in about equal intakes of P and Ca. A high incidence of urinary calculi was reported in young lambs fed a ration containing 0.56% Ca and 0.61% P (Jones and Dawson, 1976).

Two papers of particular interest on the subject of etiology of calculi are those of Hoar et al (1969) and Packett et al (1968). In the research carried out by Hoar and others, lambs were fed either 0.14 or 0.28% Ca and 0.28 or 0.55% P, either with or without 2% Na bicarbonate. The incidence of calculi increased as the P level increased with little apparent effect of the Ca level. The addition of the bicarbonate resulted in many more calculi at the 0.28% P level, possibly due to a higher urinary pH. Data presented on serum values indicated that P levels were generally increased by feeding 0.55% P, and that serum Ca levels tended to be depressed, thus showing that low Ca high P serum was indicative of a calculogenic diet. Other data suggest that elevated levels of blood Mg and P and lower Ca levels are indicative of an increased probability for calculi development and that metabolic conditions resulting in renal retention of Mg and increased Ca and P excretion lead to calculi formation (Crookshank et al, 1967; Lalov et al, 1971). Urine volume generally increased as the diets became more calculogenic, indicating that concentration of urine solutes was an unlikely

factor in calculi formation. The beneficial effect of high dietary Ca level (1.2%) in high P diets (.57%) was confirmed by Hoar et al (1970). Adding 1% KCl did not affect the incidence of calculi, but resulted in larger calculi (120 vs 83 mg). However, the effect of KCl is inconsistent, since beneficial effects were reported from KCl at 1 or 2% in protecting against phosphatic calculi in sheep fed diets with 0.5% P (Emerick et al, 1972). Feeding of Na bicarbonate increased urine pH, and markedly affected the incidence of stones (Hoar et al, 1969). In more recent research Huntington and co-workers (1977) fed high concentrate diets with 2 or 4% Na bentonite or 2 or 4% $NaHCO_3$. Both buffers had some effect on blood Ca (reduced) and Mg (increased) and 19% of the lambs fed the bicarbonate died from obstructive calculi or had calculi when slaughtered. Low urine pH has been implicated as a causative factor in stone formation by other reports (Bushman et al, 1968), although there are also numerous exceptions (Packett et al, 1968; Emerick et al, 1972).

The research reported by Packett et al (1968) involved feeding a calculogenic diet with supplements of Na citrate, Ca citrate, vitamin D_3, or Ca carbonate. Ca citrate was quite effective in preventing calculi, whereas the Na citrate had no apparent effect. Both vitamin D and Ca carbonate increased the incidence of calculi. Wethers on calculogenic diets were characterized by high serum Mg and P, low serum Ca, and high concentrations of urinary Mg and P. Non-affected animals excreted more P and Mg via the urine and retained less Mg and P and had lower serum Mg and P levels. The wethers given vitamin D showed the same trends in serum minerals, but differed in urinary excretion, the excretion of Mg being considerably higher than on any of the other diets whereas the K excretion was the lowest.

The data available at this point indicate that urine pH is a factor in some cases, but not in all. A high level of urinary P has been implicated on many occasions which may be complicated with high Mg excretion. The fact that diets promoting a high urinary excretion of P can become non-calculogenic with administraion of acid-forming salts indicates that there must be some interdependence between pH and P levels as suggested by Hoar et al (1969).

Miscellaneous Factors

Silica urolithiasis, as indicated previously, may be an important problem, particularly in the northern great plains of the USA and Canada and some areas in Australia (Nottle, 1976). In these areas, calculogenic forages may have very high levels of silica as does the urine of cattle consuming such forage (Bailey, 1967). As pointed out by Bailey, the concentration of silica in urine may be 2-3X that of a saturated solution. In these instances research (Bailey, 1967, 1969) has shown that the feeding of 4% NaCl or oral or intraruminal administration of water, which increased urine volume, resulted in fewer calculi in experimental animals. Consumption of 300 g of salt per day prevented formation of siliceous calculi in 300 kg calves (Bailey, 1973, 1976), but feeding of NH_4Cl did not affect water intake or formation of siliceous calculi (Bailey, 1976). Thus, the formation of siliceous calculi would appear to be affected by urine concentration, a different situation than in the case of phosphatic calculi. Data published by Forman and Sauer (1962) indicated that pH may also be a factor. They found that sheep fed grass hay from a problem area produced urine of a very low pH (ca. 5.5) as well as a low volume of urine. The grass hay in question had less Na, K, Ca and Mg than other hays causing no problem. Emerick et al (1959) failed to show any increase in calculi when feeding supplementary Na silicate.

Nottle (1976) observed that calculi from grazing animals in Western Australia were of four different types—silica or three different $CaCO_3$ types. Other information on animals grazing legumes suggests that calculi are primarily of silica or $CaCO_3$ (Trueman and Stacy, 1969). In one case where lambs were fed alfalfa hay, tubular precipitation of salts occurred although no calculi were formed (Davis et al, 1969). Some of the early data indicated that diethylstilbestrol treatment was apt to cause calculi in lambs (Bell et al, 1954; Udall and Jensen, 1958). These experiments involved the use of 15-30 mg implants. However, when using smaller implants (3 mg) more typical of current recommendations or when feeding stilbestrol (2 mg/day), Emerick and Embry (1964) found that hormone treatments did not increase the incidence of calculi. With beef cattle it is generally felt by many nutritionists that stilbestrol is not a predisposing factor. However, sediments containing equaol and 4'-0-methyl equol, which have estrongic activity, have been isolated from the urine of sheep grazing subterranean clover (Nottle and Beck, 1974; Nottle, 1975). A number of other

substances were found in the sediments (Nottle, 1975, 1976).

Crookshank et al (1965) reported that pelleting of a calculogenic diet resulted in an increased incidence of calculi in sheep. This was accompanied by an increased urinary excretion of P and decreased Mg and K. In one comparison pelleting of a non-calculogenic diet did not increase the incidence of calculi.

Preventive Measures

Although the causes of calculi formation are not completely understood at this time, there is enough information to indicate clearly that the severity of the problem can be reduced considerably. The information available on Ca and P dietary levels shows, for lambs at least, that P levels should be maintained near the requirement, i.e., about 0.3% of the diet. An appropriate Ca level would appear to be approximately 0.4% of the diet, although more complete information is required in order to give a firm recommendation. At any rate, the Ca:P ratio should be greater than 1:1.

For feedlot animals the inclusion of large quantities of NaCl (4-10%) has been reported to be effective in preventing calculi in sheep (Elam et al, 1957) and in cattle (Whiting et al, 1958); however, this amount of salt would certainly be expected to reduce feed intake and animal performance. Lesser amounts have not been as effective as other treatments. Feeding salt with protein supplements has helped reduce the incidence of siliceous calculi in grazing cattle (see previous section).

Various degrees of success in preventing calculi have been reported by feeding a variety of mineral salts which will result in a more acidic urine. For example, Crookshank et al (1960) found that both NH_4Cl and phosphoric acid were effective. NH_4Cl is effective in preventing phosphatic calculi (Udall and Chen Chow, 1965; Crookshank, 1966; Bushman et al, 1967, 1968; Crookshank, 1970), but not for siliceous calculi (Bailey, 1976). Neither is aluminum sulfate effective against siliceous calculi (Bailey, 1977). NH_4Cl appears to be effective by reducing urine pH and by increasing intestinal absorption (Braithwaite, 1972) or resorption from bone (Vagg and Payne, 1970) and increasing excretion of Ca and Mg (Bushman et al, 1967, 1968; Braithwaite, 1972; Horst and Jorgensen, 1974; Yano and Kawashima, 1975). In some cases $CaCl_2$ has been found to be equal to NH_4Cl (Bushman et al, 1967, 1968). The use of Ca citrate (Packett et al, 1968) might also be feasible under some conditions.

352

A deficiency of vitamin A has been suggested at various times as a possible factor in calculi formation; there appears to be no conclusive proof of this (Kaushal et al, 1972) but some evidence suggests that a vitamin A deficiency may be a predisposing factor (Vasudevan and Dutt, 1970). The use of antibiotics has also been suggested as a preventative.

Measures to insure an adequate intake of water, especially during the winter months, might be effective, particularly when siliceous calculi are the primary concern. The feeder should also be careful to remove buffers from the diet if calculi are a problem.

Treatment

Treatment of affected animals has been, almost without exception, of a surgical nature. Gera et al (1972) reported the successful treatment of eight cases of urolithiases in bullocks by urethomy and leparocystomy. Perhaps, acid-forming minerals might be expected to result in some solubilization of stones in the bladder or kidney, but it is not to be expected that stones lodged in the urethra could be dissolved in time to provide relief. Muscle relaxants have been used with some degree of success when obstruction is partial. A frequent surgical procedure used on feedlot animals is to perform a urethrotomy, an operation which severs the penis and exteriorizes the stump to allow for urine excretion (Jensen and Mackey, 1965).

References Cited

Magnesium Tetany

Allsop, T.F. and J.V. Pauli. 1975. Proc. N.Z. Soc. Animal Prod. 35:170; Aust. J. Biol. Sci. 28:475.

Bartlett, S. et al. 1954. Brit. Vet. J. 110:3.

Bartlett, S. et al. 1957. J. Agr. Sci. 49:291.

Birch, J.A. and K.M. Wolton. 1961. Vet. Rec. 73:1169.

Blaxter, K.L., B. Cowlishaw and J.A.F. Rook. 1960. Animal Prod. 2:1.

Blood, D.C. and J.A. Henderson. 1968. Veterinary Medicine, 3rd ed. Williams & Wilkins Co.

Bohman, V.R., A.L. Lesperance, G.D. Harding and D.L. Grunes. 1969. J. Animal Sci. 29:99.

Burau, R. and P.R. Stout. 1965. Science 150:766.

Burns, K.N. and R. Allcroft. 1967. Brit. Vet. J. 123:340,383.

Burt, A.W.A. and D.C. Thomas. 1961. Nature 192:1193.

Camp, B.J., J.W. Dollahite and W.L. Schwartz. 1968. Amer. J. Vet. Res. 29:2009.

Campbell, R.W. 1972. Aust. Vet. J. 48:440.

Care, A.D., D.B. Ross and A.A. Wilson. 1965. J. Physiol. 176:284.

Chicco, C.F., C.B. Ammerman, W.G. Hillis and L.R. Arrington. 1972. Amer. J. Physiol. 222:1469.

Christian, K.R. and V.J. Williams. 1960. N.Z. J. Agr. Res. 3:389.

Crookshank, H.R. and F.H. Sims. 1955. J. Animal Sci. 14:964.

Crowley, J.P. 1966. Irish Vet. J. 20:222.

Dobson, A., D. Scott and I. McDonald. 1966. Res. Vet. Sci. 7:94.

Draycott, A.P., M.J. Durrant and S.N. Bennett. 1975. J. Agr. Sci. 84:475.

Field, A.C. 1961. Brit. J. Nutr. 15:287.

Fontenot, J.P., R.W. Miller, C.K. Whitehair and R. MacVicar. 1960. J. Animal Sci. 19:127.

Fontenot, J.P., M.B. Wise and K.E. Webb, Jr. 1973. Fed. Proc. 32:1925.

Forbes, A.J. 1972. Aust. Vet. J. 48:444.

Frye, T.M., J.P. Fontenot and K.E. Webb, Jr. 1975. VPI & SU Res. Div. Rep. 163:80.

Frye, T.M., J.P. Fontenot and K.E. Webb, Jr. 1977. J. Animal Sci. 44:919.

Furukawa, R., Y. Kariya, H. Matsumoto and Y. Ogura. 1976. Bul. Natl. Grassld. Res. Inst. 9:69.

Garces, M.A. and J.L. Evans. 1971. J. Animal Sci. 32:789.

Geelen, M.J.H., D.L. Van Rheenen, H.J. Hendricks and L. Seekles. 1967. Nutr. Abstr. Rev. 37:956.

Grace, N.D. and G.F. Wilson. 1972. N.Z. J. Agr. Res. 15:72.

Grunes, D.L., P.R. Stout and J.R. Brownell. 1970. Adv. Agron. 22:331.

Hall, R.F. and R.A. Reynolds. 1972. Amer. J. Vet. Res. 33:1711.

Harmon, B.W. et al. 1974. J. Animal Sci. 39:239 (abstr).

Hartmans, J. (ed.) 1973. Tracing and Treating Mineral Disorders in Dairy Cattle. Centre for Agr. Pub. & Documentation, Wageningen, The Netherlands.

Head, M.J. and J.A.F. Rook. 1955. Nature 176:262.

Hemingway, R.G., N.S. Ritchie and N.A. Brown. 1965. J. Agr. Sci. 64:109.

Hemingway, R.G., N.S. Ritchie, A.R. Rutherford and G.M. Jolly. 1963. J. Agr. Sci. 60:307.

Henry, R.R., W.H. Smith and M.D. Cunningham. 1977. J. Animal Sci. 44:276.

Herd, R.P. 1966. Aust. Vet. J. 42:369.

Hjerpe, C.A. 1968. Cornell Vet. 58:193.

Horvath, D.J., J.R. Todd and R. Weiss. 1971. Amer. J. Vet. Res. 32:1851.

House, W.A. and R.J. Bird. 1975. J. Animal Sci. 41:1134.

House, W.A. and H.F. Mayland. 1976. J. Animal Sci. 43:506,842.

House, W.A. and D. Van Campen. 1971. J. Nutr. 101:1483.

Hvidsten, H., M. Odelien, R. Bauerug and S. Tollersrud. 1959. Acta. Agr. Scand. 9:261.

Jolley, L.C. and D.D. Leaver. 1974. Aust. Vet. J. 50:98.

Kariya, Y. et al. 1976. Bul. Natl. Grassld. Res. Inst. 9:63.

Kemp, A. 1958. Neth. J. Agr. Sci. 6:281.

Kemp, A. 1960. Neth. J. Agr. Sci. 8:281.

Kemp, A., W.B. Deijs, O.J. Henakes and A.J.H. Van Es. 1961. Neth. J. Agr. Sci. 9:134.

Kemp, A., W.B. Deijs and E. Kluvers. 1964. Neth. J. Agr. Sci. 14:290.

Kemp, A. and J.H. Geurink. 1967. Agr. Digest. 12:23.

Kennedy, G.S. 1968. Aust. J. Biol. Sci. 21:529.

Kunkel, H.O., K.H. Burns and B.J. Camp. 1953. J. Animal Sci. 12:451.

Larvor, P. 1976. Cornell Vet. 66:413.

Larvor, P. and C. Violette. 1970. Nutr. Abstr. Rev. 40:1135.

Leffel, E.C. and K.R. Mason. 1959. Proc. Magnesium and Agr. Symposium, W. Va. Univ., p. 182.

Lentz, D.E., F.C. Madsen, J.K. Miller and S.L. Hansard. 1976. J. Animal Sci. 43:1082.

L'Estrange, J.L., J.B. Owen and D. Wilman. 1967. J. Agr. Sci. 68:165,173.

Line, C. et al. 1958. J. Agr. Sci. 51:353.

Lomba, F. et al. 1971. Zeit. fur Tierphysiol. Tierernahrung Fittermitte. 28:189.

Madsen, F.C. et al. 1976. J. Animal Sci. 42:1316.

Marshak, R.R. 1958. J. Amer. Vet. Med. Assoc. 133:539.

Mayland, H.F. et al. 1975. Agron. J. 67:411.

Mayland, H.F. and D.L. Grunes. 1974. J. Range Mgmt. 27:198.

Mayland, H.F., D.L. Grunes and V.A. Lazar. 1976. Agron. J. 68:665.

Mayland, H.F., D.L. Grunes and D.M. Stuart. 1974. Agron. J. 66:441.

McConaghy, S. et al. 1963. J. Agr. Sci. 60:313.

McIntosh, S., P. Crooks and K. Simpson. 1973. Plant & Soil 39:389.

McLaren, J.B. et al. 1975. Tennessee Farm and Home Sci. Prog. Rpt. 94:21.

Merchon, M.M. and F.D. Custer. 1958. J. Amer. Vet. Med. Assoc. 132:396.

Meyer, H. and W. Stehling. 1973. Nutr. Abstr. Rev. 43:139.

Meyer, H. and H. Scholz. 1973. Nutr. Abstr. Rev. 43:932.

Michael, D.T. 1968. Vet. Rec. 82:34.

Molloy, L.F., A. J. Metson and T.W. Collie. 1973. N.Z. J. Agr. Res. 16:457.

Moore, W.F., J.P. Fontenot and K.E. Webb, Jr. 1972. J. Animal Sci. 35:271,1046.

Mudd, A.J. 1970. J. Agr. Sci. 74:11.

Newton, G.L., J.P. Fontenot, R.E. Tucker and C.E. Polan. 1972. J. Animal Sci. 35:440.

Ohshima, K.S. Miura, S. Numakunai and M. Iwasaki. 1973. Jap. J. Vet. Sci. 35:231.

O'Kelley, R.E. and J.P. Fontenot. 1969. J. Animal Sci. 29:959.

O'Kelley, R.E. and J.P. Fontenot. 1973. J. Animal Sci. 36:994.

Parr, W.H. and R. Allcroft. 1957. Vet. Rec. 69:1041.

Pauli, J.V. and T.F. Allsop. 1974. N.Z. Vet. J. 22:227.

Reid, R.L.. A.J. Post and G.A. Jung. 1970. W. Va. Univ. Agr. Exp. Sta. Bul. 589.

Ritchie, N.S. and R.G. Hemingway. 1963. J. Agr. Sci. 61:411.

Rogers, P.A.M. and D.B.R. Poole. 1971. Irish Vet. J. 25:197.

Rook, J.A.F., C.C. Balch and C.Line. 1958. J. Agr. Sci. 51:189.

Rook, J.A.F., R.C. Campling and V.W. Johnson. 1964. J. Agr. Sci. 62:273.

Rook, J.A.F. and J.E. Storry. 1962. Nutr. Abstr. Rev. 32:1055.

Schuster, N.H. et al. 1969. Aust. Vet. J. 45:508.

Scott, D. 1969. Res. Vet. Sci. 10:121.

Scotto, K.C., V.R. Bohman and A.L. Lesperance. 1971. J. Animal Sci. 32:354.

Sims, F.H. and H.R. Crookshank. 1956. Texas Agr. Exp. Sta. Bul. 842.

Smith, R.H. 1959. Biochem. J. 71:306.

Smith, W.H., V.L. Lechtenbery and J.R. Hodges. 1974. J. Animal Sci. 39:1001. (abstr).

Smyth, P.J., A. Conway and M.J. Walsh. 1958. Vet. Rec. 70:846.

Stillings, B.R., J.W. Bratzler, L.F. Marriott and R.C. Miller. 1964. J. Animal Sci. 23:1148.

Stout, P.R., J. Brownell and R. Burau. 1967. Agron. J. 59:21.

Suttle, N.F. and A.C. Field. 1966. Brit. J. Nutr. 20:609.

Suttle, N.F. and A.C. Field. 1967. Brit. J. Nutr. 21:819.

Suttle, N.F. and A.C. Field. 1969. Brit. J. Nutr. 23:81.

Todd, J.R. 1965. Brit. Vet. J. 121:371.

Todd, J.R. 1966. Proc. 10th In'l. Grasslnd. Congr., p. 178.

Todd, J.R. and D.J. Horvath. 1970. Brit. Vet. J. 126:333.

Van't Klooster, A.T. 1965. Nutr. Abstr. Rev. 35:674.

Wilkinson, S.R. et al. 1972. In: Magnesium in the Environment: Soils, Crops, Animals & Man. Taylor County Printing Co., Reynolds, Ga.

Wilson, G.F. et al. 1969. N.Z. J. Agr. Res. 12:467.

Wright, D.E. and J.E. Wolff. 1969. N.Z. J. Agr. Res. 12:287.

Urinary Calculi

Bailey, C.B. 1967. Amer. J. Vet. Res. 28:1743; Science 155:696.

Bailey, C.B. 1969. Can. J. Animal Sci. 49:189.

Bailey, C.B. 1973. Can. J. Animal Sci. 53:55.

Bailey, C.B. 1975. Can. J. Animal Sci. 55:187.

Bailey, C.B. 1976. Can. J. Animal Sci. 56:359,745.

Bailey, C.B. 1977. Can. J. Animal Sci. 57:239.

Bell, T.D., W.H. Smith and A.B. Erhart. 1954. J. Animal Sci. 13:425.

Bhatt, G.A., S.A. Ahmed and Beneras Presad. 1973. Indian Vet. J. 50:459.

Blood, D.C. and J.A. Henderson. 1968. Veterinary Medicine. 3rd ed. Williams & Wilkins Co.

Braithwaite, G.D. 1972. Brit. J. Nutr. 27:201.

Bushman, D.H., L.B. Embry and R.J. Emerick. 1967. J. Animal Sci. 26:1199.

Bushman, D.H., R.J. Emerick and L.B. Embry. 1965. J. Animal Sci. 24:671.

Bushman, D.H., R.J. Emerick and L.B. Ebmry. 1968. J. Animal Sci. 27:490.

Crookshank, H.R. 1966. J. Animal Sci. 25:1005.

Crookshank, H.R. 1970. J. Animal Sci. 30:1002.

Crookshank, H.R. et al. 1960. J. Animal Sci. 19:595.

Crookshank, H.R., L.V. Packett and H.O. Kunkel. 1965. J. Animal Sci. 24:638.

Crookshank, H.R., J.D. Robbins and H.O. Kunkel. 1967. J. Animal Sci. 26:1179.

Davis, W.D., R. Scott, H.R. Crookshank and H.J. Spjut. 1969. J. Urol. 101:383.

Elam, C.J., W.E. Ham and B.H. Schneider. 1957. Proc. Soc. Expt. Biol. Med. 95:769.

Elam, C.J., B.H. Schneider and W.E. Ham. 1956. J. Animal Sci. 15:800.

Emerick, R.J. and L.B. Embry. 1963. J. Animal Sci. 22:510.

Emerick, R.J. and L.B. Embry. 1964. J. Animal Sci. 23:1079.

Emerick, R.J., L.B. Embry and O.E. Olson. 1959. J. Animal Sci. 18:1025.

Emerick, R.J., H.R. King and L.B. Embry. 1972. J. Animal Sci. 35:901.

Forman, S.A. and F. Sauer. 1962. Can. J. Animal Sci. 42:9.

Gardiner, M.R., M.E. Hairan, E.P. Meyer. 1966. Aust. Vet. J. 42:315.

Gera, K.L., B.M. Khanna and R.P.S. Tyagi. 1972. Indian Vet. J. 50:88.

Hoar, D.W., R.J. Emerick and L.B. Embry. 1969. J. Animal Sci. 29:647.

Hoar, D.W., R.J. Emerick and L.B. Embry. 1970. J. Animal Sci. 30:597;31:118.

Horst, R.L. and N.A. Jorgensen. 1974. J. Dairy Sci. 57:683.

Huntington, G.B., R.J. Emerick and L.B. Embry. 1977. J. Animal Sci. 45:804.

Jensen, R. and D.R. Mackey. 1965. Diseases of Feedlot Cattle. Lea & Febiger Pub. Co.

Jones, J.O. and P. Dawson. 1976. Vet. Rec. 99:337.

Kaushal, B.S., B. Dutt and B. Vasudevan. 1972. Indian Vet. J. 49:39.

Lalov, H. et al. 1971. Nutr. Abstr. Rev. 41:1403.

Lindley, C.E., E.D. Taysom, W.E. Ham and B.H. Schneider. 1953. J. Animal Sci. 12:704.

Marsh, H. 1961. J. Amer. Vet. Med. Assoc. 139:1019.

Nottle, M.C. and A.B. Beck. 1974. Aust. J. Agr. Res. 25:509.

Nottle, M.C. 1975. Aust. J. Agr. Res. 26:313.

Nottle, M.C. 1976. Res. Vet. Sci. 21:309; Aust. J. Agr. Res. 27:867.

Packett, L.V. and J.P. Hauschild. 1964. J. Nutr. 84:185.

Packett, L.V., R.O. Lineberger and H.D. Jackson. 1968. J. Animal Sci. 27:1716.

Robbins, J.D., H.O. Kunkel and H.R. Crookshank. 1965. J. Animal Sci. 24:76.

Sutherland, A.K. 1958. Aust. Vet. J. 34:44.

Trueman, N.A. and B.D. Stacey. 1969. Invest. Urol. 7:185.

Udall, R.H. and F.H. Chen Chow. 1965. Cornell Vet. 55:538.

Udall, R.H. and R. Jensen. 1958. J. Amer. Vet. Med. Assoc. 133:514.

Vagg, M.J. and J.M. Payne. 1970. Brit. Vet. J. 126:531.

Vasudevan, B. and B. Dutt. 1970. Nutr. Abstr. Rev. 40:742.

Whiting, F., R. Connell and S.A. Forman. 1958. Can. J. Comp. Med. 22:332.

Yano, H. and R. Kawashima. 1975. J. Zootech. Sci. 46:649.

Chapter 14 - Mineral Toxicity

Information has been presented on toxicity of the required mineral nutrients (except for F and Se) in Ch. 4 and 5 of this volume, so it will not be repeated here. Rather, information will be reviewed dealing primarily with the toxicity of selenium (Se), fluorine (F) with additional information on some other contaminants such as lead (Pb). Except for Se, mineral toxicity is primarily due to the contamination of the environment by man.

SELENIUM POISONING

Information on Se poisoning is presented, to some extent, in many books on animal nutrition and in most veterinary texts. The book of Rosenfeld and Beath (1964) is by far the most complete reference on the subject known to the author. Since this coverage is so complete, the material presented here will be more of a condensation of pertinent points, along with a review of some of the more recent research papers.

Selenium Accumulation in Plants

Se is accumulated by a number of plants in sufficient amounts to be toxic if consumed by livestock. Plants have been divided into two groups according to their requirement for and ability to accumulate Se (Rosenfeld and Beath, 1964). Some plant species which require Se for growth have been termed indicator plants, because they have been used in identifying Se-bearing soils. These have also been called converter plants, since some scientists feel that these plants have the ability to extract Se from some soils which is in a form unavailable to most forage plants and convert it into a form which is available to other plants. Plants that do not require Se for growth, but are able to accumulate Se, are called secondary Se absorbers (Olsen, 1978). The various indicator plants include *Xylorrhiza* spp, *Stanleya* spp, and about 24 species of *Astragalus* (Davis, 1972). The secondary accumulators include the Asters, *Atriplex*, and others.

Data presented by Rosenfeld and Beath (1964) show that the Se content of indicator plants varies widely during the season, the content generally being high in young tissues during good growing years. Data are also available to show that the organically bound Se from indicator plants is more readily taken up from the soil by other plants. Most plants have a high proportion of water soluble Se in their tissues. Organic compounds that have been isolated include selenocystathionine, methylselenocysteine, selenocystine, selenomethionine, and Se-wax complexes.

Many indicator plants have objectionable odors, especially when the Se content is high. Se, itself, is volatile and has a garlic-like odor. Other accumulator plants have been observed to be less palatable to sheep or cattle when the Se content is high; thus it is likely that animals may sometimes discriminate against potentially toxic plants if not otherwise forced to consume them.

Most plants are non-accumulators but may take up Se from the soil in amounts that may cause toxicity. Plants in this group include native range plants, grasses, and crop plants such as barley, wheat and alfalfa. Plants containing 5 ppm or more of Se are potentially toxic. The accumulator plants may, on occasion, accumulate Se up to as much as 1% (10,000 ppm). The secondary accumulators are more apt to contain up to a few hundred ppm of Se and the non-accumulators usually have <30 ppm of Se.

Se Toxicity

Se toxicity can occur as either acute or chronic poisoning (Rosenfeld and Beath, 1964). Acute toxicity results from the ingestion of a sufficient amount of seleniferous weeds, usually in a single feeding, to produce severe symptoms. The highly toxic plants are those grouped as indicator plants.

Observations show that Se affects movement and posture of the animal, which is likely to walk a short distance with an uncertain gait and then assume a characteristic stance. The head is lowered and ears drooped. The body temperature is elevated and diarrhea may be evident. The pulse is rapid and weak, respiration labored and bloating usually occurs. Prostration usually occurs before death, which is said to be due to respiratory failure. Animals may die within a few hours after consumption of the plant material. Postmortem findings include congestion, hemorrhaging, and degeneration of many organs and tissues (Rosenfeld and Beath, 1964). Experimental observations indicate that consumption of plant material

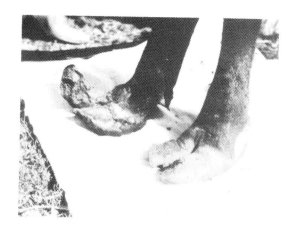

Fig. 14-1. A close-up picture of the hooves of an affected bovine showing the marked deformation that occurs in the alkali disease syndrome. Courtesy of H.E. Eppson, University of Wyoming.

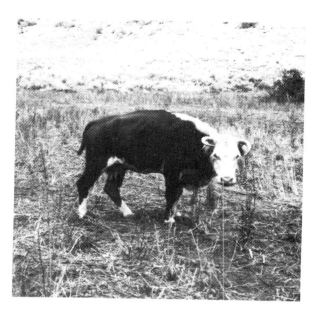

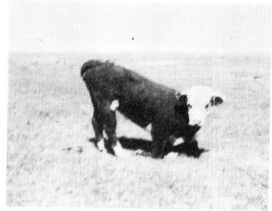

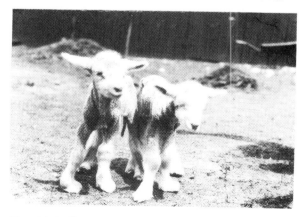

Fig. 14-2. Top. A range cow showing typical symptoms of alkali disease type of Se toxicity. Note the loss of the switch of the tail, the deformed rear hooves and the poor condition. Middle. A steer with alkali disease. Painful feet cause the animal to kneel while eating. Bottom. Lambs born to a ewe consuming seleniferous forage. Note the deformed front legs. Courtesy of H.E. Eppson, Univ. of Wyoming.

containing 400-800 ppm of Se may be fatal to mature sheep when fed in quantities of 8-16 g/kg of body weight. The lethal dose is approximately proportional to the Se content of the plants.

A chronic form of intoxification is said to result from the consumption of plant material containing 5-50 ppm of Se, most of which may be protein-bound. This syndrome, also called alkali disease, is characterized by the loss of hair and malformation and sloughing of the hooves (Fig. 14-1). This manifestation of Se toxicity is largely due to consumption of plants such as the cereals, grasses and hays. Generally, symptoms include anemia, reduced fertility, stiffness of the joints, lameness, loss of hair—particularly from the tail and hoof lesions (Fig. 14-2). The feet may be so painful that animals are sometimes seen eating in a kneeling position. Consumption of Se by pregnant ewes may result in production of lambs with malformed legs (Fig. 14-2). Although some earlier work indicated that arsenic might be a beneficial antidote, later work did not show any improvement in treated animals (Minyard et al, 1960).

A syndrome, referred to as blind staggers, has been attributed to Se toxicity, since it can be produced in animals after a number of doses by feeding plants in sufficient amounts to supply ca. 2 mg of Se/kg of body weight. The affected animals wander in circles with apparent distortion of vision, and they show anorexia, labored respiration, recumbency and death. Van Kampen and

358

James (1978) suggest that this disease is probably a result of toxic alkaloids rather than Se, as was believed to be the case in the past.

Selenium is one of the more toxic required minerals and there is little doubt that poisoning can be produced experimentally by giving oral or parenteral doses of Se compounds. This problem has developed because of the use of Se to prevent nutritional muscular dystrophy (see Ch. 5). Rosenfeld and Beath (1964) reported unpublished data on heifers, one of which was given 2.8 g of Se in 14 daily doses and the other 7.7 g over a period of 23 days. Both animals died after showing weakness, partial paralysis of the jaws and tongue, and a complete lack of appetite. They showed no tendency to walk in circles nor impaired vision, and horns, hooves, and hair were normal, as contrasted to the alkali disease syndrome. Maag et al (1960), working with cattle under feedlot conditions, found that Se was lethal when given at a rate of about 1.1 mg/kg of live wt (dosed 3X weekly). This resulted in loss of appetite, trembling of skeletal muscles, coma, and death. Signs of poisoning were seen when Se in blood exceeded 3 ppm. Severe inflammation of the GI tract and degeneration of brain tissues were reported. Feeding of half of this amount did not result in toxicity and there was no evidence of changes in hooves or hair.

In work with sheep, Kuttler et al (1961) found that a dose of Na selenate equivalent to ca. 1.8 mg/kg of live weight was lethal. In these animals no gross pathological changes were seen, other than evidence of tissue irritation with edema. Morrow (1968) found that 10 mg doses of Na selenite orally to lambs resulted in death of 7 lambs within 17 hr. Poisoning of a ewe resulted from an injection of 1 mg of Na selenite/kg of body weight. The animal became depressed and ataxic after 2 hr with progressive dyspnea. Neethling et al (1968) found that an I.V. dose of 4 mg/kg killed sheep within 20 min. and a dose of 3.4 mg/kg resulted in death in about 10 hr. Lambourne and Mason (1969) mentioned death losses of lambs resulting from an unintentionally high dose of Se (3 mg). Detailed postmortem findings were reported. Caravaggi et al (1970) reported that the LD 50 dose for lambs was 455 μg/kg of weight, when sodium selenite was given in a single intramuscular injection or 1.9 mg/kg, when given as a single oral dose. Gabbedy (1970) stated that 5 mg given parenterally or 10-15 mg orally will kill a percentage of lambs. Stressed animals were more susceptible to toxicity.

Quarterman et al (1966) observed that sub-Q injections of 15 mg of Se were severely toxic when given in winter to pregnant ewes. Furthermore, they suggested that even 3 mg might adversely affect pregnant ewes during periods of cold stress. Gardiner (1966) dosed sheep with 5 mg of Na selenite at biweekly intervals over a period of 72 wk. Some of the sheep died, but the deaths were believed to be conditioned by a concurrent Co deficiency. They suggested that a low protein intake may have made these sheep more susceptible to Se toxicity. In another long-term experiment (46 wk), Pierce and Jones (1968) indicated that dosing with 300 mcg/kg as Na selenite resulted in some reduced performance as compared to smaller doses. Rotruck et al (1969) suggested that 264 ppm in salt (ca. 2 ppm in the total diet) was sufficiently high to result in reduced gain of lambs.

Conclusions

The information discussed on Se poisoning shows that this element is quite toxic; some experiments indicating that prolonged ingestion of 2-5 ppm in the diet may result in reduced performance. Se administered parenterally can kill quickly with rather small doses on the order of 1-2 mg/kg of body wt. This information indicates a very narrow range between apparent required amounts (0.1) and toxic levels, the indicated toxic range being something on the order of 10-20 times the requirement. Some information indicates that increasing the protein intake may have some ameliorating effect on toxicity, but there is little to be done for animals with severe poisoning. The various symptoms seen when animals ingest Se of a different chemical nature (selenates, protein-bound, organic complexes) indicate a difference in metabolism, but information at this time is not available to amplify these observations.

FLUOROSIS

Fluorine has been identified as a toxic element since the early 1930's. Since that time, there have been quite a number of research papers dealing with chronic toxicity in ruminants, but there have been relatively few in the literature in recent years. In the

USA long-term experiments were carried out with beef cattle at the Tennessee Expt. Station and long-term studies on dairy cattle have been reported from the Wisconsin and Utah Expt. Stations. Further studies have been reported from Europe and Australia. Review articles of interest would include those of Shupe (1970) and Obel (1971), and Underwood (1977) has done his usual excellent job in his latest revision.

Fluoride Sources

Chronic F poisoning is a result of contamination of vegetation or water supplies as a result of effluents from factories processing steel, aluminum or other raw ores. There are some areas where fluorides in the water supplies may result in overt toxicity. Contamination may be the result of particulate material settling on plants, contamination of the soil and resultant uptake by plants, or contamination of water.

Raw rock phosphates and colloidal clays —often used as supplementary P sources for plants and animals—may contain toxic levels of F. Hodge (1964) points out that some African plants produce fluoroacetate, a highly toxic compound which characteristically produces a delayed onset of symptoms. This has been a problem to sheep and cattle ranchers. Other sources of F may include insecticides or rodent poisons. Humans may be exposed to toxic gases or dusts that may be readily taken up by the lungs.

With respect to cattle, Hobbs and Merriman (1962) found that NaF was much more toxic than raw rock phosphates. Shupe et al (1962) have compared CaF_2, NaF and high-F hays grown on contaminated soil. CaF_2 (which is less soluble) was found to be much less toxic than the other two sources, which were considered to be about equally toxic. Hodge (1964) points out that toxicity is related to solubility of the various inorganic F sources. In a more recent report F was given to steers as NaF, or the same amount of F in soil or flue dust from an aluminum plant. Retention in the bones was 3, 0.7 or 1.4 fold, respectively, of control animals (Oelschlager et al, 1971).

Clinical Symptoms of Chronic Fluorosis

In chronic fluorosis the first clinical signs are an effect on the teeth of young animals. Shupe (1970) points out that the first evidence of F poisoning is a slight mottling of teeth enamel. This is followed by a more moderate degree of mottling, discoloration and appearance of patches of chalky enamel. Teeth may also show some abrasion. More severe symptoms include a definite mottling, discoloration, hypoplasia, and hypocalcification. The enamel may be pitted and there is definite abrasion. Excessive intakes of F result in more severe lesions of this type. Teeth may be stained (vegetative stains) to the point that they are almost black (see Hobbs and Merriman, 1962). Examples of affected teeth are shown in Fig. 14-3 and

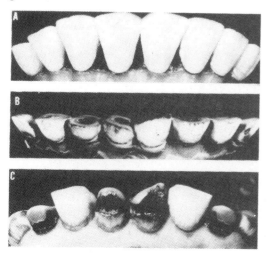

Fig. 14-3. Fluorosis. A, normal teeth. B, dental fluorosis caused by continuous ingestion of high fluorine levels. C, dental fluorosis caused by intermittent ingestion of high fluorine levels. Note the bilateral lesions. Courtesy of J.L. Shupe, Utah State University.

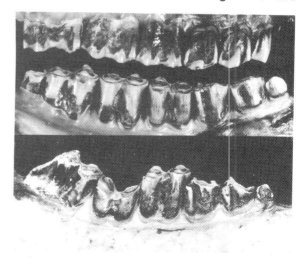

Fig. 14-4. Fluorosis. Upper picture, normal molar teeth of bovine showing sharp grinding surfaces. B, dental fluorosis resulting in excessive erosion and loss of normal table surface. Courtesy of J.L. Shupe, Utah State University.

360

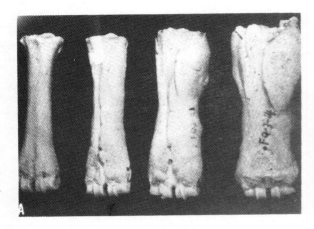

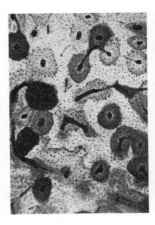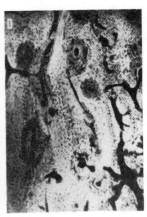

Fig. 14-5. Fluorosis. Effect of excess F intake on the metatarsal bones. Left to right, normal bone and varying degrees of osteofluorosis. Courtesy of J.H. Shupe, Utah State University.

Fig. 14-6. Effect of F on histology of the bone. Left, normal bone showing structure and various stages of remodeling activity. Right, abnormal bone structure with marked osteonal and interstitial changes. Courtesy of J.L. Shupe, Utah State University.

14-4. Note the severe wear of the molars and incisors. There is little, if any, effect on the teeth, however, if they are fully formed prior to exposure to F (Suttie and Phillips, 1959; Shupe, 1970). Severe dental fluorosis can be caused in bovine incisors by feeding F from 13-18 mo. of age (Suttie and Faltin).

As the F concentration in tissues increases, this is followed after a time by periosteal hyperostosis (see Fig. 14-5), intermittent lameness, reduced feed intake, and a reduced rate of performance (milk production, gain, etc.). After a long-term exposure to F, the skin tends to become dry, thick and non-pliable (Shupe, 1970).

Shupe (1970) points out that the bone lesions which develop may be similar to porosis, sclerosis, hyperostosis, osteophytosis, or malacia, depending upon interacting factors influencing the degree of fluorosis. The first changes seen usually affect the metatarsal, mandible and metacarpal bones. These can eventually be diagnosed by palpation. Later, lesions can be detected on the ribs. The affected bones generally appear enlarged and chalky white and have a roughened irregular periosteal surface (see Fig. 14-5). Suttie et al (1958) point out that in their studies F toxicosis was associated with a F content of compact bone in excess of ca. 5,500 ppm (ash basis) and, in cancellous bone, values in excess of 7,000 ppm. It has been shown (Suttie et al, 1958; Shupe et al, 1963) that the F content of bone may vary with the type of bone, the location within a given bone, and between

different bones of the same type in the same animal. Zipkin et al (1964) reported that F ranged from 0.1% in cows on a control ration (12 ppm) to 1.04% in cows getting 112 ppm of F. There was, however, no change in bone ash.

Abnormal osteoblastic activity is thought to cause the formation of an abnormal matrix with disorderly, defective and irregular mineralization of the bones (Fig. 14-6). In the case of joints or the spinal column, Shupe (1970) states that there may be spurring and bridging that can eventually lead to marked rigidity and malfunctioning of affected joints or a very rigid spine. In field studies, Griffith-Jones (1977) noticed a high incidence of arthritis in dairy herds which also had characteristic tooth lesions.

Chronic F toxicity is manifested almost entirely by its effects on the teeth and skeletal system with eventual effects on productivity of the animal. This is probably because F is readily taken up by bone, apparently to the extent of about 96% of body supply (Shupe, 1970), even though F is a very effective enzyme poison. Most of the relatively recent reports on bovines indicate that chronic fluorosis has no appreciable influence on milk production or growth, digestibility, reproduction, or on liver and glandular functions (Suttie et al, 1957; Suttie and Phillips, 1959; Hobbs and Merriman, 1962; Shupe et al, 1963, 1965; Stoddard et al, 1963). Studies using [45]Ca with calves indicate that 100 ppm of F in water indicated depression in amount and efficiency of Ca absorption and an elevated rate of removal from the bone (Ramberg et al, 1970). These reports indicate that little effect is seen on productivity until obvious clinical symptoms are seen. One paper (Van Rensburg and DeVos, 1966), however, indicates that a marked drop in fertility occurred in cattle before any evidence was seen of impairment of general health.

Although the soft tissues contain relatively little F, the amount can be increased about 2-3 fold by F ingestion (Suttie et al, 1958). The kidney typically has a higher concentration than most other soft tissues, possibly because urine is the major route of F excretion (Perkinson et al, 1955; Bell et al, 1961).

Toxic Levels

A number of factors makes it difficult to pinpoint precisely a toxic level of F. Shupe (1970) suggests that toxicity is a reflection of amount and duration of ingestion, solubility of fluorides ingested, age of animal, nutrition, stress factors, and differences due to individual response.

Long-term experiments with beef cattle (Hobbs and Merriman, 1962) indicated that bones concentrated F at a dietary intake of 38 ppm or more to a point that was considered to be toxic by Suttie et al (1958). In these experiments (Hobbs and Merriman), teeth of cattle getting 38 ppm of F showed definite excessive wear and marked staining. The authors reported that there was some hypertrophy of metatarsal bones of cows ingesting rations with 48 ppm or more of F, and there was decreased feed intake at this level of F. However, reproduction was not affected until levels of 78 ppm or higher were fed.

With respect to dairy cattle, Suttie et al (1957) reported typical symptoms of lameness and debilitation in cows getting 40-50 ppm of NaF. They concluded that lactating cows could tolerate 30 ppm with comparative safety, that 40 ppm was near marginal tolerance and that 50 ppm would result in fluorosis within 3-5 years. These results agree reasonably well with those reported by Shupe et al (1963) on dairy cattle. These authors found that 27 ppm of F resulted in slight mottling of teeth and periosteal hypertrophy. An intake of 49 ppm resulted in moderate to marked dental effects and moderate osteofluorosis with palpable bone lesions after ca. 4 yr. Intermittent lameness was also seen in these cows after ca. 4 yr. Thus, these results from three different experiment stations indicate that an intake of ca. 30 ppm for an extended period of time is near the limit if no adverse signs are to develop. In other work alternating treatments of 1.5 mg/kg of body weight and control ration for 6 mo. or at the 1.5 mg rate for one year did not affect growth or reproduction of heifers (Suttie et al, 1972).

Short-term ingestion of up to 200 ppm depressed consumption of a grain mix by dairy cows with only a slight effect on milk production (Suttie and Kolstad, 1977). When supplying F in water, Van Rensburg and DeVos (1966) gave heifers water with 5-12 ppm F. No adverse effects were noted in the first breeding season; in the second, 8 or 12 ppm resulted in reduced calf crop, and even 5 ppm reduced performance in all treatments by the 4th season. Defluorinated phosphate added to the water did not reduce the harmful effects, but seemed to aggravate them.

Short-term trials with much higher levels (up to 600 ppm) showed that death may result in 6-7 mo. (Hobbs and Merriman, 1962). Shupe (1970) suggests that 100 ppm of F is compatible with finishing cattle in the feedlot. The long-term experiments with female beef or dairy cattle would substantiate this conclusion. It should be pointed out that experiments with relatively high levels of F intake (100 ppm) do not indicate a sufficient placental transfer to cause any trouble in calves or do not result in a F level in milk that is outside a safe range (Shupe et al, 1963; Stoddard et al, 1963).

In studies with young animals, Chamberlain et al (1960) found that animals under 1 yr of age metabolized F more rapidly than animals about 1 yr older, particularly with respect to excretion of F. Bone concentrations were similar, although slightly higher, in the younger animals. Suttie et al (1961) started dairy heifers of 6-27 wk of age on F intakes ranging from 1-2 mg of F/kg of body wt and carried most of them through 2 lactations. In these experiments they found no influence of F on body weight. Teeth and bone changes were seen in all treatments and were especially severe in those getting 1.4 mg F/kg or higher. In other work from this laboratory, F at a rate of 2.5 mg/kg of body weight caused severe dental fluorosis when fed to heifers during their 13-15 or 16-18 mo. of life (Suttie and Faltin, 1971).

Phillips et al (1963) have investigated changes in cows after F supplementation was stopped. During a 2-yr period they found that animals mobilized and excreted a portion of the skeletal F, but the majority of it remained. No apparent improvement was shown in dental or bone lesions during this time.

Modifying Factors

When conducting studies on pasture, Newell and Schmidt (1958) found that 2-yr-old heifers could be fed up to 2.5 mg of F/kg of body wt for an extended period of time with only mild symptoms of fluorosis. Thus, this indicates a relatively marked effect of diet. Mascola et al (1974) found the F content of esophageal samples was higher than that of available forage. F content varied by season (higher in winter and spring), plant height (decreased with increased height), and from year to year.

Hobbs and Merriman (1962) reported that the feeding of aluminum sulfate reduced the F content of bones and resulted in fewer hypertrophic bone changes. Shupe (1970) mentions that other compounds such as aluminum chloride, calcium aluminate and calcium carbonate have been shown to reduce toxicity of F in animals. These may act by reducing the solubility of F in the GI tract. Although they may reduce F uptake, the best recommendation would be to reduce the F intake if it is in a range likely to be hazardous.

Acute Toxicity

Acute F toxicity is a result of consuming concentrated F sources in large amounts. This type of fluorosis is probably of much less economic importance than that which may result from chronic toxicity.

Shupe (1970) has described the symptoms that may develop. The symptoms may show up as early as a half hour after ingestion and include: excitement; high F content of blood and urine; stiffness, anorexia and reduced milk production; excessive salivation, vomiting, spasmodic urination and defecation; weakness, severe depression and cardiac failure. On postmortem cyanosis, darkly colored blood, and hemorrhagic gastroenteritis may be seen.

Conclusions

Available data on bovines indicate that long-term ingestion of F at a rate much above 30 ppm in the diet will result in symptoms of fluorosis after a period of 2-3 years. Ingestion of appreciably larger amounts (100 ppm+) can be tolerated for

time periods of several months without undue hazard. The toxic manifestations of F are exerted almost without exception on the teeth and bones, resulting in hypertrophy, softening and excessive wear of the teeth and development of hyperostosis, and lameness as a result of the effect of F on the bones and joints. Toxic bone concentrations are believed to be above 5,500-7,000 ppm, ash basis, depending on the particular bone involved.

OTHER TOXIC ELEMENTS

There are a number of elements, other than those discussed in Ch. 4 or 5, that could be toxic for ruminant animals. However, those generally considered to cause the most frequent cases of poisoning are lead and arsenic. Mercury and cadmium are toxic, without doubt, but relatively few problems occur with ruminants in practical situations. In nearly all cases problems of toxicity are the result of contamination by man through the use of poisons put out for animals or insects, ingestion of paint, sprays used on plants to control insects or diseases, defoliating agents, etc. Recent reviews on this topic include those of Bremner (1974), Neathery and Miller (1975) and Ammerman et al (1977). In this discussion reference will be made to recent papers.

Lead (Pb)

Chronic lead toxicity has only rarely been identified in ruminants, although there is reason to believe it may be more of a factor than clinical reports suggest. Blood and Henderson (1968) point out that Pb is one of the most common causes of poisoning in cattle and that the mortality rate approaches 100%. Pica—resulting from situations such as a P-deficiency—may be a predisposing factor because of the tendency of ruminants to chew and ingest a wide variety of foreign materials.

Lead has been reported to cause toxicity in sheep which were reared in an area where the sheep had access to tailings from old mine workings (Clegg and Rylands, 1966). Whether this was due to an abnormal amount of Pb in forage in the area was not stated. The ingestion of Pb resulting from licking painted surfaces is believed to be one of the more common sources of Pb. Other major sources of contamination are wastes from metal smelters, contamination of forage from combustion of leaded gasoline along highways, use of Pb in pesticides, and similar compounds. Sewage sludge usually contains considerable Pb and may contribute to soil Pb where used in large amounts. Motor oils and greases, which contain high levels of Pb after used in internal combustion engines, may be quite toxic.

Lead toxicity should be less of a problem in the future. This is likely because (at least in the USA) few paints now contain any appreciable amount (if any) of lead salts and, also, because of increasing use of non-leaded fuels in automobiles.

Lead poisoning causes severe brain lesions and irritation of the GI tract. It affects muscular coordination and red blood cell synthesis; this results in anemia. In cattle signs of toxicity include a depressed appearance and poor performance, blindness, grinding of the teeth, muscular twitching, and convulsive seizures. In sheep lead toxicity results in depression, anorexia, abdominal pain, and (usually) diarrhea. Osteoporosis has been observed in young lambs and abortions in ewes (Dollahite et al, 1975). Young animals are generally more susceptible than older animals. Clinical signs occur in cattle with a daily intake of 6-7 mg/kg of body weight (Aronson, 1972).

Chronic lead toxicity is only rarely identified (Ammerman et al, 1977). In studies with cattle, Dinius et al (1973) found no effect of feeding 100 ppm to calves for 100 days, but Keliher et al (1973) observed that 15 mg/kg of body weight (ca. 700 ppm) depressed growth after 80 days of feeding. Anemia developed after 42 days on this level of lead. With sheep Carson et al (1973) found that daily consumption of 2.3 or 4.5 mg of lead/kg of weight for 27 weeks resulted in increased packed cell volume and hemoglobin; Fick et al (1976) found that levels up to 1000 ppm for 84 days did not affect feed consumption, weight gain, feed conversion, or digestibility but they thought that the 1000 ppm might eventually be toxic based on the amount of Pb which accumulated in the tissues. Morrison et al (1977) and Quarterman et al (1977) have shown that the level of S affects survival. In one case lambs given 200 ppm of Pb survived for only 6 weeks when the S (as sulfate) was 0.07%; survival increased to 30 weeks when S level was 0.38%. When lambs were given diets with 400 ppm Pb they died in 5 weeks or less if Ca and S content was low. When diets were supplemented with Ca and S or were low in P, they survived for up to 10 mo. Male lambs given 400 ppm Pb also survived longer when the S level was increased from 0.07 to 0.38% of the diet.

Feeding lead will result in accumulation in kidney, heart and skeletal muscles as well as other tissues such as bone and brain (Fick et al, 1976). Blood levels of 0.35 ppm and clinical signs are satisfactory for diagnosis of toxicity (Buck, 1970). Moderate amounts (0.05-0.2 mg/l.) of lead may be found in milk of cows, but milk level rapidly returns to normal after withdrawal of lead from the diet (Sapetti et al, 1973).

The source of lead greatly affects toxicity. With lead arsenate (found in phenothiazine), Bennett and Scwartz (1971) observed that the minimal lethal cumulative dose for sheep was 417 mg/kg (over an 11 mo. period). In cattle Kelliher et al (1973) found that the toxic dose of lead sulfide was about 3-fold that of either lead carbonate or lead acetate.

Studies with monogastric species show that absorption of lead from the GI tract is low, although Fick et al (1976) demonstrated that absorption (amount) increased with increased dosage. Other studies with monogastric species indicate that low dietary levels of Ca and P or vitamin D result in lower accumulations of Pb in tissues such as the liver (Ammerman et al, 1977). Treatment of Pb toxicity generally involves infusions of Ca-EDTA which forms a complex with the Pb and increases its excretion.

Other Mineral Elements

Although elements such as arsenic may be important toxins in some restricted areas, much less arsenic is used in sprays and insecticides than in the past. In one situation Reagor (1973) concluded that arsenic was the most common heavy metal poison for ruminants in Texas, probably because it was used in herbicides and cotton defoliants in that area.

There is little reason to believe that other elements such as mercury or cadmium are important toxins for ruminants (Ammerman et al, 1977). Research data have been accumulated on mercury (Ansari et al, 1973; Sell and Davison, 1973; Wright et al, 1973; Neathery et al, 1974; and Stake et al, 1975) and on cadmium (Doyle and Pfander, 1974; Neathery et al, 1974; Wright et al, 1977).

There has been some interest in radio-isotopes, particularly in elements which may be in fallout from nuclear explosions (Bell et al, 1971) or as possible contaminants from nuclear power plants. Among others these include ^{131}I, ^{90}Sr, [109]Cd and [134]Cs. Papers dealing with ^{131}I have been mentioned in Ch. 5. Reports giving data on ^{90}Sr uptake by bone and transfer to milk include those of

Bohman et al (1966), Hardy and Rivera (1968) and Kahn et al (1965). Johnson et al (1968) have investigated the excretion of [134]Cs and ^{137}Cs by lactating cows, and Miller et al (1967, 1968, 1969) have studied absorption, excretion and output in milk of [109]Cd.

References Cited

Selenium Toxicity

Caravaggi, C., F.L. Clark and A.R.B. Jackson. 1970. Res. Vet. Sci. 11:146;12:501.

Davis, A.M. 1972. Agron. J. 64:751,823.

Gabbedy, B.J. 1970. Aust. Vet. J. 46:223.

Gardiner, M.R. 1966. Aust. Vet. J. 42:442.

Kuttler, K.L., D.W. Marble and C. Blincoe. 1961. Amer. J. Vet. Res. 22:422.

Lambourne, D.A. and R.W. Mason. 1969. Aust. Vet. J. 45:208.

Maag, D.D., J.S. Orsborn and J.R. Clopton. 1960. Amer. J. Vet. Res. 21:1049.

Minyard, J.A., C.A. Dinkel and O.E. Olson. 1960. J. Animal Sci. 19:260.

Morrow, D.A. 1968. J. Amer. Vet. Med. Assoc. 152:1625.

Neething, L.P., M.M. Brown and P.J. DeWet. 1968. J.S. African Vet. Med. Assoc. 39:25.

Olsen, O.E. 1978. In: Effect of Poisonous Plants on Livestock. Academic Press, New York.

Pierce, A.W. and G.B. Jones. 1968. Aust. J. Exp. Agr. & Animal Husb. 8:277.

Quarterman, J., C.F. Mills and A.C. Dalgarno. 1966. Proc. Nutr. Soc. 25:xxiii (abstr).

Rosenfeld, I. and O.A. Beath. 1964. Selenium. Geobotany, Biochemistry, Toxicity and Nutrition, Academic Press, New York.

Rotruck, J.T. et al. 1969. J. Animal Sci. 29:170 (abstr).

Van Kampen, K.R. and L.F. James. 1978. In: Effects of Poisonous Plants on Livestock. Academic Press, New York.

Fluorine

Bell, M.C., G.M. Merriman and D.A. Greenwood. 1961. J. Nutr. 73:379.

Chamberlain, C.C., S. Hansard and C.S. Hobbs. 1960. J. Animal Sci. 19:1253 (abstr.).

Hobbs, C.S. and G.M. Merriman. 1962. Tennessee Agr. Expt. Sta. Bul. 351.

Hodge, H.C. 1964. In: Mineral Metabolism, Vol. 2, part A. Academic Press, New York.

Mascola, J.J., K.M. Barth and J.B. McLaren. 1974. J. Animal Sci. 38:1298.

Newell, G.W. and H.J. Schmidt. 1958. Amer. J. Vet. Res. 19:363.

Obel, Anna-Lisa. 1971. Acta. Vet. Scand. 12:151.

Oelschlager, W., K. Loeffler and L. Opletalova. 1971. Nutr. Abstr. Rev. 41:1498.

Perkinson, J.D., et al. 1955. Amer. J. Physiol. 182:383.

Phillips, P.H., J.W. Suttie and E.J. Zebrowski. 1963. J. Dairy Sci. 46:513.

Ramberg, C.F. et al. 1970. J. Nutr. 100:981.

Shupe, J.L. 1970. In: Bovine Medicine and Surgery. American Veterinary Publications, Inc.

Shupe, J.L. et al. 1963. Amer. J. Vet. Res. 24:964.

Shupe, J.L., D.A. Greenwood and J. Lieberman. 1965. J. Amer. Med. Assoc. 192:26.

Shupe, J.L., M.L. Miner, L.E. Harris and D.A. Greenwood. 1963. Amer. J. Vet. Res. 23:777.

Stoddard, G.E., et al. 1963. J. Dairy Sci. 46:720;1094.

Suttie, J.W., J.R. Carlson and E.C. Faltin. 1972. J. Dairy Sci. 55:790.

Suttie, J.W. and E.C. Faltin. 1971. Amer. J. Vet. Res. 32:217.

Suttie, J.W., R. Gesteland and P.H. Phillips. 1961. J. Dairy Sci. 44:2250.

Suttie, J.W. and D.L. Kolstad. 1977. J. Dairy Sci. 60:1568.

Suttie, J.W., R.F. Miller and P.H. Phillips. 1957. J. Nutr. 63:211.

Suttie, J.W. and P.H. Phillips. 1959. J. Dairy Sci. 42:1063.

Suttie, J.W., P.H. Phillips and R.F. Miller. 1958. J. Nutr. 65:292.

Underwood, E.J. 1977. Trace Elements in Human and Animal Nutrition. 4th ed. Academic Press, New York.

Van Rensburg, S.W. and W.H. DeVos. 1966. J. Vet. Res. 33:185.

Zipkin, I., E.D. Eanes and J.L. Shupe. 1964. Amer. J. Vet. Res. 25:1595.

Other Toxic Minerals

Ammerman, C.B., S.M. Miller, K.R. Fick and S.L. Hansard II. 1977. J. Animal Sci. 44:485.

Ansari, M.S. et al. 1973. J. Animal Sci. 36:415.

Aronson, A.L. 1972. Amer. J. Vet. Res. 33:627.

Blood, D.C. and J.A. Henderson. 1968. Verterinary Medicine (3rd ed.). Williams & Wilkins Co.

Bell, M.C. and L.B. Sasser. 1971. J. Animal Sci. 32:371. (abstr).

Bennett, D.G. and T.E. Schwartz. 1971. Amer. J. Vet. Res. 32:727.

Bohman, V.R., C. Blincoe, M.A. Wade and A.L. Lesperance. 1966. J. Agr. Food Chem. 14:413.

Bremner, I. 1974. Quart. Rev. Biophys. 7:75.

Buck, W.B. 1970. J. Amer. Vet. Med. Assoc. 156:1468.

Cannon, H.L. and J.M. Bowles. 1962. Science 137:765.

Carson, T.L., G.A. Van Gelder, W.B. Buck, and L.J. Hoffman. 1973. Clin. Toxicol. 6:389.

Clegg, F.G. and J.M. Rylands. 1966. J. Comp. Pathol. 76:15.

Dinius, D.K., T.H. Brinsfield and E.E. Williams. 1973. J. Animal Sci. 37:169.

Dollahite, J.J. and W.H. Pfander. 1974. Nutr. Reprts. Internat. 9:273.

Fick, K.R. et al. 1976. J. Animal Sci. 42:515.

Gireev, G.I. and A.F. Rakhmatulin. 1967. Vet. Bul. 37:47.

Hardy, E.P. and J. Rivera. 1968. J. Dairy Sci. 51:1210.

Johnson, J.E., G.M. Ward, E. Firestone and K.L. Knox. 1968. J. Nutr. 94:282.

Kahn, B., I.R. Jones, C.R. Porter and C.P. Straub. 1965. J. Dairy Sci. 48:1023.

Kelliher, D.J. et al. 1973. Ir. J. Agr. Res. 12:61;259.

Miller, W.J., et al. 1967. J. Dairy Sci. 50:1404.

Miller, W.J., D.M. Blackmon, R.P. Gentry and F.M. Pate. 1969. J. Dairy Sci. 52:2029.

Miller, W.J., D.M. Blackmon and Y.G. Martin. 1968. J. Dairy Sci. 51:1836.

Morrison, J.N., J. Quarterman and W.R. Humphries. 1977. J. Comp. Path. 87:417.

Neathery, M.W. et al. 1974. J. Dairy Sci. 57:1177.

Neathery, M.W. and W.J. Miller. 1975. J. Dairy Sci. 58:1767.

Quarterman, J., J. N. Morrison, W.R. Humphries and C.F. Mills. 1977. J. Comp. Path. 87:405.

Sapetti, C., E. Ardunino and P. Durio. 1973. Folia Vet. Latina 3:74.

Sell, J.L. and K.L. Davison. 1973. J. Dairy Sci. 56:671. (abstr).

Stake, P.E. et al. 1975. J. Animal Sci. 40:720.

Wright, F.C. et al. 1977. J. Agr. Food Chem. 25:293.

Wright, F.C., J.S. Palmer and J.C. Riner. 1973. J. Agr. Food Chem. 21:414.

Chapter 15 - Livestock Poisoning by Plants

By Lynn F. James

Poisonous plants rank high among the causes of economic loss to the livestock industry (Marsh, 1958; Schmitz et al, 1968; James, 1978). Plant-associated losses include deaths, chronic illness and debilitation, photosensitization, abortion, and birth defects. Ranges and pastures infested with poisonous plants mean increased costs and problems such as fencing, decreased forage utilization, altered grazing programs and, in some instances, supplemental feeding programs. Poisonous plants may also interfere with the development of proper grazing programs (James et al, 1969).

Three to 5% of the livestock grazing the western ranges are adversely affected by poisonous plants. Indeed, it has been estimated that 8.7% of the nutritionally sick animals on these ranges are ill as a result of eating poisonous plants (NAS, 1968). Poisonous plants obviously warrant the concern of the livestock industry.

Approximately 75% of the land area of the western USA is rangeland. The forage on these areas can best be utilized by ruminants which can convert this forage into food and fiber for human consumption. Because range forage is renewed each year without tillage, fertilization, or mechanical harvesting, such production of food and fiber is not heavily dependent on energy from fossil fuel. This renewable resource, which can produce large quantities of a high quality food and fiber, must be wisely and efficiently used, especially in light of world population changes and predictions of greater food needs. Poisonous plants are a serious impediment to use of grazing lands in the USA as well as other range areas in the world (Dwyer, 1978).

HISTORY OF POISONOUS PLANT PROBLEMS IN THE USA

Poisonous plants were probably of minor importance in the USA until the early pioneers started settling the area known as the range states (17 western states). The economic impacts of poisonous plants became all too apparent with the establishment of an extensive system of animal agri-culture based upon the utilization of the native forage.

Reports of ergotism in cattle and milk sickness (due to *Eupatorium rugosum,* white snakeroot) began in the early 1800's. Later in the same century, problems of poisoning from various other plants became obvious. Among the more important of these were locoweed poisoning (certain species of *Astragalus* and *Oxytropis*), bottom disease associated with *Crotalaria* spp., larkspur poisoning from the *Delphinium* spp., lupine poisoning from the *Lupinus* spp., and sneezeweed poisoning (*Helenium* spp).

CAUSES OF LIVESTOCK POISONING BY PLANTS

The reasons for livestock being poisoned by plants are many and varied. It is generally believed that grazing animals are rarely poisoned by the plants they normally eat (Stoddart et al, 1949). Poisoning problems are more likely to occur when animals encounter a shortage of their usual, non-poisonous forage. However, several poisonous plants are readily grazed by livestock at certain times. Among the more notable of these are larkspur, locoweed, halogeton, and lupine. Most poisonous plants kill animals only if eaten in large amounts over a short period of time. However, some poisonous plants can actually form a useful part of the animal's diet when properly grazed. Lupine in the diet of sheep is a good example.

Animals frequently are inadvertently managed to produce hunger or thirst, either of which may cause them to overgraze poisonous plants (Marsh, 1958). Trucking or trailing into or through areas infested with poisonous plants may lead to poisoning. Salting in areas infested with poisonous plants can induce death. In each of the above described situations, animals may face an abundance of poisonous plants under conditions conducive to the grazing of these plants.

Cattle and sheep can vary in their responses to poisonous plants due to management procedures as well as physiological differences. In much of the country, sheep are kept in large flocks and are moved from place to place as deemed necessary by the shepherd. In contrast cattle are often left to move freely about a range, limited only by fences and natural barriers, and are free to search out the necessities of life as they feel the need. Biological differences allow sheep and cattle to metabolize toxins from plants differently. Sheep, for example, can graze larkspur with little probability of intoxication, while cattle are poisoned on relatively small amounts.

PLANT POISONS

Certain plants are toxic because they produce and contain within their tissues one or more compounds that can have a detrimental effect on the biological systems of an animal (Radeleff, 1970). Some poisons are relatively non-toxic as they occur in the plant but are metabolized to a toxic form within the animal body; for example, nitrate in a plant is converted to nitrite in the rumen of an animal. Nitrite is much more toxic than nitrate (Kingsbury, 1964; Ch. 17, Vol. 1). Dosage is also relevant when defining a poison. Small amounts of a toxic material may be metabolized or excreted and cause no damage, while larger amounts may be harmful. Many potentially poisonous plants are grazed without apparent ill effect under normal conditions. Poisoning occurs when an animal consumes large quantities of the plant, especially if over a short period of time.

Classification of Poisons
Various methods have been used in classifying poisons (Clarke and Clarke, 1967). These include effects of the poison upon the body and the chemical structure of the poison. Systems using the effects of the toxin upon the body take into account responses such as anoxia, depression, coma, and others. A poison may have an irritating or corrosive action on areas of contact or it may cause injury to body cells. Poison may also selectively damage body organs or systems; i.e., urinary, nervous, etc.

Systems using the chemical structure of the toxin as the basis for classification place compounds with similar chemical characteristics or with other similarities in a single category such as alkaloids, glycosides, and oxalates.

Whatever the system, it is an attempt to define the action of the poison and place poisons in categories that will make them easier to understand and work with. Those interested in a detailed discussion of categorization are referred to books by Kingsbury (1964), Everist (1974), or Clark and Clarke (1967).

Modes of Actions of Poisons
Apart from materials that injure or destroy tissue, i.e., acids, alkali, and irritants, it is generally believed that toxic compounds exert their effects by altering enzymatic processes that are responsible for the normal maintenance of living cells. For example, cyanide inhibits oxidation by inactivating the enzyme, cytochrome oxidase, and oxalate exerts some of its effects by interfering with the activity of succinic dehydrogenase in the citric acid cycle.

Factors Affecting Toxicity
Many factors modify the toxic effect of a given plant on a particular animal. Toxicity itself varies with the kind of toxin and the level to which that toxin accumulates in plant tissue. For example, certain alkaloids of water hemlock are extremely toxic and only a very small amount can be lethal. In contrast low levels of oxalate are not considered harmful although high levels are but oxalate-producing dangerous to animals.

Toxicity can also vary with the plant's stage of growth. Larkspur, for example, is typical of plants that are most toxic during the young, vegetating stage of growth with toxicity decreasing as they mature, while halogeton exemplifies plants that become more toxic as they mature. Stage of growth seems to have little effect on the toxicity of plants such as the locoweeds. Some plants lose their toxicity when dried; others maintain their toxicity even after they have dried up. These can cause problems when harvested in hay. Thus, plants vary in toxicity with species, stage of growth, and potentials for toxin accumulation.

Animal responses to plant poisons are also variable, depending on species, physical condition, the dose or amount of poisonous plant consumed, and the rate of consumption. Susceptibility to poisoning of one species of animal does not necessarily mean susceptibility in other species. For example, cattle are relatively susceptible to larkspur poisoning, while sheep are only slightly susceptible. Both sheep and horses are poisoned on the locoweeds but horses are the most easily poisoned of the two.

These differences are based not only in physiology but in forage preferences.

In general, animals in good condition are more resistant to intoxication than are animals in poor condition. Such variability in resistance is particularly apparent relative to plants containing nitrate, cyanide, and oxalate (Everist, 1974).

Rate of consumption can be crucial. Animals can graze many kinds of poisonous plants without overt harm if they do so slowly. Intoxication occurs when they graze too much of the plant rapidly. Sheep can be fed diets of nearly 100% halogeton without harm if they eat the materials slowly over several hours; yet death occurs if they eat much smaller amounts in 30 minutes. When animals graze poisonous plants slowly, the toxin is diluted with other material in the GI tract and absorbed more slowly, allowing time for metabolism and excretion. Plants that have cumulative effects provide a notable exception to the rule concerning slow grazing. The best example of this is the locoweed, which must be grazed for at least thirty days before a toxic effect is produced. In general, cumulative, when used relative to poisonous plants, refers to the effect on the animal, not to an accumulation of the plant toxin in the animal.

The chemical characteristics of the plant toxins have a very important bearing on toxicity of the plant. Some plant toxins are lethal at very low levels, while others require much larger amounts. Some toxins are readily metabolized in the animal body, while others are not metabolized to any extent (Kingsbury, 1964).

Effect of Plant Toxins on Livestock

The effects of plant toxins on animals are as varied as are the toxins and the situation under which intoxication takes place. The primary effect of poisoning is acute intoxication and death, but this is not always the outcome. The animal, on consuming a poison, may become either temporarily or chronically ill, or it may evidence any number of other phenomena. In acute intoxication, problems develop rapidly and progress quickly to recovery or death. In chronic poisoning, the intoxication arises slowly and insidiously and persists for a long time or indefinitely (Smith and Jones, 1961).

Chronic illness may involve damage to a specific organ such as the liver or to systems such as the nervous system. Certain toxins can disrupt metabolic processes and may cause symptoms such as a vitamin defi-

ciency or a comparable disturbance. Some plants are now thought of as being carcinogenic.

In recent years plant toxins have been recognized as important causes of reproductive problems. Certain plant toxins have been shown to cause birth defects, embryonic and fetal deaths, and abortions. The estrogen found in certain plants has adversely affected sexual activities and reproduction in some livestock. The locoweeds and plants of the *Astragalus* and *Oxytropis* genera depress spermatogenesis, oogenesis, and general sexual activity in sheep, cattle, and horses.

Under certain conditions the consumption of some plants can cause photosensitization or hypersensitivity to light (Clare, 1952). Photosensitization is a condition characterized by erythema (inflammatory edema). Photosensitization may be either of two types: primary, which results when the photodynamic agent from the plant comes directly and unchanged from the plant; and secondary, or hepatogenic photosensitization, which results when the liver is damaged and certain normal breakdown products of digestion cannot be properly eliminated. Photosensitization occurs primarily in the unpigmented areas of an animal's body. Dark skinned animals do not show typical symptoms but may be affected when exposed to massive doses of the photodynamic agent.

PLANT TERATOGENS AND TOXINS AFFECTING REPRODUCTION

There are a number of causes of congenital malformations. The more common include radiation, nutritional deficiencies, or excesses of drugs or chemicals, viruses, plants which are natural sources of teratogens, and heredity. Early in history it was thought that most birth defects were of genetic origin (James, 1977). Now, however, the importance of plants as potential sources of teratogenicity is being recognized. Several plants (including certain species of *Veratrum, Lupinus, Astragalus,* and *Lathyrus*) have been shown to have tetratogenic properties.

The variety of possible causes of congenital malformations can make it difficult to determine which malformation arises from which etiological agent. A genetically based anomaly is established at the time of fertilization, while an aberration resulting from environmental factors must arise from a stimulus applied during the period of embryonic differentiation. A dosage of a toxin too small to cause signs of poisoning in the dam may cause damage to the fetus. Genetically inspired degenerations may duplicate the appearance of those that are environmentally induced.

Man and most animals are largely herbivorous, or at least depend to a great extent directly upon plants for their existence. The health and well-being of adult animals, as well as of a developing embryo or fetus in the case of pregnancy, are influenced by diet.

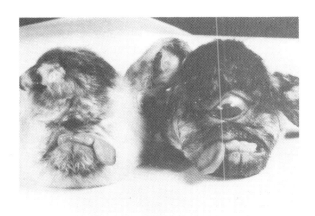

Fig. 15-2. Malformed lambs resulting from the maternal consumption of veratrum on the 14th day of gestation.

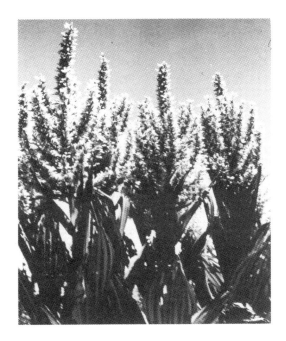

Fig. 15-1. Veratrum californicum, (western false helebore) grows in alpine meadow areas in the western United States.

Veratrum californicum, or western false hellebore (Fig. 15-1), a plant growing in wet mountain meadow areas above 6,000-ft elevations in certain areas of the west, causes cyclopian and related cephalic malformations in lambs born to ewes that ingest the plant on the 14th day of gestation (Fig. 15-2) (Binns et al, 1963; Keeler, 1975). The problem has occurred primarily in southwestern Idaho, where the incidence has varied from less than 1% to more than 25% of the lambs born in a band of sheep. Sheep seem to graze the veratrum quite readily in these areas.

The syndrome is characterized by the following, which occur in varying degrees in affected lambs: cyclopia, anopthalmia, hydrocephalus, harelip, cleft palate and a

proboscis protruding out above the eye. If a pregnant ewe consumes veratrum between her 28th and 30th days of gestation, the lamb(s) may be born with shortened metacarpal or metatarsal bones (Binns et al, 1972).

If the ewe is carrying twins or a single malformed fetus, she may go into prolonged gestation rather than giving birth at the proper time, in which case the lamb(s) may continue to grow in utero. Lambs weighing as much as 14 kg have been taken from ewes that experienced prolonged gestation. The normal birth weight of a lamb is about 3.6 kg. Survival of malformed lambs is dependent upon the severity of the cranial malformation.

Signs of intoxication are rare in ewes producing malformed lambs, but sheep under range conditions may become intoxicated from grazing this plant. Signs of poisoning include salivation, weakness and incoordination, prostration, depressed heart action, and dyspnea. The veratrum plant contains 50-60 different alkaloids, nearly all of which are toxic to animals, but only three are teratogenic. These are the steroidal alkaloids 11-deoxyjervine, jervine and 3-glucocyl-11 deoxyjervine (Keeler, 1975). Research has provided the livestock industry a practical solution to this problem: lamb malformations can be avoided by preventing ewes from grazing the V. californicum during their critical stages of gestation. This simply requires altering the grazing program.

Lupinus spp. over the years have gained notoriety as an important poisonous plant for sheep (Fig. 15-3). In recent years certain species of lupine have been shown to cause

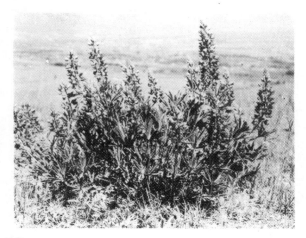

Fig. 15-3. *Lupinis serecea* (lupine) which grows in all the western states has not only been the cause of the death of thousands of sheep but also skeletal deformities in calves.

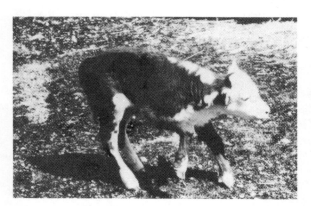

Fig. 15-4. A crooked calf resulting from the maternal consumption of lupine between the 40th and 70th days of gestation.

a condition known as crooked-calf disease. The disease is evidenced when cows ingest such lupines between their 40th and 70th days of gestation (Fig. 15-4). This condition occurs in nearly all of the western states and Alaska with the incidence varying from 0 to 35% (Shupe et al, 1967).

Crooked-calf disease is characterized by malformations of the legs, back and neck, and occasionally by a cleft palate. Affected calves appear to be normal otherwise. The joints are generally immobile because of a malalignment and malpositioning of the articular surfaces and the limbs are usually rotated laterally. These animals do not recover and should not be confused with those having contracted tendons, whose joints are all in proper alignment and without lateral or medial rotation. Joints of calves

with contracted tendons can be extended with pressure, whereas the joints of lupine-deformed calves cannot (Shupe et al, 1967).

The crooked-calf condition is related to the alkaloid anagyrine which occurs in certain lupines (Keeler et al, 1977). The anagyrine content of these species varies with the plant's stage of growth, the content being especially high during the early vegetating stages and again during the seed stage. The incidence of the crooked-calf condition can be markedly reduced by adjusting the breeding season and/or the grazing season to prevent cows from grazing young growing lupine during their 40th to 70th days of gestation (Keeler et al, 1977). A number of various mineral supplements have been recommended for the prevention of this condition, but these have not proven efficacious in preventing this malady.

Ingestion by the dams of locoweeds (certain species of *Astragalus* and *Oxytropis*) may cause malformation and abortion of fetuses (Fig. 15-5). The resultant skeletal malformations may include any or all of the following: curvature and rigidity of the joints, flexure of the carpal joint, hypermobility of the stifle joints, aplasia of the mandible, and greatly increased incidence of contracted tendons (James et al, 1967a). Many lambs born to ewes poisoned on locoweed are small and weak at birth and fail to survive. There also appears to be a higher than usual death rate in normal appearing lambs that are born to locoweed-poisoned ewes (Balls and James, 1973).

Ewes fed locoweed between their 90th to 120th days of gestation produced fetuses

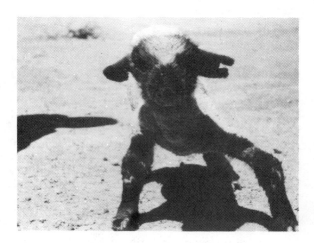

Fig. 15-5. A deformed lamb resulting from the maternal consumption of *Astragalus lentigenosus* between the 60th and 90th days of gestation.

with enlarged hearts, spleens and thyroids. Bones of lambs from these ewes appeared to be osteoporotic. Fetal edema was present in some cases (James, 1972a). More than 60% of the ewes in bands poisoned on locoweed may abort at any time during their gestations.

Sexual desire and spermatogenesis of the male and estrus and oogenesis of the female are suppressed in locoweed poisoning (Van Kampen and James, 1971; James and Van Kampen, 1978). If such animals are removed from the plants, these functions return.

Various species of the locoweeds grow on most western ranges. There is a great year-to-year variation in the growth of this group of plants (Barnaby, 1964). The toxin is not known.

Pinus ponderosa (ponderosa pine), when consumed by cows during the last trimester of their gestation, can cause abortions (Stevenson et al, 1972; James and Call, 1977). Pine needles generally become available to cows from slash from the lumber industry, windfalls, or as dried needles that have fallen from the trees. Abortions may begin within 48 hr after the needles have been ingested and continue for up to 2 weeks after the cows are removed from the pine needle source. These abortions are characterized by weak parturition contractions, excessive uterine hemorrhage, incomplete dilation of the cervix, and the presence of a characteristic nauseating odor. Premature filling of the udder and swelling of the external genital organs have also been noted in cows that have consumed pine needles and later aborted. Calves aborted near term may survive. A persistently retained placenta is a constant finding, and affected cows may develop septic metritis following the abortion. Death may occur if animals are not properly treated. The abortions occur primarily in late fall, winter, and early spring and are nearly always associated with such conditions as sudden change in weather, sudden access to needles, changes in feed, or hunger (Stevenson et al, 1972). Skeletal malformations have been associated with the experimental feeding of pine needles to ewes between their 60th and 90th days of gestation (Call and James, 1976). Ponderosa pine grows in all western states and western Canada. The severity of this problem varies considerably within areas where ponderosa pine grows.

When cows ingest *Conium maculatum* (poison hemlock) between their 40th and 70th days of gestation, their calves show skeletal malformations very similar to those seen in lupine-induced crooked calves (Keeler, 1974). Epidemiologic studies suggest that this hemlock is also responsible for birth defects in swine. The teratogenic compound in this plant is coniine. Poison hemlock grows throughout the United States.

Gutierrezia microcephela (broom snakeweed) has been an important cause of abortion in cattle in southwestern USA (James and Johnson, 1976; Sperry et al; Radeleff, 1970). Cows affected by this plant may abort in various stages of gestation or may produce living but underweight and weak calves. The placenta is commonly retained. Pregnant cows grazing snakeweed may have premature udder development and swelling of the external genitals. Symptoms of snakeweed poisoning in cattle and sheep include listlessness, anorexia, sometimes hematuria, and nasal discharge. Snakeweed growing on sandy soils is reported to be much more toxic than that growing on so-called hard soils. Broom snakeweed grows on dry range areas from Texas to California and north into Colorado and Idaho. Heavy stands of this plant are indicative of overgrazing. The toxin is thought by some investigators to be a saponin.

Field cases of abortion in sheep and cattle have been observed in animals that have ingested *Juniperus osteosperma* (juniper). Experimental feeding of this plant has also caused abortions in sheep (Johnson et al, 1976). Other plants that cause abortions or birth defects include *Senecio jacobaea*, some *Lathyrus* and *Indigofera* spp, and *Brassica* (Keeler, 1975). Species like *Tetradymia* that cause animals to become very sick may cause abortion. Other plant species will undoubtedly be incriminated as causes of birth defects and abortions as time goes on. A number of plants have been shown to contain estrogens that may affect fertility in livestock grazing them (Cox, 1978).

PLANTS CAUSING PHOTOSENSITIZATION IN LIVESTOCK

Tetradymia glabrata (little leaf horsebush, Fig. 15-6), and *T. canescens* (grey horsebrush) are two of the principal photosensitizing plants of western United States. *Tetradymia* grows in the arid portions of all eleven western states. These plants are responsible for a condition in sheep known as bighead, and caused the deaths of thousands of sheep during the first half of the 20th century. Both

372

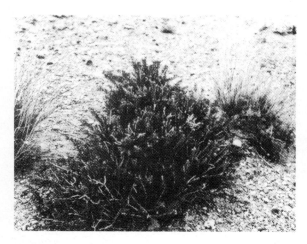

Fig. 15-6. *Tetradymia glabrata* or little leaf horsebush, is a desert shrub that can cause photosensitization in sheep.

plants cause hepatogenous photosensitization (Johnson, 1974; Jennings et al, 1978).

Bighead poisoning is characterized by uneasiness, itching and sometimes swelling of the head, and thickening of the lips and ears. The ears droop because of fluid accumulation. Fluid seeps from the skin and forms scabs on the face. As the skin becomes necrotic, the scabs peel off. Swelling does not occur in all cases. Affected sheep show anorexia, depression, incoordination, rapid weak pulse, coma and death. Abortions may occur in pregnant ewes. Photosensitization and swelling occur only if the sheep have been fed or have grazed *Artemisia nova* (black sage) or some species of big sage like *A. tridentata* prior to ingesting *T. grabrata*. The sagebrush is apparently a predisposition factor. The treatment of animals poisoned on *Tetradymia* consists primarily of placing them where they can be protected from the sun.

Cymopterus watsonii (desert parsley) produces a primary photosensitization. The photosensitization is marked by reddening of the exposed areas of the body such as the nose, external genitalia, and udder. This is followed by the formation of blisters, scabbing and soreness. Desert parsley usually grows early in the spring during the lambing season. The photosensitization results in the orphaning of lambs because affected ewes' udders and teats become exceedingly sore. This plant grows in desert areas and therefore dries up early so that it is a problem only during a short period in the spring (Binns et al, 1964).

Tribulus terrestris (puncture vine) and *Agave lecheguilla* (lechuguilla) both can

cause photosensitization of the hepatogenic type and *Hypericum perforatum* (St. Johnswort) and *Fagopyrum sagittatum* (buckwheat) cause photosensitization of the primary type (Clare, 1952; Kingsbury, 1964).

Except for problems with the plants indicated, photosensitization rarely involves large numbers of animals. However, photosensitization from undetermined causes is frequently seen in an occasional animal. Some clovers (*Trifolium* species) are thought to be involved in these cases of photosensitization (Kingsbury, 1964).

PLANTS HAVING CARCINOGENIC EFFECTS ON LIVESTOCK

Carcinogenic materials have not received a great deal of attention relative to livestock. Cancer is not generally considered to be of great importance in animals as most livestock are disposed of before they become aged. In addition no necropsy is performed nor is histological work done on most of the large animals that die. Therefore, many carcinogenic problems probably go undetected. Two plants should be mentioned in relation to cancer: pyrrolizidine alkaloid-containing plants and *Pteridium aquilinium* (bracken fern). The bracken fern produces bladder tumors and the pyrrolizidine-producing plants cause microscopic changes in the liver suggestive of carcinogenesis.

PLANTS INTERFERING WITH REQUIRED NUTRIENTS

Since *Equisetum* spp (horsetail) contains a thiamin-destroying substance, it can be successfully treated with thiamin. This poisoning occurs primarily in horses when *Equisetum* is fed in the hay. However, cases of poisoning in sheep have been reported.

Species of *Equisetum* grow throughout the United States as a weed in moist fields and meadows. Several compounds have been isolated from it that have at some time been suggested as the toxic principle. Although this plant is of little importance as a poisonous plant, the toxic effects are of interest.

Bracken fern, *Pteridium aquilinium* (Fig. 15-7) causes signs of intoxication in horses similar to that produced by horsetail. Bracken poisoning in the horse can also be successfully treated with thiamin (Kingsbury, 1964). Bracken fern is a cumulative

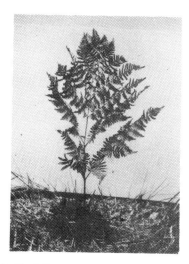

Fig. 15-7. *Pteridium aquileneum* (bracken fern) grows on wooded hillsides. Plants of this genus are world-wide in distribution.

poison in cattle. They must graze considerable amounts of the bracken for 2-4 weeks to produce toxic effects. The signs of poisoning come on rapidly and include fever, anorexia, depression, difficult respiration, salivation, nasal and rectal bleeding, hematuria, and hemorrhage of the mucous membranes. Species of *Pteridium* are world-wide in distribution. Animals seldom graze bracken fern if adequate other forage is available. The poisonous principle is unknown.

Some vegetation growing on soils high in molybdenum can become toxic (see Ch. 5). Mo in forage can exert its effect on animals in two ways: a low level can promote copper accumulation and the eventual development of symptoms of Cu poisoning; high levels cause a depletion of Cu reserves in the animal body and an ultimate Cu deficiency. Soils containing in excess of 5 ppm Mo are considered dangerous.

PLANTS CONTAINING PYRROLIZIDINE ALKALOIDS

The pyrrolizidine alkaloids occur in several plants and are poisonous to all classes of livestock. Plants that occur in the USA that contain pyrrolizidine alkaloids are *Senecio, Amsinckia, Echium, Heliotropium* and *Crotolaria* (Kingsbury, 1964).

The description of intoxication given will be that associated with *Senecio jacobaea* (tansy ragwort). Animals poisoned on other plants containing pyrrolizidine alkaloids generally respond in a similar fashion, with variation in response being associated principally with dose and the time required for intoxication to take place (Hooper, 1978).

Senecio jacobaea is a problem primarily to cattle and horses. It causes a chronic, cirrhosis-like condition of the liver which may lead to death of the animal several months after the tansy has been eaten. This makes the poisoning difficult to diagnose (Hooper, 1978).

Young animals eating 4-7% of their total daily diet of prebloom tansy for 20 days may be expected to develop signs of poisoning and die within six month's time. Older animals may tolerate more. The time of grazing to death depends upon the amount of plant consumed and the rate at which it is consumed (Johnson, 1978b). The signs of poisoning include: lethargy, anorexia, watering eyes, diarrhea or constipation, general body weakness, aimless wandering and apparent blindness. Cattle may develop a somewhat sweetish odor. The abdominal cavity may fill with water. Death may occur within only a few days after signs appear.

Senecio jacobaea is a weedy biennial plant which grows in woodlands, pastures, and hay fields of the coastal northwest USA. It is generally unpalatable to livestock. *S. longilobus* and *S. riddelli* are woody perennials growing in the drier range areas of the southwest. Herbal tea made from *S. longilobus* is commonly drunk by some American Indians and Mexican-Americans and deaths from this tea have been reported in young children (Anon., 1977). There are indications that the pyrrolizidine alkaloid can be found in the milk of cows grazing tansy and in the honey of bees foraging on the plant (Dickinson, 1978).

Amsinskia intermedia (fiddleneck) grows in some of the semiarid regions of Idaho, California, Oregon, and Washington. The seeds of this plant are a troublesome contaminant of wheat (Kingsbury, 1964). Such contaminated grain could be toxic. *Crotalaria* species grow primarily in the south and central midwest. *Echium plantagineum* grows in limited areas in California. *Heliotropium europeum* occurs sparingly in the southeastern states from Florida to New Jersey.

Selenium-Accumulating Plants

Selenium (Se) is accumulated by a number of plants in sufficient amounts to be toxic if consumed by livestock. This is an important problem in some areas. Refer to Ch. 14 for further details.

Nitrate

Nitrate is accumulated by several plants at high enough levels to be toxic. Several crop plants such as oat, hay, corn, and sorghum can accumulate nitrate at potentially toxic levels. Weeds, especially among the *Amoranthaceae, Chenopidiaceae, Cruciferae, Compositae,* and some other genera can, under the proper conditions, accumulate hazardous levels of nitrate. Plants containing more than 1.5% nitrate (as KNO_3 by weight) may prove fatal to livestock (Kingsbury, 1964). Nitrate poisoning can occur from the ingestion of nitrogen fertilizer and from water containing high levels of nitrate. Treatment of some plants with 2,4-D may cause increased production of nitrate and also increase palatability. Further details on nitrate toxicity are given in Ch. 17, Vol. 1.

CYANIDE-PRODUCING PLANTS

Cyanogenetic glycosides, under certain conditions, can accumulate in some plants at levels that render them toxic. The intact glycoside is relatively non-toxic. The toxicity comes from the HCN component following hydrolysis. This component is produced in excessive amounts in the plant during periods of drought, frost, or other conditions that might stress the plants. Hydrolysis of the glycoside can also take place in the rumen (see Ch. 17).

Plants most likely to develop appreciable amounts of cyanide are the *Sorghum* spp, Johnson grass and sudan grass; *Triglochin* spp, arrowgrass (Fig. 15-8); *Prunus* spp, cherries (Fig. 15-9), and others.

The release of the cyanide from the plant material in the stomach requires a certain amount of water, thus drinking water may prompt a quick release of the cyanide. HCN exerts its effect by inhibiting the action of the respiratory enzyme, cytochrome oxidase; therefore, HCN poisoning constitutes asphyxiation at the cell level (Conn, 1978).

HCN is a very potent toxin which affects primarily ruminants. The HCN is hydrolyzed in the rumen, freeing the cyanide which is the toxic constituent (see Ch. 17). The amount of toxin needed to cause death varies with the rate of consumption and the relative rate of absorption and detoxification by animal tissues. The signs of poisoning are nervousness, abnormal respiration, trembling, blue coloration of mucous mem-

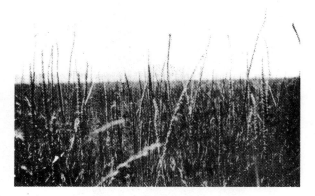

Fig. 15-8. *Triglochin* spp. (arrowgrass) is a perennial grasslike plant that grows in wet saline pasture areas. Under conditions of stress this plant may contain toxic amounts of cyanogenetic glycosides.

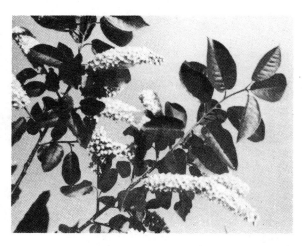

Fig. 15-9. *Prunus virginian* (chokecherry) is a small perennial tree that grows in moist areas on hillsides and canyon slopes. It also can contain toxic amounts of cyanogenetic glycosides.

branes, staggering, convulsions, coma, and death. Death may occur anywhere from 50 minutes to a few hours following the ingestion of a lethal dose of the toxic plant materials (Kingsbury, 1964). Awareness of the cyanide-producing potential of various plants and avoiding those plants during dangerous periods is the best means of prevention.

OXALATE-PRODUCING PLANTS

Oxalate-producing plants are worldwide in distribution. The two principal oxalate-producing plants in North America are: *Halogeton glomeratus* (Fig. 15-10) (halogeton), and *Sarcobatus vermiculatus* (Fig. 15-11) (greasewood). Both of these occur in

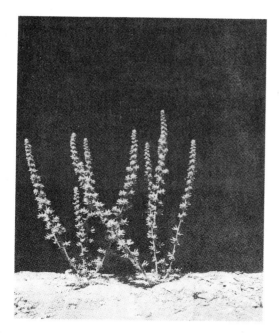

Fig. 15-10. Halogeton is the principle oxalate-producing plant of the west. It is an annual that grows in the colder, saline arid areas of the west.

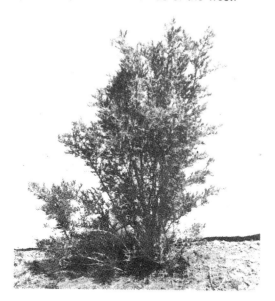

Fig. 15-11. *Sarcobatus vermiculatus* (greasewood) is a perennial oxalate-producing shrub which grows on the colder, arid, saline desert areas of the west.

the colder, saline, arid and semi-arid regions of the intermountain west. Both plants belong to the Chenopodiaceae family, which are readily grazed by cattle and sheep. They have caused a large number of deaths of sheep (Fig. 15-12) and occasional deaths in cattle (Cook et al, 1953).

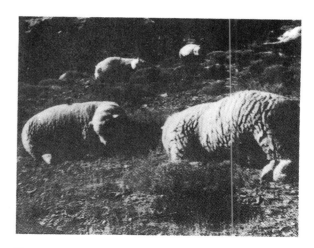

Fig. 15-12. A few of 1200 sheep that died during a 24-hour period from halogeton poisoning.

Halogeton usually contains between 12 and 18% oxalate on a dry weight basis, but may go as high as 36%; greasewood contains less. The oxalate content varies with factors such as site, stage of growth, moisture, and leaching.

Oxalate produces its toxic effect in three ways. It may be absorbed into the blood where it combines with Ca, resulting in a hypocalcemia. Ca oxalate crystals accumulate in the rumen wall and kidneys where they interfere with proper function and oxalate may interfere with energy metabolism by interfering with the enzymes, succinic and lactic dehydrogenase (James, 1972). There is evidence that animals respond differently to sodium oxalate than to acid potassium oxalate (James, 1972, 1978).

When oxalate is consumed by a ruminant, it combines with Ca to form insoluble Ca oxalate and is excreted in the feces. It can be degraded by the rumen microorganisms and absorbed from the rumen into the bloodstream where it may exert its toxic effect (James et al, 1967b; James, 1972b; Allison et al, 1976).

The signs of halogeton poisoning include depression, weakness, salivation, coma and death. The heart rate increases and there is stasis of the digestive tract. Death usually occurs between 4 and 12 hours after a lethal dose of the plant is consumed; however, some sheep may linger on for 2 or 3 days before death (Van Kampen and James, 1969a; James, 1972b; Littledike et al, 1976).

Oxalate poisoning appears to be an all or nothing situation, i.e., the animal either eats enough to kill it or there is very little effect.

Sheep can consume large quantities of halogeton with no ill effects if it is consumed over an extensive period of time. Poisoning occurs when the plant is consumed rapidly. This usually happens when the animal is hungry, so the problem of halogeton poisoning is principally one of management. There is no effective treatment for halogeton poisoning in sheep and cattle (James, 1972b).

Minimization of oxalate poisoning can be accomplished by using the following rules: (1) Move sheep slowly into areas containing heavy stands of oxalate-producing plants to allow the rumen microorganisms time to become conditioned to the oxalates. (2) Prevent hungry sheep from grazing heavy stands of halogeton. This can be accomplished by supplying animals with adequate feed and water at all times. (3) Develop a grazing plan to provide for proper preparation of sheep to graze problem areas (James and Johnson, 1970; James et al, 1970, James and Cronin, 1974). The various Ca mineral mixtures containing Ca which have been recommended for the prevention of oxalate poisoning in the past have not provided the protection from oxalate poisoning that was once thought possible (James and Binns, 1961; James and Johnson, 1970; James et al, 1970).

Syndromes of *Astragalus* Poisoning

The *Astragalus* species are involved in four separate syndromes of intoxication. They are as follows: (1) Se-accumulating *Astragalus* species; (2) nitro-bearing *Astragalus* plants —acute intoxication; (3) nitro-bearing *Astragalus* plants—chronic intoxication; and (4) locoweed poisoning (*Oxytropis* and *Astragalus* species are involved in this type of intoxication).

The nitro-bearing *Astragalus* plants include the various varieties of *A. miser, A. emoryanus, A. terapterus, A. canadensis,* and a number of others (Williams and James, 1978). This group of plants occurs throughout the western states and western Canada (MacDonald, 1952). Consumption of these plants by cattle and sheep can result in acute or chronic intoxication, depending upon the rate of consumption. The toxic compound in these plants is 3-nitro-propionic acid or 3-nitro-propanol (Stermitz et al, 1969, Stermitz, 1978). The level of this toxin in the plant is highest during the early stages of growth and declines as the plant matures.

Acute intoxication is characterized by nervousness, weakness, rapid pulse, coma,

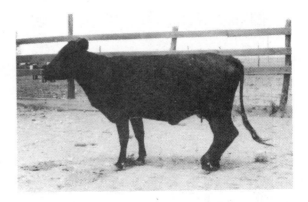

Fig. 15-13. A cow that was poisoned on *Astragalus emoryanus*. Note positioning of hind legs, especially the ankles.

convulsions and death. This type of intoxication is quite similar to larkspur poisoning in cattle. The time from consumption of the plant to death is short (Williams and James, 1978).

Chronic poisoning associated with the consumption of the nitro-bearing *Astragalus* plants is characterized by huskiness of the voice, labored respiration, and posterior paralysis (Fig. 15-13). The early signs of chronically poisoned cattle are called crackerheels. Crackerheels are characterized by knocking of the hocks and dew claws together when the animal walks, thus producing a clicking sound. If the animal is allowed to continue grazing the plant, the disease progresses from the interference of the hind legs when walking to goose-stepping and eventual posterior paralysis which progresses anteriorly (MacDonald, 1952; Williams and James, 1978). Death will eventually result. Exertion can cause sick animals to die. The lesions are of a permanent nature, principally emphysema and permanent nerve damage. Morbidity and mortality can be extensive (Williams et al, 1976).

The final syndrome of *Astragalus* poisoning to be discussed here results from livestock grazing plants such as *A. lentiginosus, A. pubentissimus,* and *Oxtropis serecea* (Fig. 15-14). There are about 13 species of locoweeds. Locoweed poisoning is a chronic type of intoxication (James et al, 1967a). The animals must graze the plant over about a 30-day period before signs of poisoning are observed. The consequences of animals grazing locoweed include: habituation, emaciation, neurological disturbance, and reproductive disturbances.

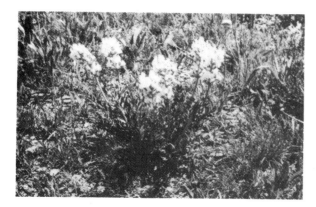

Fig. 15-14. *Oxytropis serecea.* One of the locoweeds growing in western United States.

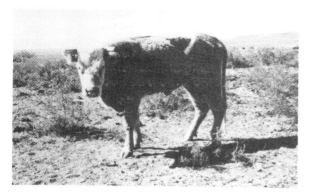

Fig. 15-15. A cow that has been poisoned on locoweed. Note the gaunt, emaciated appearance and the lusterless look in her eyes.

Most locoweeds are not especially palatable but when they are green and other forages are dry, they are readily grazed (James et al, 1969). When an animal starts to graze this plant, they will graze it at the exclusion of other forage. This is termed habituation.

Signs of locoweed poisoning include depression, dullness, excitement when disturbed, and loss of sense of direction. Symptoms may disappear when animals are removed from the plant, only to appear under stress conditions. Once an animal becomes poisoned on locoweed, it does not recover (Van Kampen and James, 1969b). If an animal starts grazing locoweed and continues to do so, it will become severely poisoned, emaciated, and will eventually become recumbent and die (Fig. 15-15).

The locoweed toxin damages the central nervous system, resulting in neurological disturbances. As a result of these disturbances, animals are often referred to as locoed animals. The changes resulting in this particular condition is called locoweed poisoning. Loco is a Spanish word meaning crazy. The toxin(s) in locoweed are not known.

LUPINE

Lupine poisoning has long been considered one of the serious poison plant problems in sheep. Many thousands of sheep have died from grazing this plant (Kingsbury, 1964). Lupine poisoning generally occurs when hungry sheep are moved into areas where there are dense stands of lupine.

There have been in excess of 80 species of lupine described in the United States and lupine can be found growing on most western ranges. There is considerable variation in toxicity among species. Some are non-toxic. In fact, many sheepmen consider lupine, especially in the seed stage, to be an excellent sheep feed.

The signs of poisoning include nervousness, depression, difficult breathing, twitching of muscles, loss of muscular control, salivation, convulsions, coma and death. Once a sheep is poisoned on lupine and shows signs of intoxication, it should be left alone. Death occurs rapidly after the sheep eat a lethal dose.

HEMLOCK POISONING

Hemlock is used as the common name of two poisonous plants of different genera— water hemlock (*Cicuta maculatum*) and poison hemlock (*Conium maculatum*). Water hemlock is probably the most toxic plant that grows in the United States. Poisoning from this plant has occurred in both man and animals (Kingsbury, 1964; Anon., 1968).

Water hemlock is a wetland plant that is usually found growing on stream banks or other wet places. The plant has a strong carrot-like odor that has been associated with the toxin, although the toxin has not definitely been isolated. All parts of the plant are toxic, but the tuberous root is especially so. The above-ground parts lose their toxicity as the plant matures. Various species of *Cicuta* (water hemlock) occur throughout the USA.

The signs of poisoning include muscle twitching, rapid pulse, rapid breathing, tremors, convulsions, dilation of pupils, salivation, coma and death. Death may occur

378

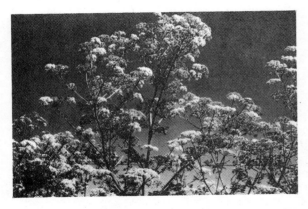

Fig. 15-16. *Conium maculatum* (poison hemlock) grows in moist areas. It may be between four and ten feet tall. It has a repulsive mousy odor.

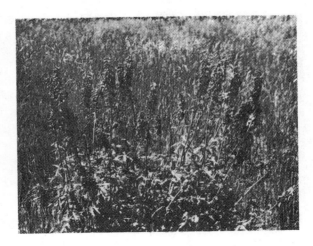

Fig. 15-17. *Delephenium occidentali* (tall larkspur) is a perennial plant that grows in moist areas on mountain hillsides, under aspen and other favorable sites.

shortly after signs of poisoning appear. *Conium maculatum* or poison hemlock (Fig. 15-16) has been discussed as a cause of birth defects in cattle in another section of this chapter.

Although poison hemlock is widely distributed throughout the USA, it is not notorious as a poisonous plant. It is distasteful to livestock and unpleasant to humans because of its mousy odor (Kingsbury, 1964; Anon., 1968). This plant contains at least five different alkaloids, the principal one being coniine. These alkaloids are volatile and are lost on drying.

Poison hemlock is, however, poisonous to all classes of livestock. Signs of poisoning usually occur shortly after ingestion of the plant. These signs include nervousness, trembling, ataxia, especially involving the lower or hind limbs, dilation of pupils, weakened and slowed heartbeat, coldness of extremities, coma and death.

LARKSPUR

Larkspur poisoning is one of the principal causes of death in cattle grazing the western ranges. These perennials belong to the genera *Delphinium* (Kingsbury, 1964; Anon. 1968). In the west, the larkspurs are divided by height as tall or low. The tall larkspurs grow at higher elevations and include species such as *D. barbeyi*, *D. occidentale*, and *D. glaucum* (Fig. 15-17). The low larkspurs grow at lower elevations and include species such as *D. nelsonii* and *D. andersonii*. Larkspur is quite palatable to cattle and is readily grazed at all stages of growth.

The larkspurs owe their toxicity to a number of alkaloids. The toxicity of these

plants decreases as they mature, and will vary considerably among species. Signs of larkspur poisoning occur shortly after a lethal amount of the plant has been consumed. Signs of poisoning include nervousness, staggering, nausea, salivation, twitching muscles, bloat, rapid irregular heart action, and the animal may suddenly collapse. Cattle dying from larkspur poisoning are often found lying on their brisket. Externally induced excitement intensifies the signs of poisoning and may increase the probability and speed of death.

Tall larkspur are a climax species, so they are expected to be found growing on the better range areas. The plants can be controlled, however, by spraying two successive years with the herbicide 2,4,5-T (Cronin, 1974).

MILKWEED

Asclepias spp (milkweed) grows throughout the USA and Canada. The milkweeds are perennials and derive their name from the thick white sap that oozes from the cut stem or leaf of the plant. Milkweeds have been generally divided into two groupings: the narrow leaf milkweeds and the broad leaf milkweeds. They are of very low palatability and consumed only when animals are excessively hungry, or when milkweeds are incorporated into hay. The more important of the milkweeds are: *A. labriformis* (Fig. 15-18), *A. subverticulatus*, *A. eriocarpa*, and *A. facicularus*. All milkweeds should be considered potentially dangerous until

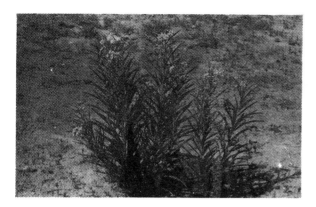

Fig. 15-18. *Asclepias labriformis* (milkweed) Milkweeds grow in dry areas. A white gummy sap seeps from broken stems and leaves.

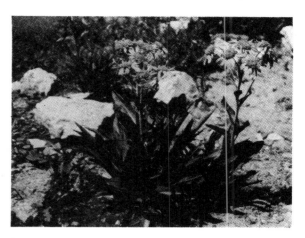

Fig. 15-19. *Helenium hoopesii* (sneezeweed) is a perennial herb that is toxic principally to sheep.

proven otherwise (Kingsbury, 1964; Benson et al, 1978).

All classes of livestock can be affected by milkweeds, with sheep and cattle being particularly susceptible. The listed milkweeds are toxic at less than 0.5% of the body weight. Death can occur quite quickly after the plant is consumed. Signs of poisoning include: loss of muscular control, staggering, spasms, bloating, rapid weak pulse, difficult breathing, and death. Losses can best be prevented by not exposing hungry livestock to these plants.

SOME TOXIC PLANTS OF THE FAMILY COMPOSITAE

Hymenoxys odorata (bitterweed), *Hymenoxys richardsonii* (pingue), and *Helenium hoopesii* (sneezeweed) all belong to the same family of plants. They apparently possess at least one common toxin, a sesquiterpene lactone, and they also resemble each other in the way they cause poisoning in livestock (Hertz, 1978). They primarily affect sheep (Kingsbury, 1964; Sperry et al, undated).

H. odorata is an annual growing primarily in the southwestern part of the USA. It is probably the most serious problem faced by sheep producers of that area. Most people feel that it is the result of overgrazing. Bitterweed is apparently not normally liked by sheep, but they can develop a taste for it. Intoxication by bitterweed is a chronic condition. Sheep must graze the plant several days before signs of poisoning occur. Acute intoxication can occur but rarely does.

Bitterweed contains an irritant to the digestive tract. Animals grazing on bitterweed lose their appetite, the rumen stops

functioning, and they may show signs of poisoning. They lose weight rapidly and tend to lag behind the herd. Green material may appear around the mouth. Animals that are not severely poisoned may recover if given proper feed and water. However, those having advaced signs continue to lose weight and waste away. At present there is no satisfactory way to treat poisoned animals. Preventive proper range and pasture management seem to be the best solution. Sheep should not be allowed to graze bitterweed-infested pastures continuously, but should be rotated so they can have access to bitterweed-free forage.

Hymenoxys richardsonii (pingue) is a perennial shrub inhabiting the more arid areas of the west at elevations of 4,000 to 10,000 feet (Fig. 15-19). Its toxic principle and effect upon sheep is similar to that of *H. odorata*.

Helenium hoopesii (sneezeweed) is a herbaceous perennial growing in western mountains at elevations between 7,000 and 10,000 feet. Its toxic principle and effects upon sheep resemble those of bitterweed and pingue.

A number of other species of *Helenium* grow throughout the USA. *Gutierrezia microcephala* (snakeweed) is a perennial shrub growing from Texas to California and north to Colorado and Idaho. It grows in the dryer desert areas.

Sheep and cattle in the southwest have been poisoned from grazing this plant (Sperry et al); the most common result of grazing this plant is abortion. Cows grazing snakeweed early in pregnancy may abort and those near term may give birth to small, weak calves. Cows that abort commonly have a retained placenta. In a significant number of cases the cow dies following the abortion. Cows grazing snakeweed may display a premature swelling of the external genital organs and a filling of the udder. Signs of poisoning in cattle and sheep include listlessness, anorexia, rough hair coat, diarrhea, vaginal discharge, and often hematuria. Snakeweeds are more toxic when growing on sandy soils.

OAK POISONING

Quercus spp (oak) is a problem through a large portion of the western states. The oaks vary from shrubs not more than 3 feet high, to large trees (Kingsbury, 1964; Panciera, 1978). The two primary oaks are *Q. gambeii*, which grows in the intermountain area, and *O. harvardii*, found in much of the southwest.

Oak poisoning occurs primarily in cattle that eat the buds and early leaves. The diet must exceed 50% oak browse before poisoning occurs. Danger of poisoning lessens as the leaves mature, but intoxication can still occur. The signs of poisoning include a gaunt, tucked up appearance, constipation often followed by diarrhea, weakness, tendency to stay near water, reluctance to move, emaciation, dark colored urine, and collapse.

DEATH CAMAS

Zygadenus spp (death camas) are found primarily west of the Mississippi river in the USA (Anon., 1968). The principal species are *Z. particulitis, Z. nuttallii, Z. graminceus,* and *Z. venenosus.* Death camas grows best on sandy plains and rocky foothills. It is seldom found growing above 8,000 feet. It has grass-like leaves and a bulbous root. These plants start growing early in the spring, providing green forage earlier than most plants. Poisoning usually occurs early in the spring while death camas is starting its growth and before other plants have started to grow. Death camas is toxic to all species of livestock, but sheep are most commonly poisoned. Signs of poisoning include rapid respiration, salivation, nausea, weakness, convulsions, and coma. Severely poisoned animals usually die. There is no known treatment for death camas poisoning.

MECHANICAL INJURY

Some plants that are not toxic can cause discomfort or stress because of their physical properties. These include plants with awns, barbs or other parts that may penetrate the skin or the mucous membrane of the mouth. Awns from certain grasses that get into the wool of sheep and work their way in to penetrate the skin can be especially troublesome. Awns or barbs may occasionally accumulate in some of the crevices of the mouth and cause sores which may become infected.

REDUCING LIVESTOCK LOSSES DUE TO POISONOUS PLANTS

There is no known treatment for animals poisoned on most poisonous plants. Even when treatment is available, affected animals are usually in remote places and are reached too late to apply the treatment. When poisoned animals have recovered enough to be handled, treatment should be for the visible symptoms.

In general, prevention of loss from poisonous plants is a problem of range and livestock management. Proper diagnosis is essential to identifying the specific plant involved. Under range conditions livestock may ingest large quantities of poisonous plants in a short period of time. Such animals may not exhibit typical signs of lesions characteristic of poisoning, or even more likely, they may never be observed.

Following a few simple rules can do much to decrease the probability of livestock poisoning by plants (Anon, 1968). To protect animals from poisoning: learn to identify the poisonous plants and the properties and conditions under which these can be dangerous to livestock; develop a grazing plan designed to improve the range in order to avoid poisonous plant problems (graze at the proper time and don't overgraze); do not allow animals that are hungry or under stress to graze in areas infested with poisonous plants; provide adequate feed and water for the livestock; be especially careful when grazing newly introduced livestock on the range; provide adequate salt and other supplements as needed; and control poisonous plants where feasible.

References Cited

Allison, M.J., E.T. Littledike and L.F. James. 1977. J. Animal Sci. (in press).

Anonymous. 1968. USDA Bul. 327.

Balls, L.D. and L.F. James. 1973. J. Amer. Vet. Med. Assoc. 162:291.

Barnaby, R.C. 1964. Atlas of North American Astragalus. New York Botanical Gardens, Bronx, NY.

Benson, J., J. Seiber, R.F. Keeler and A.E. Johnson. 1978. In: Effects of Poisonous Plants on Livestock. Academic Press, New York.

Binns, W., L.F. James, J.L. Shupe and G. Everett. 1963. Amer. J. Vet. Res. 24:1164.

Binns, W., L.F. James and W. Brooksby. 1964. Vet. Med. Small Animal Clinician 59:375.

Binns, W., R.F. Keeler and L.D. Balls. 1972. Clin. Tox. 5:245.

Call, J.W. and L.F. James. 1976. J. Amer. Vet. Med. Assoc. 169:1301.

Clarke, E.G.C. and M.L. Clarke. 1967. Garner's Veterinary Toxicology. 3rd ed. Williams and Wilkins Pub. Co., Baltimore.

Clare, N.T. 1952. Rev. ser. #3, Commonwealth Bur. Animal Health, Commonwealth Agr. Bureau, Farnham Royal, Bucks, England.

Conn, E.E. 1978. In: The Effects of Poisonous Plants on LIvestock. Academic Press, New York.

Cook, W. and L.A. Stoddart. 1953. Utah Agr. Expt. Sta. Bul. 364.

Cox, R.I. 1978. In: The Effects of Poisonous Plants on Livestock. Academic Press, New York.

Cronin, E.H. 1974. J. Range Mgmt. 27:219.

Dickerson, J.O. 1978. In: Effects of Poisonous Plants on Livestock. Academic Press, New York.

Dwyer, P. 1978. In: Effects of Poisonous Plants on Livestock. Academic Press, New York.

Everist, S. 1974. Poisonous Plants of Australia. Angus and Robertson Publishers, Sydney, Australia

Herz, H. 1978. In: Effects of Poisonous Plants on Livestock. Academic Press, New York.

Hooper, P.T. 1978. In: Effects of Poisonous Plants on Livestock. Academic Press, New York.

James, L.F. 1972a. Amer. J. Vet. Res. 33:835.

James, L.F. 1972b. Clin. Tox. 5:221.

James, L.F. 1977. World Rev. Nutr. Dietet. 26:208.

James, L.F. 1978. In: Effects of Poisonous Plants on Livestock. Academic Press, New York.

James, L.F. and W. Binns. 1961. Proc. West. Sec. Amer. Soc. Animal Prod. 12:LXVI.

James, L.F. and J.E. Butcher. 1972. J. Animal Sci. 35:1233.

James, L.F., J.E. Butcher and K.R. Van Kampen. 1970. J. Range Mgmt. 23:123.

James, L.F. and J.W. Call. 1977. Cornell Vet. 67:294.

James, L.F. and E.H. Cronin. 1974. J. Range Mgmt. 27:424.

James, L.F. and A.E. Johnson. 1970. J. Amer. Vet. Med. Assoc. 154:437.

James, L.F. and A.E. Johnson. 1976. J. Range Mgmt. 29:356.

James, L.F., J.L. Shupe, W. Binns and R.F. Keeler. 1967a. Amer. J. Vet. Res. 28:1379.

James, L.F., J.C. Street and J.E. Butcher, 1967b. J. Animal Sci. 26:1438.

James, L.F. and K.R. Van Kampen. 1971. Amer. J. Vet. Res. 32:1253.

James, L.F., K.R. Van Kampen and G. Staker. 1969. J. Amer. Vet. Med. Assoc. 155:525.

Jennings, P.W., et al. 1978. In: Effects of Poisonous Plants on Livestock. Academic Press, New York.

Johnson, A.E. 1974. Amer. J. Vet. Res. 35:1583; Can. J. Comp. Med. 38:406.

Johnson, A.E. 1978a. Amer. J. Vet. Res. (in press).

Johnson, A.E. 1978b. In: Effects of Poisonous Plants on Livestock. Academic Press, New York.

Johnson, A.E., L.F. James and J. Spillett. 1976. J. Range Mgmt. 29:278.

Keeler, R.F. 1974. Clin. Tox. 7:195.

Keeler, R.F. 1975. Lloydia 28:56.

Keeler, R.F., L.F. James, J.L. Shupe and K.R. Van Kampen. 1977. J. Range Mgmt. 30:97.

Kingsbury, J.M. 1964. Poisonous Plants of the United States and Canada. Prentice Hall, Inc. Englewood Cliffs, New Jersey.

Littledike, E.T., L.F. James and H. Cook. 1976. Amer. J. Vet. Res. 37:661.

MacDonald, M.A. 1952. J. Range Mgmt. 5:16.

Marsh, H. 1958. Newsom's Sheep Diseases. 2nd ed. Williams and Wilkins, Baltimore.

NAS. 1968. Nat. Acad. Sci. Pub. No. 1685. Washington, D.C.

382

Panciera, R.J. 1978. In: Effects of Poisonous Plants on Livestock. Academic Press, New York.

Radeleff, R.D. 1970. Veterinary Toxicology. 2nd ed. Lea & Febiger, Philadelphia, Pa.

Schmitz, E.M., B.N. Freeman and R.E. Reed. 1968. Livestock Poisoning Plants of Arizona. Univ. of Ariz. Press, Tucson.

Shupe, J.L., L.F. James and W. Binns. 1967. Amer. Vet. Med. Assoc. 151:191-197; 151:198-203.

Smith, H.A. and T.C. Jones. 1961. Veterinary Pathology. 2nd ed. Lea & Febiger, Philadelphia, Pa.

Sperry, O.E., J.W. Dollahite, G.O. Hoffman and B.J. Comp. Undated. Tex. Agr. Expt. Sta. Bul. B-1028.

Stermitz, F.R., F.A. Norris and M.C. Williams. 1969. J. Amer. Chem. Soc. 91:4599.

Stermitz, F.R. 1978. In: Effects of Poisonous Plants on Livestock. Academic Press, New York.

Stevenson, A.H., L.F. James and J.W. Call. 1972. Cornell Vet. 52:519.

Stoddart, L.A., A.H. Holmgren and C.W. Cook. 1949. Utah Agr. Expt. Sta. Sp. Rpt. No. 2.

Van Kampen, K.R. and L.F. James. 1969a. Amer. J. Vet. Res. 30:1779.

Van Kampen, K.R. and L.F. James. 1969b. Path. Vet. 6:413.

Van Kampen, K.R. and L.F. James. 1971. Path Vet. 8:193.

Williams, M.C., L.F. James and A. Bleak. 1976. J. Range Mgmt. 28:260.

Williams, M.C. and L.F. James. 1978. In: Effects of Poisonous Plants on Livestock. Academic Press, New York.

Chapter 16 - Effect of Environmental Stress on Nutritional Physiology

By David R. Ames

INTRODUCTION

Stress may be defined in terms of many varied physiological and behavioral responses. Undoubtedly, the term, environmental stress, may have different meanings depending on the context of its use and the previous experience of the interpreter. In this chapter environmental stress refers to physical and/or psychological aspects of the animal's surroundings that restrict its ability to achieve maximum performance.

Fortunately, ruminants have the ability to perform (i.e., grow and reproduce) even though they routinely encounter many stressful situations. This ability is documented by the presence of ruminants in both arctic and tropical regions, the ability of ruminants to survive both blizzard and drought, and the successful production of animals on the open range or in closely confined areas. Yet, level of performance during environmental stress is less than maximum.

Environmental stress in ruminants changes nutritional physiology including variation in nutrition requirements, efficiency of nutrient utilization, digestibility of feedstuffs, and other more subtle effects which affect environment-nutrition interaction. For ruminants to more completely realize their full production potential will require a clear understanding of environmental effects on nutritional physiology.

Material included in this chapter will deal with normal, healthy animals exposed to a variety of environmental stresses. Discussions will be directed towards an understanding of the environment and its effects on nutritional physiology. Classical physiological responses dealing with non-nutritional aspects will receive less discussion. Those interested in more detail regarding the effects of environmental stresses on general physiological responses should refer to books by Folk (1966), Hafez (1968) and Esmay (1969).

THERMAL STRESS

Thermal stress is unique among environmental variables affecting ruminants. First, it impinges directly upon homeostatic mechanisms which maintain a constant body core temperature. Second, the energetic efficiency of ruminants is altered by thermal stress in terms of energy retention, digestibility, and nutritional requirements. Third, the thermal environment is highly variable and is a major environmental factor affecting ruminants.

The basic relationship between an animal and the thermal environment begins with the animal's thermal neutral zone (TNZ, see Ch. 8). This zone in ambient temperature, sometimes termed the "comfort zone" for humans, may be defined in several ways for animals (Mount, 1974). This author prefers to define thermal neutrality as the thermal environment in which the animal's health is optimum and growth rate is maximized; this terminology will be used for discussion in this chapter.

Ambient temperatures below the TNZ are termed cold stress and temperatures above the TNZ, heat stress. Critical temperature, which is often used in discussing animal-environment relationships, is defined as the lower limit of the TNZ and is typified by the ambient temperature below which an animal must increase rate of heat production to maintain constant body core temperature. Some writers refer to an upper critical temperature defined as the upper limit of the TNZ and typified by increased rate of evaporative heat loss. Because critical temperature is a point rather than a zone in ambient temperature, it is a commonly used term in the literature to describe animal thermal environment.

It is important to understand that TNZ, critical temperature, cold stress, and heat stress maintain a consistent relationship with each other even though the animal's TNZ may change. In other words, critical temperature always refers to the lower limit of the TNZ, and cold stress is simply defined as ambient temperatures below the critical temperature. The dimension of the TNZ is variable, but Webster (1974) suggests about a 5°C range. Ames et al (1975) have estimated a 10°C range of TNZ for cattle on full feed when thermal neutrality is based on maximum performance.

In assessing the magnitude of thermal stress for animals exposed to thermal extremes, the ambient temperature should be related to the animal's specific thermal neutral temperature. For example, a temperature of 5°C for an animal with a critical temperature of 0°C. The same situation would exist with heat stress. However, it must be emphasized that 10°C cold stress does not necessarily approximate 10°C heat stress in terms of physiological response, performance response, or any other system of evaluating thermal stress.

Thermal neutrality is a description of ambient conditions and should be established in terms of effective ambient temperature. Effective temperature is defined as the cooling or heating power of the environment (i.e., wind, humidity, temperature) described in terms of dry bulb temperature. While dry bulb temperature is of major importance in describing thermal stress, the effect of combinations of dry bulb temperature with wind, humidity, and other climatic factors contributes to total thermal environment. For example, during cold stress wind-chill effect has long been recognized in humans, yet its effect on animals has been more or less overlooked. Ames and Insley (1975) studied the effect of wind-cold combinations on rate of heat loss in cattle and sheep and found that the relationship between cold and wind is not the same as that reported for bare-skinned animals (humans) by the US Weather Bureau; instead it is specific for animals with hair or wool.

Effective temperature during heat stress is mainly a function of the combination of dry bulb temperature and relative humidity, because animals must make maximum use of evaporative heat loss during heat stress. When relative humidity is high, rate of evaporation is lowered, consequently, the detrimental effect of the humidity-temperature combination is more pronounced.

Although TNZ and critical temperature are rather simple concepts, their establishment for specific animals is complicated because of difficulties in establishing accurately the effective temperature from various combinations of dry bulb temperature, wind, humidity, and radiation, and because there are three major animal variables that influence TNZ and critical temperature. These are discussed in subsequent paragraphs.

In general terms insulation is a barrier to heat flow and for animals refers to the rate at which sensible heat is lost or gained from the environment. Insulation in livestock is provided by tissue insulation; external insulation, which is provided by hair or wool; and the insulatory value of the air interface, which is provided by the thin layer of air surrounding the animal. These insulatory barriers are additive in nature with total insulation of major importance in establishing an animal's critical temperature. For example, a lamb with 5 cm of fleece may have a calculated critical temperature of -5°C effective temperature; the same lamb may have an effective critical temperature of 15°C when shorn, because of the decrease in total insulatory value.

The intake of metabolizable energy/unit of metabolic size is linearly related to the rate of heat production (Lofgreen and Garrett, 1968; see Ch. 8). As intake increases, there is a linear increase in rate of heat production, resulting in a lower critical temperature. Hence, animals on high planes of nutrition and consequent high levels of heat production have a lower TNZ compared with similar animals receiving maintenance level of nutrition. Muscular activity, whether it be for the sake of securing food and water or for other reasons, increases the rate of heat production and, therefore, lowers the TNZ and critical temperature.

Factors which determine critical temperature in ruminants work in combination, which leads to wide differences in predicted critical temperatures for ruminants of varying insulation, plane of nutrition and exercise. This does not presume that estimates of critical temperatures are not possible or that they cannot be calculated, but it does explain the variability noted in estimates from different sources. Table 16-1 lists estimated critical temperature for specifically described cattle and sheep. As evident from Table 16-1, a wide variation in critical temperature is given for different insulatory values and planes of nutrition. It must be mentioned that the basis for defining the critical temperature may also be different.

Additional research is needed to allow for more standardized estimates of critical

Table 16-1. Estimates of critical temperatures for cattle and sheep.

Specie	Description	Critical Tempera-ture, °C	Basis	Source
Sheep	· Shorn, maintenance feeding	25	Minimum heat prod.	Ames (1969)
Sheep	Shorn, full feed	15	Maximum performance	Brink & Ames (1975)
Sheep	5mm fleece, maintenance	25	Calculated	Blaxter (1967)
	5mm fleece, fasting	31	,,	,,
	5mm fleece, full feed	18	,,	,,
	1mm fleece, maintenance	28	,,	,,
	10mm fleece, maintenance	22	,,	,,
	50mm fleece, maintenance	9	,,	,,
	100mm fleece, maintenance	-3	,,	,,
Cattle	8 mm hair			
	Fasting	18	,,	,,
	Maintenance	7	,,	,,
	Full feed	-1	,,	,,
Cattle	Full feed	13	Maximum performance cal-culated (where intake and heat loss are independent of temperature)	Ames et al (1975)
Cattle	Calves			
	New born	9	,,	Webster (1974)
	One month old	0	,,	,,
	Fat stock			
	0.8 kg gain/day	-36	,,	,,
	1.5 kg gain/day	-36	,,	,,
	Beef cow maintenance	-21	,,	,,
	Dairy cow			
	Dry, pregnant	-14	,,	,,
	2 gallon/day milk prod.	-24	,,	,,
	8 gallon/day milk prod.	-40	,,	,,

temperature so that ruminants of different descriptions can be appropriately defined in terms of existing effective temperature. A thorough understanding of the relationship of an animal and the thermal environment is necessary before describing effect of thermal environment on nutritional physiology. Too often terms such as hot and cold are impressions of the investigator rather than a description of thermal state of the animal.

HEAT STRESS

Heat stress is defined as ambient effective temperature above the animal's TNZ. Physiologically, heat stress is characterized by increased respiratory rate, peripheral vasodilation, increased evaporative heat loss, and increased basal metabolic heat production

(Armstrong et al, 1960; Blaxter et al, 1959, 1966; Brook and Short, 1960; Ames et al, 1968, 1970, 1971).

Voluntary Feed Intake

From a nutritional viewpoint a reduction in voluntary intake during heat stress is well known. Vohnout and Bateman (1972) reported reduced intake of cattle in environments where chamber temperatures of 36°C daytime and 27°C nighttime were compared to 27°C daytime and 17°C mean night temperatures. Gengler et al (1969) found no difference in feed intake between 18°C and 35°C unless intraruminal temperature was raised by an internal heating coil. When intraruminal temperatures of 43°C and 51°C were combined with ambient temperatures of 18°C, feed intake was significantly reduced.

These authors reported increased water intake at ambient temperatures of 35°C, compared with that of 18°C. Roy et al (1969) found reduced intake of growing cattle when temperature increased from mean values of 18°C to 34°C measured under natural climatic conditions where mean relative humidity ranged from 38 to 75%. Brink (1975) found that voluntary intake in shorn lambs fed in climate chambers was depressed as temperature rose above critical temperature (15°C). Bhattacharya and Hussain (1974) reported that high ambient temperatures coupled with high humidity during the day, reaching a maximum of 32°C and 98%, respectively, reduced ad libitum intake in sheep, with depression most severe when the diets contained high levels of roughage. However, a later report from this laboratory (Bhattacharya and Uwayjan, 1975) showed conflicting results when temperature was coupled with low humidity. The diversity of those findings supports the need to discuss results in terms of effective temperature rather than separating the effects of temperature and humidity during heat stress.

McDowell et al (1976) reported depressed intake by lactating dairy cows during summer. They cautioned that humidity may affect intake as much as temperature, which again lends support to the need for use of effective temperatures during heat stress. They also pointed out the role of fluctuating temperatures during heat stress, stating that under normal conditions low nighttime temperatures may counteract daytime highs. The impact of fluctuating temperatures and the validity of mean daily temperature, when the standard deviation of daily temperature is high, deserve more study. This is particularly important in the design of confinement systems, where constant temperatures may not result in patterns of feed intake similar to those established during fluctuating temperatures developed under natural conditions. Several authors (Olbrich et al, 1973; Moran, 1976) point to differences between breeds or types of cattle and their response to heat stress. In effect, these differences are probably due to differences in thermal neutral temperature and, therefore, do not reflect actual differences in response to a similar magnitude of heat stress. For example, for *Bos indicus* species of cattle, which have the genetic ability to evaporate moisture from the skin's surface more effectively than *Bos taurus* breeds, the effect of 35°C ambient temperature may not be comparable with the same climatic conditions for a British breed of cattle whose capability to evaporate heat from the skin is much lower. In effect, these two individuals have different thermal neutral temperatures and 35°C represents a different magnitude of heat stress in each case.

Effect on Digestibility

Although some of the available information relating ration digestibility to heat stress does not agree, most data tend to support the hypothesis that digestibility is increased during heat stress. In many cases this results from decreased voluntary intake rather than from a direct effect of increased effective ambient temperature. Brink (1975) used shorn lambs fed in controlled environmental chambers to determine the effect of ambient temperature on the digestibility of ration components. This study showed increased digestibility of DM, CP, and NFE as temperature rose from 15°C to 35°C (critical temperature was 13°C). CF digestibility increased when temperature rose from 15°C to 30°C, but was not increased at 35°C. No difference was found in EE digestibility during heat stress. Bhattacharya and Hussain (1974) also reported that during heat stress sheep rations had lower digestibilities except for CF and NFE. They found that higher roughage (75%) rations were most affected. Perhaps variations in findings relating heat stress to ration digestibility are altered by roughage to concentrate ratio. Obviously, more knowledge is needed for different rations.

Effect on Nutrient Requirements

The effect of thermal environment on nutrient requirements is not well documented for ruminants; although information relative to non-ruminants, and for poultry in particular, suggests the need to adjust nutrients to match the environment. Several reports (Graham et al, 1959; Ames, 1969; Whittow and Findlay, 1968) point to increased heat production during heat stress in ruminants. Most attribute increased levels of heat production either to the work of panting and sweating or to the Q_{10} effect associated with elevated body core temperature. Of course, any increase in heat production during heat stress results in increased energy requirement for maintenance (NE_m) as represented in Fig. 16-1).

In growing animals protein requirement is likely reduced during heat stress because of concurrent depression in growth rate, which may be attributed to limited availability of

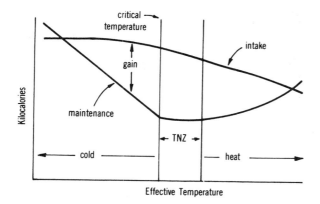

Fig. 16-1. Schematic diagram showing the relationship of intake, energy for maintenance (NE_m), and energy for gain (NE_g) as a function of effective temperature. The descriptive terms, cold, heat, TNZ, and critical temperature (C_t) are also included.

energy for growth. Using calculated estimates of protein requirements, Ames and Willms (1977) have shown that reducing protein for growth in proportion to expected reduction in gain does not reduce growth rate in heat-stressed cattle. Brink (1975) found similar results with lambs fed reduced protein levels during heat stress in environmentally controlled chambers. While temperature alters energy for maintenance, temperature does not alter the protein requirement for maintenance (Brink and Ames, 1977).

Water requirement is increased during heat in response to increased evaporation. Maloiy and Taylor (1971) found that domestic goats and sheep depend on water and require as much as 8% of their body weight daily during heat stress. That does not appear to be the case for feral desert-dwelling ungulates.

Mineral losses during sweating are common in some animals, but there is little information to suggest that sweating by ruminants increases their mineral requirement during heat stress. This might be expected because volume of sweating in ruminants is much less than in other species (i.e., humans, horses), and the secretions are from apocrine glands and are apparently lower in mineral concentrations. With respect to vitamins, Page et al (1959) reported that steers had increased loss of vitamin A when exposed to thermal stress.

It is certain that heat stress in ruminants alters their requirements for energy and protein; however, much must be done to determine the quantitative changes that specify magnitudes of heat stress for those

two nutrients. This topic could be a very productive area of research.

Performance in terms of both average daily gain and milk production is lower during heat stress in both cattle and sheep (Johnson et al, 1962a; Knox and Handley, 1973; Dowell et al, 1976; Brink, 1975). Computer simulations of performance during heat, using intake and energy prediction formulas, also indicate lowered levels of performance with increasing magnitude of heat stress (Butchbaker et al, 1973; Teter, 1973). While these data suggest reduced nutrient retention during heat stress, they are at best an indirect method of determining the effect of heat on nutrient retention. Most likely, lowered nutrient retention is a function of reduced feed intake and increased NE_m which would then alter the calorie:protein ratio (assuming protein for maintenance is not temperature dependent). Retention of protein and energy would in turn be dependent on calorie:protein ratio above maintenance levels. As explained by Knox and Handley (1973), variation in NE_m is critical to the expected growth (nutrient retention) of cattle.

Though little specific work has been done relative to nutrient retention during heat stress, Brink (1975) has found that N retention during heat stress (35°C) is lower than in TNZ. Roy et al (1969) found similar reductions in protein retention and Ames and Brink (1977) reported a lower protein efficiency ratio during thermal stress (Fig. 16-2). The effect of temperature on energy retention of lambs was lower at 35°C as compared to either 23°C (assumed TNZ) or 0°C (Soderquist and Knox, 1967).

Metabolic Effects

Metabolic changes associated with heat stress are complicated with concurrent changes in feed and water intake, increased evaporative water loss, and other adjustments to heat stress. Consequently, it is difficult to attribute changes in rumen activity and blood constituents to heat stress per se. Weldy et al (1964) reported a negative relationship with temperature and hematocrit for cows in heated chambers compared with controls exposed to lower ambient conditions. Findlay (1954) suggested that higher hemoglobin is associated with greater adaptability to heat and that heat stress appears to increase the amount of circulating hemoglobin. Roussel et al (1972) found that serum albumin, β-globulin, α-globulin, and

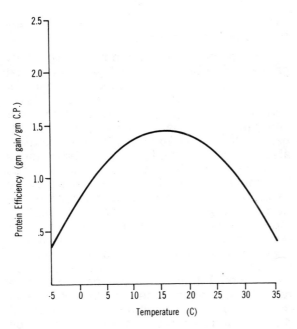

Fig. 16-2. Effect of ambient temperature on protein efficiency ratio of cows when critical temperature is 15°C.

the A:G ratio decreased as seasons progressed from cool to hot. In addition, they found that the commonly recognized milk fat depression during heat stress was positively correlated with serum albumin percentage and A:G ratio and negatively correlated with total serum protein, serum globulin and γ-globulin percentages. Yousef and Johnson (1965) reported that in lactating cows hot temperature (32°C) resulted in lower blood acetate and Mg and an increase in blood P. No effect was noted for blood Na. Weldy et al (1964) concluded that total rumen VFA was lowered in cows subjected to hot environments; likewise, Moody et al (1967) concluded that rumen VFA's were depressed by hot temperatures. Gengler et al (1969), using intraruminal heating coils, also found lower ruminal VFA concentrations at high ambient temperatures, but could not explain these changes by increasing ruminal temperature. Attebery and Johnson (1969) reported depressed rumen activity in terms of amplitude and frequency of rumen contractions during heat (38°C).

Ration Effect

It is well known that plane of nutrition, as well as composition of the diet, can aggravate heat stress. This phenomenon is explained logically by increased metabolic heat production associated with increased consumption and known as heat increment of feeding (HIF). This heat is in addition to heat produced from normal metabolic functions (see Ch. 8). There is, however, another approach to the relationship of ration and heat stress which should be mentioned. When animals exposed to heat consume feed (particularly feedstuffs with higher HIF's) they show signs of aggravated heat stress. That results from a lowered TNZ which obviously increases the magnitude of heat stress. The fed animal, therefore, suffers from heat stress at a lower temperature compared to a fasted animal or one fed at a lower level. Hence, the ration effect on severity of heat stress is logically explained on the basis of a lowered thermal neutral temperature.

A summary of heat increment values for representative roughages, concentrates, and fat (Table 16-2) reveals some interesting values regarding the relative HIF of various feedstuffs. By calculating HIF for maintenance rations and growing rations as noted at the bottom of Table 16-2, it is noted that HIF values for concentrates are higher/kg of feed compared to roughages and that HIF represents a greater percentage of ME value of the feedstuff for roughages compared to concentrates. Typically, roughages are credited with having higher HIF because roughages are normally consumed in greater quantity than concentrates, and HIF represents a larger percentage of ME for roughages compared to concentrates. These facts must be clearly understood when adjusting rations to utilize HIF during thermal stress. Little has been done to explore the value of using animal fat in diets during thermal stress, however, HIF values

Table 16-2. Heat increment of feeding of various feedstuffs.

Feed	Maintenance		Growing ration	
	Kcal/kg[a]	% ME	Kcal/kg[b]	% ME
Corn	1.01	30	1.41	42
Milo	1.14	38	1.42	47
SBM	1.01	32	1.36	44
Oats	1.02	37	1.43	52
Barley	.87	29	1.76	58
Mean	1.01	33.2	1.47	48.6
Alfalfa Hay	.86	40	1.19	56
Straw	.71	40	1.13	64
Native Hay	.74	40	1.14	62
Beet Pulp	1.00	38	1.29	49
Corn Silage	.97	38	1.26	49
Mean	.85	39.2	1.20	56.0
Animal Fat	.09	1.9	1.07	22.9

[a]HIF = ME - NE
[b]HIF = ME - (.5 NE + .5 NE)

Table 16-3. Effect of heat increment level of performance of steers during heat.[a]

Item	Heat increment level		
	High	Medium	Low
Number of steers	18	18	18
Days fed	112	112	112
Initial weight, lb	742	735	728
Daily feed intake, lb	20	21.16	21.61
Daily weight gain, lb	2.99	3.07	3.11
Feed/lb gain, lb	6.91	6.89	6.95

[a] From Lofgreen (1974).

for fat (Table 16-2) are much lower than for other feedstuffs. That would be an advantage during heat and has been reported to improve performance of swine during heat stress (Stahly et al, 1977).

Manipulating rations is a practical solution to minimizing the effect of heat. Lofgreen (1974) confirmed the validity of formulating rations for relief of heat stress by lowering HIF of the ration while keeping the NE constant. These adjustments are accomplished by reducing the roughage content of the rations, adding dried beet pulp, and increasing fat content. Results of trials with steers fed rations adjusted for HIF during heat stress are shown in Table 16-3. Moose et al (1969) found that low concentrate rations (35%) had lower HIF than high concentrate rations (70% concentrate) when fed to lambs. They also found that at temperatures above 23°C, HIF can seriously impair the efficiency of rations containing higher percentages of roughage. Rea and Ross (1961), in trials with growing lambs, concluded that lambs gain more in warm temperatures when given rations of 60% concentrate as compared to 40% concentrate. Stott and Moody (1960) found that low roughage rations fed cows during the summer were superior for milk production although milk fat percentage was depressed. Rainey et al (1967) also noted improved milk production for cows fed higher concentrate to roughage (65-35) rations during the summer. Many authors report that milk fat percentage is lowered when high concentrate rations were fed. That apparently is true when rations are adjusted to higher concentrates during summer.

In conclusion, heat stress depresses voluntary feed intake, particularly diets that are high in fiber. While digestibility may be higher during heat, both average daily gain and milk production are lowered. Nutrient requirements are altered during heat stress. Ration changes designed to reduce HIF have been suggested as a method of partially alleviating heat stress.

COLD STRESS

Effect on Voluntary Intake

While it is widely reported and often observed that voluntary intake is inversely related to ambient temperature, there is little reported evidence relating increased feed intake to decreasing temperature below the critical temperature. Soderquist and Knox (1967) reported that DM intake by lambs was high at 0°C compared to 23°C, and McDowell et al (1976) reported increased feed intake of lactating cows during cold stress. Brink (1975) reported increased DM consumption by lambs, whose critical temperature was 13°C, to be statistically higher at 10, 5 and 0°C, but no further increase was noted at -5°C. Those data show clearly that voluntary intake is increased above thermal neutral values during mild cold, but that a limit in voluntary intake was reached before animals were severely cold stressed. The magnitude of cold stress reached when voluntary intake approaches its maximum probably depends on the type of ration being fed and is a function of whether intake is controlled by physical or chemical mechanisms (see Ch. 11).

Digestibility

Several authors (Blaxter and Waiman, 1961; Young and Christopherson, 1974; Ames and Brink, 1977; Christopherson, 1976) indicate lowered DM digestibility during cold. In the studies mentioned, these findings did not derive results from changes in temperature (where mild vs. severe heat stress data is interpreted as evidence of effects of cold), but were legitimate effects of cold stress. The examples of depressed digestibilities are shown in Table 16-4. Often increased intake is credited with lower DM digestibility during cold, but Ames and Brink (1977) showed that a decrease in DM digestibility was attributed to temperature alone. When increased intake during cold was considered in combination with decreased digestibility (Fig. 16-3), it is evident that advantages of increased intake by ruminants during cold would be partially offset by lower digestibility. For example, increased consumption/unit of metabolic size from 10°C to 0°C was 5.3%, but with decreased digestibility, the net increase in DE was only 2.7%. Christopherson (1976), who conducted

Table 16-4. Effect of cold on dry matter digestibility:

Species	Ration	ΔDig/ΔT	Source
Sheep	Alfalfa pellets	0.27	Young & Christopherson (1974)
Sheep	Grain and alfalfa pellets	0.40	,, ,,
Calves	Grain and chopped alfalfa hay	0.27[a]	,, ,,
Calves	Grain and chopped hay	0.21	Christopherson (1976)
Steers	Grain and chopped hay	0.08	,,
Sheep	Grain and alfalfa pellets	0.14	Ames & Brink (1977)

[a] Mean of two values.

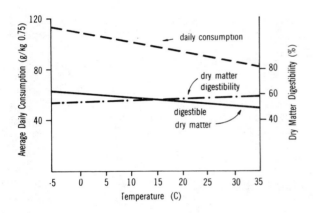

Fig. 16-3. Effect of ambient temperature on daily consumption and dry matter digestibility by ruminants.

extensive studies of digestibility during prolonged cold with both sheep and cattle, also found a temperature effect independent of level of intake. He reported that DM digestibility had a 0.31%, 0.21% and 0.08% decline/degree C cold stress for sheep, calves and steers, respectively. The greater magnitude of effect for smaller animals can be expected since larger surface area/unit of mass in smaller animals increases the effect of each degree of cold stress, but not necessarily per unit of surface area.

Data also indicate lowered N digestibility of ruminants exposed to cold (Graham et al, 1959; Blaxter and Waiman, 1961; Brink, 1975; Christopherson, 1976). Christopherson (1976) found N digestibility lower for calves fed outdoors in Canada. Brink and Ames

(1976) reported lower CP digestibility during cold compared with heat, but no consistent decrease as cold stress became more severe. They also reported increases in both EE and NFE during severe cold (-5°C when critical temperature was 13°C).

Nutrient Requirements

During cold exposure, rate of heat loss above thermal neutral values and, as a consequence, heat production must increase to maintain body temperature. Increased heat production results from shivering, increased plane of nutrition, and acclimation via increased basal metabolic rate controlled by thyroid activity; to some extent non-shivering thermogenesis is also a result of adrenal involvement. Several authors (Blaxter, 1967; Graham et al, 1959; Bennett, 1972) have documented increased heat loss during cold, while others (Brink and Ames, 1975; Knox and Handley, 1973) have measured reduced performance during cold and cited increased requirement for NE_m as the underlying reason for reduced performance.

Although other nutrient requirements (primarily protein) are eventually altered during cold, it is the increased requirement for NE_m that is the basis for these changes. The magnitude of increased NE_m is a function of those variables responsible for rate of sensible heat loss; namely insulation, temperature gradient, and surface area. Figure 16-4 indicates the rate of increased NE_m as a percentage of true maintenance (i.e., 131 Kcal/$W^{0.75}$ or that level of ME intake in which heat production equals ME intake)

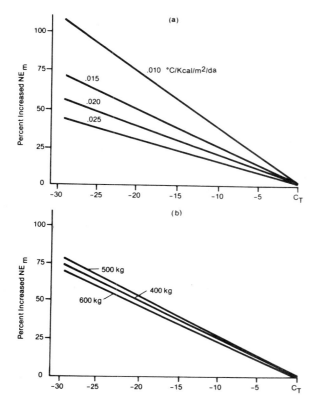

Fig. 16-4. Percentage increase in NE_m for animals of varying insulation (a) and size (b) where x axis is temperature below critical temperature (C_t) in degrees centigrade.

(Lofgreen and Garrett, 1968) for animals of constant size but different insulation and at different magnitudes of cold (Fig. 16-4a) and for animals of constant insulation but of different sizes at different magnitudes of cold (Fig. 16-4b). Table 16-5 lists the expected increase in NE_m per degree C of cold stress for cattle of different sizes and insulations. In both cases magnitude of cold is linearly related to increased NE_m. This is based on the fact that thermal gradient (in this case core temperature and ambient temperature) has a linear relationship with rate of sensible heat flow as described by the relationship: $I = \dfrac{T_1 - T_2}{H_f}$ where I is insulatory value, $T_1 - T_2$ is thermal gradient and H_f is subsequent heat flow. Surface area is a function of body size and is greater/unit of weight for small compared to large animals. Since heat production (maintenance) is a function of $W^{0.75}$ in nonstressed adult animals and surface area, which is related to heat loss, is a function of $W^{0.66}$, energy for maintenance increases at a greater rate/ degree of cold for small than for large animals (Fig. 16-4a). This premise is exemplified by Bergman's Law which indicates that larger animals are more adapted to colder climates and smaller animals (greater surface area/unit of mass) more logically appropriate for warmer climates. Study of

Table 16-5. Increased NE_m during cold for cattle.

Insulation °C/Kcal/m/day	Weight kg	$W^{0.75}$	Surface[a] area, m²	Fasting[b] %Inc/C°	Fed[c] %Inc/C°
.010	200	53.2	2.88	7.03	4.13
.015	,,	,,	,,	4.69	2.76
.020	,,	,,	,,	3.52	2.07
.025	,,	,,	,,	2.81	1.65
.010	300	72.1	3.67	6.61	3.89
.015	,,	,,	,,	4.41	2.59
.020	,,	,,	,,	3.30	1.94
.025	,,	,,	,,	2.64	1.55
.010	400	89.4	4.36	6.33	3.72
.015	,,	,,	,,	4.22	2.48
.020	,,	,,	,,	3.17	1.86
.025	,,	,,	,,	2.53	1.49
.010	500	105.7	4.99	6.13	3.60
.015	,,	,,	,,	4.09	2.40
.020	,,	,,	,,	3.07	1.80
.025	,,	,,	,,	2.45	1.44
.010	600	121.2	5.57	5.97	3.51
.015	,,	,,	,,	3.98	2.34
.020	,,	,,	,,	2.98	1.75
.025	,,	,,	,,	2.39	1.40

[a]$A = .120 W^{.600}$; [b]Use $NE_m = 77$ Kcal/wt$^{0.75}$; [c]Use $NE_m = 131$ Kcal/wt$^{0.75}$

Table 16-5 suggests that maintenance requirements for energy during cold should be appropriately adjusted according to size, insulation, and magnitude of cold to assure a more accurate determination of the maintenance energy requirement.

Protein requirement for the growing animal during cold is logically altered because of the relationship of energy and protein above maintenance levels. It is generally accepted that the protein:calorie ratio above maintenance levels should remain constant for animals of similar composition. As mentioned previously, cold increases NE_m requirements and, consequently, restricts available NE_g. Therefore, to maintain constant calorie:protein ratio, protein above maintenance level must be reduced.

When protein is available in excess, it is probably used only as an energy source (Albanese, 1959). This view is supported by lowered protein efficiency ratio during cold as reported by Ames and Brink (1977; Fig. 16-2) and during heat Willms (1977). Trials with cattle during cold (Ames, 1976) have shown that performance is not lowered when protein is reduced in proportion to the decline in expected gain, which suggests lowered protein requirements during cold, resulting from reduced NE_g and not from changes in protein maintenance. Preston (1966) has reported protein for maintenance values for cattle and sheep to be 2.79 g/$W^{0.75}$ Work by Brink and Ames (1977) would indicate that thermal state does not alter protein for maintenance in sheep. It has been shown that exposing cattle and sheep to severe cold does not increase protein catabolism (Graham et al, 1959).

There appears to be no evidence supporting change in mineral or vitamin requirements during cold. Most studies suggest decreased water intake.

There is limited information relating energy and protein retention in non-ruminants to ambient temperature, and there are very few reports of similar information for ruminants. In most cases nutrient retention must be inferred from performance data, which are more plentiful (Knox and Handley, 1973; Christison and Milligan, 1974; Ames et al, 1975). Graham et al (1959) measured energy retention of sheep exposed to different temperatures and found that at a medium level of feeding, lambs stored 2000 Kcal/day at thermal neutrality (33°C), but lost 150 Kcal/day during cold (8°C). Ames and Brink (1977) measured N retention during cold and found significantly lower values compared to thermal neutrality. They also noted reduced protein efficiency ratio during cold.

Metabolic Changes

Most newborn mammals have quantities of brown adipose tissue which is responsive to norepinephrine, allows for nonshivering thermogenesis, and is considered necessary for survival during cold exposure (Alexander and Williams, 1968). In lambs this tissue disappears at a relatively young age (Jenkinson and Thompson, 1968); it is apparently active only when newborn lambs are exposed to cold. Histological examination of adipose tissue from newborn calves has revealed no brown fat.

Cold exposure has been shown to increase blood glucose levels in both cattle (Olsen and Trenkle, 1973; Young, 1975) and sheep (Basset and Alexander, 1971; Halliday et al, 1969). In sheep this increase in plasma glucose concentration is thought to contribute to increased metabolism, particularly in animals chronically exposed to cold (McKay et al, 1974). Halliday et al (1969) reported that glucose levels in sheep increased initially, but fell toward the end of acute exposure, suggesting that they used relatively less carbohydrate and more fat for energy during cold. This is supported by Blaxter (1967), who noted increased catabolism of fat during cold exposure with no appreciable increase in either carbohydrate or protein catabolism.

Increased blood levels of free fatty acids are commonly observed in cold-stressed ruminants. Slee and Halliday (1968) exposed sheep to severe cold (60°C below the critical temperature) and noted free fatty acid concentrations at 200 microequiv./l. However, mild cold exposure (3-8°C below the critical temperature) and moderate exposure (25°C below the critical temperature) did not change free fatty acid levels, compared with thermal neutrality. Slee and Halliday (1968) concluded that large increases in free fatty acid level were a normal response to acute cold exposure, noting that animals failing to increase free fatty levels during cold showed poor resistance to cold. Panaretto (1968) underfed four very fat ewes for a month and then exposed them to 3°C. In this experiment three of the four ewes died, but prior to death, urinary losses of K were great. In ewes that were not underfed, however, Sykes et al (1969) found that exposing them to 8°C caused a reduction in plasma Mg, but had no effect on their blood Ca, Na or K. Panaretto

(1968) also found that, with respect to N compounds, undernourished ewes showed marked protein catabolism for 24 to 28 hr before death; urinary N and creatinine excretion were high. Others (Halliday et al, 1969; Roussel et al, 1972) have reported increased circulating levels of serum proteins while Blaxter (1967) observed no increase in protein catabolism during cold. The crux of this seemingly contradictory data probably stems from two major variables among experiments; namely, level of feed intake and severity of cold exposure. It is conceivable that only in situations where the combination of cold and intake is such that energy intake is inadequate to meet maintenance needs and fat catabolism does not meet excessive demands for energy then protein is catabolized. While this is logical, it should receive further study.

One factor that may affect concentration of blood constituents during cold is hemoconcentration. Young (1975) reported increased hematocrit in cold exposed cattle, while data reported by Bailey (1964) and Mears and Groves (1969) indicated increased Mg and P after cold exposure. As noted previously, Sykes et al (1969) indicated that increase in K was thought to be due to hemoconcentration during cold.

Ration Effect

An animal's nutritional requirements change noticeably during cold, especially energy. Several authors have suggested increased maintenance needs for energy during cold; however, few have offered any system for matching rations to the thermal environment. One possibility which may have virtue is the use of feedstuffs of relatively high HIF values during cold. Often one hears suggestions on the HIF value of roughage vs. concentrate feeds, implying added value of roughage feeds during cold. The fact that HIF is a much higher percentage of ME in roughages compared to concentrates (Table 16-2) is important when it is considered that calories from HIF of a roughage may be less expensive than those from a concentrate source. Consequently, from an economical standpoint, energy costs could be reduced during cold by increasing roughages and decreasing concentrates in rations. Moose et al (1969) has reported that feeds with high HIF during cold have a sparing effect on net energy for production, thus allowing their use for gain. Various models have been developed to blend rations of different HIF's to improve

performance during cold stress. These models predict economic advantages for altering rations during cold.

In conclusion, cold stress is typified by increased voluntary intake and requirement for maintenance energy. Lower ration digestibility is widely reported during cold stress. Blood levels of free fatty acids and glucose are elevated during cold; however, acclimation to cold exposure is readily noted in most blood measurements. Performance is lowered during cold stress because of limited NE$_g$ resulting in reduced protein efficiency ratio. Adjusting diets during cold is suggested as a practical method of more efficiently utilizing available feedstuffs.

HUMIDITY

During heat stress ruminants must rely on evaporative heat loss to maintain constant body temperatures. Consequently, high humidity in combination with heat (high effective temperature) produce animal responses commensurate with those noted during heat stress. Johnson et al (1962b) reported decreased milk production of cattle exposed to elevated relative humidity when dry bulb temperatures are above 65°F (Fig. 16-5). They also report a positive relationship between temperature-humidity index (THI) and depression in milk production (Note: THI = 0.55 dry bulb + 0.2 dew point + 17.5) with higher producing cows most affected. Cargill and Stewart (1966) found that milk production declines when THI value exceeds 75. Klett and Schilling (1969) reported reduced feedlot performance of cattle exposed to higher humidity. Johnson et al (1963) reported lowered feed intake as humidity rose when temperature was above 80°F.

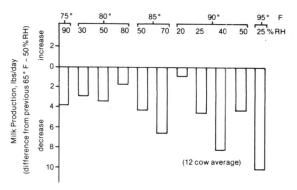

Fig. 16-5. Average difference in milk production of 12 cows from previous 65°F, 50% R.H. level. From Johnson et al (1962).

Table 16-6. Rate of gain and feed conversion for beef animals in tests with artificial rainfall.[a]

		No rain	Rain
1969	Gain, lb/day	3.13	2.67
	Lb feed/lb gain	7.00	8.44
1970	Gain	3.02	2.85
	Feed/gain	6.27	6.61

[a] From Morrison et al (1970).

They found an inverse relationship between TDN consumption and THI.

Relative humidity during cold stress is of minor importance until it reaches 100% which occurs during rain or when ambient temperature falls below the dew point. These occurrences have a major impact on external insulation usually resulting in elevated critical temperature and consequently increasing magnitude of cold stress. Stokes (unpublished data) found near total destruction of the insulatory value of cattle hair when wetted and Morrison et al (1970) reported reduced performance of feedlot cattle when artificial rain was provided (Table 16-6). These workers point out that, while it is probable that prolonged rain will reduce performance, some of the observed effects may be attributed to muddy lot conditions.

SOUND STRESS

Studies are limited which specifically describe the influence of the audio environment on ruminants. However, substantial data exist for other animals (Welch and Welch, 1970), suggesting a number of physiological responses to sound which may alter the nutritional physiology of the ruminant. Most discussions relating sound and ruminants deal with the effect of the sonic boom on growth and efficiency of feedlot animals and with milk production of the dairy cow. In all instances (Casaday and Lehmann, 1967; Bond et al, 1963; and Parker and Bayley, 1960) there was no long term effect of sonic booms on performance of farm animals with acclimation evident within one week. More recent work (Arehart and Ames, 1972) indicates lamb performance can be altered by both type and intensity of sound. Harbers et al (1975) reported lower dry matter intake by lambs exposed to high sound levels (75 and 100 dB compared to 45

dB). They also reported increased water intake and urinary output for lambs that were subjected to intermittent noise as compared to continuous sound. Arehart and Ames (1972) noted no difference in intake of lambs exposed to different intensities of continuous music, but did report an increase in DM intake with intermittent noise of 75 and 100 dB intensity as compared with 45 dB.

Harbers et al (1975) reported higher digestibility coefficients for sheep exposed to intermittent sound compared with continuous sound. CF digestibility was lower for lambs subjected to continuous music, but sound intensity did not affect digestibility. They found that when N intake was held constant, no differences were evident in fecal and absorbed N values suggesting that N metabolism is not influenced by auditory stimuli. Rumen motility was not affected by either sound level or sound type although individual variation was evident (Harbers et al, 1975). Arehart (1970) measured oxygen consumption of lambs exposed to various sound intensities and noted variable values with no consistent effect of audio environment.

MISCELLANEOUS FACTORS

There are reports suggesting that light may alter the nutritional physiology of ruminants. Murrill et al (1969) studied effect of corral lighting on milk production and feed intake of Holstein cows and concluded that light has little, if any, value during summer and limited value during longer periods of darkness during winter. Feed intake of beef steers was not improved by feedlot lighting (Boren et al, 1965) and weight gain of lambs is apparently not influenced by light (Hoersch et al, 1961). Feeding behavior is affected by presence of light with darkness resulting in less grazing and more rumination (Gordon, 1964; see Vol. 1).

Effect of ionizing radiation on livestock has been reviewed by Byrne and Bell (1973). These authors suggest that loss of appetite and consequent reduction in performance could result from whole body γ irradiation or ingestion of feedstuffs contaminated with β radiation. Damaged digestive tracts of irradiated animals would probably alter normal digestive activity.

Although ammonia appears to depress feed intake in the pig and possibly requirement for protein in chicks, information is not available relating ammonia level to reduced protein requirement in ruminants. Drummond et al (1976) found that air containing 75 ppm ammonia reduced intake of lambs and increased feed required/lb of gain. Knowlton et al (1969) have reported decreased DM intake and digestibility by sheep exposed to air environments containing up to 18% CO_2. DM intake was not altered at 4% CO_2 compared to controls, but was lower at 8, 12, 16 and 18%. Nutrient digestibility decreased in 16 and 18% CO_2 environments.

Smith (1972) has predicted that gravity adds approximately 25% to the energy requirement of the chicken. For larger animals Kleiber (1969) has estimated the energy requirement is gravity dependent. While this may be of little practical concern, it appears that gravity increases energy requirement for maintenance from 25 to 40%, depending on animal size.

SOCIAL OR PSYCHOLOGICAL STRESSES

Information relating social and psychological stress to nutritional consequences is minimal. In response to traditional stress, some animals may increase metabolic heat production, serum free fatty acids, blood glucose, and other nutritionally related measurements, but the effect of psychological stress on intake, digestibility, rumen function, and nutritional requirements is not well known. Eating behavior of cattle of varying social rank has been observed by Schake and Pickle (1971), who reported that submissive heifers utilized the least time consuming a liquid supplement and grain ration. The authors report that the consequence of that behavior could be dramatic, because heifers in most apparent need of feed were the least successful in attaining feed. Heifers in the submissive group had less finish and lighter weights than those in the dominant social rank. Social rank apparently did affect water intake, but salting time was inversely related to time used to consume feed. Overfield et al (1976), who studied "stressed" feeder cattle, reported improved performance when natural protein (SBM) was fed compared to urea based supplements. They also suggest some value of B-complex vitamins for stressed calves.

One factor involved with both intake and requirement for food is exercise or its absence. In a practical sense many writers have suggested reduced NE_m for confined animals compared to those raised under range conditions. This observation is substantiated by Blaxter (1967) who suggests 10% increase in fasting maintenance energy requirement for sheep and 15% for cattle. He quickly points out that wide differences may exist because of terrain, distance traveled and other factors. Schake and Riggs (1969) report that confined cows walk approximately 1/10 the distance recorded for range cows. Larsen (1963) reported information showing the effect of social dominance on distance traveled to obtain food (Fig. 16-6). He indicated that animals low in the social order would be forced to travel farther to obtain food to avoid being molested by more dominant animals. This would increase maintenance requirement and reduce efficiency of production.

EFFECT OF ENVIRONMENTAL MODIFICATIONS

Because of the depressing effect of stressful environments on animal performance and efficiency, various procedures are used to modify existing conditions to enhance animal production. While most of these modifications such as sprinkling, windbreaks, shades, etc., simply create a new effective environment, results are usually not reported in this manner. There is considerable interest in environmental modification ranging from simple construction of windbreaks to complete environmental control. The effect of various environmental modifications on nutritional physiology is usually measured in terms of performance differences.

Shades will reduce the incidence of solar radiation as much as 30%. Responses of cattle to shades are variable when measured in terms of feed intake, average daily gain or milk yield depending on location. Studies in southern California, Arizona, Florida and Louisiana have indicated improved performance with shade, but reports from midwestern states (Henderson and Gleaser, 1968) show no advantage from use of shades. Bond and Laster (1974) subjectively established threshold values that indicate need for summer shades as: mean maximum air temperature above 32°C, mean minimum air temperature above 21°C, or mean daytime radiant heat load above 700 Kcal/m²/hr. Garrett (1963) suggested a positive value of shades at locations with more than 500 hr with air temperature above 29.5°C. Pontif et al (1974) found that shade increased feed consumption and daily gain in Louisiana, and Roman-Ponce et al (1977) measured a

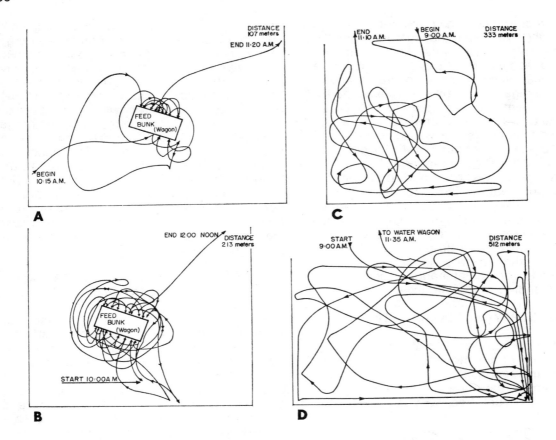

Fig. 16-6. A,B, feeding pattern of cows at a bunk. In A the cow occupies high position in dominance order while in B it is a high-producing small cow with a low position in the dominance order. She takes every opportunity afforded her to eat. C, dominant cow able to graze unmolested. D, grazing behavior of a cow at the low end of the dominance order. Note the wandering pattern of grazing while she is searching for a spot to graze unmolested. From Larsen (1963).

10.7% increase in milk yield of cows provided with shade in Florida. Bond and Laster (1974) observed that animals without shade spent more time eating and less time resting, but found no difference in feed intake of feedlot cattle in Nebraska.

Forced air movement, which enhances rate of evaporation, has been successfully used in southern California (Bond et al, 1967) to improve performance and in Louisiana it increased feed intake and gain for cattle (Pontif et al, 1974). These authors also note that use of shades and fans in combination is superior to either shades or fans alone.

Increased evaporative heat loss using sprinklers to alleviate heat stress has been successful when response is measured in daily gain (Kelly et al, 1955) and milk yield (Seath and Miller, 1948). Morrison et al (1973) reported increased feed intake and gain for cattle sprinkled for 1 min. every 30 min. when ambient temperature was above 27°C in southern California. These workers found sprinkling to be as beneficial as a refrigerated barn maintained at 24°C. Arizona workers reported improved micro-climates for feedlot cattle using sprinklers in combination with shade, but they found no change in feed intake or performance measurements (Wiersma et al, 1972). They point out that while use of sprinklers or foggers is aimed at increasing evaporative heat loss, they also increase relative humidity which lowers rate of evaporation.

Evaporative cooling systems have been extensively studied (Brown et al, 1973). These studies show that feed intake is increased in cooled dairy cows in Mississippi, but that milk yield and milk fat % is not consistently improved.

Webster (1970) suggested a 4% reduction in energy costs for cattle protected from the wind in Canada. Bond and Laster (1973) tested the influence of windbreaks on feedlot cattle in Nebraska during the winter and found no difference in daily gain for cattle provided with windbreaks compared to cattle in open lots. They did observe lowered feed intake in cattle with wind protection. Activity observations indicated that windbreaks located 200 ft from the bunk area resulted in cattle spending less time feeding.

References Cited

Albanese, A.A. 1959. Protein and Amino Acid Nutrition. Academic Press.

Alexander, G. and D. Williams. 1968. J. Physiol. 198:251.

Ames, D.R. 1969. Ph.D. Thesis, Michigan State Univ., East Lansing.

Ames, D.R. 1976. J. Animal Sci. 42:1342 (abstr).

Ames, D.R. and D.R. Brink. 1977. J. Animal Sci. 44:136.

Ames, D.R. and D.R. Brink and R.R. Schalles. 1975. J. Animal Sci. 41:262,264 (abstr).

Ames, D.R. and L.W. Insley. 1975. J. Animal Sci. 40:161.

Ames, D.R., J.E. Nellor and T. Adams. 1968. J. Animal Sci. 27:1784 (abstr).

Ames, D.R., J.E. Nellor and T. Adams. 1970. J. Animal Sci. 31:80.

Ames, D.R., J.E. Nellor and T. Adams. 1971. J. Animal Sci. 32:784.

Ames, D.R. and C.L. Willms. 1977. 69th Annual Meeting Amer. Soc. Animal Sci., p 52 (abstr).

Arehart, L.A. 1970. M.S. Thesis, Kansas State Univ., Manhattan.

Arehart, L.A. and D.R. Ames. 1972. J. Animal Sci. 34:994.

Armstrong, D.G. et al. 1960. J. Agr. Sci. 55:395.

Attebery, J.T. and H.D. Johnson. 1969. J. Animal Sci. 29:734.

Bailey, D.B. 1964. Can. J. Animal Sci. 44:68.

Bassett, J.M. and G. Alexander. 1971. Biology of the Neonate 17:112.

Bennett, J.W. 1972. Aust. J. Agr. Res. 23:1045.

Bhattacharya, A.N. and F. Hussain. 1974. J. Animal Sci. 38:877.

Bhattacharya, A.N. and M. Uwayjan. 1975. J. Animal Sci. 40:320.

Blaxter, K.L. 1967. Energy Metabolism of Ruminants. 2nd ed. Hutchinson and Co. Pub.

Blaxter, K.L., N.M. Graham, F.W. Wainman and D.G. Armstrong. 1959. J. Agr. Sci. 52:25.

Blaxter, K.L., N.M. Graham and F.W. Wainman. 1966. Brit. J. Nutr. 20:283.

Blaxter, K.L. and F.W. Wainman. 1961. J. Agr. Sci. 56:81.

Bond, T.E., C.F. Kelley and N.R. Ittner. 1967. Agricultural Engineering, p 208.

Bond, T.E. and D.B. Laster. 1973. Amer. Soc. Agr. Eng. Paper No. 73-425.

Bond, T.E. and D.B. Laster. 1974. Amer. Soc. Agr. Eng. Paper No. 74-4536.

Bond, J., C.F. Winchester, L.E. Campbell and J.C. Webib. 1963. USDA Tech. Bul. No. 1280.

Boren, F.W., R. Lipper, E.F. Smith and D. Richardson. 1965. Kan. Agr. Expt. Sta. Bul. 483.

Brink, D.R. 1975. M.S. Thesis, Kansas State Univ., Manhattan.

Brink, D.R. and D.R. Ames. 1975. J. Animal Sci. 41:264.

Brink, D.R. and D.R. Ames. 1976. Sheep Day Report of Progress 263. Kan. Agr. Expt. Sta., p 22.

Brink, D.R. and D.R. Ames. 1977. 69th Annual Meeting Amer. Soc. Animal Sci., p 223.

Brook, A.H. and B.F. Short. 1960. J. Agr. Res. 11:557.

Brown, W.H., J.W. Fuquay, W.H. McGee and S.S. Iyengar. 1973. Amer. Soc. Agr. Eng. Paper No. 73-404.

Butchbaker, A.F., M.D. Paine and R. Shirley. 1973. Amer. Soc. Agr. Eng. Paper No. 73:424.

Byrne, W.F. and M.C. Bell. 1973. Biomedical and Environmental Research of U.S.A.E.C., Extension Service of U.S.D.A. and Defense Civil Preparedness Agency. RCD-3. April, 1973.

Cargill, B.F. and R.E. Stewart. 1966. Trans. Agr. Eng. 9:749.

Casady, R.B. and R.P. Lehmann. 1967. National Sonic Boom Evaluation Office Report NS BE-1-67.

Cristison, G.I. and J.D. Milligan. 1974. In: Energy Metabolism of Farm Animals. Univ. Hohenheim, Stuttgart, p 39.

Christopherson, R.J. 1976. Can. J. Animal Sci. 56:201.

Drummond, J.G., S.E. Curtis, J.M. Lewis and F.C. Hinds. 1976. Sheep Res. 1976. Univ. of Illinois, p 143.

Esmay, M.L. 1969. Principles of Animal Environment. AVI Publishing Co.

Findlay, J.D. 1954. Meteric. Mono. 2:19.

Folk, G.E. 1966. Introduction to Environmental Physiology. Lea and Febiger.

Garrett, W.N. 1963. Amer. Soc. Animal Sci. Symposium Paper.

Gengler, W.R. et al. 1969. J. Dairy Sci. 53:434.

398

Gordon, F.G. 1964. Nature 204:798.

Graham, N.M., F.W. Wainman, K.L. Blaxter and D.G. Armstrong. 1959. J. Agr. Sci. 52:13.

Hafez, R., A.R. Sykes and J. Slee. 1969. Animal Prod. 11:479.

Harbers, L.H., D.R. Ames, A.B. Davis and M.B. Ahmed. 1975. J. Animal Sci. 41:654.

Henderson, H.E. and M.R. Geasler. 1968. Amer. Soc. Animal Sci. Invited paper presented
   Nov. 29, 1968 Chicago, Ill. Review Paper AH-BC-48. Michigan Agr. Expt. Sta.

Hoersch, T.M., E.P. Reineke and H.A. Henneman. 1961. J. Animal Sci. 20:358.

Jenkinson, D. and G.E. Thompson. 1968. J. Physiol. 198:88.

Johnson, H.D., A.C. Ragsdale, I.L. Berry and M.D. Shanklin. 1962b. Mo. Agric. Res. Bul. 791.

Johnson, H.D., A.C. Ragsdale, I.L. Berry and M.D. Shanklin. 1963. Mo. Agric. Res. Bul. 846.

Johnson, J.C., B.L. Southwell, R.L. Givens and R.E. McDowell. 1962a. J. Dairy Sci. 45:695
   (abstr).

Kelley, C.F., T.E. Bond and N.R. Ittner. 1955. Agr. Eng. 36:173.

Kleiber, M. 1969. In: Energy Metabolism of Farm Animals. Oriel Press.

Klett, R.H. and P.E. Schilling. 1969. J. Animal Sci. 28:147 (abstr).

Knowlton, P.H., W.H. Hoover and B.P. Poulton. 1969. J Animal Sci. 28:554.

Knox, K.L. and T.M. Handley. 1973. J. Animal Sci. 37:190.

Larsen, H.J. 1963. J. Animal Sci. 22:1134 (abstr).

Lofgreen, G.P. 1974. 13th Calif. Feed. Day, p 81.

Lofgreen, G.P. and W.N. Garrett. 1968. J. Animal Sci. 27:793.

Maloiy, G.M.O. and C.R. Taylor. 1971. J. Agr. Sci. 77:203.

McDowell, R.E., N.W. Hoover and J.K. Camoens. 1976. J. Dairy Sci. 59:965.

McKay, D.G., B.A. Young and L.P. Milligan. 1974. In: Energy Metabolism of Farm Animals.
   Univ. Hohenheim, Stuttgart, p 39.

Mears. G.J. and T.D. Groves. 1969. Can. J. Animal Sci. 49:389.

Moody, E.G., P.J. Van Soest, R.E. McDowell and G.L. Ford. 1967. J. Dairy Sci. 50:1909.

Moose, M.G., C.V. Ross and W.H. Pfander. 1969. J. Animal Sci. 29:619.

Moran, J.B. 1976. J. Agr. Sci. 86:131.

Morrison, S.R., R.L. Givens, W.N. Garrett and T.E. Bond. 1970. Calif. Agric. 24:6.

Morrison, S.R., R.L. Givens and G.P. Lofgreen. 1973. J. Animal Sci. 36:428.

Mount, L.E. 1974. In: Heat Loss from Animals and Man. Butterworths.

Murrill, F.D., R.N. Erde, R.O. Leonard and D.L. Bath. 1969. Amer. Dairy Sci. Assoc. June 22-25.

Obrich, S.E., F.A. Martz and E.S. Hilderbrand. 1973. J. Animal Sci. 37:574.

Olsen, J.D. and A. Trenkle. 1973. Amer. J. Vet. Res. 34:747.

Overfield, F.R., D.L. Hixon and E.E. Hatfield. 1976. Beef Cattle Day. Univ. of Illinois AS 6721.

Page, H.M., E.S. Erwin and G.E. Nelms. 1959. Amer. J. Physiol. 196:917.

Panaretto, B.A. 1968. Aust. J. Agr. Res. 19:273.

Parker, J.B. and N.D. Bayley. 1960. USDA, ARS 44-60:22.

Pontif, J.E., W.A. Nipper, A.F. Loyacano and H.J. Braud. 1974. Livestock Environment. Amer.
   Soc. Agr. Eng., p 305.

Preston, R.L. 1966. J. Nutr. 90:157.

Rainey, J., J.E. Johnston and J.B. Trye. 1967. J. Dairy Sci. 50:966. (abstr).

Rea, J.E. and C.V. Ross. 1961. J. Animal Sci. 20:949 (abstr).

Roman-Ponce, H. et al. 1977. J. Dairy Sci. 60:424.

Roussel, J.D., K.L. Koonce and M.A. Pinero. 1972. J. Dairy Sci. 55:1093.

Roy, C.R., M.V.N. Rao and D.P. Sadhu. 1969. Indian J. Dairy Sci. 22:248.

Schake, L.M. and R.E. Pickle. 1971. Beef Cattle Res. in Texas, p 28.

Schake, L.M. and J.K. Riggs. 1969. J. Animal Sci. 28:568.

Seath, D.M. and G.D. Miller. 1948. J. Dairy Sci. 31:5.

Slee, J. and R. Halliday. 1968. Animal Prod. 10:67.

Smith, A.H. 1972. J. Animal Sci. 35:635.

Soderquist, H.G. and K.L. Knox. 1967. J. Animal Sci. 26:930.

Stahly, T.S., G.L. Cromwell and D.D. Kratzer. 1977. 69th Annual Meeting Amer. Soc. Animal
   Sci., p 108 (abstr).

Stott, G.H. and E.G. Moody. 1960. J. Dairy Sci. 43:871 (abstr).

Sykes, A.R., A.C. Field and J. Slee. 1969. Animal Prod. 11:91.

Teter, N.C., J.A. DeShazer and T.L. Thompson. 1973. Trans. of Amer. Soc. Agr. Eng. 16:740.

Vohnout, K. and J.V. Bateman. 1972. J. Agr. Sci. 78:413.

Webster, A.J.F. 1974. In: Heat Loss From Animals and Man. Butterworths.

Webster, A.J.F., J. Chumecky and B.A. Young. 1970. Can. J. Animal Sci. 50:89.

Weldy, J.R., R.E. McDowell, P.J. Van Soest and J. Bond. 1964. J. Animal Sci. 23:147.

Whittow, G.C. and J.D. Findlay. 1968. Amer. J. Physiol. 214:94.

Wiersma, F., D. Ray and C. Roubicek. 1972. Amer. Soc. Agr. Eng. Paper No. 72-424.

Willms, C.L. 1977. M.S. Thesis, Kansas State Univ., Manhattan.

Young, B.A. 1975. Can. J. Physiol. Pharm. 53:947.

Young, B.A. and R.J.Christopherson. 1974. International Livestock Environment Symposium. Amer. Soc. Agr. Eng., p 75.

Yousef, M.K. and H.D. Johnson. 1965. J. Dairy Sci. 48:1974.

Chapter 17 - Effect of Miscellaneous Stresses on Nutrition

STARVATION

Starvation, as defined by Webster's New World Dictionary, means to die from lack of food or to suffer or become weak from hunger. Fasting generally implies a complete lack of food and in human terminology it is usually used to mean a voluntary deprivation of food. In the discussions on this subject that follow, the second definition of starving will be used as a general description of the situation for animals—a condition varying from a submaintenance diet to complete fasting.

Many wild ruminant species are periodically subjected to periods of inadequate nutrient consumption, ranging from a condition of semistarvation to complete fasting for time intervals ranging from a few hours to several days. Domestic ruminants, particularly range animals, may also be subjected to starvation during heavy snowfalls or during extreme droughts and very young animals may be subjected to severely restricted food consumption, if their dam gives an inadequate amount of milk.

Starvation often occurs concurrently with various environmental stresses such as heat or cold stress, drought and water deprivation, heavy snowfalls or other severe weather disturbances, during transit on vehicles, as a result of anorexia related to nutritional deficiencies, diseases of various types, parasitism, following surgery or other treatments and so forth. Thus, these other stresses may compound the effects of starvation and result in severe problems for the affected animals.

It is obvious that submaintenance diets will result in loss of body weight, reduced production, adverse effects on reproduction, etc. The severity will depend on the duration and degree of undernutrition as well as complications resulting from other stresses. A good illustration of this is shown in data reported by Panaretto (1968) in an experiment in which ewes were underfed for a month and then subjected to temperatures of 21 or 3°C. Those at 21° survived in good shape, but 3 of 4 ewes died when subjected to 3° temperatures.

Effect on the Rumen

When ruminants are deprived of food, the numbers of rumen microorganisms decline very rapidly. Quin et al (1951) showed this indirectly by measuring gas production from glucose in vitro. Inoculum obtained from sheep showed less gas production as starvation was prolonged. In addition to a decline in glucose or cellulose digestion, Nesic (1961) reported that protozoa disappeared completely from the rumen fluid of sheep starved for 3-4 days. Warner (1962) observed that *Entodenia* protozoa species were lost in sheep starved four days. *Oscillospira* spp of bacteria also disappeared and total bacteria counts declined to less than half of the prestarvation counts. Long term studies (27 days) have demonstrated that both bacteria and protozoal species decreased in fasted sheep (Hershberger and Cowan, 1972). In studies with game species, Pearson (1969) noted that no protozoa species were found in antelope which died around haystacks of alfalfa. In studies with confined white-tailed deer which were fasted, Hershberger and Cowan (1972) noted a decrease in protozoal numbers. De Calesta et al (1974) have studied the effect of starvation on rumen bacteria in mule deer. Data (Table 17-1) show that total counts declined drastically along with rumen volume in starved deer. The decline in numbers of rumen bacteria was affected by time as well as access to feces, but in vitro digestion of alfalfa was not markedly different, perhaps because the fermentations were carried on for 48 hr.

Robertson and Thin (1953) as well as Brown and Shaw (1957) found that starvation of lactating cows for 5 days resulted in a sharp drop in rumen VFA levels. Fowle and Church (1973), when working with goats, found that total VFA levels dropped from a concentration of ca. 115 μM/ml after 2 days of starvation (see Fig. 17-1). Starvation for several days did not depress total VFA any further; acetic and butyric acids were most affected but there was little effect on concentrations of valeric, isovaleric or isobutyric acids. Several other papers show the depressing effect of starvation on rumen VFA (Zelenak et al, 1972; Sasaki et al, 1974;

Table 17-1. Bacterial counts, rumen volume, rumen pH and in vitro dry matter digestion in starved mule deer.[a]

Treatment	Days starved	Bacterial culture counts[b] (x 10^8)		Rumen volume, ml	Rumen pH	In vitro DMD of alfalfa, %
		per ml	total			
1[c]	0	34.6 ± 7	2067 ± 404	5980 ± 237	6.1	66
2[c]	20-29	37.4 ± 40	535 ± 501	1605 ± 431	7.1	64
3[c]	16-22	2.9 ± 0.9	28 ± 21	1251 ± 915	7.2	69
4[c]	31-47	0.9	36	1936 ± 1535	7.2	58

[a]From DeCalesta et al (1974)
[b]Based on bacteria which grew in an agar medium roll tubes.
[c]1, control; 2, access to water, soil and feces; 3, access to water and sterilized soil; 4, access to water.

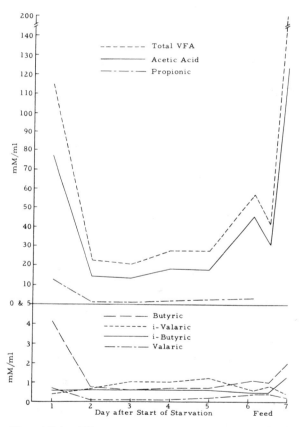

Fig. 17-1. Effect of starvation on rumen VFA production of goats. Note the marked decline by day 2 in concentration of total acids and of acetic and butyric acids. From Fowle and Church (1973).

Munchow et al, 1976; and Hashizume et al, 1976). Munchow et al found that there was a continuous increase in molar proportions of acetic, isobutyric and isovaleric acids and Hashizume et al reported an increase in molar proportion of acetic and n-valeric acids. In wild species, Dean et al (1975) and Hershberger et al (1972) noted decreased total VFA.

Numerous other changes have been observed to occur in the rumen. Starvation results in an increase in rumen pH to values on the order of 7.5-8 by 5-7 days. Total N, urea, amino acids and ammonia decrease rapidly. Methane production decreases very rapidly during the first 3-4 days and contents of the rumen become more fibrous as the more soluble and digestible components are digested. P and Na increase and Mg, Ca and K decline. In vitro studies show reduced digestibility of cellulose or alfalfa hay (Coop, 1949; Meiske et al, 1958; Juhasz, 1963; Leibholz, 1970; Hershberger and Cowan, 1972; Zelenak et al, 1972; Fowle and Church, 1973; Sasaki et al, 1974; Hasizume et al, 1976; Cakala and Albrycht, 1977).

With respect to rumen motility, even short term fasting (20 hr) results in a reduced rate and amplitude of rumen contractions (Attebery and Johnson, 1969). Nesic (1961) has shown that fasting of sheep for 6 days resulted in weak contractions at about half the normal rate. Reid (1963) has made extensive studies on the effect of fasting (see Ch. 6, Vol. 1), data indicating weak and irregular contractions on prolonged fasting.

Hecker and co-workers (1964) have studied sheep deprived of food or food and water for as long as 8 days. Their results indicated a rapid decrease in rumen fluid volume during the first 2-3 days and a gradual loss thereafter. In sheep starved for 4 days, rumen fluid losses accounted for about half of body weight losses. Gupta (1967) reported that rumen contents of sheep or goats became more liquid after 24 hr without feed. The weight losses in 24 hr were: rumen, 35% and omasum, 40%. Quin et al (1951) have also shown that the dry matter in rumen contents decreased in sheep starved for 4 days.

Starvation of the Young Ruminant

During conditions of submaintenance intake or fasting, it is obvious that the animal must catabolize body tissues in order to maintain body temperature and provide for the various vital functions. Depending upon the tissue reserves available, this may result in catabolism of adipose tissue and body proteins initially with minimal catabolism from the limited supply of carbohydrates. As the adipose tissues are depleted, proteins will provide more and more of the energy needed.

In studies with young calves, Blaxter and Wood (1951) showed a constant decline in the heat production of young calves. Detailed investigations on these calves showed a very high loss of urinary N, average excretion amounting to 250 mg/kg BW/day, much higher than for mature animals. The increased excretion of urinary N was primarily accounted for by excretion of more urea, ammonia and creatine than by normal calves. Urinary excretion of S also increased. This is a finding that might be expected in any situation resulting in excessive catabolism of body proteins. Urinary Cl, K, Na and Ca fell during starvation but there was no evidence of excessive bone catabolism. Neither was there evidence of acidosis or ketonuria during starvation, although a slight ketosis was seen during realimentation. Dalton (1966, 1967) has shown that young calves have the ability to excrete hyperosmolar urine when deprived of food or food and water. He reported increased hematocrits, plasma urea and Cl in calves. Johnson et al (1966) showed that the glycogen content and fresh weight of the liver were reduced. Total liver content of crude protein, water and glycogen decreased.

Starvation of Adult Ruminants

In the case of adult ruminants, fortunately, food reservoirs in the reticulo-rumen and omasum should tend to delay the onset of starvation as compared to monogastric species. However, it is also likely that recovery may be delayed while the rumen microbial population becomes reestablished.

In addition to losses in body weight, numerous other qualitative and quantitative changes occur in affected tissues. Hight and

Barton (1965) found that partial starvation reduced the content of muscle protein and fat in the leg, loin, and rib of sheep carcasses. Prolonged undernutrition reduced the weight of the heart. Suzuki (1965) reported that the percentage of muscle declined in starved animals, with the loss being greater in muscles of the better cuts. Starvation reduced diameter of muscle fibers and the glycogen content of muscle. Butterfield (1966) found that dissectible fat decreased 70% in steers on a semi-starvation diet, much of the loss being in subcutaneous fat. Dissectible muscle decreased 21%, however, the actual weight of muscle lost was 1.18X the fat lost. In long term studies with cattle, Price (1977) observed a marked decrease in the proportion of fat, but he estimated that muscle loss was 32% greater than fat loss in bulls and 25% less than fat loss in steers during the same period. Other data on the bulls indicated greater loss of carcass weight and lesser loss of offal weight than for steers. In long term studies with sheep, Farrell and Reardon (1972) found that the fat content was markedly less in undernourished sheep and the water content in the fat-free empty body was greater than for controls. Lindsay et al (1977), using A-V differences, have shown that the arterial concentration for most amino acids was lower in starved than in fed sheep. They calculated that total α-amino acid loss was about 4.4 g/day, equivalent to a break down of about 30 g/day of muscle protein.

With regard to other physiological changes, Hashizume et al (1976) noted that the respiratory quotient dropped to 0.7 after 8 days of starvation from prestarvation levels of 0.83-0.93. A value of 0.7 indicates that fat was supplying nearly all of the energy for metabolism. The findings suggested that the starved cows were in a post absorptive state by the 4th day. Heat production from 4-8 days averaged 1.47 Kcal/kg$^{0.75}$ in 30 min., a value which was 78% of resting heat production (1.88 Kcal/kg$^{0.75}$). Over a shorter time period (96 hr), Vercoe (1970) estimated that protein oxidation accounted for 22-26% of the fasting heat production in different breeds of cattle. In other studies where cattle were deprived of feed and/or water, Rumsey and Bond (1976) determined that deprivation for 96 hr reduced rectal temperature by 1.5%, respiration rate by 47% and heart rate by 19%. The packed cell volume was increased, indicating dehydration.

Although body reserves of protein and fat may be seriously depleted during starvation, this is generally not the case for the mineral nutrients. Hyden (1961) and Leibholtz (1970) both reported, for example, that salivary secretion was reduced in animals deprived of food; thus this would tend to conserve those minerals secreted in saliva. Data from a variety of sources show that serum Ca may fall during starvation (White et al, 1956; Christian and Williams, 1960; Fowle and Church, 1973). Information indicates that inroganic P levels may first increase and then fall during starvation (White et al, 1956; Christian and Williams, 1960; Herd, 1966), although Rumsey and Bond (1976) observed an increase of 43% in serum P after a 96 hr fast. They also noted an increase of 12 and 23% for Na and K, respectively. Other data (Williams and Christian, 1959) indicate that underfeeding had no effect on plasma P, Ca or Mg.

Information on blood glucose is somewhat inconsistent (see Ch. 12), but the bulk of it indicates that blood glucose is depressed and glucose metabolism occurs at a slower rate in starving animals. For example, Munchow et al (1976) found that blood glucose declined after 24 hr of fasting, remained low for 2 days and then was normal on the 4th day of fasting.

Blaxter and Wood (1951) noted that there was no acidosis or ketosis in starved calves. Other reports indicate increased plasma ketones in older animals that have been starved, particularly in the case of pregnant ewes or lactating cows (see Ch. 12). Munchow et al (1976) found that acetoactic acid was increased 4 fold in starved cows and Emmanuel and Nahapetian (1975) found that starvation increased blood levels of β-hydroxybutyrate and acetoacetate in rams. Blood pyruvate levels may also increase during starvation (Robertson et al, 1960).

Plasma lipids, free fatty acids and cholesterol may be expected to increase with starvation (Masters and Horgen, 1962; Jackson et al, 1966; Saba et al, 1966). Munchow et al (1976) noted an increase of 40-fold in free fatty acids in starved cows, and Jackson and Winkler (1970) noted an increase of 2-fold in starved mature ewes by the 4th day of fasting. They also noted some differences in mobilization of different fatty acids from adipose tissues, with palmitate being removed more rapidly during the first 4 days.

Plasma urea may remain relatively constant in the early stages of starvation, but falls sharply in later stages (Masters and Horgen, 1962; Saba et al, 1966; Leibholz, 1970). Blood proteins may not change greatly but certain changes have been observed in amino acids. Although Sasaki et al (1974) and Slater and Mellor (1977) did not note a decrease in plasma amino acids, reports from other laboratories on studies with sheep show that total plasma amino acids decline, usually with a greater decrease in essential amino acids and the ratio of essential to non-essential amino acids tends to decrease (Leibholz, 1970; Joassart, 1977; Lindsay et al, 1977).

With respect to urinary excretion by older animals, N components will usually increase (Masters and Horgen, 1962; Meyer et al, 1955, 1962). During long periods of sub-maintenance intake on diets low in protein, the urinary excretion of N may reach relatively low levels, probably as a result of adaptation (Meyer et al, 1962). The feeding of readily available carbohydrates during such stress will have a N-sparing effect (Meyer et al, 1962; Gupta, 1967). Vercoe (1970) noted that urinary urea decreased and creatinine increased during a 96 hr fast in cattle. Total N, urea and creatine excretion increased as fasting heat production increased. Jensen et al (1951) and Dale et al (1954) have shown a marked decrease in excretion of P. No disturbance in the acid-base balance of blood was seen although ketones in plasma and urine increased during starvation. Martin (1969) reported little change in excretion by sheep in phenylacetic acid or creatinine, but found reduced excretion during starvation of other urinary components such as hippuric acid and total aromatic acids. Hashizume et al (1976) observed that urine of cows became acidic by the 4th day of starvation.

Fasted cows tend to develop a fatty liver. Reid et al (1977) found that hepatic uptake of free fatty acids increased 2 to 3-fold (6 day fast). In fed cows there was a net liver production of triglycerides which decreased and became a net uptake during fasting. Histological changes were also described. In livers from starved animals, Manns (1972) found a rapid accumulation of neutral fat and a low glycogen content. No marked differences were noted in a number of common liver enzymes although Martin et al (1973) found a substantial reduction in glucose-6-phosphatase.

The periods of time that ruminant animals may survive fasting can, at best, only be estimated roughly. This is so because of the marked effect of other stressing factors such as temperature, etc. It might be of interest to mention that Otsuka and Nakajima (1959) reported starving goats for 34 days without losses and Suzuki (1965) starved sheep for 10-46 days without losses. Gerstell (1942) starved a deer in good condition at temperatures ranging from -12 to 14°C; the deer survived for 14 days. DeCalesta et al (1975) found that mule deer survived 16-47 days when mean temperatures were 9°C. Thus, it is obvious that resistance varies considerably in different animals.

Realimentation of Starved Animals

The reaction of an animal when food is offered after a period of fasting or underfeeding is of interest and concern since body tissues may have been depleted of some nutrients and the usual digestive mechanisms are probably not functioning at the normal rate. Since rumen fermentation and numbers of rumen microorganisms drop off drastically during fasting, it is to be anticipated that some time will be required to build the rumen population back to its normal level.

Quin (1951) demonstrated that fasting sheep for 2-4 days resulted in a slower in vitro utilization of glucose or cellulose as compared to fed sheep and Meiske et al (1958) concluded that in vitro rumen cellulose digestion did not return to normal until 3-4 days after feeding steers which had been fasted for 3 days. Warner (1962) found that total bacterial numbers returned to normal within 2-3 days in sheep starved for 4 days.

With regard to rumen VFA, Coop (1949) concluded that production was normal within 18 hr after refeeding of sheep starved for 1-4 days in spite of the fact that feed consumption was not back to normal for several days and rumen pH was not normal—it dropped on refeeding and was low for 2 days.

Fowle and Church (1963) also noted that rumen VFA increased very rapidly after refeeding (see Fig. 17-1). Rumen lactic acid was moderately high.

When starved deer were refed (Hershberger and Cowan, 1972), it was observed that bacterial and protozoal numbers, lactic acid and total VFA concentration increased rapidly as did in vitro digestion of cellulose or alfalfa. Rumen pH decreased as might be expected. Rumen function was considered to be normal within 2 weeks following refeeding either hay or concentrate (sheep). Hashizume et al (1976) also concluded that rumen function had returned to normal after 10 days of refeeding (cows).

Data of Quin et al (1951) indicated that rumen water content was normal within 24 hr after refeeding. When sheep were fed a low protein grass hay, appetite returned to normal "immediately after starvation," but, with a diet of alfalfa hay or low protein hay plus casein, sheep were slower to attain normal consumption. The authors concluded that this represented the time for the animal to adapt to the protein in the diet. Juhasz (1963) found that cows starved for 2-3 days were back on full feed in 2 days and in 3 days when given half feed. With ewes Weeth et al (1959) found that ewes would eat a ration with 75% grass hay and 25% barley. Fasted ewes would not eat a ration with 15% tallow and 85% grass hay, although this was consumed when offered before fasting. Data on goats (Fowle and Church, 1973) indicate that at least 4 days were required for a return to a normal appetite (Table 17-2). In experiments in which wethers had been maintained at submaintenance levels for some time, Keenan and McManus (1970) observed that feed consumption increased slowly during the first 4 weeks after feed restrictions were

Table 17-2. Feed consumption of goats followed a fasting period of 5 days.[a]

Diet	Days after end of fasting						
	1	2	3	4	5	6	7
Chopped orchardgrass hay, g	138	115	208	298			
Chopped alfalfa hay, g	121	220	275	364			
Alfalfa pellet, g	140	77	212	340			
Pellet, 45% barley & 55% alfalfa hay, g	60	59	143	259			
Barley pellet, g	18	62	84	161	251	284	225

[a] From Fowle and Church (1973)

removed. Sheep which had been severely restricted ate less food during the first 2 weeks and no more during the second 2 week period than those sheep fed at a maintenance level. They noted that the process of adaptation to unrestricted feeding was associated with an increase in the net rate of disappearance of VFA from the rumen.

The information which has been presented on refeeding suggests that animals fasted for any appreciable period of time are likely to come back on feed slowly over a period of several days. There is information to show that rumen microorganisms recover rather rapidly, but there is a dearth of information on the function of other organs after a period of fasting. Does it take some time for the abomasum, small intestine and liver to recover and renew normal functions? There is some information on some non-digestive enzymes in liver and other tissues, but apparently none (certainly recent information) on important enzymes in the GI tract.

One might anticipate digestive disturbances known to occur following drastic ration change (see Ch. 17, Vol. 1). Blaxter and Wood (1951) did mention that diarrhea was seen in calves given half or full rations after 4 days of fasting. In work with goats it has been shown that goats can be refed on a variety of feedstuffs without apparent problems, when they were previously adapted to low-quality grass hay. Furthermore, the energy intake was similar regardless of the diet, with the exception of a 100% barley pellet which required 5-6 days for normal feed intake (Table 17-2). Similar although very limited information is available on mule deer (Dean, 1973). In this case deer were starved and then refed on alfalfa hay or fresh grass or rolled barley with no apparent signs of illness. The fact that fasted animals do not gorge themselves is, no doubt, the reason that there are relatively few problems on refeeding.

In view of the large N losses shown to occur in starving ruminants—particularly in young animals—one might anticipate that refeeding with more protein than normal might be desirable. This may well be advisable in underfed animals (Meyer et al, 1962), but would not appear to have any immediate beneficial effects in animals subjected to fasting for several days since the data on Quin et al (1951) indicated a delay in return to normal feed intake when added protein was fed to sheep. Obviously, the body tissues must be replenished if the animal's performance is to return to pre-

fasting levels, but a gradual increase in protein intake is probably to be recommended along with a moderate to low intake of readily available carbohydrates. Since serum Mg drops and urinary excretion of P and S may be high, it would seem that sources of these nutrients should definitely be considered when refeeding starved or underfed ruminants. Limited data indicate that high-fat diets are not to be recommended.

DIARRHEA

Diarrhea affects ruminant anmals of all ages but is much more severe in the preruminant animal prior to the establishment of normal rumen functions. Death losses may be high and of those animals which survive severe cases, many may be so affected that they become an economic liability. The incidence of diarrhea varies greatly from season to season and from farm to farm. Of the many different non-nutritional factors that may cause diarrhea, Hull (1972) points out that those usually affecting cattle less than two years of age are parasitism, chronic bovine viral diarrhea-mucosal disease (BVD-MD) and the malabsorption syndrome. Those usually confined to cattle more than 2 years of age are Johne's disease and lymphosarcoma. Details on parasites are given later. Diarrhea associated with BVD-MD may be intermittent. Affected cattle are unthrifty and do not gain weight. Cattle often have a dry, scaly coat. They are anemic. The rumen is usually atonic and filled with fluid. In the malabsorption syndrome affected cattle constantly pass soft feces and the condition is often associated with calfhood diarrhea. Chronic parasitism may also cause secondary malabsorption. Cattle affected with Johne's disease have severe watery diarrhea and weight loss but continue to eat vigorously. The condition is usually noticed after imposition of stress and all cases eventually terminate in death. Lymphosarcoma with abomasal involvement can cause chronic diarrhea.

In the preruminant animal, severe diarrhea is primarily related to conditions that allow the development of bacteria or viruses and their toxins in the GI tract. Nutrient deficiencies such as avitaminosis A may cause profuse diarrhea in young animals. In older animals an outright Cu deficiency or one precipitated by excessive Mo can be a problem (see Ch. 5). Other causes include the ingestion of plant and mold toxins and parasitic infections such as coccidiosis and stomach or intestinal worms.

Further reading on this subject that might be of interest would include papers by Roy (1969), Radostits (1975) and Fisher and Martinez (1975).

Predisposing Conditions

It is well recognized that colostrum has a protective action in young mammals with respect to diarrhea and other diseases caused by invasive microorganisms. Colostrum is able to exert its protective functions to the fullest only if ingested early in the life of the young animal while the gut is still permeable to the globulins in colostrum (see Ch. 9, Vol.1; Roy, 1964). However, the feeding of colostrum past this absorptive period (up to 24 hr) still has some protective value against organisms which cause diarrhea (Roy et al, 1955; Roy, 1964), perhaps because of localized action in the gut.

A number of rather recent studies show, in general, that calves which have low blood levels of globulin are more susceptible to septicemia from *E. coli* organisms. However, they may still have diarrhea and the evidence suggests that colostrum may prolong survival although not offering much protection to septicemia (Fey, 1971; Logan and Penhale, 1971; Penhale et al, 1971; Shaw, 1971; Fisher, 1973).

Smith (1965) has pointed out that the first bacterial organisms to colonize the GI tract of the young calf are *Escherica coli*, various streptococci and *Clostridium welchii*. The lactobacilli then develop and become the most numerous organisms in the stomach and small intestine. This sequence of development seems likely to be related to pH in these areas. At birth the pH in the abomasum is relatively high, but drops as the abomasum starts to function, thus encouraging the lactobacilli to grow since they thrive in acidic conditions. Roy (1969) has cited data from a thesis by Ingram regarding the development of bacteria in the gut of the young calf. This information indicated within 5.5 hr after birth that *E. coli* are restricted mainly to the ileum and the large intestine. By 8.5 hr after birth they are found in the abomasum at a level of 10^3/ml. In the duodenum the viable *E. coli* count reaches a peak at 1-4 days of age, and in normal healthy calves it declines to a very low level at 10 days of age, presumably because of the increasing dominance of the lactobacilli. In the case of calves with severe *E. coli* infections, counts may be as high as 10^7-10^8/ml in the duodenum at 10 days of age.

Data from a variety of different sources (cited by Reisinger, 1965; Roy, 1969) indicate that *E. coli* infections are the predominant cause of death in young calves. Smith (1971) found that the only significant abnormality in the alimentary flora of calves dying of septicemia was the presence of high numbers of *E. coli* in the small intestine. Reports from England indicate that salmonella infections must be reckoned with also, since they caused about as many death losses as did *E. coli*. In a recent study on 59 beef herds in Canada, Acres et al (1977) found that enterotoxic *E. coli* were present in 31.4% of the cases of diarrhea primarily from calves under 5 days of age. In calves from several days to one month of age, reo-like viruses were the predominant pathogenic organism. Salmonellae, IBR, BVD, and Pl$_3$ viruses were not isolated in any of 33 herds examined.

The deaths that occur from bacterial infections may be a result of localized infection and/or septicemia. These pathogenic organisms are known to produce potent endo- or exotoxins which cause varying degrees of illness or death. They may cause damage to the epithelial tissues of the GI tract, allowing the entry of invasive strains. In other cases the highly potent toxins may be so quickly absorbed that illness and death result from toxemia without bacteremia or diarrhea (Reisinger, 1965).

The development of toxemia and diarrhea, even in the presence of a high population of pathogenic organisms in the environment, is highly related to the nutrition and digestive physiology of the young animal. Information on this subject is discussed in a later section.

Effect of Diarrhea on the Animal

Fecal Excretion and Digesta Passage. Severe diarrhea, as might be anticipated, is apt to cause marked changes in the excretory patterns of affected animals. Blaxter and Wood (1953) have reported information resulting from extensive analyses on feces of scouring calves used in various metabolic experiments. Some of their data are shown in Table 17-3.

Blaxter and Wood (1953) mentioned other facts regarding these scouring calves that might be of interest. They found that passage of digesta through the GI tract took about 48 hr in normal calves but only 6 hr in

Table 17-3. Fecal excretion of various components by normal and scouring calves.[a]

Fecal component	Normal calves (a)	Calves with diarrhea (b)	Ratio, b:a
Water, g	51.0	927	18.2
Dry matter, g	12.5	93.5	7.5
Lipids			
Total fat, g	4.1	37.4	9.1
Neutral fat, g	1.5	10.6	7.0
Soaps, g	1.9	8.3	4.4
Free fatty acids, g	0.7	18.5	26.4
Volatile fatty acids, ml 0.1 N acid	164	1056	6.4
Crude protein, g	5.5	41.0	7.5
Minerals			
Ash, g	1.5	10.6	7.1
Ca, meq	21.6	98.8	4.6
Mg, meq	11.4	24.0	2.1
Na, meq	5.0	41.6	8.3
K, meq	2.2	39.9	18.1
P, meq	21.0	94.0	4.4
Coliform count x 10^8	118	2907	24.6
Fecal pH	6.8	6.0	

[a] From Blaxter and Wood (1953)

scouring calves. Average fecal weight was about 20-fold that of normal calves, but was as high as 40-fold in severely affected individuals. Digestibility fell, sometimes to as low as 40%. Increased fecal losses were seen in fat-soluble vitamins. Purine N, presumed to be of bacterial origin, rose from nil in normal calves to 270 mg/day in scouring calves. Na and K urinary losses declined only slightly even though fecal losses of these elements were very high. In other work Michel (1971) found that excretion of free amino acids and amines was increased 10 to 100-fold in calves with diarrhea. He points out that intestinal degradation of amino acids such as lysine would result in lower biological value of the diet, a factor which would compound the effects of reduced absorption. He also suggests that the various biological amines (volatile amines, cadaverine, putrescine, etc.) which are produced by microorganisms in the gut, are a consequence of the diarrhea and may have little toxicity for the host animal.

It is apparent from these data that an animal with severe diarrhea is losing a tremendous amount of undigested material plus the excretion of metabolites from body tissues. Blaxter and Wood suggested that the diarrhea arises from a primary disturbance high in the intestinal tract which, in turn, gives rise in the lower gut to large quantities of undigested food that provides a suitable medium for bacterial fermentation. They also suggested that the increase in the number of small molecules in the lower gut (from fermentation activity) would result in an increased osmotic pressure within the lumen of the gut which would cause water and electrolyte infiltration. Acid irritation of the mucosa along with loss of protective muscus would make invasions of bacteria easier, as well.

Fayet (1969) has reported limited data on calves with diarrhea which indicated that total fecal excretion (volume) was increased about twice and total fecal dry matter was about the same as that of normal calves. In calves with diarrhea, feed intake and urinary volume decreased. Fecal Na excretion was increased to about the extent found by Blaxter and Wood, but fecal K was only about 2.8X that of normal calves. Other papers giving data on fecal volume include those of Lewis and Phillips (1972), Thornton and English (1972) and Fisher and Martinez (1975).

Mylrea (1968) has studied the flow of digesta in the intestines of calves with salmonellosis, abomasitis and non-specific scours. The calves used had cannulas in various sites in the small intestine. Although the calves were afflicted with a variety of ailments, the results generally indicated that abomasal emptying was retarded in calves in which the disorders were developing, the pattern being abnormal and the pH of the chyme did not show the usual increase due to feeding. In calves with salmonellosis and well developed abomasitis, the passage of PEG and pH changes were essentially normal although the volume of chyme was increased but rarely more than 2-fold that of normal calves. However, the volumes and quantities of substances analyzed for that were recovered from the ileum were usually more than twice normal, and, in severe scouring, were up to 34 times the normal quantities. Analyses for reducing substances indicated greater quantities passing out of the small intestine in calves with salmonellosis (146% of controls) or non-specific scouring (228%). Other constituents for calves with salmonellosis and non-specific scouring were increased as shown: N, 3-6; lipids, 1.5-5; Na, 2.5-15; and K, 4.3-11 times. Thus, these data indicate a marked reduction in absorption or increased excretion into the gut of scouring calves. Data on the rate of passage confirmed that of Blaxter and Wood in that passage rate was greatly increased in scouring calves, but Mylrea's data showed that this was probably due to shorter retention time in the large intestine and resultant more frequent defecation rather than a shorter passage time in the small intestine.

Tagari and Roy (1969) found that diarrhea in one calf resulted in an increased pyloric outflow, an increased outflow of undigested protein from the abomasum, and a high pH value of 5.1. In the ileal effluent the volume of contents and quantity of N were increased.

Water and Nutrient Losses

Changes in fecal or urinary concentration of nutrients or electrolytes do not allow a good overall evaluation of body losses. Lewis and Phillips (1972) have conducted balance studies with normal and diarrheic calves (Table 17-4). Note that Ca was the only component measured that did not change from a positive to a negative balance. Thus, these values give a better indication of the severity of diarrhea on the young animal than do analyses on feces. With regard to

other components, Grys and Malinowska (1974) found increased levels of intestinal Fe and decreased levels of Na and Mo in the jejunum or liver. Little change was observed in jejunal Mg, Ca or Mn, but inorganic P was increased slightly. The content of K, total P, and Ni were not influenced.

Total body water in calves with diarrhea may be expected to decrease (Dalton, 1964; Watt, 1967). Phillips et al (1971) found a marked increase in the half life of body water in calves with diarrhea. Fayet (1969) concluded that total body water was not markedly changed in calves with diarrhea, but extracellular volume decreased considerably as did blood volume. Cellular water, on the other hand, increased. Fayet (1971) reported the following changes in body water for normal and diarrhetic calves: total body water, 76.5 and 74.0; extracellular fluid, 50.2 and 35.0; intracellular water 26.6 and 39.0.

With regard to urinary excretion of water, Fisher and De LaFuente (1972) found that diarrhetic calves reduced water excretion, apparently to compensate for large fecal losses. In further work from this laboratory (Fisher and Martinez, 1975), it was found that there was no difference between total fluid output of healthy and diarrhetic calves when fluid input was maintained. In these experiments increased fecal losses were compensated by reduced urinary losses (see Table 17-5). These authors point out that the effect of diarrhea on the calf depends on

Table 17-4. Water* and electrolyte† balance of calves.[a]

	Normal	Diarrheic	No. of calves normal-diarrheic
Total water	+ 22.3 ± 5.6	- 72.3 ± 8.8	8-8
Insensible water	- 16.8 ± 0.7	- 16.8 ± 0.7	7-7
Sodium	+ 8.4 ± 2.5	- 235.2 ± 45.8	6-8
Potassium	+ 28.8 ± 9.6	- 65.5 ± 15.0	8-8
Chloride	+ 20.4 ± 11.8	- 280.4 ± 65.8	8-6
Calcium	+ 121.6 ± 30.6	+ 22.1 ± 7.9	3-3
Magnesium	+ 7.4 ± 3.0	- 5.7 ± 0.4	3-3
% Body wt. change/day	+ 0.9 ± 0.4	- 7.9 ± 1.8	8-8
Hr. of study	98.2 ± 17.7	38.5 ± 2.3	8-8

[a] From Lewis and Phillips (1972)

* In g per kg body weight per day (mean ± S.E.).

† In mg per kg body weight per day (mean ± S.E.).

Table 17-5. Daily water balance in calves affected with enteric colibacillosis.[a]

| Item | Healthy | Diarrhetic calves | |
		Surviving	Dying
	- - - - mg/kg BW - - - -		
Water in milk	87.3	81.7	70.5
Metabolic water	5.0	5.0	4.9
Total	92.3	86.7	75.4
Water losses			
Insensible	23.8	27.6	27.6
Urinary	57.2	34.2	25.4
Fecal	4.7	25.0	38.9
Total	85.6	86.8	92.0
Actual water balance	6.7	- 0.1	-16.6

[a] From Fisher and Martinez (1975)

whether fluid intake is maintained, the manner in which diarrhea is induced, and on the doses of the infectious agents.

Blood and Fluid Changes. Changes in blood metabolites of scouring calves have been investigated in a number of laboratories. Some fairly typical results are shown in Table 17-6. These data show a minor decline in plasma Na and Cl, a decrease in plasma volume, and a marked increase in plasma urea. Other papers showing similar results include those of Roy et al (1959), Watt (1967), Fayet (1969), Lewis and Phillips (1973), and others.

Tennant et al (1968) found that blood glucose was quite low in calves with *E. Coli* diarrhea as did Lewis et al (1975); the latter authors also noted that plasma lactate was quite high in some calves. Michel (1971) observed that plasma glucose increased 2-3 days before the beginning of diarrhea. Depending on the severity of the diarrhea, the blood glucose returned to normal or decreased. Bywater and Penhale (1969) observed depressed lactase activity in the intestinal mucosal tissues of calves after scouring. Demigne and Remesey (1978) observed that blood glucose was lower initially in sick calves but rose to higher levels than in normal calves and remained at higher levels (max time 21 days). Other blood components that were higher were: lactic acid, alanine, urea and free fatty acids.

Tennant et al (1968) found that plasma proteins tend to be high. However, Thornton et al (1972) noted little variation in total serum proteins or fibrinogen, but diarrhetic calves tended to have increased serum albumin and α-globulin and decreased γ-globulin concentrations. Only calves which developed severe dehydration showed an increase in blood urea N and packed cell volumes that exceeded the normal range.

In other studies Fayet (1971) observed a decrease in plasma osmolality which decreased from 294 in healthy calves to 287 mosmol/l. in scouring calves; these changes were accompanied by dehydration. Fisher and McEwan (1967) found that there was no significant change in oxygen-carrying capacity of the blood of calves with diarrhea, but there was marked acidosis and a marked lowering of myocardial K which decreased from 223 to 169 mg/100 g of muscle. Extracellular K was normal or high, results which were similar to those of Lewis and Phillips

Table 17-6. Effect of diarrhea on blood components of calves.[a]

| Item | Normal calves | Calves with diarrhea | |
		Survived	Died
Plasma			
Na, meq/l.	142	129	129
K, meq/l.	5.1	5.1	6.1
Cl, meq/l.	100	92	94
Volume, ml/kg body wt	66	59	57
Blood urea, mg/100 ml	16	41	91
Blood pH	7.4	7.3	6.9
Plasma bicarbonate, mM/l.	29	22	9

[a] From Fisher (1965)

(1973). These authors suggest that this change in muscle ions may cause a decrease in membrane potential causing weakness, lethargy and giving rise to cardial arrhythmias, which were observed in calves with diarrhea (Fisher and McEwan, 1967). Acid infusions caused similar effects (arrhythmias) on the heart.

Dalton (1968) has shown that the young calf can readily excrete large amounts of excess fluid. When systemic acidosis was induced, the major renal response was an increased ammonia excretion but titratable acid excretion was little different from controls (Dalton and Phillips, 1969). Michel (1971) reported marked increases in urinary excretion of P and urea in scouring calves and Tsvetkov (1972) found that the buffer capacity of urine increased during diarrhea. Titratable acidity increased by 6-12 days of age.

Dietary Factors and Diarrhea

Farmers and husbandrymen, as well as many nutritionists and veterinarians, believe that overfeeding calves is a predisposing factor in the development of diarrhea. While this may very likely be the case when the background infection of virulent strains of *E. coli* is high (Roy, 1964, 1969), research evidence (Mylrea, 1966; Burt and Irvine, 1970) indicates that overfeeding is not apt to greatly increase the incidence of diarrhea in young calves, when the level of infection is low. In practical situations on the farm, Willoughby et al (1970) point out that the incidence of diarrhea is usually the highest during the stabled period, when milk substitutes are fed and when little attention is paid to the amount of milk being fed.

A series of experiments with a large number of calves at the National Institute for Research in Dairying in England (Shillam et al, 1962; Shillam and Roy, 1963) showed that the quality of milk in the diet of the young calf was of primary importance with respect to the development of *E. coli* infections. Heating of skim milk to the point that the proteins were denatured was very detrimental and resulted in a much higher incidence of diarrhea. Associated with the denaturation of the whey proteins was a reduction of ionizable Ca, release of SH groups, poor clotting ability of rennet, and a reduced digestibility of the protein. The biological value of the protein was not changed, however. Other work from this station (Tagari and Roy, 1969) has shown that the pyloric outflow from calves fed over-

heated milk was higher in pH. Small pieces of clot passed out of the abomasum, whereas that from other milk was clear. The overheated milk resulted in less undigested milk protein in the pyloric outflow. A reduced flow of NPN after feeding occurred about 3 hr after, whereas the other milk reached peak flow of NPN shortly after feeding. The results from this as well as other experiments would, then, indicate that the high pH and poor digestibility of overheated milk in the abomasum make a marked contribution to the growth of pathogenic organisms in the upper small intestine. Roy (1969) has cited other evidence indicating that there is a negative relationship between the N percentage in the feces and the dry matter content of feces, which is a rough measure of the severity of diarrhea.

The inclusion of carbohydrates such as sucrose and starch in the diet of young ruminants may cause diarrhea, at least partly due to the fact that the ruminant apparently produces no sucrase enzyme and amylolytic activity at a young age, especially, is very low (see Ch. 9, Vol. 1 for further details). Slagsvold et al (1977) have observed that increasing the lactose content of milk replacers by ca. 30% resulted in increased frequency of diarrhea the first 10-12 days in all young calves.

The physical nature of the diet has also been shown to have some effect on diarrhea in calves fed milk replacers. Roy (1969) points out that young calves given solid food generally have a lower incidence of diarrhea than those on liquid diets. He mentions also that skim milk will result in the production of feces with a higher dry matter content than many milk replacers. Gorrill and Nicholson (1969) found that liquid diets with added fibrous materials (sawdust, purified wood cellulose, oat hulls), especially oat hulls, increased fecal dry matter and reduced the incidence of scouring, but had no affect on growth, digestibility or N retention.

Roy (1969) points out that in older cattle diarrhea may be associated with the ingestion of diets high in proteins or peptides. It has been suggested that such diets allow the migration of bacteria from the large to the small intestine, causing autointoxication as a result of the amines and toxins produced.

Diarrhea associated with clostridial infections (enterotoxemia) in older animals has been associated, in at least one instance, with the ingestion of diets high in readily available carbohydrates. It is assumed that a high level of starches or sugers in the duodenum provides a favorable environment for these organisms to grow (Bullen and Battey, 1957). In this research it is of interest that the authors found a marked hypoglycemia in a sheep with enterotoxemia while those that developed acidosis had normal blood glucose concentrations.

Treatment of Scouring Calves

It is not the intent of this section to attempt to outline appropriate medications for calves with diarrhea, other than to point out that representative information (Mylrea, 1968) has shown that various of the infective bacteria respond differently to different antibiotics. For those readers interested in further detail, Reisinger (1965) has discussed drug therapy. More recent data from Europe suggest good responses to some glucocorticoids which have some mineralocorticoidal activity (Dovrak, 1971).

With respect to treatments other than drugs or antibiotics, the literature that has been reviewed indicated clearly that most calves with diarrhea are dehydrated; that they have probably lost large amounts of body proteins and electrolytes, particularly Na, K and Cl; and that blood glucose may be low. A number of different reports (Fisher and McEwan, 1967; Watt, 1967; Carter, 1969; Melichar and Masek, 1971; Edwards and Williams, 1972; McLean and Bailey, 1972; Wilgenbusch and Sextion, 1971) indicate a good response from treatment with fluids containing NaCl and/or NaHCO₃. This would help to alleviate the acidosis likely to be present and would aid in replenishing body Na supplies. In view of the fact that blood K may be high even though cellular K is low, care in use of K would be indicated. However, administration of I.V. and oral NaHCO₃ would tend to build up serum Na and should drive some of the serum K back into the cells, thus allowing subsequent treatment with K salts. Subcutaneous administration of K salts might be the preferred means of administration along with oral and I.V. Na salts. Carter (1969) suggests that about half of the needed solutions should probably be administered via stomach tube or with a catheter passed down the nostril and the other half given via I.V. drip administration. He suggests solutions with 1 level tablespoon of NaCl and one of NaHCO₃/gal of water for such purposes. Other formulas have been given by Wilgenbusch and Sexton (1971).

Glucose should also be a useful treatment, since blood glucose may be low and it is certain that the calf is in need of energy. Watt (1967) suggests that the most effective treatment of several tried was administration of bovine plasma along with solutions to replace electrolytes and a 5% glucose solution to replace water lost from the tissues. Reisinger (1965) also suggests blood transfusions, but preferably from a donor other than the calf's dam so that a different source of antibodies is obtained.

Administration of vitamins A and E is frequently recommended and many veterinarians routinely administer B-complex vitamins on the assumption that the gut may have been sterilized by drugs and that rumen or gut microorganisms may not be supplying the usual amount of B vitamins. European data suggest that vitamin C levels in plasma are quite low and that it should be given to scouring calves parenterally because of poor absorption (Salageanu et al, 1972).

Conclusions

Diarrhea in ruminants may be a major economic problem to all producers, but may be an especially severe problem in young animals such as young dairy calves or, in many cases, young beef calves. Published data indicate that *E. coli* infections are the major cause of diarrhea and that infections may develop very rapidly, especially in young animals that have not had an adequate intake of colostrum. Milk substitutes which contain milk that has been overheated are to be avoided, since this seems to be a major factor in allowing undigested whey proteins to escape into the duodenum, thus providing a favorable medium for rapid growth and proliferation of pathogenic bacteria. Overfeeding does not appear to be a major factor, especially where the background level of infection is low. Body losses of protein, water and Na, K and Cl may be severe, indicating that these nutrients must receive consideration in treating or feeding calves with diarrhea. Appropriate therapy includes the use of buffered solutions to control acidosis, to rehydrate body tissues, and to replenish lost electrolytes.

INTERNAL PARASITES

Fortunately, since this volume was first published in 1971, more data are now available which relate the effect of internal parasites to the nutritional utilization of ruminant animals. Some information on this topic may be found in good veterinary texts such as Blood and Henderson (1968) and in a review by Miller (1968).

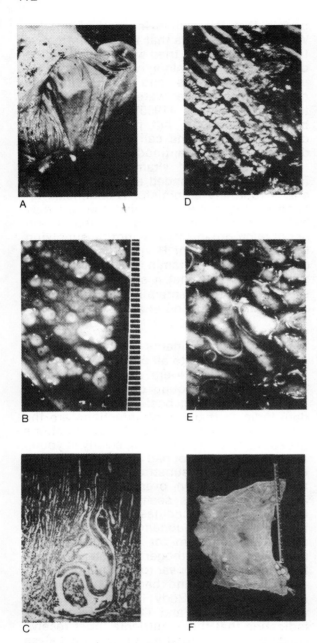

Fig. 17-2A. Examples of nematode damage to the abomasum or intestines. A. The mucosal surface of a heavily parasitized abomasum. Note thickening of mucosa and nodules. B. Closeup of abomasal surface depicted in A. Note marked alteration of normally smooth surface. C. Histologic cross section of abomasal tissue showing a developing nematode larva. Note disruption of mucosal architecture. D. Mucosal surface of abomasum heavily parasitized with the small stomach worm, *Trichostrongylus axei*. Note numerous folds and diptheritic membrane. E. Thickened mucosa of a heavily parasitized small intestine. F. An opened cecum showing nodules characteristic of damage caused by *Oesophagostomum columbianum*.

Parasites that are probably of most concern are lungworms, liver flukes, gastrointestinal nematodes and coccidia. It has been estimated that nematodes infesting the GI tract of cattle may cost American cattlemen more than $100 million a year. Sheep, of course, are continually bothered by stomach worms, and it is well recognized that constant effort is required to keep the parasite burden down, so that performance is not adversely affected.

According to Miller (1968), parasites may affect the host in a number of ways: by damaging or consuming the host's tissues and thus reducing their absorptive capacity; absorbing the host's food; sucking the host's blood and tissue fluids; causing mechanical obstruction of blood and lymphatic vessels or other vital channels; causing wounds through which other antagonistic organisms can enter; secreting or excreting into the host various harmful substances such as hemolytic and digestive enzymes, possibly antienzymes and anticoagulants; and introduction into the host of other species of parasites.

Effect of Parasites on the Animal

Information on many of the internal parasites (Blood and Henderson, 1968) indicates that most heavily parasitized animals are anemic; many are edematous; and diarrhea is frequently seen although this varies with species of animal and parasite. Ross and Dow (1965) have described the lesions seen in the abomasum of calves infected with *Ostertagia*. The abomasum was found to be hemorrhagic and many of the glandular cells were degenerated (see Fig. 17-2). A subsequent report (Ross and Todd, 1965) showed that the abomasum of heavily infected calves had a very high pH, values in the range of 6.2-8.5 being found in infected animals as opposed to 3.6-4.4 in control animals. In studies with sheep infected with *O. circumcincta*, sheep with abomasal pouches were used to evaluate the nature of the response (McLeay et al, 1973; Anderson et al, 1976). The main body of the abomasum could not maintain normal acidity which rose to pH 7 or higher, but acid secretion in the pouches increased. Coupled with an increase in blood gastrin, they concluded that reduced acid production results from toxins secreted by the parasites or host tissues. Hypersecretion has been observed in pouches of calves or sheep infected with other stomach but not with intestinal nematodes (Titchen and Anderson, 1977). Ross

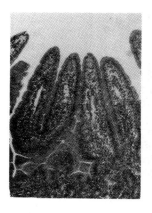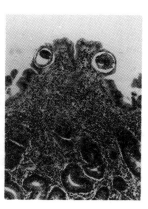

Fig. 17-2B. A. Section of normal sheep small intestine. Note long finger-like filli.
B. Section of sheep small intestine infected with *Trichostrongylus colubriformus*. Note the absence of villi. The mucosa is flat and hypertrophied. Note cross sections of the worms burrowing just under the surface epithelium. Courtesy of R.L. Coop, Moredun Institute, Edinburgh.

and Todd (1965) observed that the pepsin concentration was low, being 0.19% in infected calves as compared to 1.26-1.60 in controls. Other information showed that *Ostertagia* infection increased serum pepsinogen in lambs as early as four days after infection indicating leakage into the blood (Downey et al, 1969; McLeay et al, 1973) and that *Nematodirus battus* infection resulted in a decrease in intestinal mucosal levels of alkaline phosphatase, lactase and maltase 12-16 days after infection in lambs (Coop et al, 1972).In studies with calves infected with *Cooperia*, Dharsana et al (1976) found elevated levels of duodenal maltase and acid phosphatase, but a number of carbohydrate enzymes were not altered.

Ross and Dow (1965) also observed that congestion of the duodenum was present to varying degrees in calves that had scours prior to slaughter. Coop et al (1976) observed that *T. colubriformus* infections resulted in extensive atrophy of intestinal villi and flattening of the intestinal mucosa (Fig. 17-2B). When lambs were infected with the large intestinal nematode *Oesophagostomun columbianum*, Bawden (1970) found increased retention times of roughage in the GI tract accompanied by reduced feed consumption. Roseby (1977) has demonstrated that *T. colubriformus* infection resulted in reduced rumen content of dry matter, water and N, but these components were higher in

the abomasum, small intestine and cecumproximal colon. Transit time of markers through the tubular intestine was increased. He concluded that relatively more fermentation occurred in the large intestine of infected lambs; also, that increased leakage of serum into the gut coupled with reduced absorption resulted in less net absorption of amino acids by infected sheep. Thus, this information indicates clearly that abomasal function and, very likely, intestinal function must be markedly diminished. Abomasal digestion, particularly of protein, is probably reduced considerably by abomasal nematodes and intestinal absorption is most likely reduced as a result of damage done by intestinal nematodes. However, studies have not been done with intestinal cannulated animals to evaluate digestion in different segments of the GI tract. Furthermore, the effect of heavy parasite infections of young animals may persist for as long as a year if the animals are subjected to adverse conditions (van Adrichem and Shaw, 1977).

In animals parasitized with liver flukes, it appears that liver function must be greatly diminished if infections are severe. Severely infected animals may have fibrinous peritonitis, severe ascites (abdominal edema), and abnormal fluid in the gall bladder. In addition, plasma enzymes and liver clearance of dyes indicated severe liver dysfunction between 4 and 11 weeks after infection (Pullan et al, 1970). In one experiment infected cattle gained 8% less during the first 6 months after infection; higher levels of

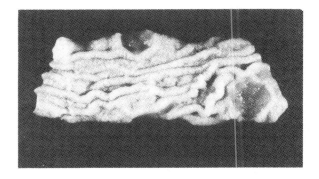

Fig. 17-2C. Sheep small intestine infected with *Trichostongylus vitrinus*. Small localized flat areas are present with no villi. Surrounding mucosa is normal. In larger magnification worms can just be seen on these flat areas, which are designated "finger-print" lesions. Courtesy of R.L. Coop. Moredun Institute, Edinburgh.

infection reduced gain by 28%. The impaired gain was believed to be due to poor feed utilization at the low level and also to reduced consumption at the higher level (Hope Caudery et al, 1977).

Effect on Blood or Tissue Metabolites

In addition to causing anemia, data from a variety of laboratories indicate that nematodes, in particular, will result in lower blood protein and, especially, lower blood albumin (Ross and Todd, 1965; Vercoe and Springell, 1969; Berry and Dargie, 1976; Coop et al, 1976; Horton, 1977; van Adrichem and Shaw, 1977). Ross and Todd found that serum albumin fell concomitantly with the packed cell volume values in infected calves. This may occur in sheep by 5-9 days after infection (Holmes and McLean, 1971). Vercoe and Springell did not find any difference in the half-life of plasma proteins even though they were depressed in animals infected with helminths, and Coop et al did not detect any effect on total blood proteins although hypoalbuminemia was evident after 3 weeks. Liver fluke infections also result in low blood albumin (Berry and Dargie, 1976).

Evans et al (1963) have shown that infections of *Haemonchus contortus* in sheep resulted in a marked rise in the concentration of K and a fall in the concentration of Na in erythrocytes, although plasma K and Na were not greatly changed. Fitzsimmons (1966) reported that *Trichostrongylus* infections in goats resulted in hemoconcentration accompanied by decreased serum, P, Ca, and Mg. In young calves Waymack and Torbert (1969) found that *Ostertagia* infections caused low serum Mg and/or low Ca as well as a decreased Ca balance.

Other studies show low blood P in parasitized lambs although little effect was noted on plasma Ca, urea or glucose (Coop et al, 1976). In this report there was evidence of arrested bone growth and osteoporosis in lambs infected with *Trichostronglyosis* nematodes. Horton (1977) has shown low blood Ca and P in infected lambs. Reveron et al (1974) also demonstrated poor bone mineralization and bone deformities in lambs infected with *Trichostronglyus* spp. Roseby and Leng (1974) reported that sheep with T. *colubriformis* infections had higher plasma urea than paired controls after 15-35 days as well as higher urinary excretion of urea; they suggested that the additional urea was apparently produced from ammonia released from amino acids in the tissues or gut. Roseby (1977) concluded that the rate of glu-

cose synthesis was higher in infected sheep because there was more recycling, but, because of lower feed intake, an overall reduction in glucose synthesis. In pregnant ewes Bennett et al (1968) found higher blood ketone levels 1-2 weeks prepartum, but there was no apparent effect on blood glucose.

Soliam (1953) observed that the livers of cattle affected with lungworms were low in vitamin A. Gardiner (1966) found that infections of a variety of stomach nematodes in sheep resulted in a decrease in liver Co. Morphological changes in the abomasum and intestines were suggested as causes for reduced uptake of Co. Eveleth et al (1953) published tentative data which indicated a reduced conversion of carotene to vitamin A in sheep infected with parasites.

Effect on Feed Utilization

There are many research reports (only a few of which will be cited) indicating that a heavy parasite burden will harm the performance of the host. Performance on pasture is generally more drastically affected that that of animals in the dry lot or those which are fed rations with appreciable quantities of concentrates (Ames et al, 1969; Utley et al, 1974; Jordan et al, 1977; Neville et al, 1977).

Research reports from a number of different laboratories generally agree that a heavy nematode burden will almost invariably result in a depressed appetite (as much as -20%) along with poor performance of both cattle and sheep. The data are less conclusive with respect to the effect on digestibility and efficiency of feed utilization. Some information shows reduced digestibility of organic matter, protein and energy; usually energy digestibility is less affected than protein. N, Ca and P balance may also be affected. Recent papers dealing with this topic include those of Vercoe and Springell (1969), Ross et al (1970), Barger (1973), Roseby (1973), Reveron et al (1974) and Horton (1977).

For a more specific example data are cited on digestibility studies of Sykes and Coop (1976, 1977). In studies with O. circumcincta (stomach nematode), they found that parasitism caused a 20% reduction in food consumption by the 2nd week which was maintained throughout the experiment of 13 weeks. Digestibility of N was reduced (see Table 17-7) but subsequently showed a gradual recovery. N balances of infected animals were lower than controls but pair feeding (both animals of a pair fed same amount) showed that reduced feed intake

Table 17-7. Effect of nematodes on digestibility by sheep.[a]

Item	O. circumcincta[b]		T. colubriformis[c]	
	Infected	Pair-fed controls	Infected	Pair-fed controls
Energy digestibility, %	53.1	54.9	55.3	55.4
DE, kj/g DM	9.0	9.3	9.4	9.4
N digestibility, %	54.7	63.8	55.9	57.0
N balance, g	2.34	2.8	0.8	2.3
Ca balance, g	0.2	1.3	-0.26	0.91
P balance, g	0.32	0.3	-0.37	0.44

[a] From Sykes and Coop (1976) [b]7-8 weeks after infection [c]6-7 weeks after infection.

rather than parasites was responsible for reduced N retention. Energy digestibility was reduced slightly. Weight gain was only 80% of controls and fat deposition was reduced. It was calculated that gross efficiency of ME for growth was reduced by 30%. Mineral deposition (Ca and P) in the skeleton was reduced by 30-50%. Similar studies with *T. colubriformis* (intestinal nematode) showed that parasitism reduced food consumption by 9% but had no effect on digestibility of energy or N although N balances were inferior to pair-fed controls. Ca and P balances were less and weight gain was markedly reduced in infected animals. Efficiency of energy utilization (ME) was calculated to be 13% as compared to ca. 25% in controls. It may be that some of the differences observed in these two studies were caused by different nematode species which affect different areas of the GI tract.

In further work from this laboratory (Sykes and Coop, 1977) lambs were reared parasite free, then half were dosed weekly with *Q. circumcincta* larva. Infected lambs were pair-fed with uninfected lambs. Infection caused a drop in feed intake (Fig. 17-3) which was maintained throughout the trial. N digestibility dropped from 60 to 44% at 2 weeks but gradually recovered, and N balance was reduced as was energy digestibility. Weight gain (Fig. 17-4) was only 80% of controls. Lambs were less efficient. Deposition of Ca and P in the skeleton was reduced to 35 and 50%, respectively, of controls. With the abomasal nematodes, protein utilization would be affected because of pepsin and pH changes. With the intestinal parasites, absorption would likely be impaired and serum loss increased from damaged tissues.

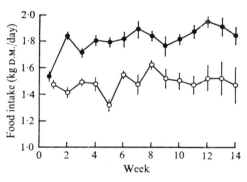

Fig. 17-3. Mean food intake of growing sheep infected with *O. circumcincta* (o) and in controls (•). From Sykes and Coop (1977).

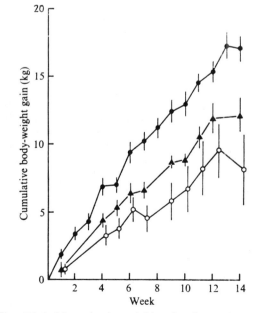

Fig. 17-4. Mean body-weight gain of growing sheep infected with *O. circumcincta* (o) and of controls fed *ad libitum* (•) or pair-fed (▲). From Sykes and Coop (1977).

In studies with cattle in which mono-zygous twins were used, van Adrichem and Shaw (1977) found that mixed worm popula-tiions (natural infections of *Cooperia, Oster-tagia* and *Oesophagostomum*) resulted in a depressed appetite for roughage throughout at least 7 months of the study. Growth was reduced when animals were housed in a stable and non-treated animals were less efficient in feed utilization. In milk produc-tion studies with monozygous twin heifers (van Adrichem and Shaw, 1977), treated animals produced significantly more milk, milk fat and fat-corrected milk than controls (6.6% more FCM) and showed an advantage in weight gains, presumably as a result of a better appetite. There was no effect of nema-todes on breeding performance or birth weight of calves.

Effect of Diet on Parasite Burden

There can be little doubt that diet has a bearing on the parasite burden of ruminant animals. For example, Weir et al (1948) found that lambs were more resistant to experimental infection with *H. contortus* when given liberal allowances of protein. Gordon (1950) also reported that sheep were more apt to throw off parasites when main-tained on dry rations adequately supple-mented with protein. Similar results have been reported for cattle on pasture which were fed added concentrate or protein (Vegors et al, 1956). Downey et al (1969) found that higher protein diets (18 v 11%) resulted in greater feed consumption by infected lambs. In further work Downey et al (1972) concluded that adequate protein in the diet may affect the animal's resistance to parasite infection. Adequate protein has also been reported to improve the performance of lambs infected with liver flukes (*Fasciola gigantica*) (Elmagdoub and Badr, 1966) but in another instance protein deficiency appar-ently did not alter resistance to infection (Deo et al, 1967). When sheep were given 6 or 13% protein and infected with flukes (*F. hepatica*), those on the lower protein developed anemia more rapidly as well as hypoalbuminaemia and weight loss and died earlier than those on 13% protein. When shifted from high to low protein diets, sheep were affected more rapidly by flukes (Berry and Dargie, 1976).

Trekeld et al (1956) and Downey (1965) have shown that Co-supplemental lambs, as opposed to those on a Co-deficient diet, had a bigger worm load of *H. contortus*. With respect to other mineral supplements, Weir et al (1948) found that the addition of trace minerals to the diet resulted in the recovery of more *Haemonchus* from the abomasum of lambs receiving the trace mineral supple-ments. Emerick et al (1957) observed that lambs fed dicalcium phosphate had a greater resistance to infection of *Haemonchus* than did non-supplemented lambs, but results of Reveron et al (1974) were inconclusive when infected animals (*T. colubriformis*) were given extra P or vitamin D or both, even though earlier experiments showed that infected lambs had severe lack of bone mineralization. In studies with flukes, Deo et al (1967) concluded that a P or trace element deficiency reduced the number of parasites, vitamin A deficiency had no effect and Ca deficiency reduced resistance to infection.

Rohrbacker et al (1958) found that milk-fed calves were less apt to have *Haemonchus* species than calves fed grain and hay along with milk; also, that weaned calves had a greater burden than unweaned calves. Vetter et al (1963) concluded that lambs fed semipurified diets excreted fewer viable eggs from *Haemonchus* than similar lambs fed natural diets. Abomasal pH was higher in lambs fed the purified (4.4 pH) than those fed the natural diets (4.0). These workers also showed that pelleted natural diets resulted in a lower egg production than the same diet fed in loose form, although the number of stomach worms recovered at necropsy were similar. Theurer et al (1965) found that lambs excreted more fertile eggs (*H. contortus*) when fed alfalfa hay than a variety of different hay-free rations. When 1% alfalfa hay was added, there was little change, but 5% added resulted in increased egg production. In studies with cattle, added fat had no effect on nematode egg counts (Utley et al, 1974).

Ciordia and Bizzel (1963) found that fewer larvae of *Trichostrongylus* were recovered from the feces of cattle fed grain as compared to grain and hay. In another study Ciordia et al (1977) observed that cattle pastured on grass fertilized with broiler litter had fewer trichostrongyle eggs at slaughter than cattle pastured on control pastures. Utech et al (1969) noted that cattle fed 'low' rations were more susceptible to infestations of the biting louse (*Damalinia bovis*) than cattle fed on 'high' rations. The authors concluded that the reduced self-grooming and later shedding of hair by the poorly-fed cattle contributed to this difference. Gordon (1964) and Goldberg (1965) did not find a marked difference in susceptibility of sheep or cattle, respectively, when fed at different planes of nutrition on the same diets. However, Gordon did notice some greater susceptibility to re-infestations of sheep so fed.

MISCELLANEOUS PLANT TOXINS

Information on a number of poisonous plants has been given in some detail in Ch. 15; therefore, it is the intent in this section to cover some factors of importance that were not mentioned in that chapter. These include mold toxicity, HCN and a few other miscellaneous problems.

Molds

All harvested grains, forage or other feedstuffs are suitable mediums for growth of a wide variety of molds provided temperature and moisture conditions allow growth to occur. Thus, feedstuffs may frequently have detectable and very substantial mold populations. The degree of visible mold infestation is not necessarily an indication of the amount of toxin present and that mold may not be apparent at all after milling or processing of food (Prior, 1975).

Surprising as it may seem, molds have been given a rather small amount of attention insofar as their production of toxins is concerned. Pier (1973) points out that about 100 fungi that grow on standing crops or feeds are known to produce toxic materials and that about 20 of these mycotoxins have been associated with naturally occuring diseases in man or animals. With the exception of a few acute forms of toxicity, Pier believes that toxicity is seldom diagnosed. Subclinical toxicity may result in lowered production, reduced weight gains, and impaired resistance to infections.

Pelhate (1967) points out that many different molds have been implicated in disease or death of ruminants. In the case of cattle, *Mucor circinelloides*, *Absidialichtheimii* and *Aspergillus flavus* were found in feed. *Hemispora stellata* was found in feed or fodder; *Scopulariopsis brevicaulis* was a dominant species in moldy hay; *Scopulariopsis canida* developed in damp, stored grain; and *Geotrichum canidum* was found in silage.

Molds may begin spoiling grain while the crop is still growing in the field. Many of the toxins are heat-stable and survive pelleting and other feed processing methods, thus the only sure method of controlling molds is to have the moisture content of the feed and the humidity where it is stored low enough to prevent growth. While various mold inhibitors are statisfactory for preserving high moisture feeds (propionic acid, for example), very little can be done to make moldy feed satisfactory for animals if it is highly contaminated (Nyvall, 1977; Pier, 1973).

For further reading on this topic, a number of reviews are available. Kingsbury (1964) has presented a brief historical review. Other papers include those of Lancaster (1969), Newberne (1972) and Harwig and Munro (1975).

Aflatoxins. Aflatoxins are toxins produced by ca. 30% of the strains of *Aspergillus flavus* and *Penicillium puberulum*. Most of the early work on acute toxicity has been related to contaminated peanut meals, but many harvested feeds stored under conditions of high humidity and temperature may be contaminated. Aflatoxins are toxic to the liver and may be carcinogenic for some species (Edds, 1973). Prior (1975) has reported that 4.2% of feed samples were contaminated with aflatoxin or Ochratoxin, so it is likely that a fair number of animals may be affected by these potent toxins, although animals often show a distaste for moldy feeds and may not eat them unless forced to do so.

With respect to ruminants, there are a number of papers reporting field cases of aflatoxin poisoning. These reports generally show that young animals (up to 6 mo. of age) are more severely affected than yearling or adult cattle (Loosemore and Markson, 1961; Clegg and Bryson, 1962; Allcroft and Lewis, 1963). Affected animals may have diarrhea, are often seen aimlessly walking in circles and may fall frequently. Ear twitching and grinding of the teeth were seen in all outbreaks on farms (Loosemore and Markson, 1961). Death usually occurred within 2 days after the first symptoms were observed and from 5-100% of calves in a herd were affected. Affected animals showed a marked loss of body condition (Clegg and Bryson, 1962) and in lactating cows a marked drop in milk production was observed (Allcroft and Lewis, 1963).

Postmortem findings indicate toxic effects on the liver resulting in centrolobular necrosis and ductal cell hyperplasia. Liver vitamin A is depleted also and serum alkaline phosphatase levels have been reported to rise up to the 12th week and then decline (Allcroft and Lewis, 1963). Other studies show a reduction in feed consumption, liveweight gain and in serum carotene and vitamin A in calves (Lynch et al, 1971). N balance may be reduced and urine volume and N excretion increased (Lynch et al, 1973). Animals may develop icterus (jaundice) of mucus membranes and serum (Rajan et al, 1973) and blood clotting time may be increased (Upcott, 1970).

Sheep are relatively resistant to aflatoxins. In one study lesions were seen in a sheep only after long term (5 years) exposure (Lewis et al, 1967). Dosage of 3-4 mg given 2X/week for 6 weeks resulted in clinical and pathological changes (Abrams, 1965). Armbrecht and Shalkop (1972) found that 2 mg/kg of body weight of aflatoxin B_1 was lethal for rams. However, a priming dose of $80 \mu g$/kg of body weight or of 50 mg of DDT/kg of body weight protected rams against a lethal dose. Young goats are also susceptible when given injected doses (Shadmi et al, 1974) as are buffaloes (Rajam et al, 1973).

Data reported by Allcroft et al (1966) indicate that the liver of sheep may have the capability of metabolizing aflatoxins. In the case of both sheep and cattle, aflatoxins may be recovered in milk and urine (Lancaster, 1969).

Although these toxins do not produce a sudden pharmacologic action such as some toxins may, the fact that liver function is seriously impaired and that exposed animals may take a long time to recover makes it obvious that aflatoxins should be avoided if possible. In young calves Lynch et al (1970) fed levels of aflatoxin B_1 ranging from 0.008 to 0.08 mg/kg of body weight for 6 weeks. At the 0.02 mg level an increase in serum phosphatase was observed. Gross lesions at postmortem included adrenal hyperplasia and loss of normal liver color. Typical histological changes in the liver occurred along with an increase in liver fat and reduced glycogen. In other studies from this laboratory (Lynch et al, 1971, 1972) calves were fed from 0 to 0.10 mg/kg of body weight for 6 weeks. Effects on performance and blood changes (noted previously) were observed by the 2nd week at 0.08 or 0.10 mg doses. Liver damage was observed at a dose level of 0.04 mg at postmortem (6 weeks). In another experiment calves were given single doses of aflatoxin. All calves survived doses of up to 1 mg/kg of body weight. Two of 3 died at dose levels of 1.2-1.6 mg and at 1.8 mg all calves died. Those that survived had a slow recovery.

In other studies with young ruminants, Rajan et al (1973) fed buffaloes or Jersey crossbred males (6 mo. of age) at a level of 20 mg of aflatoxin/kg of feed. Feed intake was reduced after 1 week and icterus was observed in 2-3 weeks. The Jerseys died after 32-68 days and the buffaloes after 30-65 days (8-9 mo. of age) and an older buffalo (30 mo.) was killed after 84 days. In a study with cattle over a prolonged period (13 mo.), Flatla et al (1971) fed diets with 204-474 ppb of aflatoxin. No clinical signs were observed and only mild liver damage was found. Animals receiving the higher level of aflatoxin gained slower and had lower feed conversion. Garrett et al (1968) found no apparent abnormalities in steers fed 100-300 ppb of aflatoxin for a time interval of 133-196 days. Higher amounts (700-1000 ppb) produced gross evidence of liver damage.

Other information published by Upcott (1970) suggests that treating calves with high dosages of vitamin A might have some protective effect against aflatoxin poisoning. Data on rumen microorganisms suggests that aflatoxin B_1 inhibits mixed cultures of rumen and *Streptococcus bovis* cultures (Mathur et al, 1976).

In most cases there is little than can be done to improve moldy feeds. Fortunately with aflatoxin, an ammoniation procedure removes the B_1 toxin and feeding trials with cows show that a metabolite, M_1, is not excreted in milk after treating contaminated cottonseed meal with ammonia (McKinney et al, 1973).

Molds Causing Photosensitivity. New Zealand sheep producers have been plagued for many years with a disease that results in a facial eczema. A long series of papers are available in the literature on this topic. In one of this series, McFarlane et al (1959) published evidence which showed that the essential pathology was the result of severe liver damage partly due to obstruction of the bile ducts. The result being that bile and its metabolites were not excreted at a normal rate. This appears to result in the accumulation in the blood and tissues of phylloerythrin, a degradation product of chlorophyll, which gives rise to the problems of photosensitivity in light colored areas of the body or in areas where the skin is thin. Percival (1959) showed conclusively that facial eczema was due to ingestion of the mold *Sporidesmium bakeri* Syd. Cultures of this fungus, when fed to lambs, produced characteristic facial eczema lesions as well as icterus and photosensitivity.

A similar type of problem has been reported in cattle in Florida (Kidder et al,

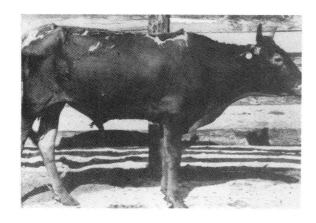

Fig. 17-5. Photosensitivity in cattle. Experimental steer showing the peeling of thin-skinned areas 30 days after the blistering took place. From Kidder et al (1961).

1961), where a mold, *Periconia minutissima* Cla., was found to grow on frosted Bermudagrass. The symptoms seen included: an empty, dejected appearance combined with excessive salivation and, sometimes, lacrimation and usually diarrhea. During the next 24-48 hr the animals could be observed licking themselves more than usual and switching their tails. The 3rd and 4th day they reach a violent head-shaking stage and repeatedly scratch the horns or polls with the hind feet or rub on posts, etc. Sunburned tissues may show up at this stage. In the next 2-3 days, blisters appear on light-colored or thin-skinned areas. Autopsy findings indicate varying degrees of icterus and liver damage. Experiments indicate it took 7-14 days exposure before the first symptoms showed up and that up to 20% might die. Treatment with Na thiosulfate was shown to be rather effective. Some good illustrations are shown in the bulletin by Kidder et al (see Fig. 17-5).

Molds on Forage. A mold, *Rhizoctonial leguminicola*, found principally on red clover forage or hay has been shown to produce an alkaloid (Rainey et al, 1965) that is toxic to cattle. This particular mold has been found on hay of apparent good quality with no visible mold (Crump and Henning, 1963). It results in excessive salivation, watery diarrhea, anorexia and frequent urination (Crump and Henning, 1963; Crump et al, 1967). Only small amounts of forage (ca. 2-6 kg) were required to stimulate salivation. Extracts, when given intra-ruminally, would produce excess salivation in less than 1 hr (Byers and Broquist, 1960, 1961). No severe symptoms

were reported in cattle, but the toxin is lethal to guinea pigs and excessive salivation was produced in sheep and several monogastric species (Crump et al, 1967).

Mohanty et al (1969) have reported studies on molded alfalfa hay when fed to cattle. Some of their results are tabulated in Table 17-8. Nineteen different species of mold were isolated from this hay, *Scopulariopsis brevicaulis* being the dominant species. They reported that the molded hay had a tobacco-like aroma and appeared to be palatable to cattle. No adverse signs were seen except some slight degree of diarrhea and rough hair coats. Cattle on moldy hay consumed more salt (232 g/day) than those on good hay (186 g/day). However, the data in the table show clearly that the feeding value of the moldy hay was reduced considerably— on the order of 25-30%. Asplund (1971) observed that hay baled at 30% moisture had lower digestibility of dry matter, N and energy but there was no evidence of discrimination when compared to good quality hay in cafeteria trials with sheep.

Table 17-8. Effect of feeding moldy hay on various parameters.[a]

Item	Good hay	Moldy hay
Dry matter intake, kg/day		
hay	7.1	6.5
total	8.8	8.2
Daily gain, kg	0.73	0.61
Feed conversion, kg	12.0	13.4
Total rumen VFA μM/ml	88.0	72.5
Rumen ammonia, mg%	23.4	15.5
Total protozoa, 1×10^5/ml	7.0	6.4
Digestibility, %		
Dry matter	63.7	53.7
Protein	76.9	53.0
Energy	63.1	54.4

[a]From Mohanty et al (1969)

Moldy silage has often been implicated in problems with ruminants. In one recent case Smith and Lynch (1973) isolated *Aspergillus fumigatus* from silage. A number of cows fed this silage had died at parturition. Some of the cows had premature, stillborn calves. Those that died showed various symptoms including liver damage; there was not, apparently, positive evidence that the moldy silage was the only toxic factor.

Molds on Grains or Other Stored Concentrates. Molds may be a serious economic problem in stored feeds if the feed is stored in a manner so that moisture level is relatively high. If the air is moist and if it is stored in containers so that heat cannot escape, heating may result. Christensen and Kaufman (1977) point out that *Aspergillus candidus* and *A. flavus* predominate when grain heats at temperatures up to 50-55°C. Above this temperature thermophilic fungi predominate and then thermophilic bacteria which may raise the temperature to 70-75°C. The combination of mold infestation, oxidation of material from the feed and long term heating drastically reduce value of the feed to say nothing of fire hazards.

There is relatively little information on poisoning of ruminants from ingestion of moldy grains (see Kingsbury, 1964). Some of the older literature reports evidence that moldy mill feed, grain, silage or forage may result in excessive hemorrhaging in cattle. Sippel et al (1954) have described field cases which occurred in cattle after ingestion of moldy corn. Deaths occurred within 3 days after the corn was first fed. Symptoms of depression and anorexia usually lasted from 1-3 days before death and were often accompanied by bloody diarrhea and bleeding from the nostrils. Further work on this problem (Burnside et al, 1957) led to the isolation of 13 fungal isolates of which *Penicillium rubrum* and *A. flavus* gave positive results for toxicity. Several isolates resulted in low plasma vitamin A. Albright et al (1964) reported death losses (20 of 29 head) in cattle fed a very moldy corn for a few days. Affected animals showed a hemorrhagic syndrome. *A. flavus, Penicillium cyclopium* and *P. palitans* were isolated from the feed. Recent reports show mold toxicity resulting from feeding moldy barley to cattle (Dyson, 1977). In this case the disease was characterized by hemorrhages, anemia, skin lesions, degenerative and inflammatory tissue changes and death in dairy cows. In another example cows fed moldy high moisture ensiled corn developed symptoms of tetany (Lynch et al, 1970). In yet another case 69 cattle in a herd of 275 died after being fed moldy cull sweet potatoes (*Ipomoea batatas*). Findings were characteristic of atypical interstitial pneumonia, and the disease could be produced experimentally by feeding cultures of *Fusarium solani* isolated from the sweet potatoes (Peckham et al, 1972).

Ergot

Ergot is a fungus (*Claviceps* spp) which infests the heads of various of cereal grains and grasses. The toxins are alkaloids which contain lysergic acid in combination with different amines. Kingsbury (1964) has reviewed the older literature on ergot poisoning, and points out that cattle, which are more subject to poisoning than other species, may show a gangrenous or a neurotoxic syndrome. He mentions several instances where very high death losses have occurred in cattle.

With respect to the gangrenous syndrome, the assumption is that this reflects a chronic poisoning. Woods et al (1966) have published a paper on this subject and have presented some excellent illustrations. In this case cattle were grazing ryegrass which was heavily infected with ergot. It was observed that it took about 10 days for the first symptoms to appear. The first symptom was lameness in the hind feet. The skin at the back of the fetlock became gangrenous and cracks formed with suppuration beneath the hard, dead skin. Separation of the hoof at the posterior aspect of the coronary band now became evident and, in some animals, extended around the horn to the front of the hoof. Later, large pieces of skin began to slough off from the back of the feet (Fig. 17-6). Lesions of various types were seen in the necrotic areas, but no lesions were seen in any place but the feet. Generally, the front

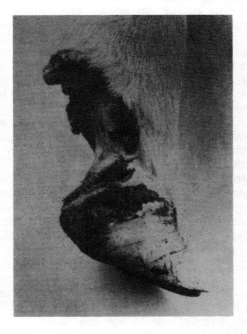

Fig. 17-6. Ergot toxicity. Hind foot lesion. Gangrenous tissue has sloughed and rupture of flexor tendons has taken place. From Woods et al (1966).

feet were less severely affected than the hind feet. Affected cows which were pregnant had normal calves or fetuses (when slaughtered). Animals that died did so from secondary causes. The primary alkaloid present was ergotamine. Other data (Goodwin, 1967) show that ergot poisoning may occur on Dallisgrass.

In other experimental studies chronic toxicity was produced in heifers and steers fed from 0.06 to 1% ergot (Dinnusson et al, 1971). The symptoms generally observed were reduced feed intake and gain, unthriftiness, increased urine excretion. In addition they were more subject to heat stress. The cattle did not shed their winter hair normally. Lameness and tender feet and legs were observed. Some were nervous and others dull and listless and recovery was not complete by 6 weeks when taken off the ergot. Skarland and Thomas (1972) reported somewhat similar results with heifers. In one trial two heifers lost 3-10 inches of their tails when fed 1.6% ergot. Heifers fed 0.2-0.8% ergot had digestive disturbances, and it was difficult to keep them on full feed.

Ergot toxicity has also been observed in cattle fed ergot infected silage made from grass (McKeon, 1971). In this instance 12 of 30 dairy cows developed gangrene of the hind legs (see Fig. 17-6) and 12 others were disposed of due to impaired production. Lameness was first observed 14 days after first feeding the silage. No abortions or gangrene of ears or tails were observed. Silage samples had 0.1% ergot (dry basis) containing 0.13% alkaloids.

Dillion (1955) has reported a case of acute ergot poisoning in cattle. These were feeder calves which had been on pasture 12 days when the first symptoms were observed. The animals stood with heads down and were trembling violently. When aroused, they started off at a rather stilted gait and then began leaping into the air, but were soon exhausted. No mention was made of death losses.

In the case of sheep, Cunningham et al, (1944) reported that typical gangrene of the extremities did not occur when ergot was given at levels which produced death. Necrosis of the tongue and ulceration in various parts of the GI tract were more typical symptoms. Clegg (1959) reported a convulsive syndrome in affected lambs on pasture. The lambs were seen to rush wildly at and through hedges and to leap into the air. They showed exceptionally violent muscular spasms. Meningitis-type lesions were seen in the brain and spinal cord.

In experimental studies with sheep, it was observed that ergotamine tartrate was considerably more toxic than ergot sclerotia. A dose of the tartrate at 0.8 mg/kg caused intestinal inflammation and hemorrhages and a dose of 1 mg/kg elicited acute responses such as coldness of the lower limbs, dyspnoea, profuse salivation and necrosis of the tongue. Hemorrhages were observed at autopsy in many of the tissues. With both the tartrate and ergot sclerotia, responses were more marked at lower temperatures (Greatorex and Mantle, 1973). In further studies with pregnant sheep (Greatorex and Mantle, 1974) when ground ergot (with 0.25% ergotamine) was fed at a rate of 0.4 g/kg of body weight, severe illness was produced; alkaloid-free ergot was not toxic at much higher levels, but similar responses were observed when ergotamine tartrate was combined with the alkaloid-free ergot. Dosage under field conditions during the 11th week of pregnancy produced illness and even death but not abortion. Dosage of animals indoors at later stages in pregnancy resulted in less acute illness but caused fetal death in 3 of 4 animals at or beyond the 3.5 mo. stage of pregnancy. It might be noted that several of these papers indicate that ergot poisoning is less likely in pastures that are closely grazed so that the seed heads are not allowed to mature and provide a place for the ergot fungus to develop.

Forage Alkaloids

A disease known in Australia as phalaris staggers results from the consumption of *Phalaris tuberosa*. It has been more of a problem with sheep than with cattle, but a paper from California (Mendel et al, 1969) reports staggers in cattle consuming canary grass (*Phalaris minor*).

Gallagher et al (1966) have described in detail the symptoms seen in affected sheep. They classify symptoms as peracute, acute and chronic, and point out that the peracute and acute syndromes may occur in the same flock within 6-12 hr of grazing toxic pasture, but the chronic syndrome takes much longer to develop. Sheep with either of the first 2 types may recover, but those showing chronic symptoms usually die due to degenerative lesions in the central nervous system. Those with the peracute form may suddenly collapse and die of heart failure. The acute stage results in prostration with convulsion spasms and extensor rigidity of the legs, similar to signs seen in tetanus. In lesser affected animals incoordination, high-stepping of the forelegs and excitability are often seen. In the chronic form persistent head nodding, ataxia or weakness of the forelegs are seen and animals may move about on their knees. Symptoms are more exaggerated in excited animals. Abnormal pigmentation may be observed in histological preparations of the brain, spinal cord, kidney or liver. Tissues showed reduced respiration rates and liver glycogen was high. Early work from Australia (Lee et al, 1957) showed that supplementation with Co was effective in providing protection, although other evidence (Moore et al, 1961) indicates this is not the case for the acute or peracute syndromes.

Ryegrass staggers occurs in sheep and cattle (Cunningham and Hartley, 1959; Clegg and Watson, 1960) in various places, but the disease is apparently less severe than phalaris staggers and few deaths have been reported. Aasen et al (1969) have isolated alkaloids from ryegrass which, when administered parenterally, caused symptoms of ryegrass staggers including the typical tetnic spasms seen in animals on pasture. In other work from Australia, Berry and Wise (1975) discuss 58 outbreaks of ryegrass toxicity in sheep and cattle on 26 properties. A variety of treatments and management methods were tried without any success. Outbreaks

occurred on pasture (79%) but also on cereal stubble, seed screenings and hay. Clinical signs were staggering, collapse, convulsions and death. Abortions occurred in pregnant sheep. Removal of affected stock from parasitized pastures with nematodes (*Anguina* spp) and bacteria (*Corynbacterium* spp) resulted in a cessation of signs and mortality within 10 days; thus it seems likely that one or both of these parasites may be the toxin producer. In other studies in New Zealand, Latch et al (1976) could not relate ryegrass staggers to fungi infections.

Fescue toxicity is another disease in which alkaloids such as peroline have been implicated (Jacobson et al, 1963). Studies on fungi associated with toxic pastures suggest *Aspergillus terreus* (Futrell et al, 1974) or other molds such as *Balansia epichloe* (Bacon et al, 1975) may be the source of the toxic alkaloids.

Fescue toxicity appears to be a problem primarily with cattle (Cunningham, 1949; Goodman, 1952; Sterns, 1953) and is, generally, more prevalent in winter and early spring. Cunningham (1949) reported that lameness may develop within 10-14 days after animals were turned out to pasture. Symptoms seen included local heat and swelling and pain in the feet and legs, and, later, development of dry, hard skin with an indented line at the junction of normal and necrotic tissue. The foot may eventually

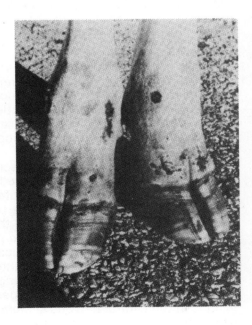
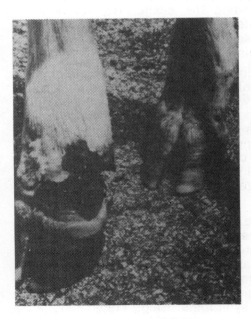

Fig. 17-7. Fescue toxicity. The picture of the hind feet of an animal on the left shows the early lesions caused by fescue toxicity. The picture on the right shows the type of lesion seen during the recovery phase. From Jacobson et al (1970).

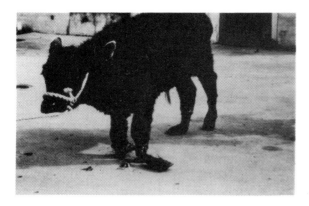

Fig. 17-8. A naturally-occurring case of fescue toxicity. Despite the loss of both front feet, the animal is in little apparent pain. Courtesy of D.R. Jacobson, University of Kentucky.

completely slough off. Extracts from some toxic plants (Walls and Jacobson, 1970) have been shown to result in a reduced heart rate and lower tail temperatures in cattle. Jacobson et al (1963, 1970) found that symptoms were seen as early as 26 days or as late as 210 days after grazing began. Incidence of toxicity ranged from 10% in some years to ca. 45% in others. Symptoms ranged from a rough haircoat to diarrhea to very slight lameness to severe necrosis of the tail or rear legs or both. Toxic extracts have been produced which cause lameness in cattle (Jacobson et al, 1963; Julien et al, 1974; Williams et al, 1975). Examples of naturally occuring symptoms are shown in Fig. 17-7 and 17-8.

In lambs given peroline monohydrochloride, crude protein and cellulose digestibility were depressed as was N retention. Rumen VFA were lower and there was some elevation of body temperature after 10 days of treatment (Boling et al, 1975).

A toxic effect has been shown on rumen microorganisms by peroline and other alkaloids from fescue; the alkaloids inhibited cellulose digestion in vitro (Bush et al, 1970; 1976). Extracts of toxic plants depressed consumption of cattle when the extracts were added to alfalfa pellets (Julien et al, 1974).

Fescue staggers are seen in some areas and tend to result in relatively high death loss after the typical manifestation of neurological symptoms. The causes remain unknown.

The occurrence of alkaloids in plants is much more widespread than might be indicated by these few brief references. Kingsbury (1964) has documented many other instances where alkaloids are found in weedy and noxious species. Nematodes which infest grasses have also been implicated as sources of toxic concentrations of alkaloids (Galloway, 1961).

Hydrocyanic Acid Poisoning

A variety of cultivated plants, particularly members of the sorghum family (sorghum, sudan grass, Johnson grass), are often offenders with respect to having lethal concentrations of cyanogenic glycosides. Many legume species as well as tame grasses, weeds, fungi, bacteria, asters and ferns also contain cyanates (Moran, 1954; Kingsbury, 1964). Linseed meal has also caused problems (Franklin and Reid, 1944; Blood and Steel, 1944) as well as white clover (Coop, 1949). In healthy plant tissue free hydrocyanic acid (HCN) is found in very low concentrations, but there may be very substantial amounts in tissues damaged by frost, wilted tissues, or those stunted by drought (Kingsbury, 1964). Ensiling decreased the HCN content (McCarty et al, 1971).

Research data indicate that intact glycosides such as amygdalin are not toxic, but become toxic after the compound is hydrolyzed to release free HCN. Damaged plants may have high concentrations of HCN. However, one reason ruminant species are more susceptible than monogastric species is that rumen microorganisms have the ability to rapidly hydrolyze these glycosides, whereas the monogastric stomach's conditions are apt to inactivate enzymes that will hydrolyze these glycosides (Moran, 1954). Coop's (1949) data show that the time required for in vitro rumen hydrolysis of lotaustralin (a glycoside in white clover) ranged from 4-22 min. for half of it to disappear.

Absorption of HCN or KCN is very rapid, data of Blakley and Coop (1950) showing that blood cyanide in sheep reached a maximum about 15 min. after dosing; although it was not back to zero level for about 5 hr. Blood thiocyanate levels took 24-48 hr to return to normal. It is probable that many of the naturally occurring cyanogenic cyanides are metabolized much less rapidly than this (Coop, 1949). The increase in blood thiocyanate is due to normal detoxification reactions, since HCN is converted by the liver to the relatively nontoxic and stable thiocyanate which then persists in the blood and other tissues for a longer period of time.

The symptoms seen in cyanide poisoning include: an early stimulation of respiration which rapidly changes to dyspnea, excitement, gasping, staggering, paralysis, prostration, convulsions, coma, and death (Kingsbury, 1964; Blood and Henderson, 1968). The most common lesions seen are dark muscle tissue, congestion or hemorrhage of the lungs, petechiation of the tracheal mucosa, and a frothy, bloody discharge from the mouth and nostrils (Moran, 1954). In animals that die rapidly, the blood is a very bright red due to its high oxygen content (Blood and Henderson, 1968). Death is due to cellular anoxia. Because of the rapid absorption of HCN from the rumen, death may occur (when HCN or KCN are given) as early as 15 min. after dosing although many animals may survive for several hr (Coop and Blakley, 1950). The first symptoms may be seen within 1-2 min. following oral dosing with HCN and in 3-7 min. after dosing with lotaustralin and severe symptoms in 5-10 and 15-25 min., respectively.

The minimum lethal dose of free cyanide given orally is about 2.4 mg/kg of body weight in sheep and about 4.5 mg/kg of lotaustralin (Coop and Blakley, 1950). Cattle appear to be slightly more susceptible than sheep (Moran, 1954). Starvation has been shown to result in a delayed reaction in sheep given lotaustralin (Coop and Blakley, 1950), but starved rams have been shown to be more susceptible to poisoning from linseed meal (Franklin and Reid, 1944). If ingested rapidly enough, an intake of 5-7 mg may be lethal to sheep. Coop and Blakley suggest that the ingestion of 7 mg of HCN equivalent as fresh clover in 15 min. would be fatal to sheep. These authors mention some data of Rose (1941) in which cattle were observed to eat sudan grass containing 0.13% HCN without problems when pastured continuously on the grass, but high mortality was observed in cattle grazing 1-2 hr/day on sudan that contained as little as 0.07% HCN. These data indicate clearly that speed of ingestion is critical; the moderate and continuous ingestion of HCN or cyanogenic glycosides allows the tissues to detoxify it at sufficient speed so that it is not harmful. Moran (1954) points out that nitrate fertilization is apt to increase the HCN content of plants. Continued ingestion of moderate levels of cyanogens—as in the case of those in white clover—results in higher levels of thiocyanate in the serum than is usually seen (Worker, 1957). Levels found in sheep (Flux et al, 1956) are in the range in which thiocyanates will cause goiter in rats and guinea pigs.

Other Plant Toxins

There are many other plant toxins or poisons that have been documented in the literature. For example, the presence of goitrongenic compounds, especially in the Brassica genera (cabbage family) is well known. Legume species—particularly red clover—also are known to have plant estrogens in concentrations that may interfere with reproduction processes in sheep (see Drane and Saba, 1968). Many plants, especially weedy species, have toxic concentrations of oxalates (see Kingsbury, 1964). Lupines are often toxic, resulting in a condition in cattle called the crooked-calf syndrome (Shupe, 1970). Thus, these as well as many others may be a problem at times for ruminant species. Further details are given on toxic species in Ch. 15.

References Cited

Starvation

Attebery, J.T. and H.D. Johnson. 1969. J. Animal Sci. 29:734.
Blaxter, K.L. and W.A. Wood. 1951. Brit. J. Nutr. 5:53.
Brown, R.E. and J.C. Shaw. 1957. J. Dairy Sci. 40:667.
Butterfield, R.M. 1966. Res. Vet. Sci. 7:168.
Cakala, S. and A. Albrycht. 1977. Nutr. Abstr. Rev. 47:777.
Christian, K.R. and V.J. Williams. 1960. N.Z. J. Agr. Res. 3:389.
Coop, I.E. 1949. N.Z. J. Sci. Tech. 31A:1.
Dale, H.E., C.K. Goberdhan and S. Brody. 1954. Amer. J. Vet. Res. 15:197.
Dalton, R.G. 1966. Vet. Rec. 79:53.
Dalton, G.R. 1967. Brit. Vet. J. 123:237.

Dean, R.E. 1973. Ph.D. Thesis, Oregon State University, Corvallis.

Dean, R.E., et al. 1975. J. Wildl. Mgmt. 39:601.

DeCalesta, D.S., J.G. Nagy and J.A. Bailey. 1975. J. Wildl. Mgmt. 38:815.

Emmanuel, B. and A. Nahapetian. 1975. J. Animal Sci. 41:1468.

Farrell, D.J., R.A. Leng and J.L. Corbett. 1972. Aust. J. Agr. Res. 23:483.

Farrell, D.J. and T.F. Reardon. 1972. Aust. J. Agr. Res. 23:511.

Fowle, K.E. and D.C. Church. 1973. Am. J. Vet. Res. 34:849.

Gerstell, R. 1972. Pennsylvania Game Comm. Bul. 3.

Gupta, D.N. 1967. Indian Vet. J. 44:942.

Hecker, J.F., O.E. Budtz-Olsen and M. Ostwald. 1964. Aust. J. Agr. Res. 15:961.

Herd, R.P. 1966. Aust. Vet. J. 42:269.

Hashizume, T. et al. 1976. Nutr. Abstr. Rev. 46:133.

Hershberger, T.V. and R.L. Cowan. 1972. J. Animal Sci. 35:266 (abstr).

Hight, G.K. and R.A. Barton. 1965. J. Agr. Sci. 64:413.

Hyden, S. 1961. In: Digestive Physiology and Nutrition of the Ruminant. Butterworths Pub. Co.

Jackson, H.D., C.A. Burtis and G.D. Goetsch. 1966. Amer. J. Vet. Res. 27:885.

Jackson, H.D. and V.W. Winkler. 1970. J. Nutr. 100:201.

Jensen, R. et al. 1951. Amer. J. Vet. Res. 15:202.

Joassart, J.M. 1977. Nutr. Abstr. Rev. 47:385.

Johnson, G., L. Hassler and K. Ostlund. 1966. Acta. Vet. Scand. 7:143.

Juhasz, B. 1963. Nutr. Abstr. Rev. 33:1039.

Keenan, D.M. and W.R. McManus. 1970. J. Agr. Sci. 74:477.

Liebholz, J. 1970. Aust. J. Agr. Res. 21:723.

Lindsay, D.B., J.W. Steel and P.J. Buttery. 1977. Proc. Nutr. Soc. 36:33A.

Manns, E. 1972. Res. Vet. Sci. 13:140.

Martin, A.K. 1969. Brit. J. Nutr. 23:715.

Martin, R.J., L.L. Wilson, R.L. Cowan and J.D. Sink. 1973. J. Animal Sci. 36:101.

Masters, C.J. and D.J. Horgen. 1962. Aust. J. Agr. Res. 13:1082.

Meiske, J.C., R.L. Salsbury, J.A. Hoefer and R.W. Luecke. 1958. J. Animal Sci. 17:774.

Meyer, J.H., W.C. Weir and J.D. Smith. 1955. J. Animal Sci. 14:160.

Meyer, J.H., W.C. Weir and D.T. Torell. 1962. J. Animal Sci. 21:916.

Munchow, H.B. et al. 1976. Archiv fur Tierr. 7:533.

Nesic, P. 1961. Nutr. Abstr. Rev. 31:113.

Otsuka, J. and T. Nakajima. 1959. Nutr. Abstr. Rev. 29:913.

Panaretto, B.A. 1968. Aust. J. Agr. Res. 19:273.

Pearson, H.A. 1969. USDA Forest Service Research Note, Rocky Mountain Forest and Range Expt. Sta., Ft. Collins.

Price, M.A. 1977. Aust. J. Agr. Res. 28:521, 529.

Quin, J.W., W. Oyaert and R. Clark. 1951. Onderstepoort J. Vet. Res. 25:51.

Reid, C.S.W. 1963. Proc. N. Aust. Soc. Animal Prod. 23:169.

Reid, I.M. et al. 1977. Proc. Nutr. Soc. 36:41A; J. Comp. Path. 87:253.

Robertson, A., H. Paver, P. Barden and T.G. Marr. 1960. Res. Vet. Sci. 1:117.

Robertson, A. and C. Thin. 1953. Brit. J. Nutr. 7:181.

Rumsey, T.S. and J. Bond. 1976. J. Animal Sci. 42:1227.

Saba, N. et al. 1966. J. Agr. Sci. 67:129.

Sasaki, M., Y. Yamatani and I. Otani. 1974. Nutr. Abstr. Rev. 44:613.

Slater, J.S. and D.J. Mellor. 1977. Res. Vet. Sci. 22:95.

Suzuki, A. 1965. Tohoku J. Agr. Res. 16:117.

Vercoe, J.E. 1970. Brit. J. Nutr. 24:599.

Warner, A.C.I. 1962. J. Gen. Microbiol. 28:129.

Weeth, H.J., C.R. Torell and D.W. Cassard. 1959. J. Animal Sci. 18:694.

White, R.R., K.R. Christian and V.J. Williams. 1956. N.Z. J. Sci. Tech. 38A:440.

Williams, V.J. and K.R. Christian. 1959. N.Z. J. Agr. Res. 2:677.

Zelenak, I., J. Varady, K. Boda and I. Havassy. 1972. Physiol. Bohemoslovaca. 21:531.

Diarrhea

Acres, S.D., J.R. Saunders and O.M. Radostits. 1977. Can. Vet. J. 18:113.

Blaxter, K.L. and W.A. Wood. 1953. Vet. Rec. 65:889.

Bullen, J.J. and I. Battey. 1957. Vet. Rec. 69:1268.

Burt, A.W.A. and S.M. Irvine. 1970. Animal Prod. 12:376.

Bywater, R.J. and W.J. Penhale. 1969. Res. Vet. Sci. 10:591.

Carter, J.M. 1969. J. Amer. Vet. Med. Assoc. 154:1168.

Dalton, R.G. 1964. Brit. Vet. J. 120:378.

Dalton, R.G. 1968. Brit. Vet. J. 124:371.

Dalton, R.G., E.W. Fisher and W.I.M. McIntyre. 1965. Brit. Vet. J. 121:34.

Dalton, R.G. and G.D. Phillips. 1969. Brit. Vet. J. 125:367.

Demigne, C. and C. Remsey. 1978. Nutr. Abstr. Rev. 48:147.

Dovrak, M. and P. Safarovsky. 1971. Veterinarian's SPOFA. 4:197.

Edwards, A.J. and L.L. Williams. 1972. VM/SAC, March.

Fayet, J.C. 1969. Nutr. Abstr. Rev. 39:1376.

Fayet, J.C. 1971. Brit. Vet. J. 127:37.

Fey, H. 1971. Ann. N.Y. Acad. Sci. 176:49.

Fisher, E.W. 1973. Ann. Rech. Veter. 4:191.

Fisher, E.W. and G.H. de LaFuente. 1972. Vet. Sci. 13:315.

Fisher, E.W. and A.A. Martinez. 1975. Brit. Vet. J. 131:190.

Fisher, E.W. and A.D. McEwan. 1967. Brit. Vet. J. 123:4.

Gorrill, A.D.L. and J.W.G. Nicholson. 1969. Can. J. Animal Sci. 49:305.

Grys, S. and A. Malinowska. 1974. Acta Microbiol. Polonica. 6:185.

Hull, B.L. 1972. J. Amer. Vet. Med. Assoc. 161:1291.

Lewis, L.D. and R.W. Phillips. 1972. Cornell Vet. 62:596.

Lewis, L.D. and R.W. Phillips. 1973. Ann. de Rech. Vet. 4:99.

Lewis, L.D., R.W. Phillips and C.D. Elliott. 1975. Amer. J. Vet. Res. 36:413.

Logan, E.F. and W.J. Penhale. 1971. Vet. Rec. 27:222.

McLean, D.M. and L.F. Baily. 1972. Aust. Vet. J. 48:336.

Melichar, B. and J. Masek. 1971. Acta Vet. Brno. Suppl. 2:117.

Michel, M.C. 1971. Ann. Biol. Anim. Bioch. Biophys. 11:304.

Mylrea, P.J. 1966. Res. Vet. Sci. 7:407.

Mylrea, P.J. 1968. Res. Vet. Sci. 9:5,14.

Penhale, W.J., E.F. Logan and A. Stenhouse. 1971. Vet. Rec. 89:623.

Phillips, R.W., L.D. Lewis and K.L. Knox. 1971. Ann. N.Y. Acad. Sci. 176:231.

Radostits, O.M. 1965. J. Amer. Vet. Med. Assoc. 147:1367.

Radostits, O.M. 1975. J. Dairy Sci. 58:464.

Reisinger, R.C. 1965. J. American Vet. Med. Assoc. 147:1377.

Roy, J.H.B. 1964. Vet. Rec. 76:511.

Roy, J.H.B. 1969. Proc. Nutr. Soc. 28:160.

Roy, J.H.B. et al. 1955. Brit. J. Nutr. 9:11.

Roy, J.H.B. et al. 1959. Brit. J. Nutr. 13:219.

Salaganeau, G., D. Curca, I. Ursu and A. Batrinu. 1972. Nutr. Abstr. Rev. 42:403.

Shaw, W.B. 1971. Brit. Vet. J. 127:214.

Shillam, K.W.G. and J.H.B. Roy. 1963. Brit. J. Nutr. 17:171;183.

Shillam, K.W.G., J.H.B. Roy and P.L. Ingram. 1962. Brit. J. Nutr. 16:267,585,593.

Slagsvold, P. et al. 1977. Acta. Vet. Scand. 18:194.

Smith, H.W. 1965. J. Path. Bact. 90:495.

Smith, H.W. 1971. Ann. N.Y. Acad. Sci. 176:110.

Tagari, H. and J.H.B. Roy. 1969. Brit. J. Nutr. 23:763.

Tennant, B., D. Harrold and M. Reina-Guerra. 1968. Cornell Vet. 58:136.

Thornton, J.R., G.G. Butler and R.A. Willoughby. 1973. Aust. Vet. J. 49:20.

Thornton, J.R. and P.B. English. 1972. Cited by Fisher and Martinez (1975). Brit. Vet. J. 131:190.

Thornton, J.R., R.A. Willoughby and B.J. McSherry. 1972. Can. J. Compl. Med. 36:17.

Tsvetkov, O.X. 1972. Nutr. Abstr. Rev. 42:399.

Watt, J.G. 1967. J. Amer. Vet. Med. Assoc. 150:742.

Wilgenbusch, L.C. and J.W. Sexton. 1971. Iowa State U. Vet. 1971. p. 153.

Willoughby, R.A., D.G. Butler and J.R. Thornton. 1970. Can. Vet. J. 11:173.

Parasites

Ames, E.R., R. Rubin and J.K. Matsushima. 1969. J. Animal Sci. 28:698.

Anderson, N., R. Blake and D.A. Titchen. 1976. Parasit. 72:1.

Barger, I.A. 1973. Aust. J. Exp. Agr. Anim. Husb. 13:42.

Bawden, R.J. 1970. Brit. J. Nutr. 24:291.

Bennett, D.G., S.D. Van DeWark and H.D. Jackson. 1968. Amer. J. Vet. Res. 29:2135.

Berry, C.I. and J.D. Dargie. 1976. Vet. Parasit. 2:317.

Blood, D.C. and J.A. Henderson. 1968. Veterinary Medicine (3rd ed.). Williams and Wilkins Co.

Ciordia, H. and W.E. Bizzel. 1963. J. Parasit. 49:44.

Ciordia, H. et al. 1977. J. Am. Vet. Res. 38:1335.

Coop, R.L., C.J. Mapes and K.W. Angus. 1972. Res. Vet. Sci. 13:186.

Coop, R.L., A.R. Sykes and K.W. Angus. 1976. Vet. Sci. 21:253.

Deo, P.G., K.C. Tandon, V. Kumar and H.D. Srivastava. 1967. Indian J. Vet. Sci. An. Hus. 37:351.

Dharsana, R.S., J.P. Fabiyi and G.W. Hutchinson. 1976. Vet. Parasit. 2:333.

Downey, N.E. 1965. Brit. Vet. J. 121:362.

Downey, N.E., J.F. Connolly and J. O'Shea. 1969. Vet. Rec. 85:201.

Downey, N.E., J.F. Connolly and J. O'Shea. 1972. Irish J. Agr. Res. 11:11.

Elmagdoub, A. and M.F. Badr. 1966. Alexandria J. Agr. Res. 14:197.

Emerick, R.J. et al. 1957. J. Animal Sci. 16:937.

Evans, J.V., M.H. Blunt and W.H. Southcott. 1963. Aust. J. Agr. Res. 14:549.

Eveleth, D.F., A.I. Goldsby, F.M. Brolin. 1953. Vet. Med. 48:441.

Fitzsimmons, W.M. 1966. Res. Vet. Sci. 7:101.

Gardiner, M.R. 1966. J. Helminthol. 40:63.

Goldberg, A. 1965. J. Parasit. 51:948.

Gordon, H.M. 1950. Aust. Vet. J. 26:46.

Gordon, H.M. 1964. Aust. Vet. J. 40:55.

Holmes, P.H. and J.M. McLean. 1971. Res. Vet. Sci. 12:265.

Hope Cawdery, M.J., K.L. Strickland, A. Conway and P.J. Crowe. 1977. Brit. Vet. J. 133:145.

Horton, G.M. 1977. J. Animal Sci. 45:891,1453.

Jordan, H.E., N.A. Cole, J.E. McCroskey and S.A. Ewing. 1977. Amer. J. Vet. Res. 38:1157.

McLeay, L.M., N. Anderson, J.B. Bingley and D.A. Titchen. 1973. Parasit. 66:241.

Miller, R.F. 1968. Presented at 2nd World Conf. on Animal Prod., College Park, Maryland.

Neville, W.E., T.B. Stewart and W.C. McCormick. 1977. J. Animal Sci. 44:1119.

Pullan, N.B., M.H. Sewell and J.A. Hammond. 1970. Brit. Vet. J. 126:543.

Reid, J.F.S., J. Doyle, J. Armour and F.W. Jennings. 1972. Vet. Rec. 90:486.

Reveron, A.E. et al. 1974. Res. Vet. Sci. 16:299,310.

Rhorbacker, G.H., D.A. Porter and H. Herlich. 1958. Amer. J. Vet. Res. 19:625.

Roseby, F.B. 1973. Aust. J. Agr. Res. 24:947.

Roseby, F.B. 1977. Aust. J. Agr. Res. 28:155,713.

Roseby, F.B. and R.A. Leng. 1974. Aust. J. Agr. Res. 25:363.

Ross, J.G. and C. Dow. 1965. Brit. Vet. J. 121:18.

Ross, J.G. and J.R. Todd. 1965. Brit. Vet. J. 121:55.

Ross, J.G. et al. 1970. Brit. Vet. J. 126:159;393.

Soliam, K.N. 1953. Brit. Vet. J. 109:148.

Sykes, A.R. and R.L. Coop. 1976. J. Agr. Sci. 86:507.

Sykes, A.R. and R.L. Coop. 1977. J. Agr. Sci. 88:671.

Theurer, R.C. et al. 1965. Amer. J. Vet. Res. 26:123.

Threkeld, W.L., O.N. Price and W.N. Lindous. 1956. Amer. J. Vet. Res. 17:246.

Titchen, D.A. and N. Anderson. 1977. Aust. Vet. J. 53:369.

Utech, K.B.W., R.H. Wharton and L.A. Wooderson. 1969. Aust. Vet. J. 45:414.

Utley, P.R., T.B. Stewart, H. Ciordia and W.C. McCormick. 1974. J. Animal Sci. 38:984.

van Adrichem, P.W.M. and J.C. Shaw. 1977. J. Animal Sci. 46:417,423.

Vegors, H.H., D.M. Baird, O.E. Sell and T.B. Steward. 1956. J. Animal Sci. 15:1199.

Vercoe, J.E. and P.H. Springell. 1969. J. Agr. Sci. 73:203.

Vetter, R.L., W.G. Hoekstra, A.C. Todd and A.L. Pope. 1963. Amer. J. Vet. Res. 24:439.

Waymack, L.B. and B.J. Torbert. 1969. Amer. J. Vet. Res. 30:2145.

Weir, W.C. et al. 1948. J. Animal Sci. 7:466.

Poisonous Plants and Fungi

Aasen, A.J. et al. 1969. Aust. J. Agr. Res. 20:71.

Abrams, L. 1965. J.S. African Med. Assoc. 36:5.

Albright, J.L. et al. 1964. J. Amer. Vet. Med. Assoc. 144:1013.

Allcroft, R. and G. Lewis. 1963. Vet. Rec. 75:487.

Allcroft, R., H. Rogers and G. Lewis. 1966. Nature 209:154.

Armbrecht, B.H. and W.T. Shalkop. 1972. Environ. Physiol. Biochem. 2:3.

Asplund, J.M. 1971. J. Animal Sci. 33:275 (abstr.).

Bacon, C.W., J.K. Porter and J.D. Robbins. 1975. Appl. Microbiol. 29:553.

Berry, P.H. and J.L. Wise. 1975. Aust. Vet. J. 51:525.

Blakley, R.L. and I.E. Coop. 1950. N.Z. J. Sci. Tech. 31A(3):1.

Blood, D.C. and J.A. Henderson. 1968. Veterinary Medicine (3rd ed.) Williams & Wilkins Co.

Blood, D.C. and J.D. Steel. 1944. Aust. Vet. J. 20:338.

Boling, J.A. et al. 1975. J. Animal Sci. 40:972.

Burnside, J.E. et al. 1957. Amer. J. Vet. Res. 18:817.

Bush, L.P., H. Burton and J.A. Boling. 1976. J. Agr. Food Chem. 24:869.

Bush, L.P., C. Streeter and R.C. Buckner. 1970. Crop. Sci. 10:108.

Byers, J.H. and H.P. Broquist. 1960. J. Dairy Sci. 43:873 (abstr.),

Byers, J.H. and H.P. Broquist. 1961. J. Dairy Sci. 44:1179 (abstr.),

Christensen, C.M. and H.H. Kaufman. 1977. Feedstuffs 49(44):39.

Clegg, F.G. 1959. Vet. Rec. 71:824.

Clegg, F.G. and H. Bryson. 1962. Vet. Rec. 74:992.

Clegg, F.G. and W.A. Watson. 1960. Vet. Rec. 72:731.

Coop, I.E. 1949. N.Z. J. Sci. Tech. 30A:277.

Coop, I.E. and R.L. Blakley. 1950. N.Z. J. Sci . Tech. 31A(5):44.

Crawford, M. 1962. Vet. Bul. 32:415.

Crump, M.H. and J.N. Henning. 1963. J. Amer. Vet. Med. Assoc. 143:996.

Crump, M.H., E.B. Smalley, R.E. Nichols and D.P. Rainey. 1967. Amer. J. Vet. Res. 28:865.

Cunningham, I.J. 1949. Aust. Vet. J. 25:27.

Cunningham, I.J. and W.J. Hartley. 1959. N.Z. Vet. J. 7:1.

Cunningham, I.J., J.B. Swan and C.S.M. Hopkirk. 1944. N.Z. J. Sci. Tech. 26A:121.

Dillon, B.E. 1955. J. Amer. Vet. Med. Assoc. 126:136.

Dinnusson, W.E., C.N. Haugse and R.D. Knutson. 1971. Farm Res. 29(2):20.

Drane, H.M. and N. Saba. 1968. J. Agr. Sci. 70:165.

Dyson, D.A. 1977. Vet. Rec. 100:400.

Edds, G.T. 1973. J. Amer. Vet. Med. Assoc. 162:304.

Flatla, J.L., E. Mordum and T. Homb. 1971. Nutr. Abstr. Rev. 41:1072.

Flux, D.S. et al. 1956. N.Z. J. Sci. Tech. 38A:88.

Franklin, M.C. and R.L. Reid. 1944. Aust. Vet. J. 20:332.

Futrell, M.C. et al. 1974. J. Environ. Qual. 3:140.

Gallagher, C.H., J.H. Kock and H. Hoffman. 1966. Aust. Vet. J. 42:279.

Galloway, J.H. 1961. J. Amer. Vet. Med. Assoc. 139:1212.

Garrett, W.N., H. Heitman and A.N. Booth. 1968. Proc. Soc. Expt. Biol. Med. 127:188.

Gibbons, W.J., E.J. Catcott and J.F. Smithcors (ed.). 1970. Bovine Medicine and Surgery. American Veterinary Publications, Inc.

Goodman, A.A. 1952. J. Amer. Vet. Med. Assoc. 121:289.

Goodwin, D.E. 1967. J. Amer. Vet. Med. Assoc. 151:204.

Greatorex, J.C. and P.G. Mantle. 1973. Res. Vet. Sci. 15:337.

Greatorex, J.C. and P.G. Mantle. 1974. J. Reprod. Fertility 37:33.

Harwig, J. and I.C. Munro. 1975. Can. Vet. J. 16:125.

Horrocks, D.A., W. Burt, D.C. Thomas and M.C. Lancaster. 1965. Animal Prod. 7:253.

Jacobson, D.R. et al. 1963. J. Dairy Sci. 46:416.

Jacobson, D.R. et al. 1970. J. Dairy Sci. 53:575.

Julien, W.E., F.A. Martz, M. Williams and G.B. Garner. 1974. J. Dairy Sci. 57:1385.

Kidder, R.W., D.W. Beardsley and T.C. Erwin. 1961. Florida Agr. Expt. Sta. Bul. 630.

Kingsbury, J.M. 1964. Poisonous Plants of the United States and Canada. Prentice-Hall, Inc.

Lancaster, M.C. 1969. Proc. Nutr. Soc. 28:203.

Latch, G.C.M., R.E. Falloon and M.J. Christensen. 1976. N.Z. J. Agr. Res. 19:233.

Lee, H.J., R.E. Kuchel, B.F. Good and R.F. Trowbridge. 1957. Aust. J. Agr. Res. 8:494.

Lewis, G., L.M. Markson and R. Allcroft. 1967. Vet. Rec. 80:312.

Loosemore, R.M. and L.M. Markson. 1961. Vet. Rec. 73:813.

Lynch, G.P. et al. 1970. J. Dairy Sci. 53:1292.

Lynch, G.P. et al. 1971. J. Dairy Sci. 54:1688.

Lynch, G.P., F.T. Covey, D.F. Smith and B.T. Weinland. 1972. J. Animal Sci. 35:65.

Lynch, G.P., D.F. Smith, F.C. Covey and C.H. Gordon. 1973. J. Dairy Sci. 56:1154.

Lynch, G.P., G.C. Todd, W.T. Shalkop and L.A. Moore. 1970. J. Dairy Sci. 53:63.

Mathur, C.F., R.C. Smith and G.E. Hawkins. 1976. J. Dairy Sci. 59:455.

McFarlane, D., J.V. Evans and C.S.W. Reid. 1959. N.Z. J. Agr. Res. 2:194.

McCarty, G., E. Gray, E.R. Shipe and L.D. Brown. 1971. Agron. J. 63:402.

McKeon, F.W. 1971. Irish Vet. J. 25:67.

McKinney, J.C. et al. 1973. J. Amer. Oil Chem. Soc. 50:79.

Mendel, V.E., G.L. Crenshaw, N.F. Baker and R. Muniz. 1969. J. Amer. Vet. Med. Assoc. 154:769.

Mohanty, G.P., N.A. Jorgensen, R.M. Luther and H.H. Voelker. 1969. J. Dairy Sci. 52:79.

Moore, R.M., G.W. Arnold and R.J. Hutchings. 1961. Aust. J. Sci. 24:88.

Moran, E.A. 1954. Amer. J. Vet. Res. 15:171.

Newberne, P.M. 1972. Clin. Toxicol. 5:439.

Nyvall, R.F. 1977. Feestuffs. July 11 issue, p. 20.

Peckham, J.C., F.E. Mitchell, O.H. Jones and B. Doupnik. 1972. J. Amer. Vet. Med. Assoc. 160:169.

Pelhate, J. 1967. Nutr. Abstr. Rev. 37:652.

Percival, J.C. 1959. N.Z. J. Agr. Res. 2:1041.

Pier, A.C. 1973. J. Amer. Vet. Med. Assoc. 163:1259.

Prior, M.G. 1975. Can. J. Comp. Med. 40:75.

Rainey, D.P., E.B. Smalley, M.H. Crump and F.M. Strong. 1965. Nature 205:203.

Rajan, A., M.K. Neir and C.G. Sivadas. 1973. Kerala J. Vet. Sci. 4:109.

Rose, A.L. 1941. Aust. Vet. J. 17:211.

Shadmi, A., R. Volcani and T.A. Nobel. 1974. Zb. Vet. Med. A. 21:544.

Shupe, J.L. 1970. In: Bovine Medicine and Surgery. American Veterinary Publications, inc.

Sippel, W.L., J.E. Burnside and M.B. Atwood. 1954. Proc. Amer. Vet. Med. Assoc. 90:174.

Skarland, A.S. and O.O. Thomas. 1972. Proc. West. Sec. Amer. Soc. An. Sci. 23:426.

Smith, D.F. and G.P. Lynch. 1973. J. Dairy Sci. 56:828.

Sterns, T.J. 1953. J. Amer. Vet. Med. Assoc. 122:388.

Upcott, D.H. 1970. Nutr. Abstr. Rev. 40:1515.

Walls, J.R. and D.R. Jacobson. 1970. J. Animal Sci. 30:420.

Williams, M. et al. 1975. Amer. J. Vet. Res. 36:1353.

Wilson, B.J. and C.H. Wilson. 1961. Amer. J. Vet. Res. 22:961.

Woods, A.J., J.B. Jones and P.G. Mantle. 1966. Vet. Res. 78:742.

Worker, N.A. 1957. N.Z. J. Sci. Tech. 38A:709.

Chapter 18 - Nutrient-Nutrient, Nutrient-Hormonal and Nutrient-Genetic Interactions

By Werner G. Bergen

INTRODUCTION

All nutrients (or metabolites) have a specific function in cellular metabolism of organisms. For instance, vitamin A plays a specific role in the maintenance of epithelial tissues but this vitamin is a relatively unstable compound and susceptible to oxidation. Without adequate vitamin E in the diet (E acts as an antioxidant) during marginal vitamin A consumption, a vitamin A deficiency can occur and, conversely, if vitamin E is adequate, vitamin A is protected from excessive oxidation and the dietary needs of this vitamin are lower. This is an example of a nutrient-nutrient interaction where a certain nutrient promotes the activity of another nutrient without specifically modulating the site of action of the latter nutrient.

Similarly, such interactions can occur between nutrients and hormones or nutrients and genetic (phenotypic) characteristics. For example, the consumption of glucose in non-ruminants or absorption of certain VFA from the rumen in ruminants enhances N (protein) accretion in growing animals. While glucose and VFA are energy sources for cellular ATP generation and ATP is obviously necessary for peptide bond synthesis, this response of glucose (or VFA) on protein metabolism is elicited by insulin, where secretion is stimulated by glucose (and VFA) and which is necessary for normal carbohydrate metabolism by the tissues. Genetic variations in the ability of animals to synthesize certain α-keto acids affects their dietary needs for essential amino acids. In mammalian systems arginine is synthesized during the urea cycle, while in poultry this metabolic pathway is absent and arginine is a dietary essential for these animals.

In this chapter a number of these types of interactions will be discussed in detail. Although emphasis will be placed on such interactions in ruminants, many pertinent examples have only been described in non-ruminants and will be included here.

NUTRIENT-NUTRIENT INTERACTION IN RUMINAL FERMENTATIONS

A number of nutrients exert modifying effects on quantitative and qualitative aspects of the ruminal fermentation beyond their usual role in general metabolism. Three major areas of such interactions will be discussed: the phenomenon of reduced roughage (fiber) digestibility by the inclusion of grains (α-linked soluble carbohydrates) or associative (interactional) effects of feedstuffs and its implication to animal performance; the interrelationship between N (NH_3-N) availability, carbohydrate fermentation and cofactors (such as S or carbon skeletons) on optimal dry matter digestion and microbial protein synthesis; the interaction of dietary ingredients and physical state (processing) on ruminal dilution rate and ruminal microbial cell growth.

Associative Effects of Feeds

It has been shown clearly that the nutritive value of a ration ingredient varies with the ration to which it is added. These associative effects of ration ingredients result in differences in the animals' metabolism as influenced by the physical and chemical makeup of the ration. The most dramatic of these interactions is the well known depressing effects of starch or any soluble α-linked carbohydrate on fiber digestibility. Upon addition of rapidly fermented concentrates to a high roughage ration, the rate of fiber digestion falls and the intake and proportional utilization of roughage is decreased (only if fed separately) (Lonsdale et al, 1971). The ruminal mechanism responsible for the depressed fiber digestibility has not been elucidated clearly but microorganisms tend to use the most readily available carbohydrates as an energy source. The cellulolytic organisms may then utilize glucose (arising from α-linked CHO) directly and the production of cellulase may be decreased. Further, the microbial population may also shift toward a higher proportion of amylolytic microorganism while the growth of cellulolytic organisms may be discouraged.

The most visible effect of the above interaction is observed in the energy metabolism and performance of growing ruminants when the proportion of concentrates and roughages are varied in ration formulations in response to costs of various feed ingredients.

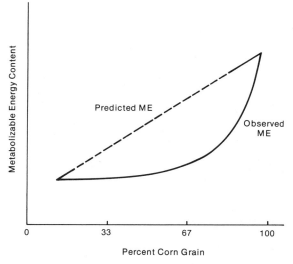

Fig. 18-1. Predicted and observed metabolizable energy value of rations fed to steers as corn grain is increased from 0 (all roughage) to 100 percent (all grain).

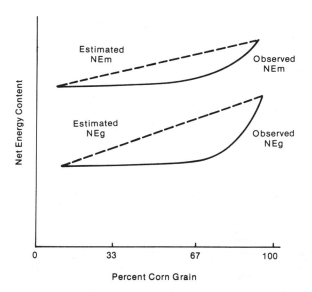

Fig. 18-2. Predicted and observed net energy value of rations fed to steers as corn grain is increased from 0 (all roughage) to 100 percent (all grain).

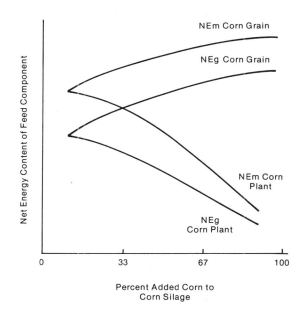

Fig. 18-3. Net energy for maintenance and gain values of corn silage - added corn grain rations.

When the NE or ME systems are used to predict ration NE or ME and performance, the calculated ration NE, ME or expected gains are not always equal to the observed values. This point is well demonstrated in Fig. 18-1, 2. Byers et al (1975) calculated the expected ME/kg of DM as increasing amounts of corn were added to a basal corn silage ration. Using individual ME values (eg. those established when feeding the feedstuff alone) for both corn silage and corn grain, the expected ME change in response to corn addition was positive and linear at each level of corn addition (Fig. 18-1). The observed ME curve did not conform to the predicted ME pattern. Rather, corn substitution up to about 50% resulted in a very small increase in the ration ME content (Fig. 18-1). A similar situation arises when predicted and observed NEm and NEg values from corn silage-corn grain rations are compared (Fig. 18-2). Finally, the contribution of the corn plant (non-grain) component to the total NEm or NEg content of corn silage-corn grain ration declined with each added increment of corn grain (Fig. 18-3). Not only does the inclusion of readily fermentable carbohydrate depress fiber digestibility, but also the pattern of fermentation end products is changed from a predominantly high acetate-low propionate to a low acetate-higher propionate pattern. This change in fermentation pattern modifies the efficiency of ME utilization such that

432

with higher propionate production the efficiency of ME utilization increases (Blaxter and Wainman, 1964). This phenomenon can be called an interactional effect of ration ingredients at the cellular level. In the conventional energy utilization scheme, $ME = NEm + Heat\ Increment\ (HI)$ (see Ch. 8). The HI of propionate and butyrate (in short trials) are usually assumed to be lower than for acetate, hence fermentations producing less acetate should yield a higher $NEm + p$.

This simple analysis of the fact that NE increases as a % of ME as the proportion of concentrate increases in grain-roughage rations is not universally shared. The difficulty lies in the HI value of acetate when measured alone or as part of a VFA mixture. The work of Blaxter and co-workers indicated a HI of 40.8, 13.5 and 18.9 Kcal/100 Kcal ME for acetate, propionate and butyrate, respectively, and HI of 17 Kcal/100 Kcal ME for a 5:3:2 Ac-Pro-But. mixture. The high HI for acetate was only noted when Ac was at least 90% (meq. basis) of the VFA mixture. Holter et al (1970), although confirming the individual HI of the VFA as reported by Blaxter, obtained a HI value of 32% (% of ME) for a 5:3:2 VFA mixture. The HI of VFA when given above maintenance were higher and shifts in acid ratios markedly affected the over-all HI. Thus the HI of 75:15:10 and 25:45:30 (Ac-Pr-But) VFA mixtures were 68 and 42 Kcal/100 Kcal ME, respectively (Armstrong et al, 1958). More recent work (Ørskov and co-workers, 1966) could not confirm the above results and their data showed that the animals' efficiency of VFA utilization for single or VFA mixtures were not greatly different. These workers speculated that the higher HI or poorer energetic efficiency of high roughage rations is due to losses within the rumen during the production of acetate rather than in its subsequent utilization.

As already noted the change in efficiency of ME utilization in rations containing all roughage to rations containing high levels of readily fermentable carbohydrates has been studied and an increase in NE as % of ME has been reported by various workers as the proportion of grain increases. Blaxter and Wainman (1964) reported that the efficiency of ME utilization increased linearly both for maintenance and fattening (Fig. 18-4) although the slope for fattening was steeper. Vance et al (1972) varied corn and corn silage in feedlot rations and found that the efficiency of ME utilization for maintenance increased linearly with each increment of corn: however, the efficiency of ME utiliza-

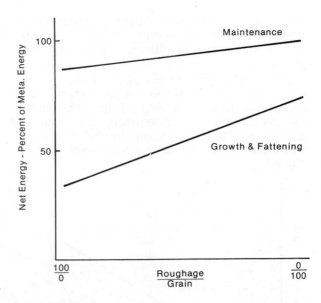

Fig. 18-4. Efficiency of metabolizable energy utilization (NE) for maintenance and gain in ruminants for rations of varying roughage to grain ratios. (Adapted from Blaxter and Wainman, 1964).

tion for growth increased in a curvilinear fashion with the most rapid increase at high corn grain content in the ration.

More recently Byers et al (1975) have shown that in feedlot cattle fed varying corn grain-corn silage rations, both NEm and NEg increased in a curvilinear manner as the ration corn content increased (Fig. 18-2). The number of animals used in this work was rather small and may have a bearing on their results. The higher efficiency of ME utilization appears to be related to the increasing propionate fermentation and hence a steadily decreasing HI component of the ME. Although the increase of energy efficiency of ME can easily be shown as the proportion of concentrate increases in the ration, the cause for this phenomenon is not yet clear cut. This discussion serves to emphasize the problem. However, the HI hypothesis seems to be the most tenable explanation of the phenomenon. If changes in NEm and NEg were linear, such information could easily be predicted from feed analysis and energy content data. However, if these changes are curvilinear, they would be much more difficult to incorporate in the NE system for gain prediction and ration balancing.

Dietary protein level also has a profound effect on DE, ME and $NEm + p$ values of feedstuffs. A protein (AA) deficiency at the cellular level will increase the HI. A protein

(NH₃-N) deficiency in the rumen will lower substantially the DE (ME) content of the feed. This situation has arisen especially with NE determinations with all corn silage rations. When unsupplemented with protein, the NEm + p per kg DM may be as much as 25-30% lower than when fed with adequate protein.

N:CHO Interrelationship

The two primary substrates for ruminal fermentation are N and carbohydrates. Although the carbohydrates are degraded and metabolized to generate ATP for the microorganisms and $N(NH_3-N)$ must be available for microbial growth, these two substrates show an interaction in that, in the absence of one or the other, microbial cell growth and feed digestion is greatly impaired. Hence, the extent of microbial growth is linked to the extent of carbohydrate fermentation (ATP), while the extent of carbohydrate breakdown is dependent upon microbial activity or growth (N utilization). A number of other substrates are necessary for optimal ruminal fermentation. Among these are a S source, possibly carbon chain precursors for a synthesis or amino acids per se and other factors. If any one of these factors is inadequate, CHO digestion and cell growth are depressed. These relationships are shown in Fig. 18-5.

Efficiency of Microbial Growth and Ruminal Outflow Rate

Growth of microorganisms, if no other factors are limiting, is dependent on the available ATP (energy) arising from degradative catabolism of energy substrates. Baudrop and Elsden (1960) showed that ATP was the common denominator between observed cell growth and substrate disappearance

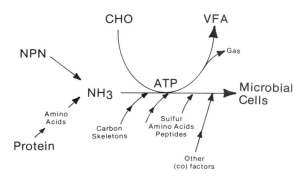

Fig. 18-5. Paths of nitrogen and carbon sources in the ruminal fermentation.

since microbial growth was directly proportional to the amount of ATP generated from the catabolism of energy substrates. Bauckop and Elsden defined the relationship between ATP and cell growth as YATP (yield of microbial dry matter as g/mole ATP). Based on their experiments with energy limiting batch cultures, these authors also concluded that YATP was a constant value for different microorganisms. Current evidence indicates that YATP is not a constant value, but can be influenced by the type of substrate for cellular growth and also by the specific growth rate (dilution rate, D) in continuous culture of a given microorganism. Gunsalus and Shuster (1961) calculated that the maximal YATP (max YATP) may be as high as 32. Stouthamer (1969) estimated that with glucose as substrate, the Y max ATP of bacteria would be 27. In contrast, if the cell starts with CO_2 as the primary C sources, the assembly of macromolecule precursors consumes energy and in this case the YATP max is around 5 (Forrest and Walker, 1971). The ATP produced by the microorganisms can be used for biosynthetic and maintenance functions. The extent to which the organism can utilize the ATP for biosynthesis will determine quantity of cells produced in any given fermentation. As indicated above, if some ATP is needed for endogenous synthesis of macromolecular precursors, the amount of ATP available for cell growth will also then be adjusted correspondingly.

Specific growth rate (or D) of microorganisms in continuous culture can regulate their growth efficency and ATP utilization. Hence at low D, YATP tend to be low, whereas at high D, YATP are much higher. Thus it is obvious, for any given ATP yield from energy substrate catabolism, more cells (or microbial protein) can be produced at higher D (Stouthamer and Bettenhausen, 1973).

Isaacson et al (1975) first demonstrated that, as the D of a continuous culture of washed rumen bacteria (glucose substrate) was varied from 2%/hr to 12%/hr, YATP increased from 6 to 15. The YATP max in this system was 19. Studies with sheep and cattle have also shown this same relationship. Cole et al (1976), Harrison et al (1975) and Kropp et al (1976) all showed that as the fractional outflow from the rumen (or passage rate) increased, microbial cell yield/100 g DOM increased (Fig. 18-6).

434

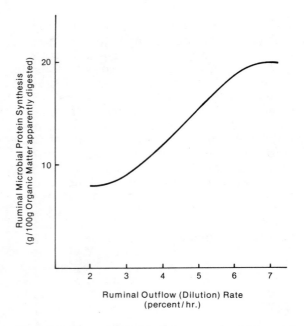

Fig. 18-6. The relationship between microbial protein yield and ruminal outflow (dilution) rate.

Ruminal outflow of digesta (D) can be influenced by the physical (particle size) and chemical (α vs β linked CHO polymers) characteristics of rations. Outflow for ground cereals would be higher than for coarse roughages. Since particle size and specific gravity govern the rate of particle removal from the rumen, ground cereal grains exit much more readily than roughages. There are, however, various so called pools or phases in the rumen. That is, there are at least a liquid phase (pool), a small particle phase (pool) and a large particle phase (pool). These phases do not leave the rumen at similar rates and the extent of microbial distribution between these phases will determine the overall efficiency of microbial growth. In a cereal based ration, most microorganisms would be found in the liquid and small particle pool; these pools have a higher D than the large particle pool. Conversely, in an animal fed largely roughages, the cellulolytics are often closely associated with the feed particles and the D for these organisms may be quite low. Various approaches have been used to modify ruminal digesta outflow and improve feed utilization. The classic case is the grinding of coarse roughages, which decreases the ruminal retention time of this feedstuff and hence increases D. When ruminal D is increased, net ruminal organic matter digestion declines, but this is a small price to pay for the enhanced overall performance of animals consuming coarse roughages.

Some feed processing methods actually increase ruminal retention time and thus enhance ruminal digestion. For example, steam flaking of corn depresses ruminal D and improves overall intraruminal starch digestion (Galyean et al, 1976) but may depress efficiency of microbial cell growth. Other procedures have been used to vary D in ruminants. Harrison et al (1975) infused artificial saliva into sheep. Whenever D was increased, α-linked glucose polymer bypass increased.

From a practical viewpoint, two ruminal processes need to be optimized. First, for any given ration the highest possible ruminal organic matter digestion is desired (especially for α-linked carbohydrate polymers). Second, it is also desirable to achieve the highest microbial protein synthesis rate. Since the efficiency of microbial protein synthesis is influenced markedly by D changes, a small compromise in reaching the first goal may increase microbial cell yield substantially. Hence, feed processing procedures, additives, or management schemes should be developed to enhance the ruminal D. The overall loss in ruminal feed organic matter digestibility is usually also rather small (3-5% decrease) in comparison to microbial protein yield changes as ruminal D is increased.

NUTRIENT - HORMONAL INTERACTIONS

To obtain growth and/or production in animals, both a supply of dietary protein and energy are required. Energy demands are set by the level of productivity and maintenance needs of animals. Concomitantly, however, an adequate source (amount and quality) of dietary protein is required for the expression of the animal's productivity. At fixed low protein intakes, increasing the dietary energy intake from inadequate to adequate will only result in a small increment of productivity (N balance). On adequate or high protein intakes, incremental increased dietary energy intake results in incremental increases in N balance (or performance). Hence, an interdependence exists between dietary protein and energy and a limitation of either will depress performance (Munro, 1964).

The overall effect of energy intake on protein metabolism is not dependent on the source of calories (eg. carbohydrate or fat;

Munro, 1964). However, dietary carbohydrates do exhibit a specific (non-caloric) effect on protein metabolism (Munro, 1964). This specific role of dietary carbohydrate relates to the resulting insulin secretion upon carbohydrate (glucose) absorption. Two major lines of evidence for a specific action of carbohydrate on protein metabolism are: the urinary N excretion of fasting animals can be lowered by carbohydrate but not by fat administration (CH_2O protein sparing effect), and the lowering of circulating blood amino acid levels after administration of glucose.

Munro (1964) has reviewed many early reports on the role of feeding carbohydrate or fat on the urinary N output in fasting human subjects, dogs, rabbits and rats. In all species tested, fat either failed to reduce the N output of that fasting animal or was much less effective than carbohydrate administered under similar circumstances. The reduced N output was due primarily to a reduction of urea-N excretion (Butler et al, 1945).

Folin and Berglund (1922) demonstrated that the carbohydrate induced depression in N output was accompanied by a lowering of plasma amino acid levels. Wiechman (1926) reported that the plasma α-amino nitrogen declined in normal fasting human subjects after a glucose load and in diabetic subjects after insulin injection. Further, Wiechman (1926) observed that amino acid levels in venous blood of untreated diabetics were higher than arterial levels. Upon insulin administration this A-V difference was nullified. The dramatic lowering of circulating plasma amino acids after glucose or insulin administration has been ascribed to the insulin mediated enhancement of muscle protein synthesis and decrease in protein turnover (Munro, 1964; Cahill et al, 1972).

A rapid, observable effect of insulin on liver protein metabolism had not been shown, although insulin enhanced amino acid incorporation into various liver preparations in vitro after prolonged incubations with the hormone (Munro, 1964). Insulin enhances incorporation of amino acids into muscle protein (translation) independently of muscle cell uptake of glucose and also enhances the uptake of some but not all amino acids into muscle cells. Further, insulin enhances the incorporation of amino acids synthesized intracellularly (Manchester, 1972).

Munro and Thomson (1953) and Lotspeich (1949) observed that insulin or glucose administration produced a transient lowering of circulating amino acid levels and also that the pattern of the amino acid decline conformed to the amino acid composition of muscle. This high apparent correlation between muscle amino acid composition and the glucose/insulin induced plasma amino acid depression pattern has been used as an indirect probe to study limiting amino acids in ruminants. The hypothesis was advanced that the essential amino acid showing the largest percent decline after glucose (or energy) administration should be the limiting amino acid of the composite protein undergoing digestion in the small intestine of ruminants. Upon ruminal starch administration (Purser et al, 1966) or venous infusion of glucose or propionate (Potter et al, 1968) to fasting sheep, a general decline in plasma amino acid levels was observed. This lowering of circulating amino acid levels can be ascribed to the resulting insulin secretion in response to rapid VFA (primarily propionate) production in the rumen after starch infusion and a direct effect on insulin secretion by glucose or propionate after I.V. infusion. Trenkle (1970) has demonstrated an insulin secretion response to VFA in ruminants.

The depression pattern results of Purser et al (1966) and Potter et al (1968) both indicated amino acids as limiting (primarily phenylalanine or isoleucine) that could really not be considered as limiting in the composite protein (microbial and by-pass) reaching the lower gut (Bergen et al, 1968). To test the use of glucose induced plasma amino acid depression directly as a tool in nutritional amino acid studies in sheep, Potter et al (1972) infused proteins with known limiting amino acids into duodenal re-entrant cannulae. The digesta (protein) from the rumen was not allowed to pass past the duodenum and was discarded. After a period of protein administration into the duodenum, glucose was administered I.V. to the sheep. Although plasma amino acids declined, the procedure did not result in the largest depression for the specific limiting amino acid for any of the test proteins. Generally, the branched chain amino acids or phenylalanine showed the greatest decline. Potter et al (1972) concluded that this approach was not suitable for amino acid studies in ruminants. Previously, in work with non-ruminants it had been established that plasma valine, leucine, isoleucine and phenylalanine showed the greatest decline after insulin/glucose infusions (Aoki et al,

1970). Curiously, these four amino acids are not among the group of amino acids whose uptake into muscle cells was specifically demonstrated by Manchester (1970).

NUTRIENT-METABOLIC RESPONSE INTERACTIONS

When a non-ruminant consumes energy above required needs (maintenance and/or production), the excess energy will be stored by the body as fat. Body fat can arise from dietary carbohydrates (also amino acid-carbon skeletons) or dietary fats. Consumption of excess calories in the form of carbohydrate induces the so called lipogenic response, which is a metabolic adaptation of liver and/or adipose tissue (species dependent) to synthesize fatty acids de novo from non-lipid precursors. The fatty acids so synthesized are then esterified with α-glycerol phosphate to form triglycerides (depot fat). The endogenously synthesized fatty acids in animal systems are generally saturated and the depot fats can be characterized as hard fat.

Dietary fatty acids, once absorbed, can be utilized directly for triglyceride synthesis. The physical characteristics (firmness) of the depot fat arising from exogenous fatty acids are markedly influenced by the fatty acid composition of the dietary fat. The classical example of the phenomenon is the feeding of rations containing high levels of vegetable oils (unsaturated fatty acids) to swine. This resulted in the so called "soft pork" syndrome. This condition can be reversed by removal of vegetable fats from the ration with a concomitant replacement with carbohydrates. The fat "hardens" as the unsaturated fatty acids are being replaced by saturated fatty acids (synthesized from carbohydrates) in the triglycerides. The continual cycle of lipid deposition and lipolysis in depot fat stores allows the hardening to proceed.

Not only do exogenous or dietary fatty acids become directly esterified into triglycerides, but the feeding of fatty acids has also a direct depressing effect on the fatty acid synthesis (lipogenesis) in liver and adipose tissue (Leveille, 1970). For de novo fatty acid synthesis to occur (lipogenesis), three components are necessary. These are the enzyme acetyl-CoA carboxylase which catalyzes the first step in fatty acid synthesis (the carboxylation of acetyl-CoA to form malonyl-CoA), the enzyme complex fatty acid synthetase which catalyzes the conversion of malonyl-CoA and acetyl-CoA in a step wise fashion to palmitic acid and the presence of reduced nicotinamide adenine dinucleotide phosphate (NADPH). The required NADPH is generated by the hexose monophosphate shunt pathway, isocitrate dehydrogenase and malic enzyme. The activities of these enzymes are elevated under so called lipogenic conditions (Leveille, 1970). All enzymes involved in fatty acid synthesis are found in the extramitochondrial (cytosolic) compartment of cells.

Acetyl-CoA carboxylase appears to play a key role in the regulation of fatty acid synthesis in animal tissues (Romsos and Leveille, 1972). The activity of the enzyme is decreased during alloxan induced diabetes and fasting and elevated upon refeeding fasted animals a fat-free, high carbohydrate diet. In addition, citrate acts as an activator and long chain acyl-CoA derivatives as an inhibitor of acetyl-CoA carboxylase activity (Romsos and Leveille, 1972). It was shown by Hill et al (1958) that as little as 2.5% of fat in the diet of rats caused measurable depression of liver fatty acid synthesis. In the fasting state, long-chain free fatty acids (FFA) are elevated in the plasma and this elevation of FFA is thought to be correlated to lower fatty acid synthesis (Mayes and Topping, 1974). Although the hypothesis that long-chain acyl-CoA can depress acetyl-CoA carboxylase activities and hence depress fatty acid synthesis appears attractive, the mechanism for this inhibition is not understood clearly. It was argued that in many of the experiments where palmitoyl-CoA depressed fatty acid synthesis, the acyl-CoA acted as a non-specific detergent (Romsos and Leveille, 1972). Goodridge (1972) was able to demonstrate that the fatty acyl-CoA effect on acetyl-CoA carboxylase was specific and also that this inhibition was completely overcome with citrate. Thus, extramitochondrial fatty acyl-CoA and citrate levels appear to play important roles (as allosteric regulators) in the regulation of lipogenesis. Finally, acetyl-CoA carboxylase is a biotin-containing enzyme and a biotin deficiency will also depress fatty acid synthesis.

The activity of the fatty acid synthetase complex can also be markedly depressed by fasting, fat feeding or alloxan diabetes. This decline in activity may be due to low supplies of malonyl-CoA, that is from the fatty acyl-CoA inhibition of acetyl-CoA carboxylase. Such a decline in substrate would then cause a decrease in the synthesis of the enzyme itself with a concomitant decline in enzyme levels. This scheme would only be operative if acetyl-CoA carboxylase is indeed the rate limiting enzyme in lipogenesis; however, this view is not shared by all workers in this area (Romsos and Leveille, 1972). It is clear that the activity of fatty acid synthetase is primarily dependent on the quantity of enzyme protein and is not extensively modulated by allosteric regulators as acetyl-CoA carboxylase. The regulatory mechanism of fatty acid synthetase synthesis and degradation, although affected by nutritional state, substrates and hormones such as glucagon and insulin has not been elucidated.

Meal size and frequency of feeding are two other factors that influence lipogenesis. The meal–fed animal must consume a large quantity of food in a relatively short time, but obviously it cannot readily utilize all the nutrients in this short time span. When animals are meal-fed (eg. one 2-hr meal/day) a low fat-high carbohydrate diet with adequate protein, a metabolic adaptation, the lipogenic response, is initiated. This involves the induction of the enzymatic machinery (in liver and/or adipose tissue) to convert carbohydrate efficiently to lipids (acetyl-CoA carboxylase, fatty acid synthetase, NADPH generation; Leveille, 1970). Meal feeding of high fat diets completely abolished the lipogenic response (Leveille, 1967), whereas meal feeding a high protein diet has a much less marked effect on lipogenesis (Leveille, 1967, 1970).

In contrast to non-ruminants, where dietary glucose is the primary precursor for de novo fatty acid synthesis, ruminants use acetate as the carbon source for de novo fatty acid synthesis. This metabolic preference for acetate as the carbon source for fatty acid synthesis has been observed in young and mature ruminants (Hanson and Ballard, 1968).

The fatty acid composition of depot fats stored in ruminants is generally not greatly influenced by dietary fatty acid composition since ruminants consume low dietary fat levels and since the ruminal microbiota hydrogenate unsaturated fatty acids (Bauman, 1976; Ch. 6). When protected lipids are fed, ruminants can consume more fat than usual and the fatty acid composition of the protected lipids may then influence (to a degree) the fatty acid compositions of triglycerides.

Animals have absolute essential amino acid and total N requirements. Amino acids consumed in excess of needs are not stored

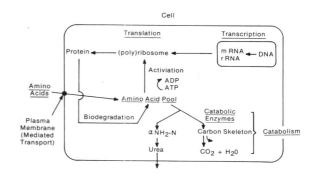

Fig. 18-7. Major pathways of cellular amino acid utilization.

as free amino acids in tissues but are degraded into keto acids and urea (from α-NH_2). The urea is excreted while the keto acids can be further catabolized to CO_2. See Fig. 18-7 for overview of AA metabolism.

Amino acids in excess of requirements can arise when animals are fed high protein diets or proteins of poor nutritional quality. Consumption of high protein diets induces a general increase in the synthesis of amino acid catabolizing enzymes. In the case of proteins of poor nutritional quality, amino acids are used to the extent allowed by the limiting amino acid intake; the remaining amino acids are then catabolized (at least deaminated) regardless of whether they were present (fed) at levels below the requirement of the animal.

Feed intake regulatory centers in the brain (for review see Rogers and Leung, 1973) appear to be sensitive to excessive amino acid concentrations (as in the case of high protein intake) or skewed (imbalanced) amino acid patterns in the blood. When non-ruminants are fed diets containing excess protein, plasma amino acids rise and food intake declines. This metabolic state also signals increased synthesis of amino acid degradating enzymes. As the activity of these enzymes increases, plasma amino acid levels decline and feed intake starts to return to a "normal" level (Anderson et al, 1969). A ration deficient in one essential amino acid also produces an aberrant blood amino acid profile characterized by an extremely low level of the deficient essential amino acid and high levels of the other essential amino acids (Harper et al, 1970). This condition causes food intake and growth depression with not much chance of recovery or adaptation as long as a ration lacking an essential amino acid is fed.

A less severe nutritional circumstance but in some respects similar to the feeding of an essential amino acid deficient diet is the feeding of amino acid imbalanced diets. Imbalanced amino acid diets can be produced by supplementing a low protein diet with all essential amino acids except the diet's limiting amino acid or by adding to a diet an excess of its second most limiting amino acid. The imbalances discussed in succeeding paragraphs were all developed by the first dietary approach. Non-ruminants fed amino acid imbalanced diets show a marked, immediate intake (3-6 hr) depression and poor growth. Further, rats given the choice between a N-free or imbalanced ration prefer the N-free ration although this type of ration cannot sustain life.

The amino acid imbalance is not just a case of a more severe amino acid limitation, since the levels of the limiting amino acid in the low protein basal and imbalanced diets are identical. Despite this, upon feeding the imbalanced diet, the plasma level of the limiting amino acid is lower than that for the basal control and the other excess essential amino acids accumulate in the plasma. This abnormal amino acid pattern is monitored by brain centers with a concomitant decrease in food intake. Somehow these brain centers judge these plasma patterns as harmful for maintaining homeostasis of the organism.

The marked decline of the limiting amino acid in plasma can be ascribed to a unique metabolic adaptation. Upon ingestion of a meal of a ration with an imbalance, the limiting amino acid as well as the surplus of the other essential amino acids are absorbed and transported to the liver by the portal vein. The excess essential amino acids stimulate liver protein synthesis so that the limiting amino acid is used with high efficiency. This efficient extraction by the liver of the limiting amino acid results in a lowered amount for utilization by peripheral tissues. The surplus essential amino acids escaping liver protein synthesis or catabolism further induce an efficient extraction of the limiting amino acid by peripheral tissue finally resulting in the aberrant plasma pattern (Harper et al, 1970).

When rats are prefed a high protein diet before exposure to an imbalanced diet, the onset of the imbalance response is delayed due to the high complement of amino acid degrading enzymes in the tissues. Prolonged feeding of an imbalanced diet will cause a decline of these enzymes as imbalanced diets generally contain low protein levels. It is not possible to induce an amino acid imbalance with a high protein diet unless the limiting amino acid of the dietary protein is present below the animal's requirement for that amino acid.

In ruminants under practical conditions, amino acid imbalances do not exist. By administration (I.V. duodenum or abomasum) of experimental protein (amino acid) sources with imbalanced amino acid patterns, a typical imbalance response (eg. depressed food intake) may be obtained. Very little is known about the induction of amino acid catabolizing enzymes in ruminants and their response to an imbalance is unclear.

NUTRIENT-GENETIC INTERACTIONS

Proteins are polymers of twenty different α-L-amino acids. The linkage between amino acids is the peptide bond. From a nutritional viewpoint the constituent amino acids of protein can be grouped into two classes: non-essential amino acids (NEAA or dispensible AA) and essential amino acids (EAA or non-dispensible AA). The NEAA are those amino acids for which organisms have retained enzymatic machinery for their synthesis while the EAA are those which can not be synthesized by the organism at all or at levels far below requirements. Hence, the EAA must be provided from exogenous (dietary) sources, but at the cellular level all AA are essential.

Type of species and physiological state influences the qualitative and quantitative pattern for amino acid requirement. For example, feeding of lysine-poor diets results in inferior weight gains in growing mammals, whereas adult mammals can maintain nitrogen equilibrium when fed such rations.

In the main the qualitative essential amino acid requirements of animal species are similar (Table 18-1). Eight amino acids (Ile, Leu, Lys, Val, Phe, Thr, Try, Met) are required by all species; fowl, young growing man and young growing rats require also histidine and arginine. The essentiality for arginine in mammals is not clear cut as arginine is generated by the urea cycle. Fowl, however, do not possess the urea cycle and have an absolute need for arginine. the quantitative arginine requirement in birds varies widely and seems to depend in part on the relative lysine intake and dietary cation and anion makeup (Nesheim, 1968; Austic et al, 1977).

Table 18-1. Qualitative essential amino acid requirements for selected species.[a]

| Essential amino acid | | | Species | | |
| | | | Rat | | |
	Fowl	Man	Young	Adult	Ruminant
Isoleucine	+	+	+	+	+
Leucine	+	+	+	+	+
Lysine	+	+	+	+	+
Valine	+	+	+	+	+
Phenylalanine	+	+	+	+	+
Threonine	+	+	+	+	+
Tryptophan	+	+	+	+	+
Methionine	+	+	+	+	+
Histidine	+	?[c]	+		+
Arginine	+	?[c]	+		
Glycine	?[b]				
Proline	?[b]				

[a] If Phenylalanine is absent from the diet, tyrosine is essential as phenylalanine is the direct precursor for tyrosine. If Methionine is absent from the diet, cystine is essential as methionine is the direct precursor for cystine.

[b] Requirement only demonstrated in young fowl.

[c] Requirement only demonstrated in young growing man.

The non-essential amino acids tyrosine and cystine represent a special case in amino acid metabolism. These amino acids can only be synthesized from their EAA precursors Phe and Met, respectively. Dietary tyrosine and cystine can be utilized directly by animals causing a sparing of their precursor EAA. From a nutritional viewpoint, Phe and Tyr and Met and cystine are often lumped together and referred to as total aromatic and sulfur AA, respectively.

The essentiality of amino acids in nonruminants has been established by direct feeding-deletion procedures, but for ruminants indirect means had to be used to establish the EAA pattern for the animal's tissues.

The basis for an indirect assessment of amino acid essentiality is the I.V. infusion of ^{14}C-compounds (such as NaAc, $NaHCO_3$) and a subsequent determination of specific activities of all amino acids in the tissues, wool or milk. The amino acids showing no (or low) ^{14}C activity are then deemed essential. Black et al (1957) and Downes (1963) injected Na $1-^{14}C$ acetate into lactating cows and ewes, respectively. Amino acids were isolated from milk proteins and also from wool. The following amino acids became labeled: glutamic acid, aspartic acid, proline, alanine, glycine, arginine, serine. These amino acids were thus non-essential; this experimental procedure could not demonstrate glutamine and asparagine (HCl hydrolysis was used) and tyrosine and cystine (Phe and Met are direct precursors) as non-essential.

There are many other genetic-nutrient interactions, as for example the requirement of ascorbic acid by primates (and a few other species such as the guinea pig). All these genetic effects on nutritional requirements in animals can be accounted for by variations in animals metabolic pathways (for organic molecules), and differences in cation (or anion) mediated processes (such as solute transport). Since the cellular needs of eukaryotic-cells are quite similar, a loss of synthetic capability for a compound results in a dietary requirement of that compound. This area has been reviewed in a recent symposium (NRC-NAS, 1975).

ROLE OF GENETICS ON THE EFFICIENCY OF GROWTH IN FEED LOT CATTLE

During growth there is an increase in the skeleton, total protein and fat. It has been established that beyond a certain body

440

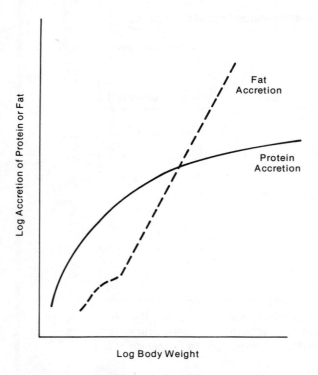

Fig. 18-8. Protein and fat accretion during growth of animals.

weight (depending on mature size of the species), fat gain becomes a large constant part of the total live weight gain (Bergen, 1974). Thus, the process of protein and fat accretion occurs simultaneously during early growth, whereas in later growth protein accretion becomes negligible (Fig. 18-8).

In the predominantly protein accretion phase of growth, the efficiency of feed conversion by cattle is quite high. This is so because for every unit of protein dry matter accretion 3 to 4 units of water are also retained by the animal. During the predominantly fat accretion phase, the efficiency of feed conversions declines markedly; however, efficiency of caloric retention is high during the fattening phase. The poorer feed: gain ratios during the fattening phase are a consequence of little or no water retention during this phase of growth.

The overall efficiency of performance in the feedlot is of considerable interest to cattle feeders. This question has always generated considerable controversy, but if this matter is analyzed in relation to Fig. 19-8 a clear picture will emerge. First, within a given size of cattle (final mature size) the younger growing animal will always be more efficient. When cattle of different mature sizes are compared at 400-500 kg, the larger (or later maturing) breed appears to be more efficient in feed conversion than the smaller breeds. However, from a physiological basis, the later maturing breed has not yet approached the predominantly fattening phase of growth and is still depositing protein and water. The above discussion may be summarized as follows: (Bergen, 1974; VanEs, 1977) (a) Fat gain becomes a large and constant fraction of weight gain beyond a certain body weight. (b) Animals with larger mature size start to fatten at a relatively greater body weight. (c) The caloric value of gain is lower over a greater body range in the larger than the smaller mature size animals and hence the larger animals have better feed efficiency (i.e., 1.0 g protein and 4 g H_2O = 5.4 Kcal, whereas 5.4 Kcal = 0.6 g fat). (d) The further the "fattening point" can be delayed the more efficient the body weight gains and lean meat production. (e) Selection based on feed efficiency (or lean body mass) will be biased towards animals of larger mature sizes. (f) Fat accretion (synthesis) is not inefficient on a caloric basis.

To compare the overall efficiency of cattle (either on energy retention or feed conversion basis) all breeds must be fed to the same physiological state or to the same overall chemical composition or finish. On this basis feedlot efficiency differences among beef breeds (straight breed and cross breed) are quite small. Straight bred Holsteins appear to be less efficient in the feedlot than beef breeds (Harpster, 1978).

References Cited

Anderson, H.L., N.J. Benevenga and A.E. Harper. 1969. J. Nutr. 97:463.

Aoki. T.T.. W.A. Muller, E.B. Marliss and G.F. Cahill. 1971. Clin. Res. 19:570.

Armstrong, D.G., K.L. Blaxter, N. McC. Graham and F.W. Wainman. 1958. Brit. J. Nutr. 12:177.

Austice, R.E., M. Okameto and R.L. Scott. 1977. Proc. Cornell Nutr. Conf., p 120.

Bauchop, T. and S.R. Elsden. 1960. J. Gen. Microbiol. 23:457.

Bauman, D.E. 1976. Fed. Proc. 35:2308.

Bergen, W.G. 1974. J. Animal Sci. 38:1079.

Bergen, W.G., D.B. Purser and J.H. Cline. 1968. J. Dairy Sci. 51:1698.

Black, A.L., M. Kleiber, A.H. Smith and D.N. Stewart. 1957. Biochem. Biophys. Acta 23:54.

Blaxter, K.L. and F.W. Wainman. 1964. J. Agr. Sci. 63:113.

Butler, A.M. et al. 1945. J. Clin. Endocrinol. 5:327.

Byers, F.M., J.K. Matsushima and D.E. Johnson. 1975. Colorado Beef Cattle Rpt., p 18.

Cahill, G.F., T.T. Aoki and E.B. Marliss. 1972. In: Handbook of Physiology, Sect. 7, Ch. 36. Amer. Physiol. Soc., Washington, D.C.

Cole, N.A., R.R. Johnson, F.N. Owens and J.R. Males. 1976. J. Animal Sci. 43:497.

Downes, A.M. 1963. Aust. J. Biol. Sci. 16:254.

Folin, O. and H. Berglund. 1922. J. Biol. Chem. 51:395.

Forest, N.W. and D.J. Walker. 1971. In: Advances in Microbial Physiology, Vol. 5. Academic Press, NY.

Galyean, M.L., D.G. Wagner and R.R. Johnson. 1976. J. Animal Sci. 43:1080.

Goodridge, A.G. 1972. J. Biol. Chem. 247:6947.

Gunsalus, I.C. and C.W. Shuster. 1961. In: The Bacteria, Vol. II. Acdemic Press, NY.

Hanson, R.W. and F.J. Ballard. 1968. Biochem. J. 108:705.

Harper, A.E., N.J. Benevenga and R.M. Wohlhueter. 1970. Physiol. Rev. 50:428.

Harpster, H.W. 1978. Michigan State Univ. Animal Hus. Mineo I.

Harrison, D.G., D.E. Beever, D.Y. Thomson and D.F. Osbourn. 1975. J. Agr. Sci. 85:93.

Hill, R. et al. 1958. J. Biol. Chem. 233:305.

Holter, J.B., C.W. Heald and N.F. Colovos. 1970. J. Dairy Sci. 53:1241.

Isaacson, H.R., F.C. Hinds, M.P. Bryant and F.N. Owens. 1975. J. Dairy Sci. 58:1645.

Kropp, J.R., R.R. Johnson, J.R. Males and F.N. Owens. 1977. J. Animal Sci. 46:844.

Leveille, G.A. 1967. J. Nutr. 91:25.

Leveille, G.A. 1970. Fed. Proc. 29:1294.

Lonsdale, C.R., E.K. Poutiainen and J.C. Taylor. 1971. Animal Prod. 13:461.

Lotspeich, W.D. 1949. J. Biol. Chem. 179:175.

Manchester, K.L. 1970. Biochem. J. 117:457.

Manchester, K.L. 1972. Diabetes 21:447.

Mayes, P.A. and D.L. Topping. 1974. Biochem. J. 140:111.

Munro, H.N. 1964. In: Mammalian Protein Metabolism, Vol. 1. Academic Press, NY.

Munro, H.N. and W.S.T. Thomson. 1953. Metabolism 2:354.

Nesheim, M.C. 1968. Fed. Proc. 27:1210.

NRC. 1975. The effect of genetic variance on nutritional requirements of animals. Nat. Acad. Sci., Washington, D.C.

Ørskov, E.R., F.D. Hovell and D.M. Allen. 1966. Brit. J. Nutr. 20:295.

Potter, E.L., D.B. Purser and W.G. Bergen. 1972. J. Animal Sci. 34:660.

Potter, E.L., D.B. Purser and J.H. Cline. 1968. J. Nutr. 95:665.

Purser, D.B., T.J. Klopfenstein and J.H. Cline. 1966. J. Nutr. 89:226.

Rogers, Q.R. and R.M.B. Leung. 1973. Fed. Proc. 32:1709.

Romsos, D.R. and G.A. Leveille. 1972. In: Advances in Lipid Research, Vol. 12. Academic Press, NY.

Stouthamer, A.H. 1969. In: Methods of Microbiology, Vol. 1. Academic Press, NY.

Stouthamer, A.H. and C. Bettenhaussen. 1973. 1973. Biochem. Biophys. Acta 301:53.

Trenkle, A. 1970. J. Nutr. 100:1323.

Vance, R.D., R.L. Preston, V.R. Cahill and E.W. Klosterman. 1972. J. Animal Sci. 34:851.

Van Es, A.J.H. 1977. Nutr. Metab. 21:88.

Wiechmann, E. 1924. Z. Ges. Exptl. Med. 44:158.

Wiechmann, E. 1926. Deut. Arch. Klin. Med. 150:186.

Chapter 19 - Purified Diets

By Gary E. Smith and L.A. Muir

Diets which might be classified as purified (i.e. synthetic, partially purified, semisynthetic) have been used in recent years, particularly the past 25 years, for a variety of purposes. They have been especially helpful in studying rumen metabolism of specific dietary components such as cellulose, starch or various nitrogenous compounds; lipid requirements, and metabolism and requirements of the various mineral elements or vitamins. If the researcher is able to utilize rather pure energy sources of energy (i.e., starch or purified cellulose), it is much easier to determine the effect of changes in the diet than when natural feedstuffs are used since nearly all natural feedstuffs are a complex mixture of many organic and inorganic compounds. The same comment applies to any specific nutrient.

Two diets with different N sources which have been used for sheep are shown in Table 19-1. Diets of this type have been proven satisfactory for moderate growth rates and for reproduction when fed to both male and female cattle for long periods of time. Thus, it follows that all required nutrients must be present or be available from water supplies. However, the reader should be aware, particularly for the mineral elements, that some (most) of the sources used probably are contaminated with traces of other elements. Ni is a case in point. Since it is now considered to be a required element, it must have been supplied by some of the chemical sources if required by ruminants.

Keep in mind that an appreciable number of the studies that have been mentioned in previous chapters have been done with purified diets. Thus, less extensive coverage of the literature will be given here than otherwise might be the case. A relatively recent review on this topic has been presented by Bunn and Matrone (1972).

Although purified diets have a number of advantages when dealing with specific dietary ingredients, there are also some disadvantages. An important one is cost, particularly for cattle because of relatively large amounts required. A second factor is that consumption of such diets is almost invariably rather low, resulting in less than normal growth rates or milk production. The low consumption may be a matter of low palatability as a result of unnatural physical texture or undesirable taste or it may be related to some modification of metabolism which may depress appetite for such diets, possibly because of less than optimum combinations of nutrients. At any rate, the researcher must be prepared to accept lower performance than with natural feedstuffs.

Nitrogen Sources

One of the more classical studies with purified diets was reported by Loosli et al (1949) in which it was demonstrated that ruminants could be fed on urea as the only source of N (see Ch. 3). Synthesis of ruminal protein was shown in this study. Since that time many different studies have been carried out with urea and other NPN sources. Although urea has been used more commonly, other N sources such as uric acid,

Table 19-1. Composition of two purified diets for sheep. [a]

Ingredient, %	Isolated soy protein	Urea
Wood pulp	30.0	30.0
Corn starch	28.6	34.8
Corn glucose	18.0	22.0
Soy protein	14.9	---
Urea	---	4.7
Minerals [b]	6.4	6.4
Soybean oil	2.0	2.0
Choline chloride	0.1	0.1
Vitamins[c]	+	+

[a] From Oltjen et al (1969)

[b] Mineral mixture in %: $CaHPO_4$, 50.0; K_2CO_3, 28.7; $MgSO_4$, 11.0; NaCl, 8.5; $FeSO_4$, 0.75; $MnSO_4$, H_2O, 0.11; $Na_2B_4O_7$, 10 H_2O, 0.36; $ZnSO_4$, 7 H_2O, 0.53; $CuCO_3$, 0.03; KI, 0.003; $CoCl_2$, 6 H_2O, 0.001; MoO_3, 0.001; Na_2SeO_3, 0.001.

[c] Vitamins provided: vitamin A, 8,800 USP units; vitamin D, 1,100 USP units; vitamin E, 21 IU/kg of diet.

biuret and urea-phosphate appear to be satisfactory (Oltjen et al, 1968).

Although many experiments have demonstrated that NPN sources can serve as the only N source in purified diets, feed consumption and performance have not been comparable to diets containing some source of natural protein. Partially or completely purified proteins such as isolated soy, casein, gelatin, blood fibrin, dried skim milk, egg albumin and others have been used with varying degrees of success. The biological values of some protein sources have been reported to be: soybean protein, 82.4; blood fibrin, 83.1; casein, 72.4; gelatin, 57.4; and urea, 83.7 (Ellis et al, 1956).

Various investigators have shown that 30-50% of the N can be supplied by urea and still have good performance (Meachum et al, 1961; McDonald et al, 1965; Oltjen et al, 1969). On the theory that amino acids might be limiting, numerous studies have been reported in which specific amino acids have been fed. However, results have not been particularly rewarding in terms of performance (Ellis et al, 1959; Harbers et al, 1961; Meachum et al, 1961; Oltjen et al, 1962; Clifford et al, 1968). Since rumen metabolism of isolated acids is relatively rapid (see Ch. 13, Vol. 1), this is not too surprising. Bypassing the rumen by giving abomasal infusions of amino acids has resulted in improved performance (Nimrick et al, 1970).

In the rumen it has been shown that purified diets with either urea or isolated soy may result in some alteration of the microbial population (Slyter et al, 1968). Slyter et al (1971) reported that ruminal urease activity was greatly reduced by feeding NPN and Maeng and Baldwin (1975) suggested that small amounts of amino acids added to urea would increase rumen microbial yields. Microbial cell yields/kg of carbohydrate digested were 139, 189, 212 and 225 g for 0, 15, 30 and 45 mg of amino acid N. They also noted that high amounts of starch increased microbial protein synthesis from labeled amino acids and reduced the amount of amino acid fermentation. Drastic reductions in protozoal numbers have been observed in cattle fed purified diets (Virtanen, 1966; Oltjen et al, 1965; Giesecki et al, 1966; Slyter et al, 1968). However, Hino and Kametaka (1974) were able to maintain protozoal populations in ruminants fed purified diets when either urea or ammonium sulfate were the sole sources of N providing that the sterol, ʋ-sitosterol, was added to the diet.

In cattle fed purified diets with NPN, it has been demonstrated that some changes occur in plasma amino acids. Steers have been shown to have lower plasma levels of leucine, isoleucine, valine and phenylalanine and increased levels of serine and glycine; calves have been shown to have low levels of the same acids plus threonine, cystine, hydroxyproline and tyrosine (Oltjen and Putnam, 1966; Oltjen et al, 1969). Abe et al (1975) suggested from their studies with mature Holstein cows that lysine would likely limit protein synthesis. Richardson and Hatfield (1978) concluded, on the basis of abomasal infusions, that methionine, lysine and threonine were the first 3 limiting (in order) amino acids for growing steers fed purified diets with urea.

Although branched-chain VFA might be expected to be limiting in the rumen (origin from branched-chain amino acids), studies with sheep have not shown any particular improvement by adding them to the diet (Cline et al, 1966; Clifford and Tillman, 1968). Data on cattle (Oltjen et al, 1971) suggest some slight improvement in N retention when urea was fed. Abomasal infusions of branched-chain amino acids also stimulated greater N retention and improved plasma concentrations.

In studies with calves fed diets with urea, uric acid or soybean meal, data obtained with re-entrant cannula showed that more of the organic matter was digested in the rumen with the urea and uric acid diets. In addition, synthesis of microbial protein was apparently greater on these two diets but more of the digesta dry matter in the duodenum was composed of amino acids with the soybean meal than with urea and the proportion of essential amino acids was also greater (Jacobs and Leibholz, 1977).

Purified diets have often been used with 12-14% crude protein. Muir et al (1972) reported that N retention and PUN values increased linearly as dietary levels of 8, 17.5 and 24% CP were fed to sheep. N retentions were 1.4, 7.5 and 10 g/day while PUN values were 9.6, 26.2 and 39.2 mg/100 ml, respectively, for these diets. Brown et al (1969) and Price et al (1969) both observed that 19% CP was more optimal than higher or lower levels for sheep. The relatively high levels for optimal performance may be a reflection of low consumption of purified diets. Cecyre et al (1973) fed purified diets containing CP equivalents of 6, 10 and 15% and measured plasma amino acids 6 hr post feeding. Total essential amino acid concentrations were 47,

73 and 73 and non-essential were 88, 110 and 105 µM/ml for the 6, 10 and 15% rations, respectively. Plasma amino acids reflected dietary N content; the authors felt that lysine was the most limiting amino acid for their particular diet.

In other studies with sheep, it has been observed that urinary citrate excretion was considerably higher than from sheep fed diets with soybean meal. Increasing the frequency of feeding from 2X to 12X/day decreased the citrate excretion; however, frequency of feeding did not affect feed intake, gain or efficiency of gain in a 44-day growth trial (Prior et al, 1972; Prior, 1976).

Other Dietary Components

A variety of different studies have been done in which different proportions of readily available carbohydrates (RAC) and cellulose have been used. Most of these suggest that sheep or cattle performance is greatest with cellulose levels on the order of 40-50% of the dry matter (Meachum et al, 1961; Oltjen et al, 1962; Smith et al, 1965; McDonald et al, 1965; Chappell and Fontenot, 1968). There appears to be some difference, depending on the N source, since Smith et al (1965) found that the level of starch or glucose was not critical in diets with isolated soy but equal parts of glucose and starch resulted in the best growth in lambs given casein. Ørskov and Oltjen (1967) noted that the proportion of acetic acid in the rumen decreased as cellulose decreased and RAC increased in the diets (typical of natural diets). The effect on rumen VFA in other studies has been variable (McDonald et al, 1965; Smith et al, 1966).

With regard to lipids, purified diets have been shown to result in softer fats and an increase in *trans* unsaturated 18:1 and 18:2 acids due to incomplete hydrogenation of dietary 18:3 acids (Tove and Matrone, 1962; Smith et al, 1969). However, there is no information at hand to show that cattle require lipids in the diet since Oltjen and Williams (1974) have fed diets with <0.02% bound lipids and did not observe any deficiency symptoms.

Purified diets have been used extensively to study mineral metabolism. The various studies have shown that levels required are somewhat similar to those for natural diets. Recommended levels for some of the trace minerals might be (ppm): B, 15; Co, 0.1; Cu, 15; Fe, 70; Mn, 20; Mo, 0.3; Se, 0.1; Zn, 50. Buffers may be more critical than in natural diets, particularly for pelleted diets, since

salivary production is reduced and this would, in turn, tend to alter rumen pH (Oltjen et al, 1965, 1969; Smith et al, 1966).

There is little question that the fat-soluble vitamins are required in purified diets (Buchanan-Smith et al, 1969; Whanger et al, 1977). With regard to the B-complex vitamins, some studies have shown improved performance and others have not. Bunn and Matrone (1972) concluded that young lambs appear to adjust to purified diets more quickly when B vitamins are included. More recently Naga et al (1975) observed symptoms of cerebrocortical necrosis in sheep that had consumed a purified diet for about 7 mo. Treatment with a B vitamin mixture or with thiamin restored the sheep to normal feed intake.

PERFORMANCE OF SHEEP ON PURIFIED DIETS

The growth rates of sheep fed purified diets containing either soy protein or casein indicate that modern diets are basically satisfactory although not equivalent to natural diets. Growth rate and feed efficiency are ca. 65% as good on NPN diets as on protein-containing diets. Nevertheless, purified diets (i.e., Table 19-1) with urea as the sole source of N will produce gains on the order of 0.2 kg/day for short-term feeding experiments (8-10 weeks) (Price et al, 1969).

On the other hand, feed intake and subsequent growth of lambs has been substandard in many studies presented in this review. For instance, Gibson et al (1968) and Smith et al (1969) reported gains of only 0.05 to 0.08 kg/day and a considerable amount of wool picking was noted (Fig. 19-1). A few lambs on these diets lost half of the wool on their body surface. Thus, it appears that further

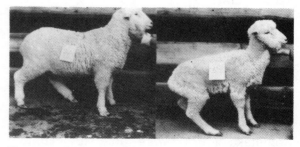

Fig. 19-1. Lambs fed purified diets. The lamb on the left received a basal diet with added corn oil while the one on the right received no corn oil. Notice the loss of wool on neck, side and flank. Courtesy of E.W. Gibson.

work is needed to develop a purified diet that will result in animal growth and feed consumption comparable to a conventional diet, if indeed this is possible.

Reproduction studies with ewes fed purified diets are limited. Matrone et al (1964, 1965) found that 5% alfalfa meal was needed to support normal reproduction when ewes were fed a casein-containing diet. The lambing percentage of the 9 ewes in the experiment was within the normal range and the lambs grew satisfactorily during lactation when alfalfa was included.

Buchanan-Smith et al (1969) used purified diets in Se-vitamin E studies when urea was the sole N source. Satisfactory reproductive performance was obtained from ewes treated with a combination of vitamin E and Se and the lambs from these ewes also grew normally. More recently, Whanger et al (1977) reported that ewes could only live 8-9 weeks on purified diets which contained neither vitamin E nor Se. However, when Se and/or vitamin E were administered, normal reproduction responses were obtained. Enzyme activities of plasma enzymes suggested that vitamin E alone is more effective in preventing white muscle disease than Se alone.

PERFORMANCE OF CATTLE ON PURIFIED DIETS

Virtanen (1969) has reviewed his extensive studies in Finland on N metabolism and reproduction in Holstein cows. Purified diets containing urea and ammonium salts as the sole source of N were adequate in maintaining a moderate level of milk production (ca. 4,000 kg/year). The composition of the milk was similar to that from cows fed natural rations. Cows fed the protein-free diet were bred and several calved more than once. Some cows did require several services to become pregnant.

Flatt et al (1969) reported that a cow fed a urea-based purified diet produced 2,630 kg of milk while her monozygotic twin fed a natural diet produced 5,435 kg (305 days). During the second lactation the cow receiving the urea diet produced about 65% as much milk as her twin. The ME was used equally well by both cows. Addition of isolated soy protein to the urea diet appeared to stimulate milk production. Decreased milk production from cows fed urea was most likely associated with reduced feed intake since efficiencies of production were comparable. In other studies there have been

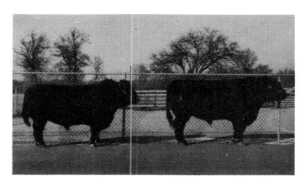

Fig. 19-2. These Angus Bulls were fed purified diets containing urea (left) or isolated soy protein (right) as the sole sources of N. Both diets supported normal reproduction. Courtesy of USDA Beef Cattle Research Center, Beltsville, Md.

problems maintaining cows on semisynthetic diets or adaptation periods have been rather long (Schwarz and Kirchgessner, 1977).

Several reproduction studies have been completed with Angus cattle at the USDA Beltsville station. Angus calves (bulls and heifers) were offered purified diets containing either urea or isolated soy or a natural diet starting at 14 days of age and were weaned onto the diets at 84 days of age. Performance of heifer calves fed the natural diet and the soy diet was similar prior to weaning while the performance of calves fed the urea diet was only 70% as great. However, after weaning the performance of heifer calves fed the soy and urea was about 70 and 30%, respectively, as great as that of calves on natural diets. Bulls fed the purified diets made considerably greater gains than heifers and utilized the urea diets more efficiently than heifers after weaning. Bulls fed urea reached puberty about 6 mo. later than heifers on soy or natural diets. Delayed puberty of heifers fed urea may have been a function of lower energy intake since several of these heifers did calve normally. Heifers raised on the urea diet and bred to bulls raised on the urea diet produced normal offspring (Fig. 19-2) (Oltjen et al, 1969; Rumsey et al, 1969).

In these studies the long term feeding of urea did not affect respiratory patterns, heart rate or EKG patterns. The hair coat of calves fed the urea diet was rough and had a dull brownish-red appearance. Cystine concentration was low while the methionine concentrations were high in the hair of calves fed urea. Thus, Oltjen et al (1969) concluded that the hair coat appearance and blood plasma amino acid pattern of urea-fed calves resembled those of African kwashiorkor subjects.

Bond and Oltjen (1973) studied the reproductive performance of two twin sets which were fed either a NPN purified diet or a natural diet after 7 mo. of age. There seemed to be only small differences in conception rate, estrous cycle, gestation length, birth weight of calves, time and weight at puberty and milk composition. In a larger study these investigators reported that heifers fed urea diets after 84 days of age reached puberty at 634 days of age whereas those fed diets with soy protein attained puberty at 364 days. Females fed the NPN diets weighed less and gave less milk at first lactation than soy-fed heifers. There were no significant effects on estrous cycle, conception rate, death rate of calves or gestation length due to diet. The effect of NPN on age to puberty most likely was associated with reduced feed intake since these heifers consumed only about 75% of NRC requirements. Nevertheless, the results from these studies clearly indicate that beef heifers can reach puberty and reproduce them when reared from an early age on NPN purified diets.

DIETS FOR PRERUMINANT CALVES

The first liquid purified diet (synthetic milk) for preruminant calves was reported in 1940, however, this diet did not support normal growth. In 1947 Wiese et al developed a liquid diet that did allow normal growth and this diet became the basis for purified diets that were used to determine nutrient requirements of the calf. This diet utilized casein for protein, cerelose for carbohydrate and lard for fat and was fortified with most essential vitamins and minerals. It was mixed to contain 13% solids and was homogenized to disperse the fat. When fed at a daily level of 2.3 kg/50 kg BW, it provided or was within 20% of all recommended nutrient levels given in the 1978 NRC except Mg, vitamin E and possibly S and B_{12}. Modifications of this diet have been reported by Blaxter and Wood (1951) and Kameoka and Tanabe (1972, 1975) among others.

References Cited

Abe, M., H. Shibui and T. Iriki. 1975. Jap. J. Zootech. Sci. 46:621.

Blaxter, K.L. and W.A. Wood. 1952. Brit. J. Nutr. 6:56.

Bond, J. and R.R. Oltjen. 1973. J. Animal Sci. 37:141.

Brown, J.A., R.A. Rippe, W.D. Price and W.H. Smith. 1969. J. Animal Sci. 29:153.

Buchanan-Smith, J.G. et al. 1969. J. Animal Sci. 29:808.

Bunn, C.R. and G. Matrone. 1972. Purified diets for ruminants. Nutr. Abstr. Rev. 42:435.

Cecyre, A., G.M. Jones and J.M. Gaudreau. 1973. Can. J. Animal Sci. 53:455.

Chappell, G.L.M. and J.P. Fontenot. 1968. J. Animal Sci. 27:1709.

Clifford, A.J., J.R. Bourdette and A.D. Tillman. 1968. J. Animal Sci. 27:1081.

Clifford, A.J. and A.D. Tillman. 1968. J. Animal Sci. 27:484.

Cline, T.R., U.S. Garrigus and E.E. Hatfield. 1966. J. Animal Sci. 25:734.

Ellis, W.C., L.M. Flynn, W.A. Hargus and W.H. Pfander. 1959. Fed. Proc. 18:2063.

Ellis, W.C., G.B. Garner, M.E. Muhrer and W.H. Pfander. 1956. J. Nutr. 60:413.

Flatt, W.P. et al. 1969. Fourth Symposium on Energy Metabolism. Oriel Press Ltd., Newcastle upon Tyne.

Gibson, E.W., G.E. Smith, L. Schwope and R.A. Field. 1968. J. Dairy Sci. 51:951.

Giesecke, P., M.J. Lawlor and K. Walsen-Karst. 1966. Brit. J. Nutr. 20:383.

Harbers, L.H., R.R. Oltjen and A.D. Tillman. 1961. J. Animal Sci. 20:880.

Hino, T. and M. Kametaka. 1974. Jap. J. Zootech. Sci. 45:223.

Jacobs, G.J.L. and J. Leibholz. 1977. J. Agr. Sci. 89:699.

Kameoka, K. and S. Tanabe. 1972. Bul. Nat. Inst. Animal Ind. 25:41.

Kameoka, K. and S. Tanabe. 1975. Jap. J. Zootech. Sci. 46:417.

Loosli, J.K. et al. 1949. Science 110:144.

Maeng, W.J. and R.L. Baldwin. 1976. J. Dairy Sci. 59:636,648.

Matrone, G., C.R. Bunn and J.J. McNeill. 1964. J. Nutr. 84:215.

Matrone, G., C.R. Bunn and J.J. McNeill. 1965. J. Nutr. 86:154.

McDonald, T.A., W.H. Smith and W.M. Beeson. 1965. J. Animal Sci. 24:896.

Meachum, T.M. et al. 1961. J. Animal Sci. 20:387.

Muir, L.A., P.F. Duquette and G.E. Smith. 1972. J. Animal Sci. 35:271.

Naga, M.A. et al. 1975. J. Animal Sci. 40:1192.

Nimrick, K. et al. 1970. J. Dairy Sci. 53:668; J. Nutr. 100:1293, 1301.

Oltjen, R.R. 1969. J. Animal Sci. 28:673.

Oltjen, R.R. et al. 1969. J. Animal Sci. 29:81,717,830.

Oltjen, R.R. and P.A. Putnam. 1966. J. Nutr. 86:385.

Oltjen, R.R., P.A. Putnam and R.E. Davis. 1965. J. Animal Sci. 24:1218.

Oltjen, R.R., R.J. Sirney and A.D. Tillman. 1962. J. Animal Sci. 21:277,302; J. Nutr. 77:269.

Oltjen, R.R., L.L. Slyter, A.S. Kozak and E.E. Williams. 1968. J. Nutr. 94:193.

Oltjen, R.R., L.L. Slyter, E.E. Williams and D.L. Kern. 1971. J. Nutr. 101:101.

Oltjen, R.R. and P.P. Williams. 1974. J. Animal Sci. 38:915.

Ørskov, E.R. and R.R. Oltjen. 1967. J. Nutr. 93:22.

Price, W.D., J.A. Brown, R.A. Rippe and W.H. Smith. 1969. J. Animal Sci. 29:170.

Prior, R.L. 1976. J. Animal Sci. 42:160.

Prior, R.L., J.A. Milner and W.J. Visek. 1972. J. Nutr. 102:1223.

Richardson, C.R. and E.E. Hatfield. 1978. J. Animal Sci. 46:740.

Rumsey, T.S., J. Bond and R.R. Oltjen. 1969. J. Animal Sci. 28:659.

Schwarz, W.A. and M. Kirchgessner. 1977. Nutr. Abstr. Rev. 47:896.

Slyter, L.L., R.R. Oltjen, D.L. Kern and J.M. Weaver. 1968. J. Nutr. 94:185.

Slyter, L.L. et al. 1971. J. Nutr. 101:839.

Smith, G.E. et al. 1969. J. Animal Sci. 29:171.

Smith, G.E., T.A. McDonald, W.H. Smith and W.M. Beeson. 1965. J. Animal Sci. 24:903.

Smith, G.E., W.H. Smith and W.M. Beeson. 1966. J. Animal Sci. 25:355; J. Dairy Sci. 49:714.

Tove, S.B. and G. Matrone. 1962. J. Nutr. 76:271.

Virtanen, A.I. 1966. Science 153:1603.

Virtanen, A.I. 1969. Fed. Proc. 28:232.

Whanger, P.D. et al. 1977. J. Nutr. 107:998,1288,1298.

Wiese, A.C., B.C. Johnson, H.H. Mitchell and W.B. Nevens. 1947. J. Nutr. 33:263.

INDEX

452